MICROBIOLOGY OF THE EYE

MICROBIOLOGY OF THE EYE

DEBORAH LOCATCHER-KHORAZO, M.D.

Formerly Director of the Laboratory of Microbiology,
Edward S. Harkness Eye Institute of Presbyterian Hospital, New York;
Assistant Professor of Microbiology,
College of Physicians and Surgeons, Columbia University,
New York, New York

BEATRICE CARRIER SEEGAL, M.D.

Professor Emeritus of Microbiology,
College of Physicians and Surgeons, Columbia University,
New York, New York

With 258 illustrations, including 4 color plates

THE C. V. MOSBY COMPANY

Saint Louis 1972

Printed in the United States of America

International Standard Book Number 0-8016-3024-X
Library of Congress Catalog Card Number 70-181594

Distributed in Great Britain by Henry Kimpton, London

Contributors

HENRY F. ALLEN, M.D.

Henry Willard Williams Clinical Professor and Head, Department of Ophthalmology, Harvard Medical School; Chief of Ophthalmology, Massachusetts Eye and Ear Infirmary, Boston, Massachusetts

JAMES H. ALLEN, M.D.

Professor of Ophthalmology, Associate Dean and Medical Director, Tulane Clinics, Tulane University School of Medicine, New Orleans; Consultant in Ophthalmology, U.S. Public Health Service Hospital, Carville, Louisiana

MARGARET BRAND, M.B., B.S. (London)

Ophthalmologist, U.S. Public Health Service Hospital, Carville, Louisiana; Associate Clinical Professor of Ophthalmology, Tulane University School of Medicine, New Orleans, Louisiana; formerly Ophthalmic Consultant, Schieffelin Leprosy Research Institute, Karagiri, S. India

DAVID H. BROWN, M.D.

Assistant Resident in Ophthalmology, Edward S. Harkness Eye Institute of Presbyterian Hospital, New York, New York

HAROLD W. BROWN, M.D., Sc.D., D.P.H., LL.D.

Professor Emeritus of Parasitology, College of Physicians and Surgeons of Columbia University; Parasitologist, Presbyterian Hospital, New York, New York

RICHARD W. DARRELL, M.D.

Instructor in Ophthalmology, Columbia University; Assistant Ophthalmologist, Edward S. Harkness Eye Institute of Presbyterian Hospital, New York, New York

ARTHUR GERARD DeVOE, M.D.

Edward S. Harkness Professor of Ophthalmology, Columbia University; Director, Edward S. Harkness Eye Institute of Presbyterian Hospital, New York, New York

ELIZABETH H. GUTIERREZ, B.A.

Registered Microbiologist of The American Academy of Microbiology; Supervisor of Microbiology, Edward S. Harkness Eye Institute of Presbyterian Hospital, New York, New York

SEYMOUR P. HALBERT, M.D.

Professor of Pediatrics, National Children's Cardiac Hospital, University of Miami, Miami, Florida

G. RICHARD O'CONNOR, M.D.

Associate Professor in Ophthalmology (in Residence) and Director, the Francis I. Proctor Foundation, University of California, San Francisco Medical Center, San Francisco, California

MARGARITA SILVA-HUTNER, Ph.D.

Associate Professor of Dermatology, College of Physicians and Surgeons of Columbia University, New York, New York

FREDERICK H. THEODORE, M.D., F.A.C.S.

Clinical Professor of Ophthalmology, Mount Sinai School of Medicine; Associate Clinical Professor of Ophthalmology, New York University Medical Center; Attending Ophthalmic Surgeon and Director, External Disease and Infections Clinic, Manhattan Eye, Ear and Throat Hospital; Attending Ophthalmologist, New York Hospital; Consultant Ophthalmic Surgeon, The Mount Sinai Hospital, New York, New York

RANDOLPH WHITFIELD, Jr., M.D.

Assistant Resident in Ophthalmology, Edward S. Harkness Eye Institute of Presbyterian Hospital, New York, New York

EMIL WIROSTKO, M.D.

Instructor in Ophthalmology, Director of Microbiology Laboratory, Assistant Ophthalmologist, Edward S. Harkness Eye Institute of Presbyterian Hospital, New York, New York

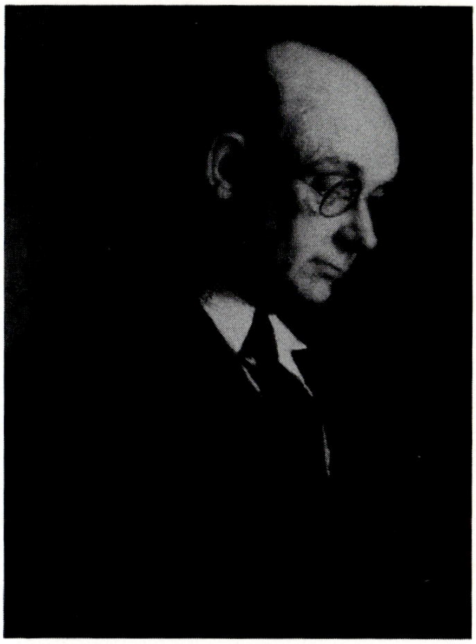

It is with pleasure that this volume is dedicated to Dr. Frederick Parker Gay, Professor and Chairman of the Department of Bacteriology, College of Physicians and Surgeons, Columbia University, from 1923 to 1939.

During forty years devoted to bacteriology Dr. Gay's researches covered many aspects of this subject. He began his experiences with infectious diseases while still a medical student at Johns Hopkins University, when he accompanied Dr. Simon Flexner on a world tour that included a study of cholera and dysentery in the Philippines. Other investigations included the relative roles of humoral and cellular mechanisms in immunity, the characterization of anaphylactic shock, the carrier state and immunity in typhoid fever, the pathogenesis and chemotherapy of infections caused by the hemolytic streptococcus, and the pathogenesis of herpesvirus infections. He was a member of many scientific societies, including the National Academy of Sciences and the Association of American Physicians.

Dr. Gay's vision of the scope and importance of infectious diseases of the eye led him to play an important role in the development of the Laboratory of Bacteriology at the Institute of Ophthalmology, Columbia-Presbyterian Medical Center. When Dr. John Wheeler became Director of the Institute of Ophthalmology he wished to establish in the Institute a laboratory for the diagnosis of eye infections and the investigation of the source, nature, prevention, and treatment of all types of such ocular disease. For this reason he sought the advice and cooperation of Dr. Gay, who was in charge of diagnostic bacteriology at Presbyterian Hospital. Dr. Gay enthusiastically supported the idea of a separate laboratory for the Institute of Ophthalmology. He recognized the special problems incident to infection of the eyes, the need for personnel trained in this field, and the great importance of rapid, accurate diagnosis and therapy. Dr. Gay also agreed with Dr. Wheeler's desire to place the laboratory in charge of a director who would participate in investigations of problems relevant to bacteriology of the eye. On this basis of cooperation the present Laboratory of Microbiology was established in 1933.

Foreword

Ophthalmology must freely acknowledge its great debt to laboratory scientists, who, though devoted to basic disciplines, have nevertheless contributed their skills to the identification of causal agents of ocular disease and, in no small measure, to their treatment. Nowhere has this been more evident than in the close relationship between microbiology and ophthalmology, a clinical specialty that was the first to diverge from the mainstream of medicine and surgery. As the specialty developed, serious students realized the necessity of firmer knowledge in certain basic areas. The first of these were anatomy and histology, followed shortly by pathology and microbiology. For many years, these were the only nonclinical fields intensively studied by the ophthalmologist in training, and it was necessary for him to travel abroad to get this knowledge. In the past few decades, although we have witnessed an explosion of information in such divergent fields as electronics, immunology, biochemistry, electron microscopy, and pharmacology, microbiology remains one of the major disciplines upon which the practicing clinician heavily depends. In good measure through the efforts of our colleagues in this field, serious complications of bacterial disease of the eye have been largely eliminated. Some progress has occurred in the treatment of mycotic invasion, and a start has been made against viral disorders. It is only a matter of time before these, too, will be controlled.

We are most fortunate that two such dedicated scientists as Dr. Locatcher-Khorazo and Dr. Seegal have devoted a lifetime to the study of microbiology, with particular reference to ophthalmic disease. It is most appropriate that the authors now present the distillation of their lifelong efforts, not only for the practical guidance of the clinician struggling with a diseased eye, but for the stimulation and, hopefully, the inducement of young clinicians to extend their interests in the fundamentals of disease.

Arthur Gerard DeVoe, M.D.

Preface

The eye, because of its location and opportunity for direct and indirect microbial involvement, offers unique possibilities for ophthalmologists concerned with clinical and experimental infection. That they have taken advantage of this opportunity is evident from the data presented by the contributors to this volume. In the text they describe many common and rare examples of infection of the eye and various prophylactic, diagnostic, and therapeutic procedures.

This book contains an analysis of the data gathered mostly in the Laboratory of Microbiology at the Edward S. Harkness Eye Institute, Columbia-Presbyterian Medical Center. In 1933 this laboratory was established under the direction of Dr. Richard Thompson, who in 1941 accepted the chairmanship of the Department of Microbiology at the University of Denver. Dr. Deborah Locatcher-Khorazo became associated with the laboratory in 1934 as Dr. Thompson's assistant and directed the laboratory upon Dr. Thompson's departure. She held this position until her retirement in 1968. In the period 1938 to 1968 over 50,000 patients and normal controls were examined in the microbiology laboratory. Thus the patterns of ocular infections were determined from the study of over 100,000 eyes. The data have been analyzed, tabulated, and compared with reports from other laboratories throughout the world.

During the laboratory's existence many members of the staff of the Eye Institute became interested in various infections of the eye and contributed valuable information regarding such diseases as trachoma, toxoplasmosis, toxocariasis, and fungal and viral infections of the eye. The composition and activity of the normal ocular flora were studied. These experiences are supplemented by three chapters—Aseptic Technique in Ophthalmology, Ocular Leprosy, and Allergy in Relation to Ophthalmology—from contributors not associated with the Columbia-Presbyterian Medical Center. This collected material, not readily available elsewhere, should prove valuable to the ophthalmologist and some microbiologists as a ready reference; it offers a potentially useful background for effective diagnosis and management of the infected eye.

The preparation of this manuscript was aided by many friends and associates both through financial assistance and in myriad other ways during the years in which the data were gathered.

Financial aid was received from Dr. Byung W. Kong, Seoul, Korea; Mr. Max Kade, of the Max Kade Foundation; Dr. Anthony Donn; Mr. and Mrs. Samuel

Kastle; Dr. Raymond L. Pfeiffer; and Dr. Algernon B. Reese.

We particularly wish to thank the past and present directors of the Institute of Ophthalmology—the late Dr. John M. Wheeler, Dr. Phillips Thygeson, and Dr. John H. Dunnington—and the present director, Dr. Arthur G. DeVoe, who made it possible to gather the data presented in this book. Dr. Harry M. Rose, Chairman of the Department of Microbiology, gave valuable assistance. The professional staff, both doctors and nurses, have offered fine cooperation in the laboratory and clinic throughout the study. Without their support the objectives could not have been realized. Dr. Konrad C. Hsu, Dr. David Seegal, and Dr. Takeo Iwamoto provided assistance in many aspects related to the preparation of the manuscript.

We are grateful to Mr. Emil G. Bethke, Mr. James Lafayette, and Mr. Edward Gonzalez for their skills in the preparation of drawings, photographs, and photomicrographs, respectively. Miss Margaret Kane and Miss Marian Johnson have provided generous administrative assistance. The staff of the record room of the Presbyterian Hospital and the libraries of the Institute of Ophthalmology and the College of Physicians and Surgeons facilitated the use of these services. Miss Elizabeth Chaffee and Mrs. Katherine Lewis, who were from the Volunteer Department, contributed secretarial help. Mrs. Nora McElligott, Mrs. Thoma Milani, and Mr. Heinz Rosskothen gave technical assistance, and Miss Regina Loewenstein and Mrs. Anita MacDonnell gave statistical assistance.

Dr. Ross M. Grey, Chairman of the Institute of Comparative Medicine and Associate Professor of Pathology, provided both space and encouragement, with the ever cheerful aid of Miss Adeline M. Elia, Administrative Assistant, and Mrs. M. E. Matthies, Senior Secretary of the Institute of Comparative Medicine.

Deborah Locatcher-Khorazo, M.D.
Beatrice Carrier Seegal, M.D.

Contents

1 Historical perspectives, 1

2 The bacterial flora of the healthy eye, 13

3 Inhibitory properties of the ocular flora, 24
SEYMOUR P. HALBERT

4 Cytology of exudates and scrapings from normal and inflamed eyes, 41

5 Bacterial infections of the eye, 63
with ELIZABETH H. GUTIERREZ

6 Postoperative infections of the eye, 77
with ELIZABETH H. GUTIERREZ

7 Aseptic technique in ophthalmology, 86
HENRY F. ALLEN

8 Ocular tuberculosis, 119

9 Ocular leprosy, 131
JAMES H. ALLEN and MARGARET BRAND

10 Allergy in relation to ophthalmology, 156
FREDERICK H. THEODORE

11 Ocular toxoplasmosis, 185
G. RICHARD O'CONNOR

12 Ocular toxocariasis, 203
HAROLD W. BROWN and DAVID H. BROWN

13 Fungal infections of the eye, 208
with ARTHUR GERARD DeVOE and MARGARITA SILVA-HUTNER

14 The Chlamydia: trachoma and inclusion conjunctivitis, 241

15 Rickettsiae in relation to infection of the eye, 253

16 Introduction to viral ocular infections, 267

17 Ocular infections caused by adenovirus and papovavirus groups, 278

18 Ocular infections caused by the herpesvirus group, 302
RICHARD W. DARRELL

19 Ocular infections caused by the poxvirus, togavirus, myxovirus, paramyxovirus, and picornavirus groups, 313
RICHARD W. DARRELL

20 Ocular syphilis, 322
RANDOLPH WHITFIELD, Jr., and EMIL WIROSTKO

Color plates

Plate 1, 46

Plate 2, 70

Plate 3, 248

Plate 4, 304

MICROBIOLOGY OF THE EYE

1
Historical perspectives

Ophthalmologists have made outstanding contributions to the early acquisition of knowledge on infectious diseases of the eye. These contributions can be appreciated better if the few landmarks they had to guide them are enumerated first. As early as 1688, van Leeuwenhoek (1632-1723), who had developed a combination of lenses to produce a microscope giving a magnification of 150×, observed spherical granules in beer yeast; and in a series of letters to the Royal Society of London he carefully drew and described recognizable infusoria, protozoa, and bacteria found in saliva and various excretions. In 1762 von Plenciz, aware of van Leeuwenhoek's findings and seeing yeasts himself, sponsored a sweeping theory that disease was caused by "contagium animatum," with a specific agent for each disease. Unfortunately, his concept was much ahead of the technical means to verify it, and little or no attention was paid to it. In 1845 von Langenbeck saw in an infected human bone what we now know to be actinomyces, and in 1850 Pollender saw large bacilli (anthrax) in blood from a sheep with splenic fever; these bacilli were grown by Koch in 1876. From this point on, a search was made for living agents producing disease; and a great number were found, though the hunt is not yet over.

Before the discovery of agents that cause infectious diseases, observant ophthalmologists supported the theory that certain eye diseases were contagious; and rules for prevention, anticipating many of today's routine precautions, were laid down. Table 1-1 includes information about some of these early observations. Charles Saint-Yves (1667-1736),[38] a much respected French ophthalmologist, had a young male patient who made a practice of washing his eyes with his urine. After this patient had contracted gonorrhea, he developed a purulent conjunctivitis. Saint-Yves had no difficulty in diagnosing the eye disease, and he is credited with having given the first exact description of ophthalmia neonatorum. He concluded that the patient had transmitted gonorrhea to his eyes. Other contributions made by Saint-Yves include the first record of what was apparently an ophthalmitis caused by herpes zoster and descriptions of ocular lesions in smallpox. He is said to have used silver nitrate "plentifully" in treating abscesses or ulcers of the eye and "probably" in treating ophthalmia neonatorum.

Carris[3] credits Quelmalz, a German physician, with having pointed out around 1785 the possible connection between "babies' sore eyes" and the discharge present in the mother's birth canal. After many years Dr. Gibson,[11] an Englishman, in 1808 confirmed the observation of Quelmalz and added that proper cleansing of the mother's vaginal canal and removing mucus from the baby's eyes might prevent the occurrence of this infection.

Joseph F. Pieringer (1800-1879),[9,17] shown in Fig. 1-1, was among the most notable of ophthalmologists. He performed empirical experiments, particularly in his

Table 1-1. Some early observations on agents responsible for ocular infections

Present designation	Clinical description	Transmission, prophylaxis, treatment	Causative agent
Gonococcal conjunctivitis	*Galen*, 132 AD, introduced term gonorrhea, "flow of seed"[42]* *Severus*, 3rd century AD, described disease of newborn with lids swollen because of abundance of matter[38]	*Saint-Yves*, 1722, described case of a young man, accustomed to wash his eyes with his urine, who transmitted his gonorrhea to his eyes[38] *Quelmalz*, 1785, noted connection between babies' sore eyes and discharge in mothers' vaginal canals[3,17] *Gibson*, 1808, recommended proper cleansing of mother's birth canal and baby's eyes to lessen chances for blindness[3,36] *Pieringer*, 1841, proved pus derived from urethral discharge produced infection when applied to conjunctiva of blind volunteers[9,17] *Credé*, 1881, introduced the extensive use of silver nitrate in eyes of newborn[3,31]	*Neisser*, 1879, described a diplococcus in urethral and conjunctival exudate[32] *Leistikow*, 1880, first cultivated the gonococcus[26] *Krause*, 1882, cultured the gonococcus and produced disease with pure culture[24]
Mycotic keratitis	*Leber*, 1879, saw corneal ulcer, greyish turbid base, in 5 days membrane from upper border lifted, had mycelial elements, hypopyon, progressive course[25]	*Leber*, 1879, contaminated corneal wounds of rabbits with culture from patient, produced similar lesions[25]	*Leber*, 1879, grew *Aspergillus glaucus* from corneal ulcer[25]
Koch-Weeks conjunctivitis	*Weeks*, 1886, reported acute epidemic mucopurulent conjunctivitis[43]	*Weeks*, 1886, demonstrated pure cultures of the bacillus-produced characteristic conjunctivitis in his own eye and those of human volunteers.[43]	*Hirschberg and Krause*, 1881, observed delicate rods in some cases of trachoma[18] *Koch*, 1883, described similar organism in some cases of Egyptian ophthalmia[23] *Weeks*, 1886, isolated the Koch-Weeks bacillus (Hemophilus aegyptius)[43]
Morax-Axenfeld angular blepharo-conjunctivitis	*Morax*, 1896, observed subacute conjunctivitis, redness at angles of lid margin, mild, bilateral[28]	*Morax*, 1896, transmitted disease to human eye; zinc sulphate used therapeutically[28] *Axenfeld*, 1897, reported finding and cultivating same organism independently[1]	*Morax*, 1896,[28] *Axenfeld*, 1897,[1] independently isolated Morax-Axenfeld diplobacillus (*Moraxella lacunata*)
Keratitis of Petit	*Petit*, 1899, described superficial serpiginous hypopyon keratitis[34]	*Petit*, 1899, showed organism not pathogenic for animals[34]	*Petit*, 1899, isolated diplobacillus of Petit (*Moraxella liquefaciens*)[34]

*Superscript numbers indicate references at end of chapter.

It might be guessed from his pioneering adventures in microbiology that Dr. Weeks had qualities of the explorer, including excellence of performance and hardihood. Dr. Knapp[22] said of him that his "modesty and superb courage were remarkable," and when asked where he would advise a young ophthalmologist to settle, he replied "wherever the competition is the keenest."[22] Certainly one can only settle for the best in such surroundings.

Harold Gifford (1858-1929) was another American ophthalmologist who brought the viewpoint of the bacteriologist to the practice of ophthalmology at a very early date. In many respects his career started in a manner similar to that of Dr. Weeks. Born in Milwaukee, Dr. Gifford received his medical degree from the University of Michigan. He went abroad for postgraduate studies in Germany and Switzerland, where he carried out early research in bacteriology of the eye. Like Dr. Weeks, he later became associated with Dr. Knapp.[19]

Dr. Gifford's studies in ophthalmic bacteriology included his important observations on the flora of the normal eye. He found potential pathogens among organisms present in the healthy eye and indicated that these might be carried into the eye following the trauma of operation. This indeed proved true. His studies on attempts at sterilization of the conjunctiva demonstrated that a sterile state could not be maintained, since the bacteria lie under the epithelium, in ducts of the glands, and in the eyelash roots.[13] Dr. Gifford's other investigations in ocular bacteriology covered a wide field. He was the first to publish a description in English (1896) of acute pneumococcus conjunctivitis and to demonstrate that the infection was transmissible by inoculation of secretions containing the pneumococci.[12] For this experiment he used the conjunctivas of his own eye and those of his assistants. He studied infections associated with the diplobacillus of Morax-Axenfeld, demonstrating this organism not only in angular conjunctivitis but also in corneal ulcers.[14] In 1910 he reported bulbar conjunctivitis caused by *Sporotrichum schenckii,* which was the first time a publication on ocular infection by this organism had appeared in English.[15] Dr. Gifford also carried out early research in experimental bacterial sympathetic ophthalmia and followed the spread of the

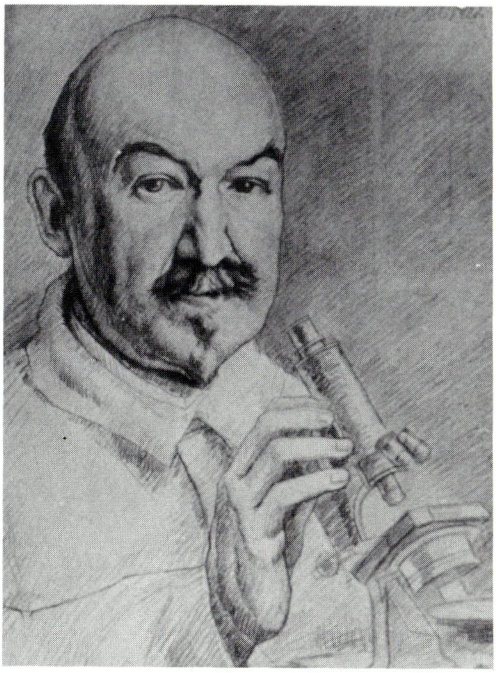

Fig. 1-7. Victor Morax (1866-1935), born in Morges on Lake Geneva, was the son of a physician who had interned at the Hôpitaux de Paris. His father had great enthusiasm for his years in Paris, and the young Victor looked forward to living in this city. In the course of his studies he acquired a passion for chemistry and a great curiosity about the pathogenic microorganisms and powerful toxins they produced. After his training at the University of Lausanne and Fribourg-en-Brisgau, a visit to Indochina focused Morax's attention on the bacteriology of the eye, which led, among other things, to his isolation of the Morax-Axenfeld diplobacillus, the causative agent of one type of conjunctivitis. His very productive scientific career was spent in his adopted country, France, and in 1900 he was nominated Ophthalmologist of the Hôpitaux de Paris. (From Duke-Elder, S.: System of ophthalmology. Diseases of the outer eye, vol. 8, part 1, St. Louis, 1965, The C. V. Mosby Co., p. 48.)

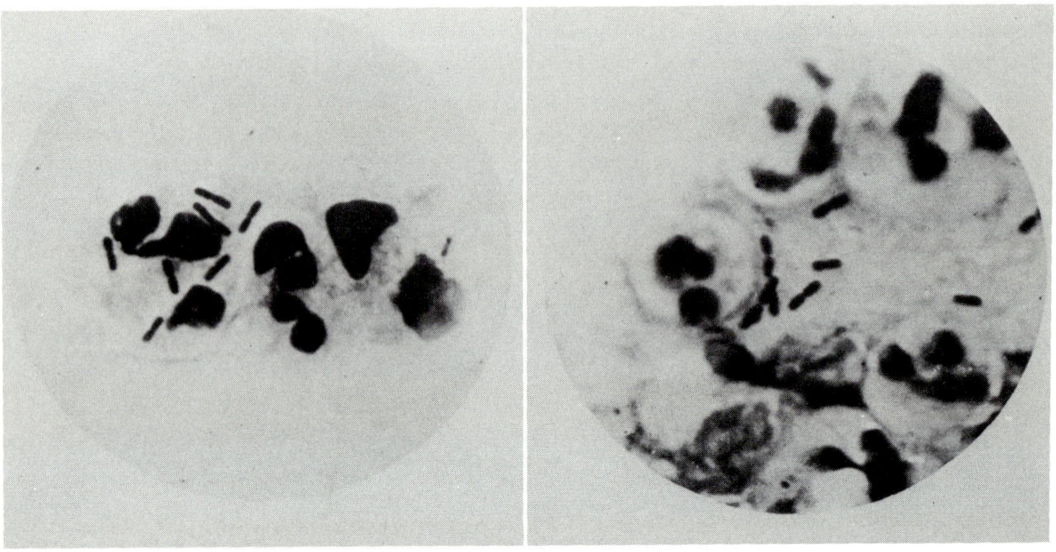

Fig. 1-8. A, Diplobacilli included in a polymorphonuclear leukocyte from conjunctival secretions in subacute conjunctivitis; **B,** diplobacilli free in the conjunctival secretions. The bacillus is now classified *Moraxella lacunata.* (From Morax, V.: Ann. Inst. Pasteur **10**:337, 1896.)

microorganisms from the inoculated eye through lymph paths into the orbit and from there to the nerve and the suprachoroidal spaces of the second eye.[19]

Victor Morax[27] (1886-1935), shown in Fig. 1-7, was born in Switzerland but received his medical education in France, where he continued to live and to contribute extensively to ophthalmology as related to bacteriology and to medicine and surgery. In 1896, while at the Pasteur Institute, independently and simultaneously with Dr. Axenfeld, Dr. Morax[28] discovered a gram-negative diplobacillus in angular conjunctivitis, which became known as the Morax-Axenfeld diplobacillus. A member of the Hemophilus group, its official name now is *Moraxella lacunata.* Fig. 1-8 is an illustration from Dr. Morax's original paper. Dr. Morax also carried out studies in cases of acute conjunctivitis, from which he isolated the Koch-Weeks bacillus. In 1901, while residing in Egypt in order to study trachoma, he observed during the acute stage of the disease multiple bacterial infections, which he considered were responsible for much of the pathology.[29,30] He continued to be closely associated with problems of trachoma and related folliculosis and established *La Revue du Trachome.*[27] He also was concerned with sympathetic ophthalmia and recommended enucleation as a precautionary measure against complications.

Theodor Axenfeld[41] (Fig. 1-9), of German origin, studied medicine at the Universities of Marburg and Berlin and bacteriology with Rubner and Fraenkel. He went from a Professorship of Ophthalmology at the University of Rostok to the University of Freiburg in 1901, where he remained for the succeeding 29 years of his life. There his Ophthalmological Institute became a mecca for students from many lands. He held the belief, revolutionary in that day, that the head of a clinic should be free from private practice in order to devote his time to teaching and research. Professor Axenfeld's research covered almost every branch in ophthalmology, but his name is kept especially in mind because of his independent discovery of the Morax-Axenfeld diplobacillus. At Freiburg Dr. Axenfeld built up the *Klin-*

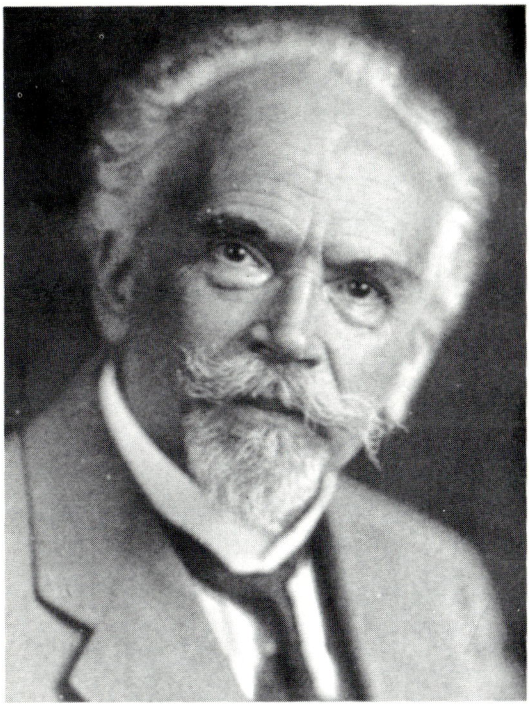

Fig. 1-9. Theodor Axenfeld (1867-1930), though born in Smyrna, obtained his early education in Bonn and his medical training at the Universities of Marburg and Berlin. The following years were spent in training in ophthalmology, pathology, and bacteriology. In 1897 he became Director of the Eye Clinic in Rostock, but moved in 1901 to Freiburg, where he remained for the rest of his life. In 1904 he published a book, *Bakteriologie in der Augenheilkunde,* which became the standard work in this field for many years. It was translated into English by MacNab in 1908. Axenfeld's presentation of his experiences during a long life devoted to the subject are still a delight to workers in this field. (From von Szily, A.: Klin. Mbl. Augenheilk. **85**(4):i-xvi, 1930.)

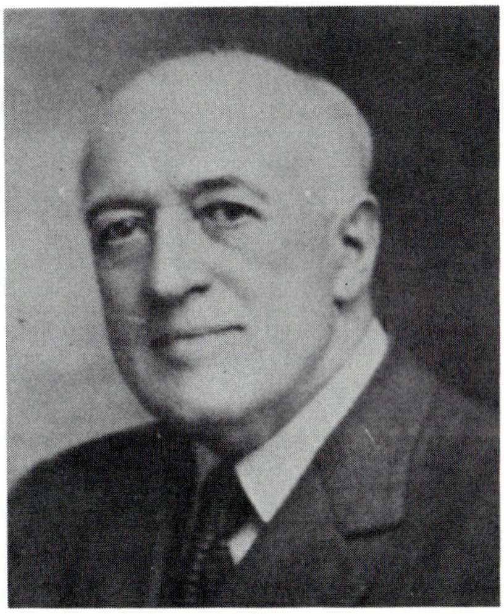

Fig. 1-10. Paul J. Petit (1875-1950), an ophthalmologist and bacteriologist, was concerned with the importance of using the bacteriologic laboratory to assist in the diagnosis of ocular disease. He was associated with Morax and with Nicolle in these endeavors. One of Petit's main interests was the cause and management of trachoma; some of his studies on this subject were carried out in Tunisia. He was Secretary General of the Ligue Contre le Trachome from 1924 to 1939. Another major interest of Petit was the identification of the possible etiologic agents of keratitis. This work led to his discovery in 1899 of a bacterium, the diplobacillus of Petit (now called *Moraxella liquefaciens*), responsible for a somewhat clinically distinctive type of keratitis. Petit was much beloved, as was gracefully said by Bailliart: "C'est un savant très modeste mais de grande valeur." (From Petit, P. J.: Rev. Int. Trachome **25**:194, 1948; legend material from Baillairt, P.: Ann. Oculist. **183**:1007, 1950.)

ische Monatsblätter für Angenheilkunde, still a leading ophthalmologic journal. The diversity of his interest in problems of eye infection was great. In 1894 he received the Graefe Prize for his "classical research" on suppurative metastatic ophthalmia. This work could still be used as a model for a complete experimental bacteriologic and pathologic examination of a disease.[41]

Mention should be made of other areas in which Professor Axenfeld contributed to bacteriology. For example, he concerned himself with studies of the etiology of serpiginous corneal ulcer, demonstrating the important role the pneumococcus plays in this disease. In 1907 he wrote a book on the bacteriology of the eye, which was translated into English in 1908 by Angus MacNab.[2] This book, which includes a consideration of mycotic and parasitic infections of the eyes, laid the foundation for the principles and techniques of ophthalmic bacteriology. Although it is more than 50 years old, the book can still be read with profit. Later monographs on trachoma and vernal conjunctivitis were written. Dr. Axenfeld kept pace with the developments in his field, and his writings are filled with records of the contributions of a great number of investigators in the same and allied fields. His own work was very stimulating to the productive research of others. Ophthalmologists are greatly indebted to Dr. Axenfeld for clarifying the relations of bacteriology to ophthalmology.

In 1899 another small gram-negative diplobacillus was isolated by Petit (Fig. 1-10) from patients with keratitis with hypopyon.[34] This organism, long known as the diplobacillus of Petit, is now classified as *Moraxella liquefaciens*. Dr. Petit was a French ophthalmologist who, as an associate of Charles Nicolle, devoted his energy to the investigation of ocular infections. He contributed much to the fight against trachoma in Tunisia[35] and collaborated with Victor Morax in a book on this subject.[30]

Trachoma has been of greatest concern to ophthalmologists and other physicians for most of recorded history. In China it dates back to about 2700 BC, and it has been described in Mesopotamia since the twentieth century BC. Celsus, in 14 AD, noted, roughness of the eyes, and Aetius of Amido, in 550 AD, described the four stages of the disease. In 1823 the ophthalmologist Werneck[17,21] transmitted the disease with follicular material to volunteers. The significance of Werneck's observation was not advanced for almost a 100 years because of the lack of techniques for carrying the studies further. Modern scientific investigation into the cause of trachoma may be said to have started with the classic observations made by Halberstaeder and von Prowazek[8,16] in 1907. When on a joint expedition to Java to study syphilis, they became interested in the conjunctivitis of trachoma, which was common there. Scrapings of the trachomatous conjunctivas revealed small granular intracellular bodies, which stained red with the Giemsa stain and lay in a blue matrix. They believed the small granular bodies to be the cause of trachoma. They were successful in producing infection typical of trachoma in the eyes of orangutans, using scrapings from trachomatous eyes. The cells in the exudates from the animals' eyes also contained foreign bodies similar to those seen in man. The illustrations that they published seemed to show both elementary bodies and inclusion bodies.

In 1912 Nicolle, Blaisot, and Cuénod[33] found that it was possible to transmit trachoma to the *Macaca inuus* and the chimpanzee with material that had been rendered bacteria free by filtration through a Berkefeld filter. In 1935 Thygeson and Proctor[40] reproduced the disease in a human volunteer with material from pooled exudates from trachomatous children. The material had been filtered through a 0.6 μg gradocol membrane filter. They showed that the filtrate was bacteria free but contained elementary bodies about 0.25 μ in diameter. Thus, at this time there was no reason to doubt that the agent that caused trachoma was filtrable but large enough to be seen at high magnification. Although fairly sophisticated methods were being developed for the cultivation of viruses and rickettsiae, the agent of trachoma escaped capture until 1957 when it was grown in China in the chick embryo by T'ang, Chang, Huang, and Wang.[39] Previous attempts to use this method had apparently failed because of the injection of penicillin with the trachoma washings into the eggs. The use of penicillin was standard procedure to eliminate bacterial contamination in viral studies, but it also eliminated the agent causing trachoma. When T'ang and his associates employed streptomycin as a bacteriostatic agent, they obtained growth of the agent causing trachoma, a microorganism belonging to the psittacosis, ornithosis, lymphogranuloma venereum group of organisms, now named *Chlamydia trachomatis* (Chapter 14). This organism has now been cultured by many investigators throughout the world.

Much is owed Dr. Ernest Fuchs (1851-1930) for his pioneer studies on keratoconjunctivitis. An Austrian ophthalmologist, Dr. Fuchs was a guide and teacher of ophthalmologists throughout the world, largely through his book *Treatise on Diseases of the Eye,* which appeared in numerous editions and translations. Dr. Fuchs[10] in 1889 gave the classical description of the clinical findings characterizing superficial punctate keratitis. Although the etiology of this condition, now called epidemic keratoconjunctivitis, was not known until the mid-1950's, Dr. Fuchs' careful delineation of the disease maintained it as a clinical entity until the specific causative agent was isolated. In 1930 Wright,[45] a professor of ophthalmology in Madras, reported on the transmissibility of this disease to man with filtered material from conjunctival scrapings, thus establishing the probable viral etiology of the disease. The agent was not identified, however, until 1955 when Jawetz, Kimura, Nicholas, Thygeson, and Hanna[20] isolated a new type of adenovirus—type 8—from patients with epidemic keratoconjunctivitis and proved this virus to be the etiologic agent of the disease (Chapter 17).

REFERENCES

1. Axenfeld, T.: Beiträge zur Aetiologie der Bindehautentzündungen, Bericht Ophthalmologischen Gesellschaft, Munich, 1897, J. F. Bergmann, p. 140.
2. Axenfeld, T.: The bacteriology of the eye, translated by Angus MacNab, New York, 1908, William Wood and Co.
3. Carris, L. H.: Preventing blindness through social hygiene co-operation, Sightsav. Rev. **4**:28, 1934.
4. Delbanco, E.: Leo Leistikow, Derm. Wschr. **66**:153, 1918.
5. Derby, G. S.: Lucien Howe: 1848-1928, Arch. Ophthal. **1**:241, 1929.
6. Duke-Elder, S.: System of ophthalmology. Diseases of the outer eye, vol. 8, part 1, St. Louis, 1965, The C. V. Mosby Co., p. 260.
7. Dunnington, J. H.: John Elmer Weeks, Amer. J. Ophthal. **32**:595, 1949.
8. Finzi, N. S.: Ludvig Halberstaedter, Brit. J. Radiol. **22**:347, 1949.
9. Friedenwald, H.: Joseph Friederich Pieringer: his methods and investigations, Johns Hopkins Hosp. Bull. **8**:191, 1897.
10. Fuchs, E.: Keratitis punctata superficialis, Wien. Klin. Wschr. **2**:837, 1889.
11. Garrison, F. H.: History of medicine, ed. 4, Philadelphia, 1929, W. B. Saunders Co., p. 578.
12. Gifford, H.: Pneumococcus of Fraenkel as a frequent cause of acute catarrhal conjunctivitis, Arch. Ophthal. **25**:314, 1896.
13. Gifford, H.: Notes on ophthalmic bacteriology, partly with reference to asepsis, Arch. Ophthal. **27**:616, 1898.
14. Gifford, H.: On the clinical importance of the diplobacillus of Morax and Axenfeld, Ophthal. Rec. **14**:511, 1905.
15. Gifford, H.: Sporotrichosis of the eyeball and eyelids, Ophthal. Rec. **19**:573, 1910.
16. Halberstaedter, L., and von Prowazek, S.: Zur Aetiologie des Trachoms, Deutsch. Med. Wschr. **33**:1285, 1907.
17. Hirschberg, J.: Charles St. Yves, S. T. Quelmalz, W. Werneck, J. Pieringer, Graefe-Saemisch Handbuch der Gesamten Augenheilkunde **14**(1):9, 203, 561, 577, 1911.
18. Hirschberg, J., and Krause, F.: Zur Pathologie der ansteckenden Augenkrankheiten, Zbl. Augenheilk. **5**:278, 1881.
19. Jackson, E.: Harold Gifford, Arch. Ophthal. **3**:217, 1930.
20. Jawetz, E., Kimura, S., Nicholas, A. N., Thygeson, P., and Hanna, L.: New type of APC virus from epidemic keratoconjunctivitis, Science **122**:1190, 1955.
21. Julianelle, L. A.: The etiology of trachoma, New York, 1938, Oxford University Press, p. 43.
22. Knapp, A.: John Elmer Weeks, Arch. Ophthal. **41**:752, 1949.
23. Koch, R.: Thätigkeit der deutschen Cholerakommission in Aegypten und Ostindien, Wien. Med. Wschr. **52**:1548, 1883.
24. Krause, F.: Die Mikkrokokken der Blennorrhoea neonatorum, Zbl. Praktische Augenheilk. **6**:134, 1882.
25. Leber, T.: Keratomycosis aspergillina als Ursache von Hypopyonkeratitis, Graefes Arch. Ophth. **25**:285, 1879.
26. Leistikow, L.: Ueber Bacterien bei den venerischen Krankheiten, Charité-Annalen, **7**:750, 1880.
27. Magitot, A.: Victor Morax, Ann. Oculist. **172**:529, 1935.
28. Morax, V.: Note sur un diplobacille pathogène pour la conjonctivite humaine, Ann. Inst. Pasteur **10**:337, 1896.
29. Morax, V., and Lakah, M.: Recherches cliniques sur l'étiologie du trachome en Égypte, Ann. Oculist. **126**:353, 1901.
30. Morax, V., and Petit, P. J.: Le trachome, Paris, 1929, Jean Morax, Éditeur.
31. Narayanrao, U. B.: Lives of great men: Carl Siegmund Franz Credé (1819-1892), Indian J. Venereal Dis. **2**:161, 1936.

32. Neisser, A.: Ueber eine der Gonorrhoe eigentümliche Micrococcusform, Zbl. Med. Wiss. **17**:497, 1879.
33. Nicolle, C., Blaisot, L., and Cuénod, A.: Le magot animal réactif du trachome: filtrabilite du virus; pouvoir infectant des larmes, C. R. Acad. Sci. **155**:241, 1912.
34. Petit, P. J.: Sur une forme particuliere d'infection cornéenne a type serpigineux, Ann. Oculist. **121**:166, 1899.
35. Petit, P. J.: Souvenirs d'une mission en Tunisie, Rev. Int. Trachome, **25**:194, 1948.
36. Posey, W. C.: The romance in the movement for the prevention of blindness, Sight-sav. Rev. **4**:83, 1934.
37. Pusey, W. A.: Albert Neisser. In The history of dermatology, Springfield, Ill., 1933, Charles C Thomas, Publisher, p. 155.
38. Shastid, T. H.: Charles Saint-Yves, Amer. Encyc. Dict. Ophthal. **15**:11496, 1919.
39. T'ang, F., Chang, H., Huang, Y., and Wang, K.: Studies of the etiology of trachoma with special reference to isolation of the virus in chick embryo, Chin. Med. J. **75**:429, 1957.
40. Thygeson, P., and Proctor, F. I.: The filtrability of trachoma virus, Arch. Ophthal. **13**:1018, 1935.
41. von Szily, A.: Theodor Axenfeld, Klin. Mbl. Augenheilk. **85**:1, 1930.
42. Vertue, H. St. H.: An enquiry into venereal disease in Greece and Rome, Guy. Hosp. Rep. **102**:277, 1953.
43. Weeks, J. E.: The bacillus of acute conjunctival catarrh, or "pink eye," Arch. Ophthal. **15**:441, 1886.
44. Weeks, J. E.: A treatise on diseases of the eye, Philadelphia, 1910, Lea and Febiger, p. 255.
45. Wright, R. E.: Superficial punctate keratitis, Brit. J. Ophthal. **14**:257, 1930.

2

The bacterial flora of the healthy eye

THE NORMAL FLORA OF THE EYE

The eye harbors bacteria from the time of birth throughout life. During his passage through the birth canal, the infant acquires some of the microorganisms in the mother's vagina. Although the dramatic example of this is *Neisseria gonorrhoeae*, causing gonorrheal conjunctivitis, the infant routinely picks up bacteria carried in the healthy vagina. Grünberger and Kofler[12] carried out a simultaneous study of the vaginal flora of the mother and the eye flora of the newly born infant. In Table 2-1, adapted from their table, it is seen that *Staphylococcus epidermidis*, *Staphylococcus aureus*, streptococci, and sometimes *Escherichia coli* were transmitted to infants' eyes during birth. The authors point out the failure of silver nitrate to influence parasitism, particularly by *S. aureus*. Franklin and Loeb[10] examined the bacterial flora of 200 infants, covering a period from 4 to 40 hours after birth. The cultures were taken following the instillation of penicillin in the eyes of 100 of the children and silver nitrate in the eyes of the others. Nevertheless, cultures revealed the presence of a variety of staphylococci, streptococci, diphtheroids, and gram-negative bacilli in 41% and 45% of the children, respectively.

Several studies of the ocular flora of healthy eyes of children as compared with adults have been reported. Khorazo and Thompson[14] in 1935 examined the normal eyes of 1,084 individuals ranging in age from birth to over 70 years. The results obtained in the various age groups are shown in Table 2-2. The bacteria commonly found in the eyes at all ages were the staphylococci and diphtheroids; streptococci

Table 2-1. Incidence of individual bacteria in birth canal of 53 mothers and in eyes of the newly born infants

Bacteria	Mothers' vaginal canal	Infants' eyes: Before treatment — At birth	Infants' eyes: After silver nitrate — 2 days	Infants' eyes: After silver nitrate — 5 days
S. aureus	26	26	28	30
*S. albus**	22	20	16	18
Streptococci	12	7	3	1
B. coli†	21	4	0	2

Data from Grünberger, V., and Kofler, E.: Uber den Keimgehalt der kindlichen conjunctiva nach der Geburt, Gynaecologia **137:**331, 1954.

**Straphylococcus epidermidis.*

†*Escherichia coli.*

Table 2-2. Bacteria recovered from normal eyes in individuals of various ages

	Age group					
	0-5	**6-14**	**15-29**	**30-49**	**50-69**	**70+**
Total cases in each age group	64	106	143	220	412	139
Staphylococcus epidermidis†	41%	39%	43%	39%	42%	45%
Staphylococcus aureus	25%	24%	24%	21%	25%	23%
Streptococcus hemolyticus	(1)*	(1)	3%	(1)	2%	(1)
Streptococcus viridans	8%	4%	2%	3%	4%	1%
Pneumococci	13%	2%	2%	3%	2%	1%
Diphtheroids	25%	24%	28%	38%	42%	45%
Mixed cultures	26%	16%	18%	19%	30%	34%
No growth	20%	23%	20%	20%	14%	12%

Data from Khorazo, D., and Thompson, R.: The bacterial flora of the normal conjunctiva, Amer. J. Ophthal. **18**:1115, 1935.
*Parentheses indicate actual numbers, not percent.
†*Staphylococcus albus.*

Table 2-3. Incidence of microorganisms cultured from conjunctivas and eyelid margins*

	1-18 years		20-35 years		40-90 years	
	Percent positive (range)†		Percent positive (range)		Percent positive (range)	
Microorganisms	**Conjunctivas**	**Eyelids**	**Conjunctivas**	**Eyelids**	**Conjunctivas**	**Eyelids**
Staphylococcus epidermidis	56–73	62–81	61–78	63–76	54–83	62–82
Staphylococcus aureus	35–38	32–45	30–41	31–44	31–45	31–47
Diphtheroids	21–23	20–24	32–39	33–43	21–34	28–43
Streptococcus viridans	1.1–2.1	0.7–2.5	0.3–0.7	0.3–0.8	0.5–5.0	0.5–5.0
Diplococcus pneumoniae	5.0–9.0	5.0–9.0	0.9–2.7	0.5–1.3	0.4–0.8	0.2–1.2
Escherichia coli	0.1–0.2	0.2–0.4	0.2–2.7	0.3–1.5	0.4–3.0	0.5–4.0
Klebsiella pneumoniae	0.6–3.0	0.6–3.0	0.3–3.0	0.3–1.3	0.2–1.2	0.2–2.2
Klebsiella ozenae	—	—	—	—	0.2–0.6	0.2–0.6
Proteus vulgaris	0.1–0.2	0.1–0.2	0.1–0.2	0.1–0.3	0.6–3.0	0.9–4.0
Proteus morgani	0.1–0.2	0.1–0.2	0.1–0.2	0.1–0.6	0.3–3.0	0.3–3.0
Proteus mirabilis	0.1–0.2	0.1–0.2	0.1–0.4	0.2–0.9	0.7–2.4	0.7–2.4
Proteus rettgeri	—	—	—	—	0.5–0.9	0.5–0.9
Neisseria catarrhalis	0.9–3.0	1.2–0.6	0.1–1.3	0.2–1.5	0.2–1.2	0.2–1.2
Neisseria sicca	0.5–0.9	0.9–2.0	0.2–2.0	0.2–3.0	0.2–1.1	0.5–1.1
Neisseria flava	—	—	0.1–0.7	0.2–0.9	0.3–1.2	0.3–1.2
Bacillus subtilis	0.6–1.3	0.5–1.3	0.7–2.3	0.8–4.0	0.2–1.8	0.6–2.6
Bacillus cereus	—	—	—	—	0.2–1.2	0.2–1.5
Bacillus megaterium	—	—	—	—	0.4–1.1	0.3–1.5
Sarcina	0.8–1.2	0.9–1.2	0.5–1.0	0.5–1.5	0.2–1.8	0.2–2.4
Micrococcus tetragenus	0.7–1.2	0.6–1.2	0.5–2.0	0.7–3.2	0.4–4.0	0.8–4.1

*From 1,024 young people 1-18 years old, 1,786 adults 20-35 years old, and 7,461 patients awaiting ocular surgery, 1952-1968. None had infected eyes. Ages 1-18 drawn from children awaiting surgery, those accompanying parents to clinic, and visiting high school students; ages 20-35 years drawn from graduate students and from some of the personnel at the Columbia-Presbyterian Medical Center, 1957-1962.
†Figures given are from the years showing the lowest and the highest incidence for each microorganism.

and pneumococci were present infrequently. The bacterial flora was not modified by the age of the subjects except for a rise in the incidence of diphtheroids in those over 50. From 1952 to 1968 Locatcher-Khorazo and Gutierrez[16] determined the bacterial flora of noninfected eyes of 10,271 individuals 1 to 90 years of age. Table 2-3 shows data from these studies in which the conjunctivas and eyelid margins of both eyes were cultured. The percent of persons carrying the individual isolated bacteria was determined for each year. Since there was considerable fluctuation in the carriage rate from year to year, the lowest percentage and the highest percentage of positive cultures obtained during the years of study are recorded. Three age groups, 1 to 18 years, 20 to 35 years, and 40 to 90 years are represented. The data confirm the preponderance of staphylococci and diphtheroids in the normal eye, an observation that is supported in reports from many other laboratories.[1,7a,15,18] Other bacteria were found in a few cases. The incidence of diphtheroids was somewhat less in the age group 1 to 18 than in the other age groups. There was no significant difference in the floras recovered from the eyelid margins and the conjunctivas.

Further analysis of the data from which Table 2-3 was constructed has given the following information: (1) there was no difference in bacterial flora between the healthy eyes of males and females; (2) the data examined month by month showed no seasonal changes in the carriage rate; (3) a scrutiny of the yearly fluctuations observed failed to indicate any significant trend in the yearly variations in the number of staphylococci and diphtheroids recovered; (4) the flora obtained from the right and left eyes was almost always identical; there was a difference in only 244 individuals out of the 7,000 tested; (5) in no instance were the cultures sterile.

The routine techniques used in the studies recorded in Table 2-3 served to isolate only aerobic bacteria. Anaerobic cultures were done, however, on 2,000 eyes. Facultative anaerobes were rarely found, and true anaerobes were not seen. Others have reported anaerobes in the normal eye.[18a] Fungi were present in a small percentage of eyes, as is described in Chapter 13.

In Table 2-4 further information is given regarding the bacterial flora cultured from the eyes of the 7,461 individuals awaiting ocular surgery. The data have been presented in such a way as to show the frequency with which the eye carries only a single organism as compared with two or more organisms. In about half of these patients, only single bacteria were isolated.

Table 2-4. Bacterial flora in eyes of 7,461 patients prior to ocular surgery, 1952-1968

Organisms isolated	Conjunctivas		Eyelids	
	Number	Percent	Number	Percent
Staphylococcus epidermidis	2,804	36.2	2,813	37.8
Staphylococcus aureus	1,295	17.3	1,310	17.6
Diphtheroids	158	2.1	69	0.9
Staphylococcus epidermidis and *S. aureus*	645	8.6	688	9.2
Staphylococcus epidermidis and diphtheroids	862	11.5	864	11.6
Staphylococcus aureus and diphtheroids	534	7.4	562	7.5
Staphylococcus epidermidis, *S. aureus*, and diphtheroids	503	6.7	500	6.7
Miscellaneous organisms in various combinations with above*	638	8.5	653	8.7

**Bacillus subtilis*, coliform bacilli, *Neisseria catarrhalis*, *N. sicca*, pneumococci, *Streptococcus viridans*, *Proteus* group, and *Sarcina*.

Table 2-5. Conjunctival flora of normal eyes from various parts of the world (expressed in percentages)

Location of study	New York, Birmingham, United States		London, England	Copenhagen, Denmark	Jerusalem, Israel	Freiburg, Germany	Peking, China	Gifu-shi, Japan	Algiers, Algeria	Freiburg, Germany
Study	Locatcher-Khorazo and Gutierrez[16]*	Cason and Winkler[6]	Smith[22]	Barfoed[4]	Bachrach and associates[3]	Doden[8]	Chang[7]	Yamazaki[24]	Orfila and Courden[20]	Axenfeld[2]
Microorganisms isolated	**7,461**	**1,604**	**5,000**	**501†**	**277**	**915†**	**100**	**564†**	**120**	**61**
Staphylococcus epidermidis	68.5	68.0	33.8	35.7	58.6	75.7	62.0	40.2	50.0	65.0
Staphylococcus aureus	42.0	7.0	7.9	7.6	6.9	6.1	2.0	5.5	25.8	11.0
Diphtheroids	28.7	33.0	31.5	32.1	39.2	76.4	18.0	27.7	32.0	83.0
Streptococcus viridans	2.5	<1.0	0.9	0.6	5.4		12.0	3.7	1.1	3.0
Streptococcus hemolyticus	—	<1.0	0.3	—	—	—	1.0	—	1.7	—
Nonhemolytic streptococci	—	—	—	—	—	—	—	—	1.7	—
Streptococcus faecalis	—	—	—	—	0.54	—	—	—	—	—
Diplococcus pneumoniae	0.3	<1.0	3.2	0.8	1.08	2.3	1.0	2.8	0.8	5.0
Gram-negative bacilli‡	5.0	<4.0	2.9	0.2	2.1	0.5	2.0	6.3	11.6	—
Gram-negative diplococci§	0.7	<1.0	2.3	—	2.16	—	—	4.5	10.8	—
Gram-positive bacilli‖	3.2	<1.0	—	0.2	2.1	—	3.0	3.5	—	—
Micrococcus tetragenus and *Sarcina*	2.6	1.0	—	—	—	—	9.0	—	0.8	1.0
No organisms found	0	23.0	47.0	44.5	32.9	8.7	9.0	13.3	3.4	—

*Superscript numbers indicate references at end of chapter.
†Eyes. Other figures indicate number of individuals examined.
‡Gram-negative bacilli: *Escherichia coli*, *Klebsiella pneumoniae*, *K. ozenae*, *Proteus vulgaris*, *P. morgani*, *P. mirabilis*, *P. rettgeri*, *Aerobacter aerogenes*, *Alcaligenes faecalis*, *Hemophilus influenzae*, Koch-Weeks bacillus, *Moraxella*, and unclassified gram-negative bacilli.
§Gram-negative diplococci: *Neisseria catarrhalis*, *N. sicca*, and *N. flava*.
‖Gram-positive bacilli: *Bacillus subtilis*, *B. cereus*, and *B. megaterium*.

The two species of staphylococci were more often found alone or in combination with each other; the diphtheroids usually were in association with one or another of the staphylococci. It is apparent from the figures that the distribution of the bacterial flora in the eyelids was essentially the same as that found in the conjunctivas.

Several studies of the flora of the healthy conjunctiva have been reported from various countries. In Table 2-5 some of these data from cities around the world are tabulated. The organisms most often present in the eye throughout these studies were those already reported, namely, *Staphylococcus epidermidis, S. aureus,* and diphtheroids. *Streptococcus viridans* and *Diplococcus pneumoniae* also were found in small numbers in all the reports. The remaining groups of bacteria listed were found by some but not all of the investigators. There were variations in the reported incidence of the three major groups, particularly of *Staphylococcus aureus;* but considering the large differences in the sizes of the sampling, in the geographic location, and in the period in time when the cultures were obtained, the uniformity of the results is quite striking. Eight of the workers have reported from 3.4% to 47% of persons with no bacteria in the eyes. The exceptions were the early studies of Axenfeld and the report of Locatcher-Khorazo and Gutierrez. This later report, covering the years 1952 to 1968, is at variance with the earlier paper by Khorazo and Thompson (Table 2-2), where 12% to 23% of the subjects appeared not to have bacteria in their conjunctivas. Experience with the techniques of eye culture has led to the adoption of a routine procedure, described later, which always gives growth of some organisms, except in patients who have just received a preoperative course of local antibiotic treatment.

SOURCES OF BACTERIAL OCULAR FLORA

The bacteria cultured from the eye usually are similar to those found on the skin and in the upper respiratory tract. Occasionally, gram-negative bacilli, more common in the gastrointestinal tract, are isolated from the eye. In contrast, bacteria commonly found in the air are rarely recovered from the eye. This may be in part because of the high content of lysozyme present in tears. This agent, first described by Fleming[9] in 1922, is an enzyme, a glucosaminidase that brings about the lysis of *Micrococcus lysodeikticus, Sarcina lutea,* and some staphylococci by acting on a hexosamine bound in a mucopolysaccharide fraction incorporated in the cell wall.[19] Some ocular bacteria themselves produce antibiotic agents that also may serve to reduce the number of certain organisms in the eye (Chapter 3).

Somerville[23] has reported cultures taken from the forehead of normal men at various ages. Staphylococci, diphtheroids, streptococci, and a miscellaneous group of less frequently seen bacteria duplicate the flora reported for the normal eye. At the Institute of Ophthalmology, Columbia-Presbyterian Medical Center (IOCPMC), cultures usually have been obtained simultaneously from the eye, nose, face, and hands. Experience has shown that when one attempts to free the eye of bacteria previous to operation, it is important to give attention to neighboring areas. The incidence of bacteria on the face has averaged *Staphylococcus epidermidis* 50%, *Staphylococcus aureus* 22%, diphtheroids 37%, *Bacillus subtilis* 3%, *Streptococcus viridans* 1.5%, *Proteus* group 2%, gram-negative diplococci 5%, and *Klebsiella pneumoniae* 1%. Although many of these organisms are found in the nose and on the hands, the highest incidence and greatest variety usually have been on the skin of the face.

Staphylococcus aureus has been the most common cause of postoperative infections; therefore, the presence of this organism on areas neighboring the eye has been tested. Table 2-6 summarizes some data gathered from 1966 to 1968. Forty-three percent of 2,379 healthy individuals who were found to carry *S. aureus* in the eye also had *S.*

Table 2-6. Incidence of *Staphylococcus aureus* in neighboring areas in relation to incidence in noninfected eyes

	Incidence of *Staphylococcus aureus*					
	Skin of face		Hands		Nose	
Noninfected eyes	Number positive	Percent	Number positive	Percent	Number positive	Percent
Carrying *Staphylococcus aureus* in conjunctivas Number: 2,379	1,026	43	949	40	921	38
Not carrying *Staphylococcus aureus* in conjunctivas Number: 2,104	398	19	735	35	714	34

aureus on the skin of the face, whereas only 19% of 2,104 individuals who did not show this bacterium in the eye carried it on the skin. The incidence of S. *aureus* on the hands or in the nose was only slightly less in the group that did not carry this bacterium in the eye. It may be that the skin of the face is an important source of contamination of the eye. S. *epidermidis* and the diphtheroids may equally well enter the eye from the skin. The nose and hands, however, also are potential areas from which the eye may acquire bacteria.

Gowen[11] made a study of the possible role the eyelids play in maintaining the flora of the eye. He noted the identity of the flora of the eye and eyelid margins and further pointed out that when the eyes are closed, the upper eyelids overlap the lower lids; thus, the upper eyelids are exposed to bacteria of the skin. Gowen believed that the eyelashes play a major role in maintaining the skin flora in the conjunctival sac and that the eyes are never devoid of staphylococci, because the source of contamination is always present.

FLORA OF CADAVERIC EYES

The bacterial flora of cadaveric eyes used for grafting has been studied by Polack and his associates[21] and by others[5,13] in order to determine changes in ocular flora of eyes after death. Methods to promote sterilization of the donor eye were tested. It may be seen from Table 2-7 that the flora is essentially the same in both cadaveric and living eyes. However, a few organisms, notably hemolytic streptococci, *Escherichia coli, Klebsiella pneumoniae, Pseudomonas aeruginosa,* and *Flavobacterium,* are present more frequently in cadaveric eyes. The density of the growth of these bacteria is also greater in the cadaveric eyes. Attempts to utilize disinfecting agents indicated the difficulty of producing sterility without injury to the tissue.

RELATIONSHIP OF NORMAL OCULAR FLORA TO INFECTIONS OF THE EYE

It is apparent from the presence of certain microorganisms in the normal conjunctiva that man often carries with him potentially pathogenic organisms in his eyes just as he may be a carrier of such bacteria in his upper respiratory tract. *Staphylococcus aureus* is the potential pathogen most frequently found. In Chapter 6 evidence is given to indicate that this organism is the commonest cause of postoperative infection and that this infection may arise from the patient's own eye.[17] *Hemophilus influenzae* and some of the gram-negative bacilli found in normal eyes, namely, *Pseudomonas aeruginosa, Escherichia coli, Proteus vulgaris,* and *Klebsiella pneumoniae,* may produce grave infections, such as corneal ulcers or postoperative complications (Chapters 5 and 6). The importance of all these organisms

Table 2-7. A comparison of the ocular flora of normal living eyes with that of postmortem donor eyes

Microorganisms isolated	Percent positive in 566 normal living eyes	Percent positive in 240 postmortem donor eyes
Staphylococcus epidermidis	69.7	71.7
Staphylococcus aureus	30.2	36.3
Diphtheroids	73.1	60.8
Pneumococci	—	0.8
Streptococcus viridans	3.7	8.3
β-Hemolytic streptococci, presumptive group A (bacitracin sensitive)	—	8.3
Neisseria catarrhalis	0.9	0.4
Escherichia coli	1.1	10.0
Proteus mirabilis	1.9	3.3
Proteus morgani	1.6	0.8
Klebsiella pneumoniae	1.4	18.8
Klebsiella ozenae	—	1.7
Pseudomonas aeruginosa	—	4.2
Bacillus megaterium	0.5	—
Bacillus cereus	—	1.7
Sarcina	0.7	2.5
Flavobacterium	—	10.8

From Polack, F. M., Locatcher-Khorazo, D., and Gutierrez, E.: Bacteriologic study of "donor" eyes, Arch. Ophthal. **78**:221, 1967.

is such that, when they are present in the eye of a patient awaiting surgery, prophylactic preoperative treatment with antibiotics has been initiated at the IOCPMC (Chapter 6).

TECHNIQUE FOR OBTAINING CULTURES FROM CONJUNCTIVAS AND EYELIDS

It seems appropriate to include the techniques employed to obtain material for culture, since this must often be performed by the ophthalmologist. The basic media used for the initial cultivation of organisms from the normal external eye is nutrient agar enriched with blood. Fig. 2-1 shows the kit that is used to obtain the material for culture. The wax pencil in the foreground is for labelling the plates in the basket. Zephiran is for cleansing the skin around the eye. The sterile forceps and the cotton on the left and the sterile saline bottle, rear right, are used to wash out any previously applied ointments or makeup. Moist, sterile swabs in test tubes containing a few drops of nutrient broth (see basket) are used to obtain cultures of the conjunctiva and eyelid, because the moistened swab lessens trauma to the patient and ensures optimal yield of bacteria. Table 2-8 presents data that show the great superiority of the moistened swab over the dry swab for cultivation of the bacteria. One of these moistened swabs is passed back and forth twice over the greater part of the lower conjunctiva, carefully avoiding the eyelid border and the eyelashes (Fig. 2-2). Fig. 2-3 shows the inoculation of the blood agar plate. The plate should be inoculated at the patient's bedside, or the material should be sent immediately to the laboratory and the plate promptly inoculated there. The swab is rubbed over the entire surface of the plate; the bottom of the plate is labelled with the individual's name, the date, and the source of the culture (such as the conjunctiva or lid margins) and is incubated overnight. The top of the swab is broken to ensure that it will not be reused. Fig. 2-4, *A* shows the ap-

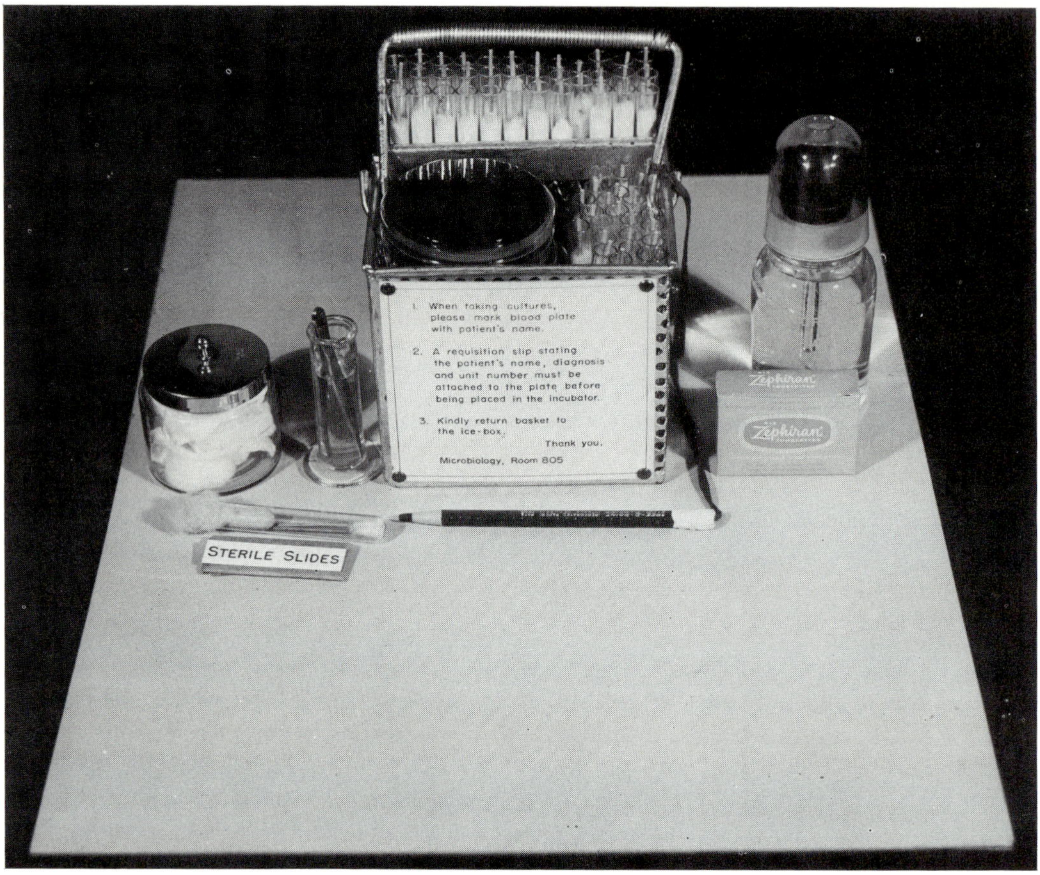

Fig. 2-1. Equipment for routine culturing of eyes.

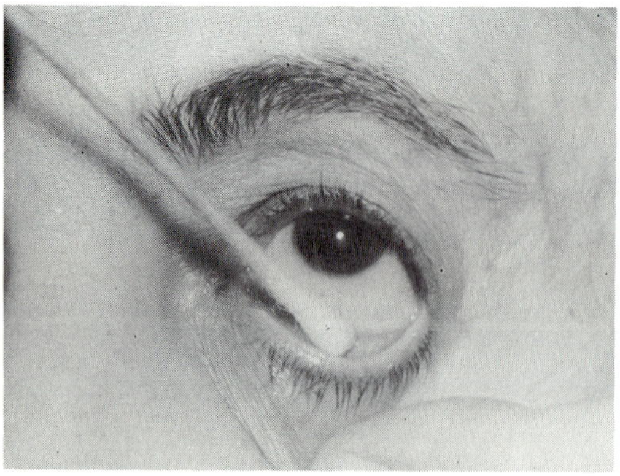

Fig. 2-2. Obtaining culture from lower conjunctiva.

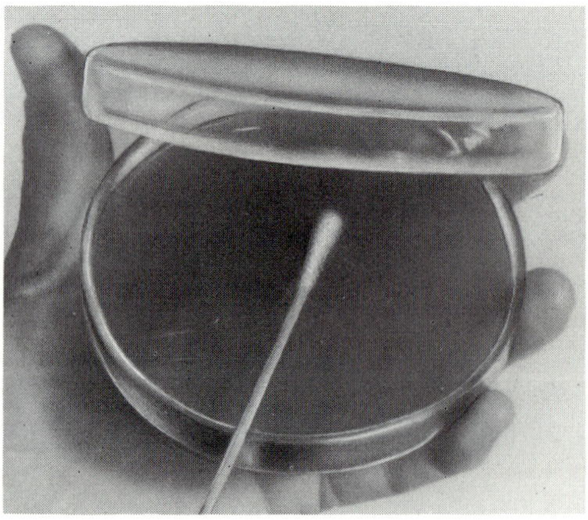

Fig. 2-3. Inoculation of blood agar plate.

Table 2-8. Comparison of cultures of conjunctiva obtained with dry and wet swabs

Case no.	Diagnosis	Dry swab	Wet swab
1	Cataract	No growth	14 colonies *Staphylococcus epidermidis* 6 colonies *Staphylococcus aureus*
2	Cataract	No growth	16 colonies *Corynebacterium hoffmannii* 14 colonies *Staphylococcus epidermidis*
3	Cataract	43 colonies *C. hoffmannii* 18 colonies pneumococci	125 colonies *C. hoffmannii* 63 colonies pneumococci 3 colonies *Staphylococcus aureus*
4	Cataract	1 colony pneumococci	23 colonies pneumococci 24 colonies *Staphylococcus aureus*
5	Cataract	110 colonies *C. hoffmannii*	120 colonies *C. hoffmannii* 32 colonies *Staphylococcus aureus*
6	Normal eye	No growth	Numerous diphtheroids 12 colonies *Staphylococcus aureus*
7	Dacryocystitis	3 colonies *C. hoffmannii*	14 colonies *C. hoffmannii* 2 colonies *Staphylococcus aureus* 6 colonies pneumococci
8	Acute conjunctivitis	6 colonies *Staphylococcus aureus*	Numerous colonies *Staphylococcus aureus* and *Hemophilus influenzae*
9	Chronic conjunctivitis	14 colonies *Staphylococcus epidermidis* 6 colonies *Staphylococcus aureus*	Numerous colonies *Staphylococcus epidermidis* 34 colonies *Staphylococcus aureus* 2 colonies *Escherichia coli*
10	Corneal ulcer	No growth	6 colonies *Staphylococcus aureus*

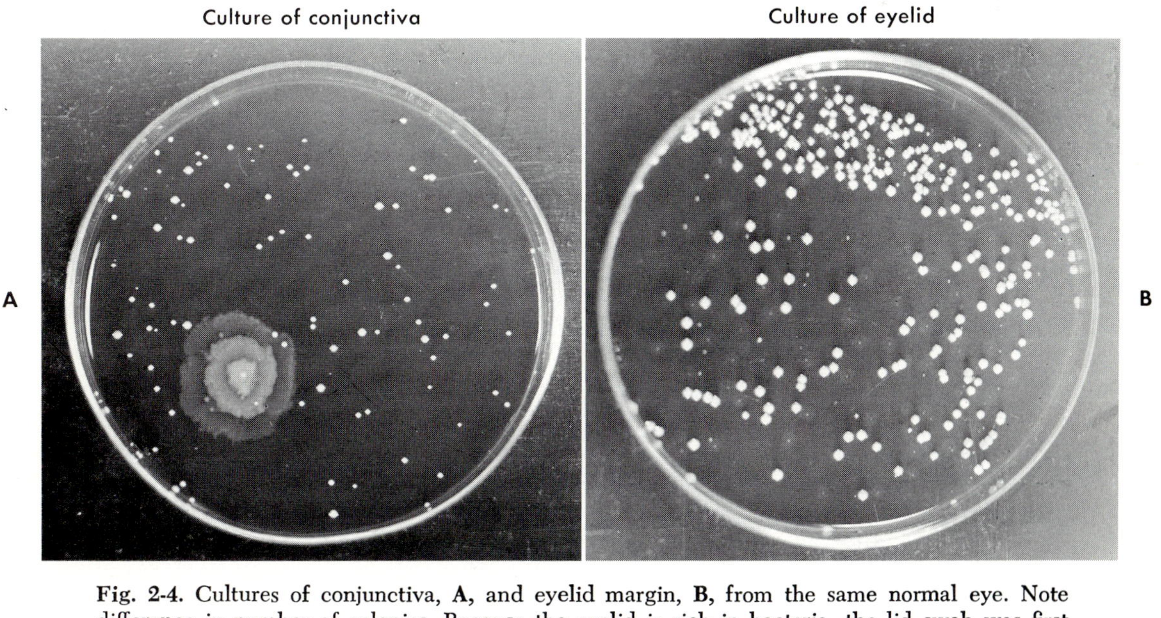

Fig. 2-4. Cultures of conjunctiva, **A,** and eyelid margin, **B,** from the same normal eye. Note difference in number of colonies. Because the eyelid is rich in bacteria, the lid swab was first passed over a portion of the upper part of the plate; then a sterile moist swab was used to complete the inoculation of the plate.

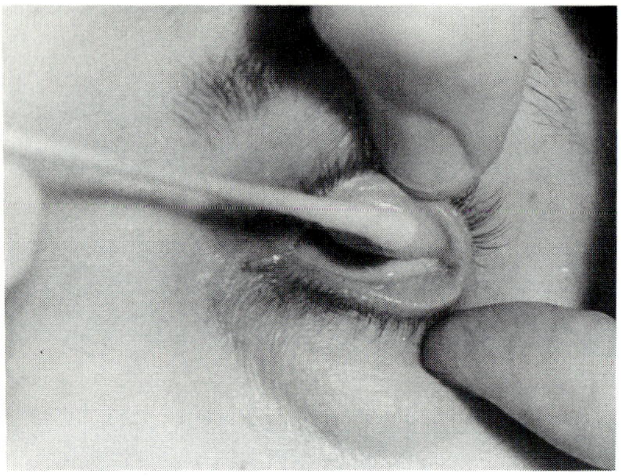

Fig. 2-5. Obtaining culture from upper conjunctiva.

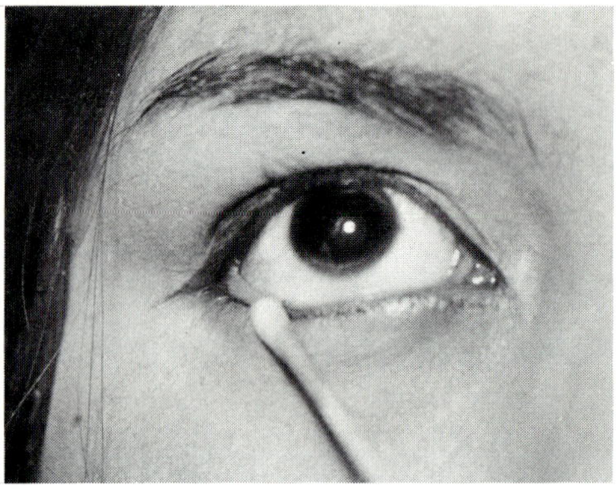

Fig. 2-6. Obtaining culture from eyelid margin.

pearance of growth on such a plate of material from a normal conjunctiva after 24 hours. Note the increased number of bacteria recovered from the eyelid of the same individual (Fig. 2-4, *B*).

Cultures from the upper conjunctiva are not usually necessary except when there is a local area of inflammation. However, the number of bacteria recovered are often more than are found in the lower conjunctiva. If cultures are negative or growth is sparse, a culture of material from the upper conjunctiva is indicated. The technique for obtaining cultures from the upper conjunctiva is illustrated in Fig. 2-5. The material is handled in the same manner as for the lower conjunctiva.

For eyelid cultures another moistened swab is applied to the outer margin of each lid (Fig. 2-6) as the eye is held open, and the material from each lid is swabbed on another blood agar plate. Growth of bacteria is usually heavier from the lid, as is seen in Fig. 2-4, *B*. When an infection is present the swab is rubbed over only one third of the plate, and a fresh sterile swab is used to spread the heavy inoculum further (Chapter 5). The entire process must be repeated for the second eye if there is any question of infection in that eye. It may also be important to obtain cultures from both normal eyes in order to determine whether there is a difference in the flora of the two eyes. Direct smears taken from normal eyes for histologic examination are not helpful, because the organisms are relatively few in number.

SUMMARY

Bacterial flora of the conjunctiva of the normal eye is remarkably constant around the world. Cultures taken from persons of all ages in many parts of the world have shown essentially the same findings, namely, that *Staphylococcus epidermidis,* diphtheroids, and *Staphylococcus aureus* are the predominant organisms. This also was true over 65 years ago, according to Axenfeld.[2] A number of other organisms, some of them potential pathogens, occur very much less frequently but nevertheless must be recognized because of their potential importance.

The source of bacteria in the eye may be the skin of the face, the upper respiratory tract, and the skin of the hands.

Eyes obtained for the eye bank carry the same flora found in life in the normal eye with a few exceptions. All bacteria are more numerous than in the living eye.

Directions are included for obtaining cultures from healthy eyes. These stress the use of moist swabs and the direct inoculation of the media at the bedside or promptly in the laboratory. Blood-enriched nutrient agar is the basic medium for primary isolation.

REFERENCES

1. Allansmith, M. R., Ostler, H. B., and Butterworth, M.: Concomitance of bacteria in various areas of the eye, Arch. Ophthal. **82**:37, 1969.
2. Axenfeld, T.: The bacteriology of the eye, translated by Angus MacNab, New York, 1908, William Wood and Co.
3. Bachrach, U., Gurevitch, J., Landau, J., and Birnbaum, D.: The flora of the normal conjunctiva of healthy people in Israel, Acta Med. Orient. **12**:10, 1953.
4. Barfoed, P.: Conjunctivas Bakterieflora. Thesis presented at Ejnar Munksgaard, Copenhagen, 1953.
5. Boberg-Ans, J., Badsberg, E., and Rasmussen, J.: Frequency of infection in donor eyes post mortem: a method of obtaining sterile eyes for corneal grafting, Brit. J. Ophthal. **46**:365, 1962.
6. Cason, L., and Winkler, C. H.: Bacteriology of the eye: normal flora, Arch. Ophthal. **51**: 196, 1954.
7. Chang, H. L.: Bacterial flora of the normal conjunctiva, Chin. Med. J. **75**:233, 1957.

7a. De Ocampo, G., Salceda, S., and de Leon, A.: Bacterial flora of the healthy conjunctiva among Filipinos, Philippine J. Surg. Surgical Spec. **20**:94, 1965.

8. Doden, W.: Vergleischende Untersuchungen über die Wirkung verschiedener Augensalben auf die Keimflora des gesunden Bindehautsackes, Klin. Mbl. Augenheilk. **131**:237, 1957.
9. Fleming, A.: On a remarkable bacteriolytic element found in tissues and secretions, Proc. Roy. Soc. London (Series B) **93**:306, 1922.
10. Franklin, H. C., and Loeb, L. N.: Bacterial flora in infants encountered at time of delivery: a study of one hundred cultures from the eyelids, Amer. J. Obstet. Gynec. **56**:738, 1948.
11. Gowen, G. H.: Source of Staphylococci on normal conjunctiva of human eye, Amer. J. Ophthal. **17**:36, 1934.
12. Grünberger, V., and Kofler, E.: Uber den Keimgehalt der kindlichen Conjunctiva nach der Geburt, Gynaecologia **137**:329, 1954.
13. Kanski, J. J.: Bacterial flora of the human conjunctiva after death, Brit. J. Ophthal. **49**:445, 1965.
14. Khorazo, D., and Thompson, R.: The bacterial flora of the normal conjunctiva, Amer. J. Ophthal. **18**:1114, 1935.
15. Khristov, G.: Bacterial flora of the normal conjunctiva and in conjunctivitis, Izv. Microbiol. Inst. (Sofiia) **7**:107, 1956.
16. Locatcher-Khorazo, D., and Gutierrez, E.: Ocular flora of 1,024 children (1-18 years old), 1,786 young adults (20-35), and 7,461 patients awaiting ocular surgery, with no known infection. Unpublished data from 1952 to 1968.
17. Locatcher-Khorazo, D., and Gutierrez, E.: Eye infections following cataract extraction with special reference to the role of Staphylococcus aureus, Amer. J. Ophthal. **41**:981, 1956.
18. Lucic, H.: Bacteriology of the normal conjunctival sac, Amer. J. Ophthal. **10**:829, 1927.

18a. Matuura, H.: Anaerobes in the bacterial flora of the conjunctival sac, Jap. J. Ophthal. **15**: 116, 1971.

19. Meyer, K.: Lysozyme, Bull. N. Y. Acad. Med. **30**:995, 1954.
20. Orfila, J., and Courden, B.: Contribution a l'etude de la flore conjonctivale normale, Ann. Oculist. **194**:892, 1961.
21. Polack, F. M., Locatcher-Khorazo, D., and Gutierrez, E.: Bacteriologic study of "donor" eyes, Arch. Ophthal. **78**:219, 1967.
22. Smith, C. H.: Bacteriology of the healthy conjunctiva, Brit. J. Ophthal. **38**:719, 1954.
23. Somerville, D. A.: The effect of age on normal bacterial flora of the skin, Brit. J. Derm. **81**(Suppl. 1):14, 1969.
24. Yamazaki, T.: Bacterial examination of conjunctival sac by thioglycolate medium and human blood agar, Acta Soc. Ophthal. Jap. **62**:1291, 1958.

3

Inhibitory properties of the ocular flora

SEYMOUR P. HALBERT

GENERAL FACTORS IN RESISTANCE TO SUPERFICIAL OCULAR INFECTION

The mechanisms involved in the resistance of the conjunctiva to superficial bacterial infections are not clearly established, but several factors appear to play significant roles. The mechanical trapping action of the eyelashes to catch fine particles of dust almost certainly has a protective function, since it is fairly well established that many airborne microorganisms are carried on such dust motes. The blinking of the eyelids and the flushing action of the tear flow also have a cleansing and protective effect. Experimental studies in which the nasolacrimal duct was tied off so that the normal flow of tears was interrupted clearly demonstrate the increased susceptibility of the conjunctiva to infection. There seems to be little question that disturbance of the nasolacrimal duct clinically results in increased incidence of superficial ocular infection.

Various chemical factors in the tear film may have protective significance. The relative importance of lysozyme as a resistance factor is not yet unequivocally established. It is conceivable that the saprophytic microorganisms that are highly susceptible to this enzyme are devoid of pathogenicity largely because of lysozyme. It is also possible that even the known pathogenic bacterial species that reveal relatively slight susceptibility to this substance might be inhibited adequately to prevent active infection. Since local antibody concentration seems to be a significant factor in certain infections, such as influenza, a knowledge of the antibody content of tears would be of some importance. However, no such data seems to be available.

POTENTIAL PROTECTIVE ROLE OF INHIBITORY OCULAR FLORA

The bulk of this chapter will be devoted to the possible role of the normal ocular flora as a protective factor in resistance to superficial conjunctival bacterial infections. As was pointed out in Chapter 2, the organisms that make up the bulk of the ocular flora are staphylococci and diphtheroids. The precise species involved and their apparent fluctuation have been discussed in Chapter 2. It is clear that they are always present in variable numbers and that they become implanted shortly after birth. Pathogenic microorganisms must multiply and invade tissues in spite of the presence of normal flora. Considerable data has accumulated demonstrating the inhibitory effects of this normal flora on pathogenic bacteria.[1-10]

In occasional instances, primary cultures of the conjunctival flora reveal inhibition of one organism by another. An example of this is shown in Fig. 3-1, which represents the growth on a blood agar plate from the

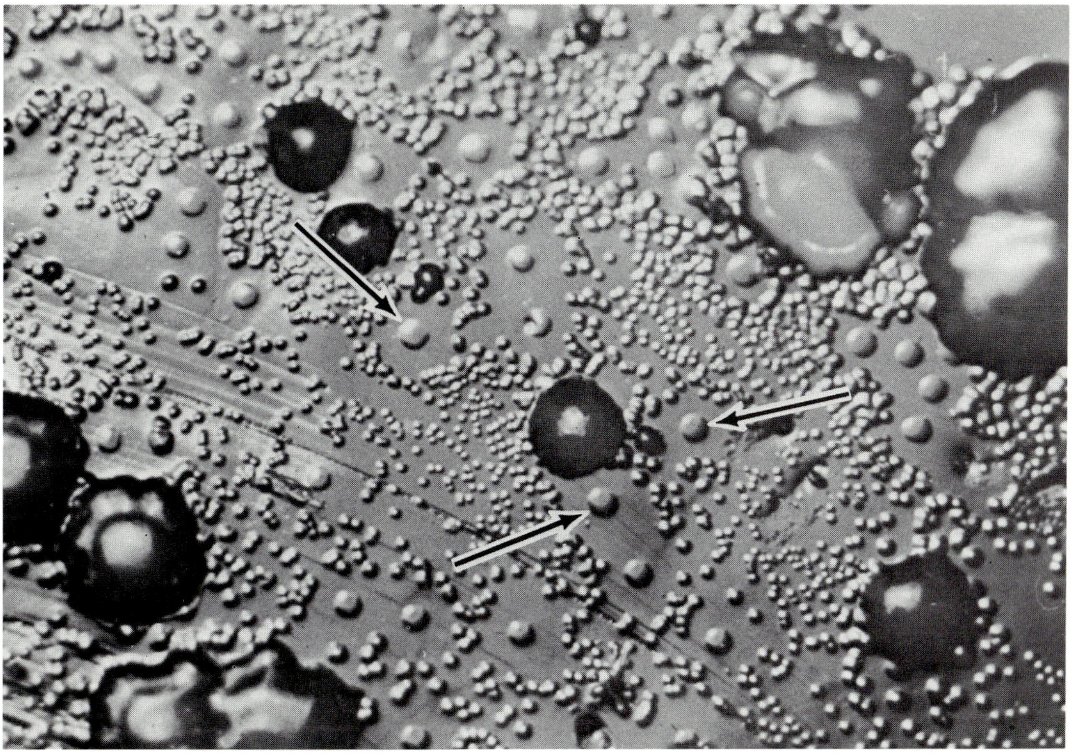

Fig. 3-1. "Spontaneous" appearance of inhibiting activity (arrows) in the original streak from the eye swab of a patient. (From Halbert, S. P., and Swick, L. S.: Amer. J. Ophthal. **35**:78, 1952.)

conjunctival swab of material from a patient with conjunctivitis. It is clear that the slightly larger translucent colonies interfered with the growth of the more numerous minute colonies of microorganisms in their immediate vicinity.

Inhibiting strains of ocular organisms can be more readily detected by other methods. When the conjunctival culture is allowed to grow for 24 hours and then the entire surface is seeded with an indicator strain by a spray technique, variable numbers of colonies can be demonstrated to have secreted inhibitors, as seen in Fig. 3-2. In this instance, the indicator organism is a strain of *Staphylococcus albus* of ocular origin, and the medium is blood agar.

Still another way of demonstrating the inhibitory effect of strains of the ocular flora consists of first growing the primary conjunctival culture and then transferring individual colonies to the surface of an agar plate already uniformly seeded with an indicator strain. Examples of results obtained with 20 colonies, each selected at random from single individuals, are shown in Fig. 3-3. In *A*, *B*, and *C* the indicator organism is a highly susceptible *Corynebacterium pseudodiphtheriticum*. It is of interest that the inhibitory activities of these strains from the same person were so variable, in spite of the fact that many of the individual colonies were otherwise indistinguishable. The striking differences in the susceptibility of different indicator strains is also shown in Fig. 3-3, *D*, where identical colonies were tested against an S. *albus* culture as well as against a *C. pseudodiphtheriticum* culture.

That the inhibitions noted resulted from secreted antibiotic substances in the case of highly active strains is revealed by the readily demonstrated activity of crude culture filtrates. The crisp inhibition zones

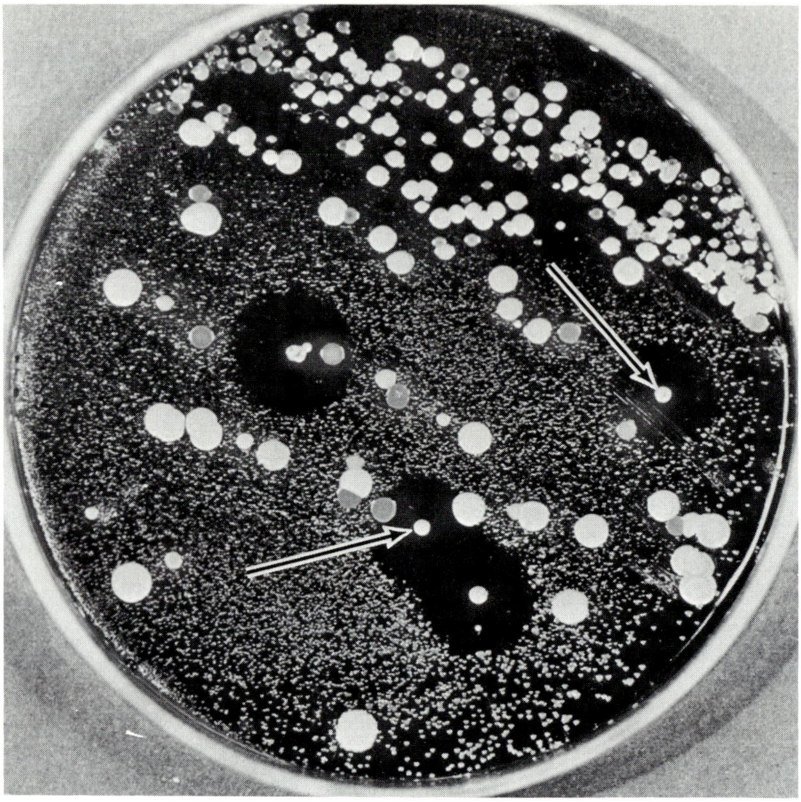

Fig. 3-2. *Staphylococcus albus* 7-6 spray-seeded onto blood agar after 48-hour incubation of original inoculum from one patient. The arrows point to highly active antibiotic-producing organisms. (From Halbert, S. P., and Swick, L. S.: Amer. J. Ophthal. **35**:74, 1952.)

produced by such filtrates from three potent organisms, 224-4, 166-4, and 303-3, are shown in Fig. 3-4. When a series of both highly and slightly inhibitory strains of ocular staphylococci were similarly tested for the secretion of antibiotics, results with the highly potent strains were always positive, although only a portion of the slightly active strains could be readily shown to secrete inhibitors. However, heat lability of the antibiotics and other factors could account for the failure to demonstrate antibiotics in a higher proportion of these latter strains. Nonactive organisms never revealed inhibitors in the crude filtrates. Some of these results are summarized in Table 3-1, where it may also be noted that the crude filtrates of many slightly active organisms produced zones of decreased opacity of the indicator organisms. When similar tests were carried out using the more sensitive indicator, *C. pseudodiphtheriticum,* about one half of the weakly inhibitory strains revealed antibiotic substances in the culture supernates. These data are shown in Fig. 3-5, which also shows the high degree of variability in the potency of the antibiotic crude filtrates.

CHARACTERISTICS OF INHIBITORY OCULAR FLORA AND THE ANTIBIOTICS THEY PRODUCE

In this study most of the inhibitory organisms of the ocular flora proved to be strains of staphylococci, although occasional active streptococci and diphtheroids were detected. A number of the staphylococcal cultures were subjected to more detailed identification tests; the results are shown in Table 3-2. It may be seen that

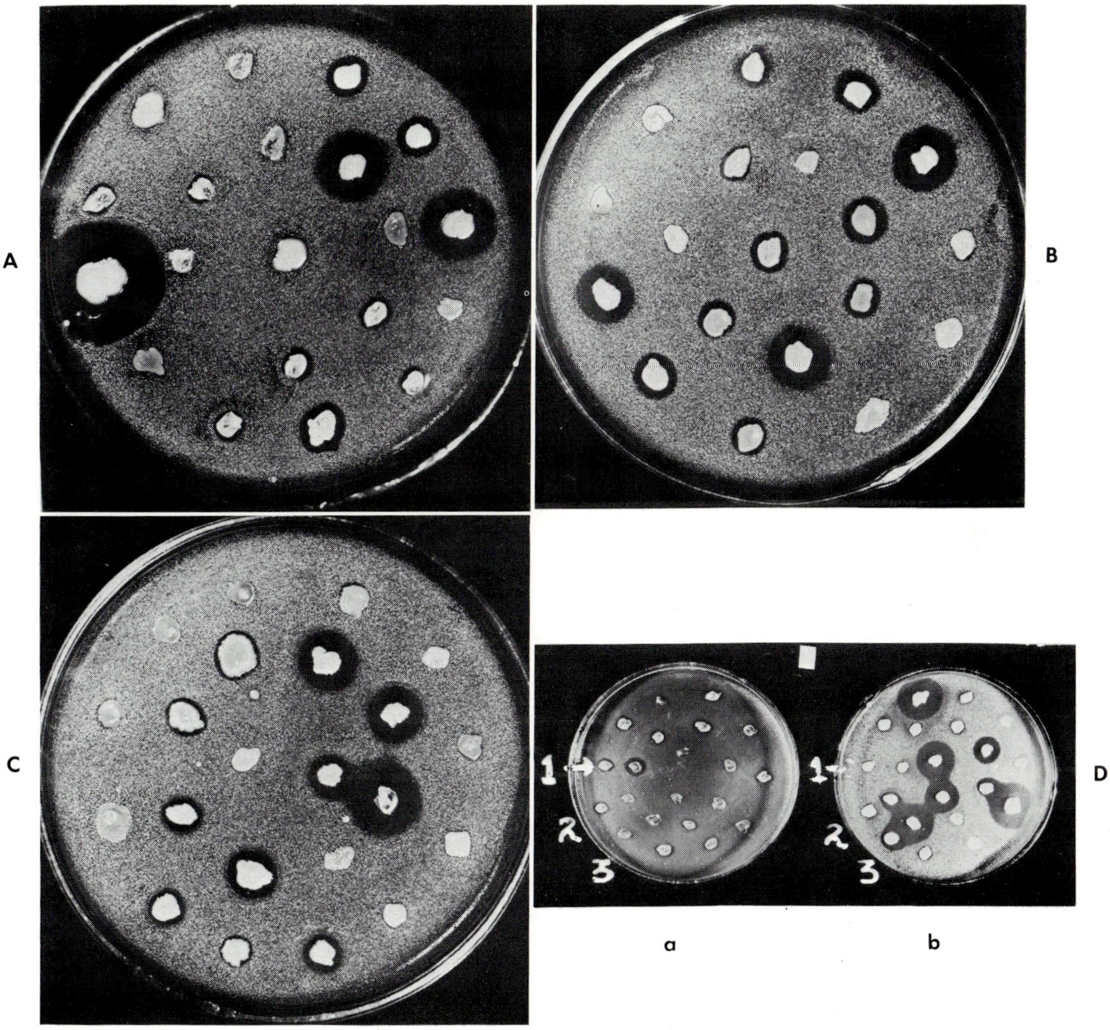

Fig. 3-3. Anitbiotic activity of sample colonies of ocular microorganisms from single individuals. **A, B,** and **C,** Tested against *C. pseudodiphtheriticum;* **D,** tested against both *S. albus* 7-6 (*a*) and *C. pseudodiphtheriticum* (*b*). In these plates the same colonies were tested against both indicators. (From Halbert, S. P., Locatcher-Khorazo, D., Sonn-Kazar, C., and Swick, L. S.: Arch. Ophthal. **58**:68, 1957.)

most of the strains were typical or atypical *Staphylococcus albus,* with occasional organisms of other *Micrococcus* species detected. It is thus clear that the inhibitory bacteria so frequently encountered in the ocular flora are derived from the most abundant species residing on the superficial eye tissues. It is also clear that the inhibitory effects are caused by the secretion of antibiotic substances.

It was found that occasional resistant variants of the indicator strains occurred with regularity upon exposure to minimal concentrations of a given antibiotic. When these resistant variants were subcultured, it was found that they were not affected by the antibiotic of the strain to which they had been exposed but that they might still be susceptible to antibiotics of other strains. In addition, investigation of the chemical and physical properties of the antibiotics produced by 22 strains of highly inhibitory ocular microorganisms demonstrated clear differences between many of them. Nine distinct groups of antibiotics could be differentiated. Some of these data are summarized in Table 3-3. Since many of the antibiotics were destroyed by the proteolytic enzymes trypsin and chymotrypsin and were precipitable by high concentrations of ammonium sulfate, it is probable that many were of polypeptide nature. Some were rather stable to heat (100° C), whereas others were destroyed by such temperatures. The fact that some were freely or partially dialyzable through Visk-

Table 3-1. Crude antibiotic production in relation to the inhibitory activity of living ocular staphylococcal cultures, tested against other staphylococci as indicators

Strains	Number of strains	Number producing active crudes (percent)	Potency of crudes: mm width*	Potency of crudes: Number of strains	Median potency (mm width)
Highly active	28	28 (100%)	0.0–3.0	3	5.0
			3.1–5.0	11	
			5.1–7.0	8	
			7.1+	6	
Slightly active	36	8 (22%)	0.0	9	—
			Zones of decreased opacity†	19	
			1.0‡–2.8	8	
Nonactive	22	0 (0%)	—	—	0

From Halbert, S. P., Swick, L. S., and Sonn, C.: Characteristics of antibiotic-producing strains of the ocular flora, J. Immun. **70**:402, 1953. © 1953, The Williams and Wilkins Co.
*Refers to the distance from the rim of the well to the edge of normal growth. The figures represent the maximum inhibition against any of the three *Micrococcus* indicator strains, 7–6, 15–1, or 13–2.
†Although no distinct inhibition was noted, the colonies surrounding these wells were of less opacity than the normal growth.
‡The edges of the inhibition zones of most of these were poorly demarcated, both with the crudes and with the living systems.

Table 3-2. Identification of a series of ocular staphylococci in relation to inhibitory activities

Biochemical pattern: Coagulase production	Mannitol fermentation	Gelatin liquefaction	NO_3 reduction	$(NH_4)H_2PO_4$ utilization	Number of strains: Highly active	Slightly active	Nonactive	Tentative identification*
0	0	+	+	0	9	30	25	"Atypical" *M. pyogenes* var. *albus*
0	+	+	+	0	8	1	2	*M. pyogenes* var. *albus*
0	+	0	+	0	1	0	2	*M. aurantiacus*
0	0	0	+	0	1	1	0	*M. epidermidis*
0	0	+	0	0	3	0	0	"Atypical" *M. candidus*
0	0	0	0	0	0	1	1	*M. candidus*
+	+	+	+	0	0	0	1	*M. pyogenes* var. *aureus*

From Halbert, S. P., Swick, L. S., and Sonn, C.: Characteristics of antibiotic-producing strains of the ocular flora, J. Immun. **70**:401, 1953. © 1953, The Williams and Wilkins Co.
*According to *Bergey's Manual of Determinative Bacteriology*, 6th edition.

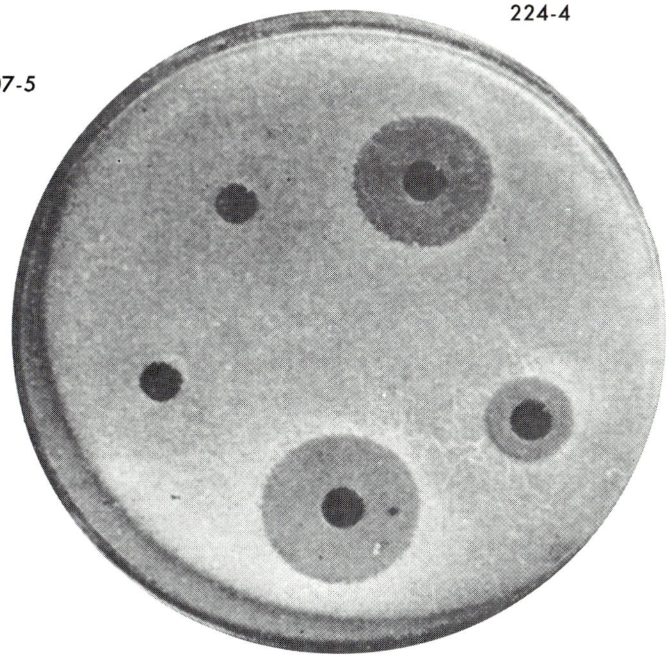

Fig. 3-4. Antibiotic activity of some crude supernates from several active staphylococci tested against strain 15-1. (From Halbert, S. P., and Swick, L. S.: Amer. J. Ophthal. 35:77, 1952.)

Table 3-3. Differentiation of the antibiotics of 22 strains of ocular microorganisms into 9 distinct groups, on the basis of tests with resistant variants of an indicator *Staphylococcus* (15-1), and chemical properties

Activity vs. resistant variants of strain 15-1	Group	Number of strains	Properties					
			Acteone precipita-bility	$(NH_4)_2SO_4$ precipita-bility	Heat stability	Dialyza-bility	Enzyme digestibility: Trypsin	Enzyme digestibility: Chymo-trypsin
Inactive vs. R_1 and R_2,	I	7	0	+†	S‡	±*	0	0
active vs. R_3 and R_4	II	1	0	+	L	±	0	0
Inactive vs. R_3 and R_4,	III	4	±	+	S	+	+†	0
active vs. R_1 and R_2	IV	2	±	+	L	+	+	0
	V	3	0	+	S	+	+	0
Active vs. R_1, R_2, R_3,	VI	2	±	0	L	0	+	+
and R_4	VII	1	±	+	L	±	+	0
	VIII	1	0	0	L	0	+	+
	IX	1	0	+	L	±	+	+

From Halbert, S. P., Swick, L. S., and Sonn, C.: Characteristics of antibiotic-producing strains of the ocular flora, J. Immun. **70**:404, 1953. © 1953, The Williams and Wilkins Co.

*+ represents free dialyzability, ± partial dialyzability, and 0 nondialyzability.

†+ represents precipitability with ammonium sulfate or acetone, or destruction by the enzyme. 0 represents failure to precipitate with $(NH_4)_2SO_4$ or acetone, or resistance to the enzyme.

‡S represents heat stability, and L represents heat lability, especially at alkaline pH levels.

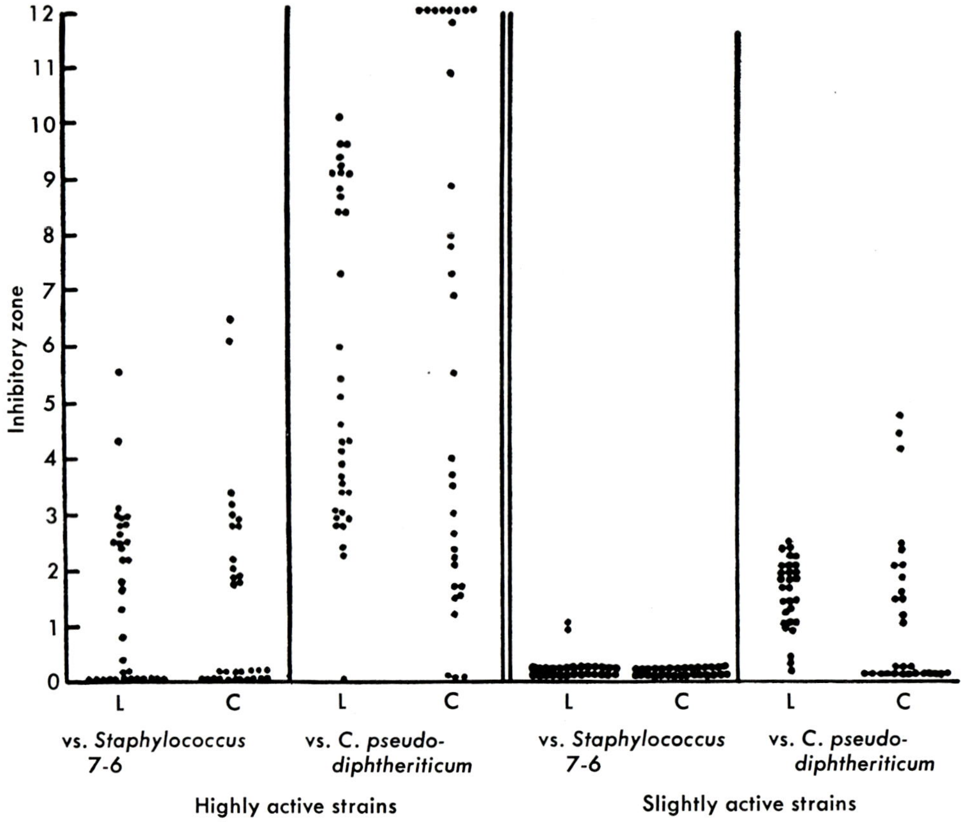

Fig. 3-5. Production of crude antibiotic solutions by sample strains of inhibitory ocular organisms. Each point represents the value obtained with one organism. *L,* Inhibition zones (in millimeters) in tests with the living antibiotic-producing strain; *C,* inhibition zones in tests with crude antibiotics from these strains. (From Halbert, S. P., Locatcher-Khorazo, D., Sonn-Kazar, C., and Swick, L. S.: Arch. Ophthal. **58**:69, 1957.)

ing cellophane membranes suggests that these antibiotics were of rather small molecular sizes.

ANTIBACTERIAL SPECTRA OF INHIBITORY OCULAR FLORA

The antibacterial spectra of these antibiotics were found to be largely limited to the gram-positive species and the neisseria. The gram-negative rods were quite resistant. Even among the gram-positive organisms, however, there was considerable variability in the susceptibility of different strains of the same species. This is clearly shown in Fig. 3-6, which shows the susceptibility of a number of bacterial species to 10 antibiotic-producing ocular microorganisms. The figure clearly indicates that differing percentages of test strains were affected by any given antibiotic and that, in general, most other staphylococci were susceptible. In the case of *Corynebacterium,* most strains were highly sensitive to the antibiotic of *Staphylococcus* 283-8, but most were resistant to strain 306-6. In addition to the organisms listed in Fig. 3-6, it was found that numerous strains of pathogenic and nonpathogenic *Mycobacterium, Neisseria,* and *Clostridium* were frequently and highly susceptible to such antibiotics. Strains of *Salmonella, Shigella, Proteus, Pseudomonas, Escherichia, Klebsiella,* and *Vibrio* were included in the Enterobac-

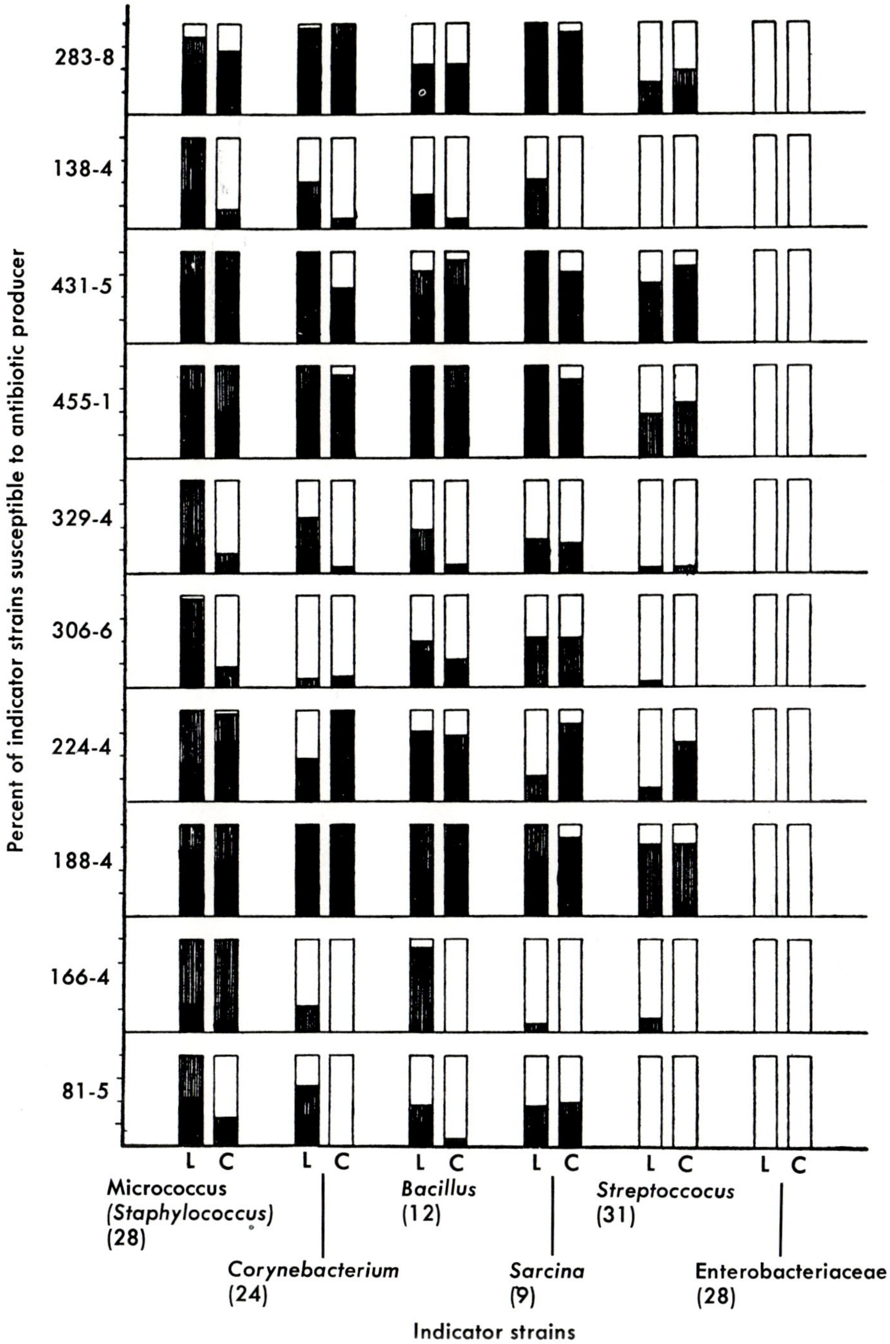

Fig. 3-6. Susceptibility of some bacterial species to a group of antibiotic-producing ocular micrococci. *L*, Tests with living microorganisms; *C*, tests with crude antibiotic derived from that strain; ( ), number of strains examined.

■ Represents percent of highly susceptible strains; that is, those being inhibited at least one half the size of the most susceptible stock indicator strains. Many showed zones much higher.

▥ Represents percent of slightly susceptible strains; that is, those being inhibited to a width of less than one half the size of the most suscpetible stock indicator strain.

□ Represents percent of resistant strains; that is, no significant inhibition noted.

(From Halbert, S. P., Swick, L. S., and Sonn, C.: J. Immun. **70**:407, 1953.)

teriaceae that were tested; these were found to be quite resistant.

CLINICAL OBSERVATIONS RELATED TO INHIBITORY OCULAR MICROORGANISMS

In a number of individuals, simultaneously sampled strains of staphylococci from the eye, nose, and skin of different patients were tested for antibiotic activities. In about one fourth of the cases the inhibitory patterns of the flora of the various tissues were strikingly different from each other. Table 3-4 shows some examples of cultures from the conjunctiva, anterior nares, and skin of the ventral surface of the hand in a series of such individuals. In patient 2 all twenty staphylococcal strains from the ocular flora produced inhibitory zones of 1.8 mm, whereas 10 such colonies from the nose and 10 from the skin had no activity whatsoever. In the remaining three fourths of patients so tested, organisms from the various tissues showed quite similar inhibitory patterns.

A series of observations were made to see if the antibiotic-producing organisms of the ocular flora could be related to superficial conjunctival infection or to inflammation. In such a study it was of some importance to characterize the microorganisms isolated from the patients with conjunctivitis and to compare them with the control group with normal eyes. When this was done in one such study, as shown in Table 3-5, it could be readily seen that no striking differences were observed between the two groups. However, only two patients with conjunctivitis revealed *Hemophilus* strains, and another two harbored diplobacilli; none of these microorganisms were found in the control eyes. These findings suggest that bacterial infections may not have been involved in the etiologies of most of the conjunctival disturbances or that the strains isolated from patients with disease differed in some subtle ways from those isolated from normal individuals.

When the patients with conjunctivitis were compared with the normal individuals with respect to antibiotic producers, no significant differences were found between the two when a staphylococcal indicator strain was used (Table 3-6). In a similar study on a different group of patients, a highly sensitive corynebacterial indicator was used. When the number of strains active against this organism from the patients with conjunctivitis were compared with the group who had normal eyes, again no differences were seen. These data are summarized in Fig. 3-7, which shows that striking fluctuations were observed in the incidence of such strains at various periods throughout the year. During March 1952, for example, about 70% of all strains tested

Table 3-4. Comparison of antibiotic activities of organisms (mostly staphylococci) of the ocular, nasal, and skin flora of single individuals

Patient	Antibiotic activity against *Corynebacterium pseudodiphtheriticum* of strains from		
	Eye	Nose	Skin (hand)
1	20 (1.2)* 0 (0)	12 (0)	4 (0.6) 6 (0)
2	20 (1.8) 0 (0)	10 (0)	10 (0)
3	15 (1.7) 5 (1.0) 0 (0)	10 (0)	2 (1.0) 8 (0)
4	20 (0)	20 (0)	7 (1.7) 2 (0)
5	11 (1.0) 9 (0)	7 (4.0) 1 (1.5) 3 (0)	10 (0)
6	20 (4.5) 0 (0)	10 (0)	—
7	20 (0)	10 (1.3) 1 (0)	—
8	12 (1.3) 8 (0)	—	15 (0)
9	20 (0)	10 (0)	10 (0)
10	20 (6.0)	10 (6.0)	11 (5.5)

From Halbert, S. P., Locatcher-Khorazo, D., Sonn-Kazar, C., and Swick, L. S.: Further studies on the incidence of antibiotic-producing micro-organisms of the ocular flora, Arch. Ophthal. **58**:73, 1957.

*The first figure represents the number of colonies; the figure in parentheses represents the zone of inhibition in millimeters.

Table 3-5. Comparison of species in the bacterial flora from patients with normal eyes and those with conjunctivitis

	Normal						Conjunctivitis					
Group	*Staphylococcus aureus**	Streptococci*	Hemophilus*	Diphtheroids*	Diplobacilli	No "pathogens"	*Staphylococcus aureus**	Streptococci*	Hemophilus*	Diphtheroids*	Diplobaccili	No "pathogens"
H	3†	0	0	0	0	20	5	0	1	1	0	10
Iota	3	0	0	0	0	17	4	1	0	(1)‡	0	15
Q	9	0	0	0	0	25	3	0	0	0	0	3
S	3	0	0	0	0	18	1	2	0	0	0	16
Y	6	4	0	1	0	23	2	(1)	0	0	0	4
Delta	1	0	0	1	0	20	5	(2)	0	0	1	12
Theta, 6th visit	0	3	0	1	0	13	3	2	1	1	1	14
Theta, 7th visit	0	4	0	1	0	14	3	5	0	4	0	9
Totals	25	11	0	4	0	150	26	10	2	6	2	83
			190							129		

From Halbert, S. P., Swick, L. S., Sonn, C., and Locatcher-Khorazo, D.: Ocular antibiotic-producing bacteria in normal eyes and in conjunctivitis, Arch. Ophthal. **51**:10, 1954.
*Only cultures showing more than 50 colonies of these microorganisms are recorded here.
†Figures represent number of patients.
‡Patients in parentheses showed two of the species indicated, usually with *S. aureus*.

Table 3-6. Comparison of patients with conjunctivitis and normal eyes, with respect to antibiotic-producing organisms of the ocular flora

	Number of patients with					
	Normal conjunctivas			Conjunctivitis		
Cottage	Highly active*	Slightly active†	Total number of patients	Highly active	Slightly active	Total number of patients
Q	1	14	34	0	3	6
Y	2	6	33	0	3	7
S	1	9	21	0	9	19
Iota	0	6	20	0	4	20
H	2	11	23	1	8	17
Delta	3	17	2	1	14	18
Theta (last 3 visits)	4	28	48	18	19	69
Totals	13	91	201	20	60	156
	(6.5%)	(45.3%)		(12.8%)	(38.5%)	
	51.8%			51.3%		

From Halbert, S. P., Swick, L. S., Sonn, C., and Locatcher-Khorazo, D.: Ocular antibiotic-producing strains of the ocular flora, Arch. Ophthal. **51**:10, 1954.
*Patients revealing any highly active strains; some had both highly and slightly active organisms.
†Patients revealing any slightly active strains; all also revealed nonactive strains.

showed some activity, whereas about 35% revealed inhibition zones of 2.0 mm or greater. During December 1952, however, only about 30% of all strains showed any inhibitory properties, and merely 3% were rather highly active. Despite the fluctuations with time, no clear differences could be observed between the group with conjunctivitis and the group with normal eyes. This lack of difference was also apparent when the number of individuals revealing *any* inhibitory strains were compared.

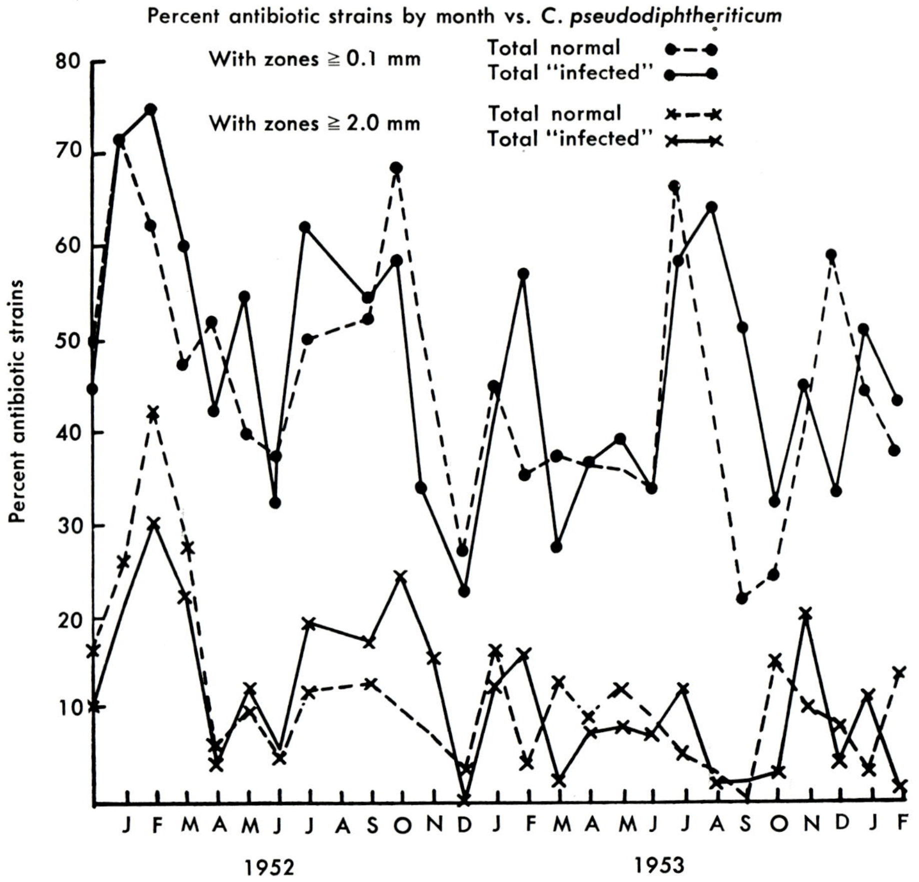

Fig. 3-7. Monthly incidence of antibiotic strains from the ocular flora during the period of observation. Each point represents the percentage of the total number of strains examined during the month. (From Halbert, S. P., Locatcher-Khorazo, D., Sonn-Kazar, C., and Swick, L. S.: Arch. Ophthal. **58**:72, 1957.)

IN VIVO SIGNIFICANCE OF INHIBITORY OCULAR MICROORGANISMS IN EXPERIMENTAL INFECTIONS

In an attempt to obtain evidence regarding the significance of these inhibitory strains in ocular resistance mechanisms, simplified experimental models were sought. Mixed infections were carried out in animals in which one member of the bacterial pair was lethally pathogenic and the other member was an ocular staphylococcus. Ocular staphylococci were chosen to represent strains both antibiotically active and nonactive against the pathogen. The virulent pathogens included a gas gangrene-producing organism (*Clostridium septicum*) and the diphtheria-producing *Corynebacterium diphtheriae.* Since superficial ocular infections would have been complicated by the presence of the normal flora of the animal itself, other routes of infection were employed.

In the case of mixed infections with *Clostridium septicum,* it was soon clear that the antibiotic activities do have in vivo biologic significance. This may be seen in Table 3-7, which summarizes the results of intramuscular infection of mice with this pathogen and mixtures of ocular staphylococci of varying antibiotic potencies. The protection against fatal outcome was

Table 3-7. Mixed infections of *Clostridium septicum* and ocular staphylococci of varying antibiotic activities in experimental infections of mice by the intramuscular route

Antibiotic group	*Micrococcus* strain*	Inhibition of *Clostridium septicum* (mm)†	Results of *Clostridium septicum* challenge with					
			10^{-4}‡			10^{-2}		
Highly active	117-3	7.1	S	S	S	S	S	S
	K1328-1	7.0	D4§	S	S	D2	S	S
	96-6	6.8	S	S	S	D3	S	S
	K88-8	5.9	S	S	S	S	S	S
	188-4	5.5	S	S	S	D2	D2	S
	K21-4	5.5	D2	S	S	D2	S	S
	K610-18	5.2	D1	D1	D1	D1	D1	D1
	K618-6	4.6	S	S	S	D2	D4	S
	455-1	4.3	D4	S	S	D4	D4	S
	K102-11	4.0	S	S	S	D1	D2	S
	K609-16	3.9	D2	S	S	D2	D2	D2
	K423-11	2.7	D2	S	S	D2	D2	D4
Slightly active	K1745-5	2.4	D1	D1	D1	D1	D1	D1
	K462-2	1.5	D2	S	S	D2	D2	S
	K36-2	1.4	D1	D2	S	D1	D4	S
	K1750-5	1.9	D1	D1	D2	D1	D1	D1
	K1771-11	0.7	D1	D2	S	D1	D1	D1
	100-5	2.9‖	D1	D1	D1	D1	D1	D2
Nonactive	191-4	0	D1	D1	D1	D1	D1	D1
	431-5	0	D1	D1	D1	D1	D1	D1
	K887-9	0	D1	D1	D1	D1	D1	D1
	K1115-19	0	D1	D1	D1	D1	D1	S
	81-5	0	D1	D1	D1	D1	D1	D1
	166-4	0	D1	D1	D1	D1	D1	D1
	303-3	0	D1	D1	D1	D1	D1	D1
	127-1	0	D1	D1	D1	D1	D1	D1
	K619-5	0	D1	D1	D1	D1	D1	D1
	K-1101-6	0	D1	D1	D1	D1	D1	D1
	K420-2	0	D1	D1	D1	D1	D1	D1
	K582-7	0	D1	D1	D1	D1	D1	D1
Controls	—	—	D1	D1	D1	D1	D1	D1
			D1	D1	D1	D1	D1	D1
			D1	D1	D1	D1	D1	D1

From Halbert, S. P., Sonn, C., and Swick, L.: Mixed bacterial infections in relation to antibiotic activities: *Clostridium septicum*–micrococcus infections, J. Immun. **73:**172, 1954. © 1954, The Williams and Wilkins Co.
*The micrococcal inocula averaged about 300 million organisms (as judged by colony counts), or 0.3 mg of bacterial cell solids. All suspensions were prepared to roughly similar concentrations.
†Millimeter width of inhibition zone of *Clostridium septicum* produced by the living micrococcal strains, assayed at the time of infection.
‡These dilutions of *Clostridium septicum* spores represented inocula of 10–100 LD_{50} and 1,000–10,000 LD_{50}, equivalent to 1,000 and 100,000 spores respectively.
§S = survived 7 days; D1 = died first day, etc.
‖This zone was very poorly demarcated.

clearly apparent when the latter organism was highly active antibiotically against the *Clostridium* strain. The complete lack of protective effect of the noninhibitory strains was also clear, as was the small increase in survival when the ocular staphylococci were slightly active.

It was also evident that this protective property was much more effective when the staphylococcal partner in these mixed

Table 3-8. Effect of heat-killed and living ocular staphylococci in mixed intramuscular infections with *Clostridium septicum* in mice

Group	Dilution of *Clostridium septicum* spore suspension											
	Experiment 1				Experiment 2				Experiment 3			
	10^{-3}	10^{-4}	10^{-5}	10^{-6}	10^{-3}	10^{-4}	10^{-5}	10^{-6}	10^{-3}	10^{-4}	10^{-5}	10^{-6}
Clostridium controls	D1	D1	D1	D1	D1	D1	D1	D1	D1	D1	D1	D1
	D1	D1	D1	D1	D1	D1	D1	D1	D1	D1	D1	D1
	D1	D1	D1	D2	D1	D1	D1	D1	D1	D1	D1	D1
	D1	D1	D1	S	D1	D1	D2	D2	D1	D1	D1	D1
	D1	D1	D1	S	D1	D1	D2	S	D1	D1	D1	D1
	D1	D1	S	S	D1	D1	D2	S	D1	D1	D1	S
	D6	S	S	S	D1	S	S	S	D1	D4	S	S
Clostridium + *Micrococcus* K88-8 (living)	S	S	S	S	D2	S	S	S	D2	D2	D4	S
	S	S	S	S	S	S	S	S	D4	D4	S	S
	S	S	S	S	S	S	S	S	S	D4	S	S
	S	S	S	S	S	S	S	S	S	D7	S	S
	S	S	S	S	S	S	S	S	S	S	S	S
	S	S	S	S	S	S	S	S	S	S	S	S
	S	S	S	S	S	S	S	S	S	S	S	S
Clostridium + *Micrococcus* K88-8 (heat-killed)	D1	D1	D2	S	D1	D3	S	D6	D1	D1	D2	D1
	D1	D1	S	S	D1	S	S	S	D1	D2	D2	D2
	D1	D1	S	S	D2	S	S	S	D1	D2	D4	S
	D2	D2	S	S	D4	S	S	S	D1	D2	D4	S
	D2	D2	S	S	S	S	S	S	D1	D2	S	S
	D2	S	S	S	S	S	S	S	D1	D4	S	S
	D2	S	S	S	S	S	S	S	S	S	S	S

From Halbert, S. P., Sonn, C., and Swick, L.: Mixed bacterial infections in relation to antibiotic activities: *Clostridium septicum*–micrococcus infections, J. Immun. **73**:175, 1954. © 1954, The Williams and Wilkins Co.

infections was living. This is shown in Table 3-8, which indicates that heat-killed staphylococci were much less protective than were the living organisms. Such data thus indicated that the staphylococcus must have been secreting an antibiotic in the in vivo environment and that this secretion inhibited the growth of the clostridia in the tissues.

That this was actually the case was demonstrated when an antibiotic from one of these ocular staphylococcal strains was partially purified and tested for its protective capacity against the *Clostridium septicum* infection. The high potency of this agent is illustrated in Table 3-9, where it may be seen that a dose of as little as 0.1 mg given intramuscularly at the infection site completely protected against as much as 1,000 LD_{50} doses of the virulent organism. A dose of the antibiotic of 1 mg given intraperitoneally also protected most of the animals against this size of challenge infection. In view of this data it seems clear that the active protective agent in the mixed infections is the staphylococcal antibiotic produced in vivo. If similar production of such antibiotics occurs in vivo on the surface of the ocular tissues, as seems reasonable, it is fair to suspect that such substances and activities are of considerable significance in superficial resistance mechanisms of the eye.

Even when the ocular staphylococcal antibiotic was administered at varying times following the infection dose, definite therapeutic effects could still be observed. The data from such an experiment are summarized in Table 3-10. It may be recalled that this infection system is usually fatal within 18 to 24 hours (Table 3-7), and a 6-hour delay in starting treatment repre-

Table 3-9. Prophylaxis of *Clostridium septicum* infections of mice by antibiotic concentrate derived from an ocular staphylococcus

Group	Antibiotic dose (mg)	Dilution of *Clostridium septicum* spores			
		10^{-3}	10^{-4}	10^{-5}	10^{-6}
Controls	—	0/18*	1/18	2/27	18/22
Staphylocococcal antibiotic,	1.0	8/8	9/11	8/8	7/8
locally intramuscular	0.5	8/8	11/11	11/11	8/8
at infection site	0.2	8/8	8/8	8/8	8/8
	0.1	8/8	7/8	8/8	8/8
Staphylococcal antibiotic,	8.0	8/8	11/11	8/8	7/8
intraperitoneal	4.0	7/8	9/11	11/11	8/8
	2.0	6/8	8/11	9/11	8/8
	1.0	6/8	4/8	7/8	8/8

From Halbert, S. P., Sonn-Kazar, C., and Swick, L.: Mixed bacterial infections in relation to antibiotic activities: the role of staphyloccal antibiotic in a *Clostridium septicum–Staphylococcus albus* infection, Antibiot. Chemother. **7**:237, 1957.

*The figures represent the number of survivors/total number injected.

Table 3-10. "Therapeutic" activity of staphylococcal antibiotic in *Clostridium septicum* infection

Group	*Clostridium septicum* spore dilution	Time (hours) following infection when antibiotic given			
		0	2	4	6
Staphylococcal antibiotic, intraperitoneal:	10^{-4}	14/15*	14/15	13/15	11/15
8 mg/0.5 ml	10^{-5}	14/15	15/15	15/15	13/15
Staphylococcal antibiotic, intramuscular,	$10^{\ 4}$	15/15	6/15	7/15	4/15
locally at infection site: 1 mg/0.05 ml	10^{-}	15/15	11/15	12/15	11/15
Controls	10^{-3}	0/15			
	10^{-4}	0/15			
	10^{-5}	3/12			
	10^{-6}	7/10			

From Halbert, S. P., Sonn-Kazar, C., and Swick, L.: Mixed bacterial infections in relation to antibiotic activities: the role of staphyloccal antibiotic in a *Clostridium septicum–Staphylococcus albus* infection, Antibiot. Chemother. **7**:237, 1957.

*The figure represents the number of survivors/total number injected.

sents a relatively long incubation period. In spite of this, large numbers of animals were cured of roughly 10 or 100 LD_{50} when the antibiotic was given locally or intraperitoneally 4 or 6 hours following infection.

The surprising potency of this type of antibiotic secreted by an ocular staphylococcus was apparent from comparative tests with clinically valuable antibiotics, such as penicillin and oxytetracycline. Some in vitro tests are summarized in Table 3-11, which shows that the staphylococcal antibiotic is somewhat more potent than either penicillin or oxytetracycline in agar plate assays, producing inhibition zones at concentrations of 0.1 μg/ml against the four pathogen indicators utilized.

When such a comparison was made in vivo on a limited scale, it was found that the ocular staphylococcal antibiotic revealed protective properties in vivo of the same order of magnitude as oxytetracycline or penicillin, using *Clostridium septicum*

Table 3-11. Comparative in vitro potency of the partially purified antibiotic of an ocular staphylococcus, and several clinically valuable antibiotics

Indicator strain	Antibiotic	Inhibition zone (μg/ml)						
		1000	100	10	1	0.1	0.01	0.001
Clostridium septicum	*Staphylococcus* K88-8	9.7†	9.5	8.3	3.1	3.0*	0	0
	Penicillin G	17.5	15.8	12.2	5.9	0	0	0
	Oxytetracycline	18.3	15.7	11.7	7.4	0	0	0
	Streptomycin	3.3	0	0	0	0	0	0
Clostridium perfringens (III)	*Staphylococcus* K88-8	8.9	7.0	6.4	4.9	3.8	3.0*	0
	Penicillin	26.5	24.9	16.9	5.3	0	0	0
	Oxytetracycline	19.3	17.1	14.6	7.4	0	0	0
	Streptomycin	4.1	2.3*	0	0	0	0	0
Corynebacterium diphtheriae (*mitis*)	*Staphylococcus* K88-8	10.0	9.2	8.5	5.5	2.5	0	0
	Penicillin	14.3	13.0	10.4	6.4	0	0	0
	Oxytetracycline	15.0	11.5	6.1	tr	0	0	0
	Streptomycin	11.3	8.2	2.2*	0	0	0	0
Corynebacterium pseudodiphtheriticum (A6485)	*Staphylococcus* K88-8	7.9	7.0	6.6	5.0	2.5	0	0
	Penicillin	20.1	15.0	10.8	3.9*	0	0	0
	Oxytetracycline	10.4	9.5	5.2	2.4*	0	0	0
	Streptomycin	10.8	7.5	2.5	0	0	0	0

From Halbert, S. P., Sonn-Kazar, C., and Swick, L.: Mixed bacterial infections in relation to antibiotic activities: the role of staphylococcal antibiotic in a *Clostridium septicum–Staphylococcus albus* infection, Antibiot. Chemother. **7**:238, 1957.
*These inhibition zones were poorly demarcated.
†The figures represent the width of the inhibition zone from the edge.

Table 3-12. Comparison of the prophylactic effects in mouse *Clostridium septicum* infections of the ocular staphylococcal antibiotic with penicillin, oxytetracycline, and streptomycin

Clostridium septicum **challenge, intramuscular**	**Control infections**	**Antibiotic**	**Antibiotic dose/mouse (mg intraperitoneal)**					
			4	**2**	**1**	**0.5**	**0.25**	**0.13**
10^{-3}	1/14* (7%)	*Staphylococcus* K88-8	15/17 (90%)	16/22 (75%)	9/13 (70%)	2/5	—	—
		Penicillin	—	6/11 (55%)	3/14 (20%)	3/7	1/5	—
		Oxytetracycline	—	6/6	11/14 (80%)	7/8	3/5	3/5
		Streptomycin	—	0/8	2/8	—	—	—
10^{-4}	2/14 (14%)	*Staphylococcus* K88-8	18/20 (90%)	17/25 (70%)	6/13 (45%)	2/5	—	—
		Penicillin	—	7/11 (65%)	7/14 (50%)	5/8	2/5	—
		Oxytetracycline	—	5/6	13/14 (95%)	6/8	4/5	5/5
		Streptomycin	—	0/8	2/8	—	—	—
10^{-5}	2/14 (14%)							
10^{-6}	8/14 (57%)							

From Halbert, S. P., Sonn-Kazar, C., and Swick, L.: Mixed bacterial infections in relation to antibiotic activities: the role of staphyloccal antibiotic in a *Clostridium septicum–Staphylococcus albus* infection, Antibiot. Chemother. **7**:239, 1957.
*Number of survivals/number of mice injected (percent survivors).

infection as the challenge system. These data are shown in Table 3-12, which indicates that the staphylococcal preparation appeared to be somewhat more efficient than penicillin and slightly less so than oxytetracycline. The comparability of all three is quite clear, however, even with the relatively small number of animals utilized.

Similar results were obtained in mixed infections using diphtheria inoculations of guinea pigs as the test system. When highly active ocular staphylococci were mixed with the subcutaneous challenge suspension of *Corynebacterium diphtheriae,* striking protection was usually obtained. All of the animals given nonantibiotic ocular staphylococci in the mixture succumbed

Table 3-13. Mixed *Staphylococcus*-diphtheria infection in guinea pigs (subcutaneous)

Ocular *Staphylococcus* component	Antibiotic activity of *Staphylococcus* vs. *Corynebacterium diphtheriae*	Antibiotic group	Results of mixed infections		*Staphylococcus* controls, survivors/total injected
			Survivors*/total injected	Percent	
None, diphtheria alone	—	—	0/20	0	—
None, diphtheria antitoxin	—	—	18/20	90	—
K88-8	8.4†	—	11/11	100	2/2
K609-16	8.3	—	7/8	90	4/4
K102-11	8.1	—	7/7	100	2/2
117-3	8.1	I	16/16	100	8/8
K423-11	7.4	—	7/7	100	2/2
K618-6	7.2	—	7/8	90	3/4
K17-5	7.0	I	10/12	85	6/6
K610-18	6.9	—	8/8	100	4/4
431-5	6.5	V	0/8	0	4/4
188-4	6.4	I	8/8	100	3/4
100-5	6.0	I	7/8	90	4/4
455-1	4.4	II	9/12	75	6/6
290-7	4.1	IX	0/8	0	3/4
191-4	2.4	VII	0/16	0	10/10
224-4	2.1	III	0/8	0	4/4
212-1	2.0	—	0/4	0	2/2
81-5	1.0	VII	0/8	0	4/4
127-1	0	—	0/8	0	3/4
280-3	0	—	0/8	0	4/4
223-1	0	—	0/8	0	4/4
217-1	0	—	0/8	0	3/4
K887-5	0	—	0/3	0	—
K582-7	0	—	0/3	0	—
K595-1	0	—	0/3	0	—
K1758-2	0	—	0/4	0	2/2
K1084-17	0	—	0/3	0	—
K1796-1	0	—	0/4	0	2/2
K661-1	0	—	0/3	0	—
K609-1	0	—	0/4	0	2/2

From Halbert, S. P., Sonn-Kazar, C., and Swick, L.: Mixed bacterial infections in relation to antibiotic activities: staphylococcal-diphtheria infections of guinea pigs, Arch. Ophthal. **57**:718, 1957.
*Survival time used was 14 days.
†The figures represent the zone of inhibition of the mitis strain used for infection. They are average values of a number of assays.

Table 3-14. Mixed diphtheria—ocular staphylococcal infections by the intratracheal route

Infective mixture	Results of mixed infections		Results of control staphylococcal infections	
	Experiment 1	Experiment 2	Experiment 1	Experiment 2
Diphtheria and buffer	D1 D2 D2 D2 D4	D1 D2 D2 D2	—	—
Diphtheria and antitoxin	D2 D2 S* S S	D13 S S S	—	—
Diphtheria and antibiotic *Staphylococcus* 117-3	D1 D2 D3 S S	D6 S S S	S S S S S	D2 S S S
Diphtheria and nonantibiotic *Staphylococcus* 127-1	D1 D1 D1 D1 D2	D1 D2 D2 D3	S S S S S	S S S S

From Halbert, S. P., Sonn-Kazar, C., and Swick, L.: Mixed bacterial infections in relation to antibiotic activities: staphylococcal-diphtheria infections of guinea pigs, Arch. Ophthal. **57**:720, 1957.
*S = survived one month.

like the controls. These data are shown in Table 3-13, which also shows that the slightly active organisms were without protective effect with this challenge diphtheria dose.

In an attempt to obtain results somewhat more analogous to the situation that might occur in the natural habitat of the organisms involved, mixed infections were carried out by the intratracheal route on a limited scale in guinea pigs. These data are summarized in Table 3-14, where it may be seen that mixture of the challenge dose of diphtheria organisms with antibiotic-producing staphylococci resulted in significant protection against fatal outcome, roughly comparable to that found with antitoxin treatment.

In summary, the accumulated data are strongly suggestive that the antibiotic properties of numerous organisms of the ocular flora have significance in the resistance of the eye to superficial bacterial infections and are another protective factor of this tissue against disease.

REFERENCES

1. Dujardin-Beaumetz, E.: Action antibiotique d'une variete staphylocoque a l'egard des bacilles gram-positifs et acido-resistants, Compt. Rend. Soc. Biol. **110**:1210, 1932.
2. Halbert, S. P., Locatcher-Khorazo, D., Sonn-Kazar, C., and Swick, L. S.: Further studies on the incidence of antibiotic-producing micro-organisms of the ocular flora, Arch. Ophthal. **58**:66, 1957.
3. Halbert, S. P., Sonn, C., and Swick, L. S.: Mixed bacterial infections in relation to antibiotic activities: *Clostridium septicum*-micrococcus infections, J. Immun. **73**:169, 1954.
4. Halbert, S. P., Sonn-Kazar, C., and Swick, L. S.: Mixed bacterial infections in relation to antibiotic activities: the role of staphylococcal antibiotic in a Clostridium septicum–Staphylococcus albus infection, Antibiot. Chemother. **7**:235, 1957.
5. Halbert, S. P., Sonn-Kazar, C., and Swick, L. S.: Mixed bacterial infections in relation to antibiotic activities: staphylococcal-diphtheria infections of guinea pigs, Arch. Ophthal. **57**:716, 1957.
6. Halbert, S. P., and Swick, L. S.: Antibiotic-producing bacteria of the ocular flora, Amer. J. Ophthal. **35**:73, 1952.
7. Halbert, S. P., Swick, L. S., and Sonn, C.: Characteristics of antibiotic-producing strains of the ocular flora, J. Immun. **70**:400, 1953.
8. Halbert, S. P., Swick, L. S., Sonn, C., and Locatcher-Khorazo, D.: Ocular antibiotic-producing bacteria in normal eyes and in conjunctivitis, Arch. Ophthal. **51**:7, 1954.
9. Scrivener, C. A., Myers, H. I., Moore, N. A., and Warner, B. W.: Some antagonistic activity of bacteria from the human oral cavity, J. Dent. Res. **29**:784, 1950.
10. Su, T. L.: Micrococcin: an antibacterial substance formed by a strain of micrococcus, Brit. J. Exp. Path. **29**:473, 1948.

4

Cytology of exudates and scrapings from normal and inflamed eyes

HISTORICAL NOTES

Cellular response reflects some degree of inflammation in the eye and often reveals the presence of infection. Cytologic examinations of smears from exudates and scrapings obtained from the conjunctivas, corneas, or eyelids may contribute to differential diagnosis in various ocular infections. Before bacteria were known as causative agents of disease, interest in the cells of ocular exudates existed, and Werneck[12,25] in 1839 wrote letters about the microscopic examination of exudates from normal and inflamed eyes to Dr. Florent Cunier, who later published these after Werneck's death.

In the early records on eye infections one finds that ocular smears and scrapings have been studied extensively. Leber[16] in 1879 wrote about a patient who had developed an ulceration of the cornea, and hypopyon, following an injury received from a small chaff of oats while working with a threshing machine. Microscopic examination of a smear from a light gray membrane over the ulcer, lifted out from the upper border, revealed packed masses of mycelial elements of a fungus that proved to be *Aspergillus glaucus*. Hirschberg and Krause[11] in 1881 obtained smears from the conjunctiva and urethra of an adult with gonorrhea, and, as may be observed in Fig. 4-1, the micrococci were present in or on both epithelial cells and polymorphonuclear cells. The Koch-Weeks bacillus was first described by Koch, who saw the organism in an exudate from a patient with trachoma. Kamen[15] in 1899 reported finding Koch-Weeks bacilli on or in epithelial cells (Fig. 4-2) from a patient with conjunctivitis caused by this organism. Schaudinn and Hoffmann[23] in 1905 identified *Treponema pallidum* as the etiologic agent of syphilis, and Aubineau[2] in 1907 described a chancre of the lower lid. Ulcer scrapings spread on a cover glass and stained with gentian violet showed many spirochetes (Fig. 4-3). Long before the etiologic agent of trachoma was isolated, Halberstaedter and von Prowazek[8] described small masses in the cytoplasm of epithelial cells found in conjunctival smears from patients with trachoma; these masses stained blue or violet with Giemsa stain. An example of one such inclusion is seen in Fig. 4-4. Axenfeld,[3] who contributed the definitive text on ocular microbiology in the first decade of this century, stated that "the mere examination of a film gives a great deal of information, and it is absolutely necessary, in dealing with external and internal disease, that the material should be collected at suitable stages in the disease." He also advised the exercise of greater caution in obtaining material from the cornea or infiltrated tissues, since scrapings can loosen the tissue, resulting in further spreading of the infection.

An early extensive study comparing the

presumptive diagnosis of bacterial infections of the eye, made from examinations of exudates and scrapings, with the diagnosis made by cultivation of the bacteria, is that reported in 1912 by Browning.[5a] One thousand consecutive cases of conjunctival infection were examined simultaneously by direct smear and by culture. The presumptive diagnosis made from smears was particularly accurate in infections caused by

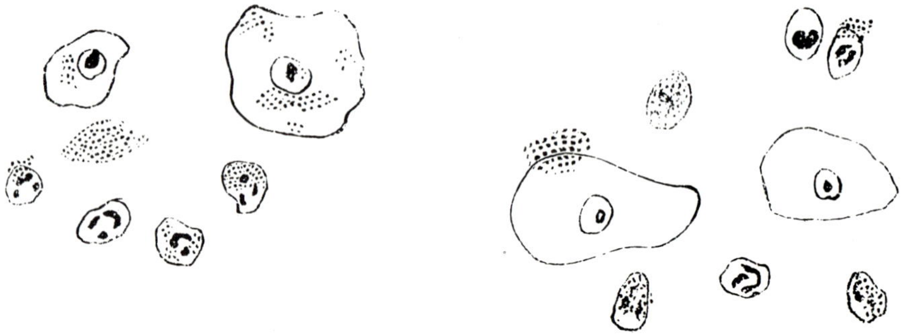

Fig. 4-1. Smears from a case of gonorrhea with eye infection in a male. The micrococci are seen in or on the epithelial and polymorphonuclear cells as well as lying free in smears from both the urethra (left) and eye (right). (From Hirschberg, J., and Krause, F.: Zbl. Augenheilk. **5**:272, 1881.)

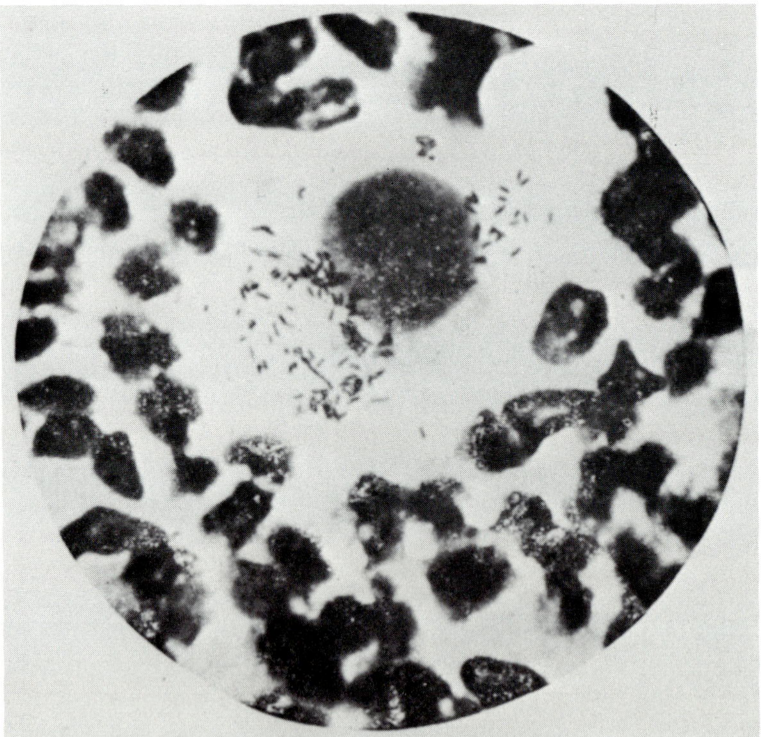

Fig. 4-2. Smear from exudate from a patient with conjunctivitis caused by the Koch-Weeks bacillus, showing numerous organisms on or in an epithelial cell. (From Kamen, L.: Zbl. Bakt. Parasit. Infekt. [Jena] **25**:449, 1899.)

gonococci, pneumococci, streptococci, the bacillus of diphtheria, and *Diplobacillus pneumoniae* (*Klebsiella pneumoniae*). McKee[19] in the same year also reported on the usefulness of scrapings in cases of ophthalmia neonatorum. He found that although cultivation of pus from the conjunctiva of suspected gonococcal infections might give negative results, when a scraping was prepared in such a way that the

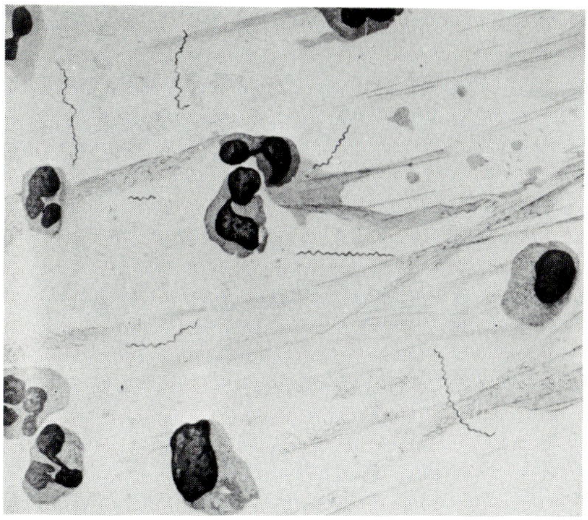

Fig. 4-3. Spirochetes and polymorphonuclear neutrophils in a smear from a scraping of a chancre of the lower lid. (From Aubineau, E.: Ann. Oculist. 138:16, 1907.)

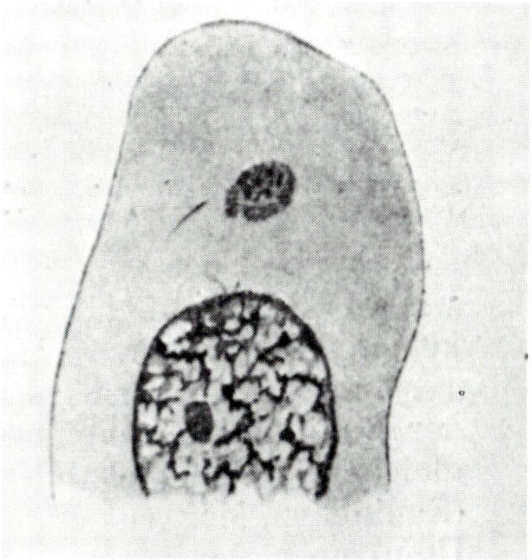

Fig. 4-4. Trachoma bodies seen in the cytoplasm of an epithelial cell in the first stage of the disease. (From Halberstaedter, L., and von Prowazek, S.: Deutsch. Med. Wschr. 33:1285, 1907.)

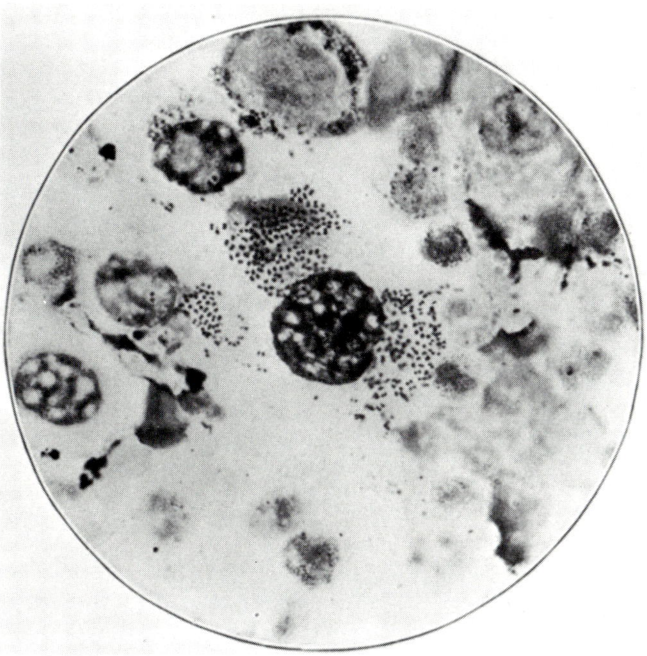

Fig. 4-5. A smear obtained from a case of ophthalmia neonatorum shows numerous gonococci in or on epithelial cells. (From McKee, H. A.: Ophthal. Rec. 21:5, 1912.)

epithelial cells were examined, masses of bacteria similar in morphology to gonococci were found. With the aid of an ear curette the palpebral conjunctiva was gently stroked, and the material was spread carefully over a glass slide and stained with Giemsa stain. Epithelial cells filled with biscuit-shaped diplococci, as shown in Fig. 4-5, were seen. The scraping containing the epithelial cells was cultured and yielded a profuse growth of gonococci. McKee concluded that the method for preparing films showing epithelial cells would demonstrate the presence of gonococci in many cases where smears of exudates yielded negative results; he did not commit himself to the relation of the microorganisms to the epithelial cells. McKee's illustrations indicate the possibility that the gonococci were colonizing in the epithelial cells.

In 1921 Lindner[17] reported that certain microorganisms directly attacked epithelial cells and in early stages of infection might be confined within the cells and be absent or sparse in the secretions until the infection was well established. Lindner considered microorganisms that thrive and multiply on living epithelial cells and confine themselves mainly to the superficial epithelium as epithelial parasites. He recognized only six such organisms: *Neisseria gonorrhoeae, Neisseria meningitidis, Diplococcus pneumoniae, Hemophilus Koch-Weeks, Hemophilus influenzae,* and *Corynebacterium diphtheriae.* Lindner believed the steps of conjunctival infection were as follows: the microorganisms localize on the normal conjunctival epithelial cells where they multiply and adhere. From this point the microorganisms spread over the conjunctiva as a result of the movements of the eyelids, establishing new foci of infection. The toxins that they produce diffuse into the tissue, and by virtue of the dissecting effect of edema these toxins may penetrate even further. In the second stage the epithelial layer is elevated and exfoliated, but the microorganisms are still on the surface. Fig. 4-6 illustrates a smear of an epithelial scraping from the bulbar conjunctiva in one of Lindner's patients who had pneumococcal conjunctivitis.

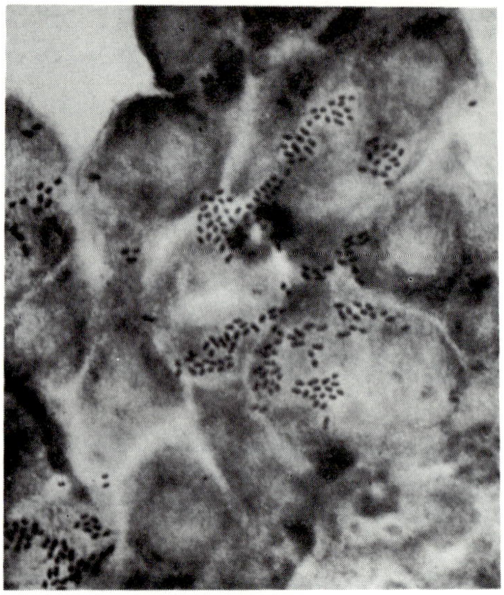

Fig. 4-6. Pneumococcal conjunctivitis, early stage. Epithelial scraping from the conjunctiva of the lower lid on the second day of infection in a 19-year-old girl. The scraping demonstrates the organisms on the epithelial cells. (From Lindner, K.: Graefes Arch. Ophth. **105**:758, 1921.)

Howard,[14] working in Lindner's laboratory, confirmed Lindner's observations; and while studying gonococcal, pneumococcal, and Koch-Weeks infections, he noted that the conjunctival epithelial cells had phagocytic characteristics (Fig. 4-7). The conjunctival epithelial cells not only phagocytized the bacteria but often immediately disgested them in the same manner characteristic of the leukocytes. He observed that the epithelial cells were not affected during phagocytosis and believed the phagocytic action of the young epithelial cells was probably one of the most important defense mechanisms against those pathogens that actively invade epithelium.

CYTOLOGY OF NORMAL OCULAR SCRAPINGS

The first recorded observations of the appearance of cells scraped from normal conjunctivas may have been those of Werneck.[25] He found in adult subjects epithelial cells in various stages of normal aging.

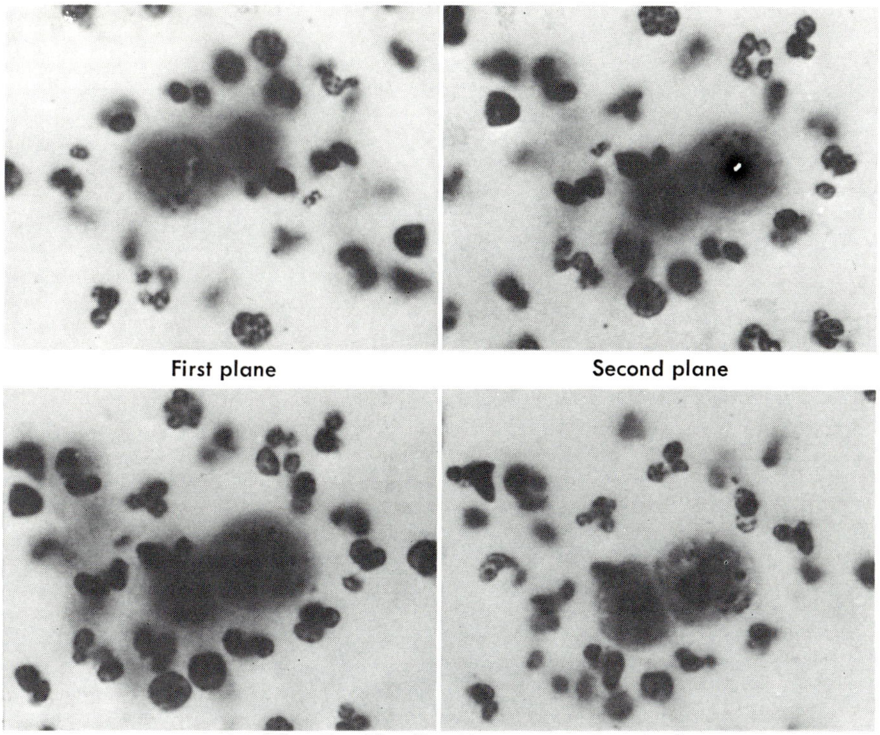

Fig. 4-7. Gonorrheal conjunctivitis in newborn, ninth day. Scrapings from palpebral conjunctiva. Phagocytosis by epithelial cell of 25 to 30 gonococci. Photographs taken in different planes show some microorganisms at different levels in the cell. (From Howard, H.: Amer. J. Ophthal. 7:909, 1924.)

Leukocytes were seen only in scrapings from inflamed eyes. Norn[21] recently has studied the cytology of conjunctival fluid in the newborn as well as in children and adults. Lymphocytes were not normally present in the newborn but were demonstrable in all children from 3 to 10 years of age; after this age the number of lymphocytes decreased gradually, and in the eye of the normal adult it was rare to see other than epithelial cells. Agarwal and Malhoutra[1] also have compared the appearance of conjunctival scrapings from normal individuals of various ages and have pointed out that the epithelial cells may be polyhedral as well as round. They found a small percentage of goblet cells that we, however, have not encountered in the normal eye. These authors also describe variations in the appearance of the epithelial cells associated with the menstrual cycle. De Azevedo[7] has made a comparison of the character of the epithelium of the normal eye as seen in histologic preparation with that seen in smears. Illustrations of the histology of the eye in health and disease are to be found in the textbook by Hogan and Zimmerman.[13] A description of the cells of the normal as well as diseased conjunctiva has been given by Liotet and Iris.[18]

In our experience with adults the normal epithelium from the conjunctiva is composed of cells that, when stained with Giemsa stain, show a single violet-colored nucleus surrounded by a light blue zone of cytoplasm (Plate 1, *A*). There is some variation in the size and shape of the epithelial cells, which may be in part because of the depth of the scraping. In addition to the normal epithelial cells, many scrapings con-

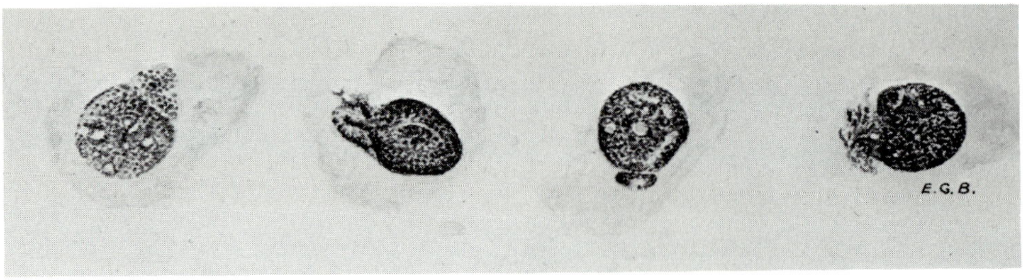

Fig. 4-8. Four epithelial cells showing a variety of so-called pseudoinclusion bodies, which are actually disrupted nuclear material sometimes seen in smears of scrapings from normal individuals.

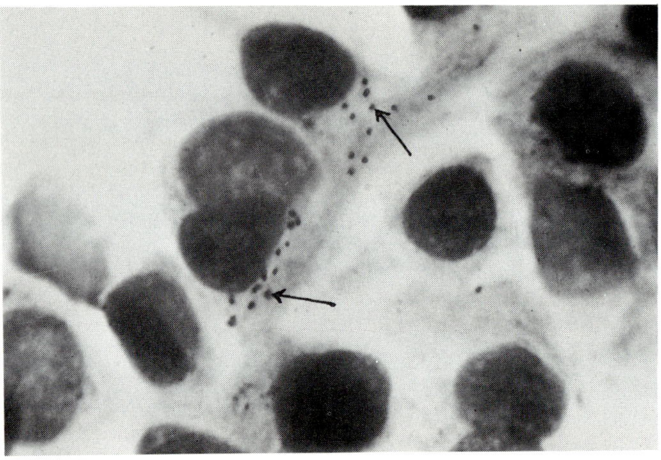

Fig. 4-9. Normal epithelial cells, some with "green granules" (arrows). (Giemsa stain.)

tain a few cells that show an abnormality caused by a fragmenting nucleus (Fig. 4-8). A superficial similarity to some viral inclusions has led to the designation pseudoinclusions, but this term does not indicate disease. Another variation of the normal epithelial cell is illustrated in Fig. 4-9, which shows intracellular granules that stain green with Giemsa stain. These occur most frequently in Orientals and people with dark complexions and are not associated with disease. Similar intracellular granules staining dark blue may be observed in normal epithelial cells. They sometimes are mistaken for viral cytoplasmic inclusions but are nonspecific and of no diagnostic value.

Goblet cells, though normal to the conjunctiva of the eye, are rarely seen in scrapings from the normal eye, since they occur mainly in the fornices. Plate 1, *B* illustrates these cells, which increase in numbers in keratoconjunctivitis sicca.

It is important in preparing scrapings of the conjunctiva to avoid obtaining material from the lid margin. Keratinized epithelial cells, which are abnormal when occurring in the conjunctiva, may be found normally on the lid margins. In addition, scrapings from lid margins may contain *Pityrosporum orbiculare,* staphylococci, and diphtheroids. The latter two organisms are present in the normal conjunctiva but usually not in sufficient numbers to be seen readily in conjunctival scrapings.

Structures identified as the female sex chromatin may be present in different ocular tissues. These structures were origi-

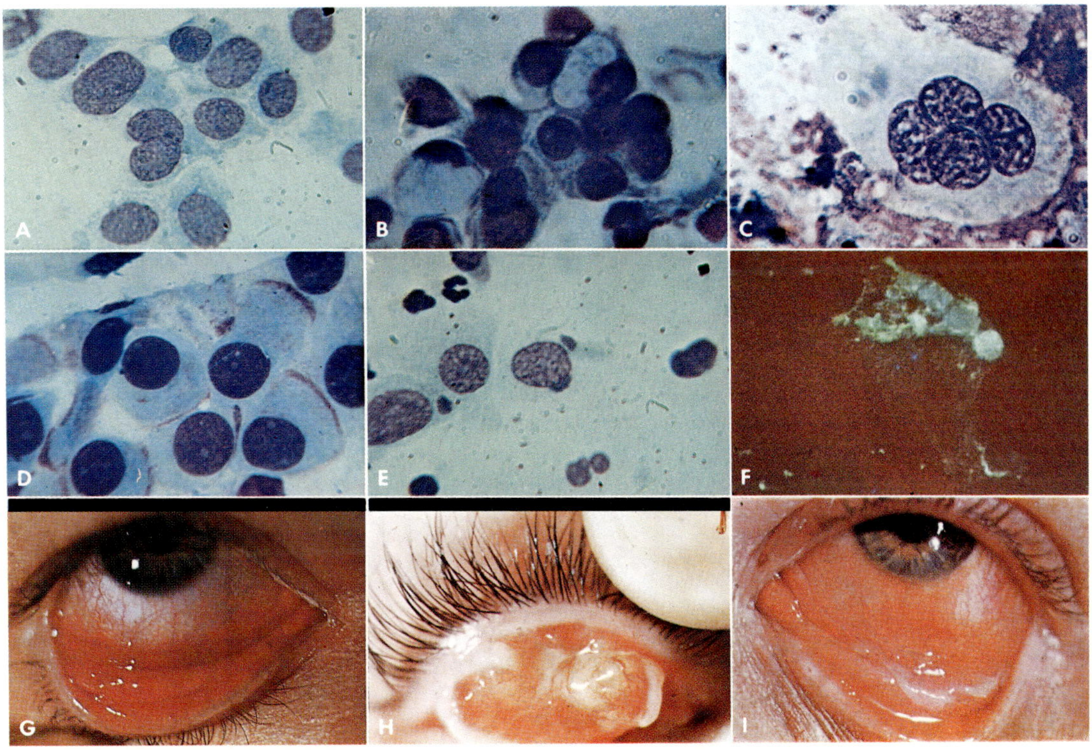

Plate 1. A, Normal epithelial cells. (Giemsa stain.) **B,** Two goblet cells with clear cytoplasm seen among epithelial cells in the early stage of keratoconjunctivitis sicca. (Giemsa stain.) **C,** Multinucleated epithelial cell from a scraping of a corneal ulcer caused by herpes simplex infection. (Giemsa stain.) **D,** Lavender keratin granules in epithelial cells in chronic conjunctivitis. (Giemsa stain.) **E,** Scraping of conjunctiva from a patient with acute trachoma. Two cytoplasmic inclusions in center epithelial cell and one in cell on left. (Giemsa stain.) **F,** Corneal scraping stained with fluorescein-labeled antibody to herpes simplex. The viral antigen is stained green. **G,** Acute bulbar conjunctivitis caused by *Staphylococcus aureus.* **H,** Membranous conjunctivitis caused by *Streptococcus hemolyticus.* **I,** Membranous conjunctivitis caused by *Corynebacterium diphtheriae.*

nally detected by Barr and Bertram[4] while studying accelerated nucleoprotein synthesis in the neurons of cats. They observed that these peculiar structures were intranuclear and lay adjacent to the large nucleoli in nerve cells of the cat. It has been shown that this chromatin mass was related to sex and could be demonstrated in the nuclei of most tissue cells from females, both human and animal, when stained with basic dyes or preferably with the Feulgen stain. Thus sections of tissues of unknown origin may be identified as to sex. Moore and Barr[20] made scrapings from the epithelial oral mucosa and detected the sex chromatin in the epithelial cell nucleus of females, whereas a similar chromatin mass was absent in males. Pedler and Ashton[22] have demonstrated that structures identified as the female sex chromatin are found in nuclei of conjunctival, ciliary, and corneal epithelium, in stromal cells of the iris and ciliary body, in the layers of the retina, and in the ganglion cells where the chromatin masses are well defined. They concluded that it is evident that sex may be determined as accurately from the epithelium of the cornea as from that of the skin. Fig. 4-10 shows sex chromatin masses in nuclei of corneal cells.

When trying to apply the Papanicolaou method of studying cytology to ophthalmology, de Azevedo[6] also found the presence of characteristic sex chromatin in the exfoliated epithelial cells of the conjunctiva. Conjunctival epithelial scrapings were made with a sterile de Wecker's iris spatula, and the material obtained was stained by Papanicolaou's method.

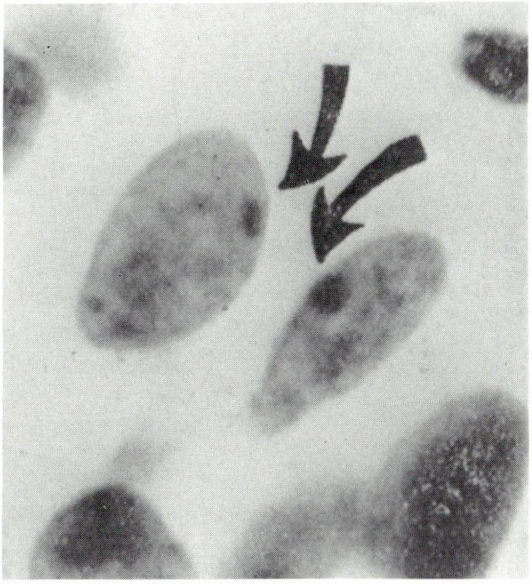

Fig. 4-10. Female sex chromatin mass (arrows) in nuclei of epithelial cells from a corneal scraping. (From Pedler, C., and Ashton, N.: Brit. J. Ophthal. **39**:364, 1955.)

Table 4-1 summaries some of the variations seen in epithelial cells of normal adult conjunctivas.

CELLS FOUND IN SMEARS AND SCRAPINGS IN INFLAMED CONJUNCTIVAS AND CORNEAS

In inflamed eyes the epithelial cells seen in scrapings from normal eyes are replaced in whole or in part by various polymorphonuclear leukocytes, lymphocytes, large mononuclear cells, plasma cells, and ab-

Table 4-1. Various intracellular granules found in epithelial cells seen in scrapings from normal eyes

Pseudoinclusion bodies	Intracellular free green pigment	Intracellular free blue granules	Sex chromatin
Extrusion of nuclear material into cytoplasm through a break in nuclear membrane	Present in cytoplasm in individuals with dark complexion	Present in cytoplasm in about 12% of smears from normal individuals; not to be confused with viral inclusions	Present in the nuclei of exfoliated epithelial cells; in females only

normal epithelial cells, a process giving expression to pathologic changes.

Polymorphonuclear neutrophils, because of their phagocytic ability, play an important role in resistance to infection and present the first line of defense. These cells are concerned primarily with phagocytosis of bacteria in the acute phase of infection. The ingestion of bacteria by polymorphonuclear cells is variable, however, since some virulent strains, such as group A *Streptococcus hemolyticus,* may be totally resistant to phagocytosis. The polymorphonuclear neutrophil exhibiting no phagocytic activity against spirochetes was well illustrated by Aubineau[2] in 1907 (Fig. 4-3); whereas Fig. 4-11 shows active phagocytosis by neutrophils in a scraping from a case of gonococcal conjunctivitis.

Even where there is rapid or complete phagocytosis by the polymorphonuclear cells, the infecting parasite may multiply within the leukocyte. Dead phagocytized bacteria lose their shape and staining properties.

Allergic reactions in the eye are notable for an exudate that usually contains *eosinophils* and sometimes *basophils* in addition to the usual polymorphonuclear neutrophils. For example, according to Thygeson,[23a] basophilic cells may be found in considerable numbers in one kind of allergic reaction, vernal catarrh, if the numbers of eosinophils are small. A few basophils also may be seen in some mild subacute ocular infections. The eye of a patient with follicular swelling caused by vernal catarrh is illustrated in Fig. 4-12.

Small *lymphocytes* are about the size of an erythrocyte or slightly larger with a single, sharply defined, round, dense violet nucleus surrounded by a varying amount of delicate, pale blue cytoplasm when stained with Giemsa stain. The cytoplasm, however, may form only a fine rim around the nucleus. Larger lymphocytes usually contain a more abundant zone of cytoplasm. Unlike the polymorphonuclear neutrophils, the lymphocytes do not exhibit phagocytosis.

Some acute infections of presumed viral origin are characterized by the presence of

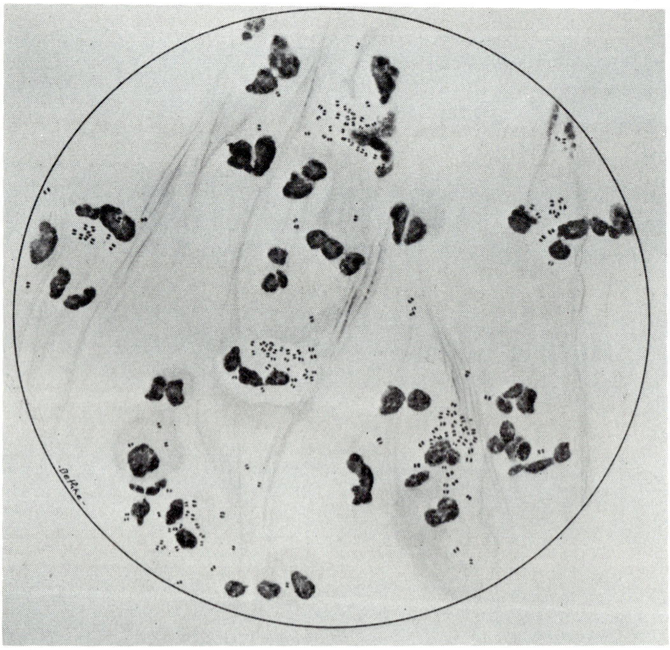

Fig. 4-11. Gonococcal conjunctivitis. Phagocytosis by polymorphonuclear cells.

lymphocytes (Fig. 4-13). Lymphocytes, usually in small number, are found also in the conjunctival scrapings from patients with various chronic ocular infections.

The large *monocyte* (macrophage) is the largest cell of the leukocytic series seen in ocular scrapings. It contains a single nucleus, which stains less deeply than the lymphocyte, and which may be round or irregularly oval. The zone of cytoplasm surrounding the nucleus of the monocyte is wider than that of the small lymphocyte. Mononuclear cells are phagocytic and engulf not only bacteria but also debris and whole cells. Monocytes are an important part of cellular reaction in ocular infections, and they may be the predominating cell in certain infections, such as pharyngoconjunctival fever. They are also found in the later stages of inflammation or infection.

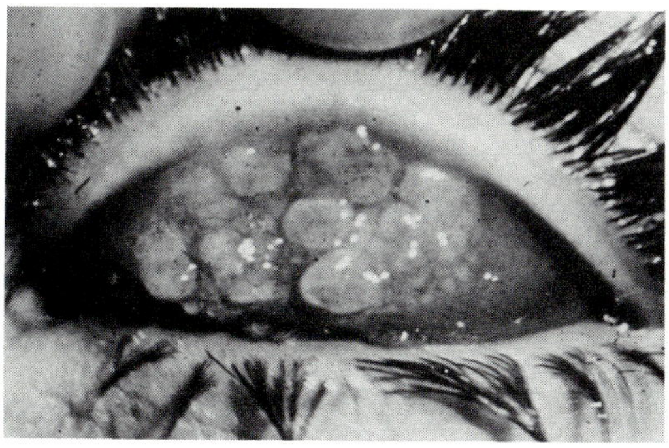

Fig. 4-12. Vernal conjunctivitis. Note follicular swelling.

Plasma cells, somewhat larger than lymphocytes, have a characteristic eccentric nucleus with distinctive distribution of chromatin, as shown in Fig. 4-14, *1.* The cytoplasm is opaque, abundant, and stains blue. These cells are found in chronic infections of the eye, notably in trachoma, where they occur in large numbers. Thygeson[24] reports that they are present in 40% of all scrapings from trachomatous eyes, whereas they are seen in only 0.5% of scrapings from nontrachomatous cases. So far as is known, the function of the plasma cells is the production of antibodies. Fig. 4-14 also shows an atypical large mono-

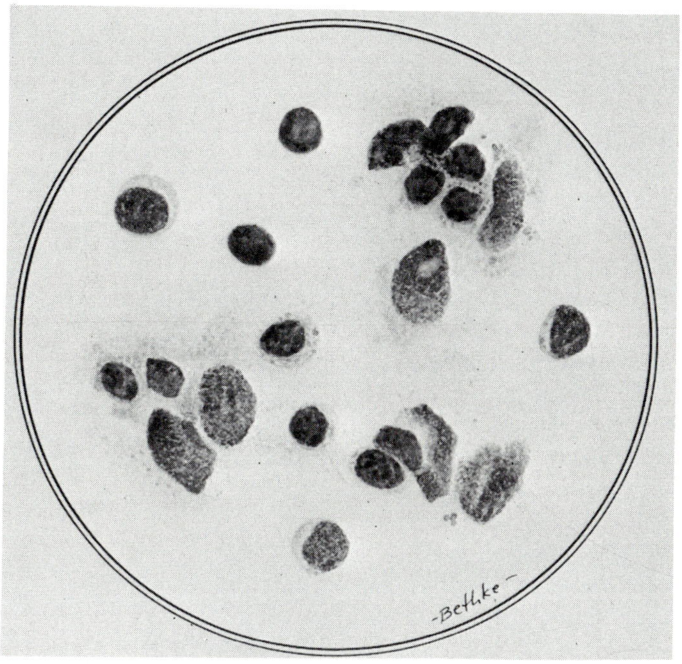

Fig. 4-13. Lymphocytes in conjunctival scrapings from a patient suspected of having a viral infection.

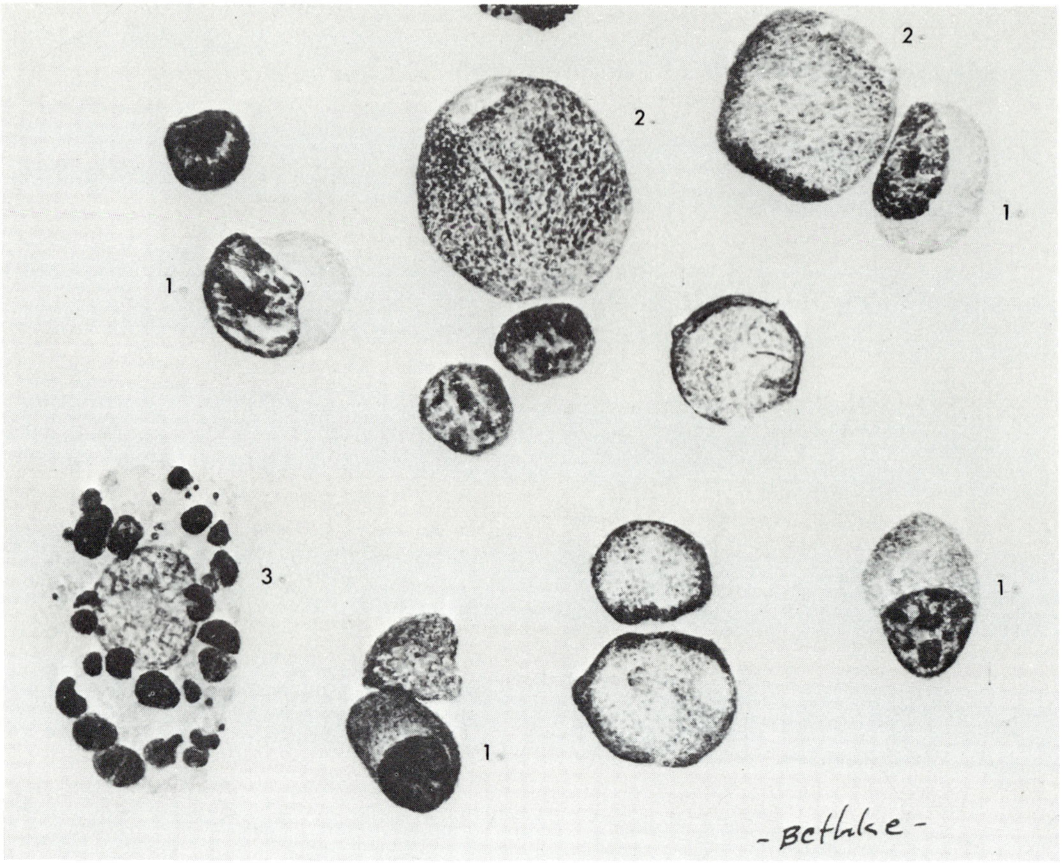

Fig. 4-14. Illustration of cells seen in a follicular expression from the conjunctiva in a case of trachoma. *1,* Plasma cells; *2,* large mononuclear cells; *3,* phagocytic macrophage.

nuclear cell (*2*) and a macrophage involved in phagocytosis (*3*).

The *multinucleated epithelial cell* is found in scrapings from eyes with certain viral infections, notably in eyes with herpetic corneal ulcers. Plate 1, *C* shows one such cell found in a corneal scraping from a patient with herpetic keratitis. Damaged epithelial cells may be found in conjunctival scrapings from cases of chronic inflammations of the eye, which are so varied as to include inflammation caused by vitamin A deficiency, keratoconjunctivitis sicca, and some chronic diseases of bacterial or viral origin. One such cell abnormality is that seen in keratoconjunctivitis sicca, where the cytoplasm contains keratin granules. Vacuoles in these epithelial cells may be few or numerous, and since they do not

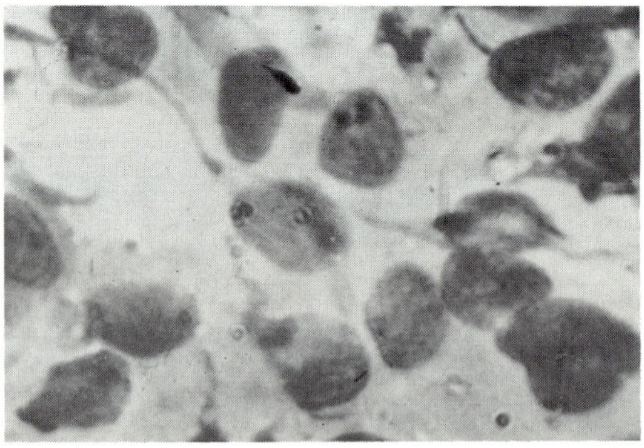

Fig. 4-15. Vacuolated epithelial cells seen in a smear of a conjunctival scraping from a patient with keratoconjunctivitis sicca. There are also strands of mucus.

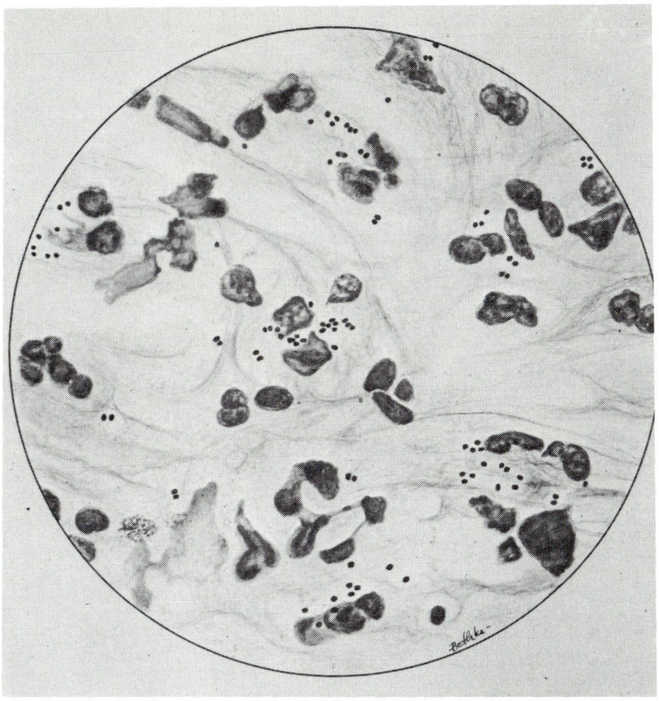

Fig. 4-16. Conjunctival scraping from a patient with conjunctivitis caused by *Staphylococcus aureus*. Note absence of phagocytosis. (Gram stain.)

stain, they appear as clear round spaces (Fig. 4-15). Cells containing keratin granules are also found in some long-standing cases of chronic conjunctivitis (Plate 1, *D*).

ACUTE BACTERIAL INFECTIONS OF THE CONJUNCTIVA AND CORNEA

Before the era of antimicrobic agents, acute bacterial infections ran a relatively protracted course, and much was to be learned from observations of cytologic changes during the disease. In the present era so many acute infections are readily controlled that few run their natural course, and some that were common years ago now are rarely encountered. Today one seldom sees a patient with ocular infection who has not already received antibiotic treatment prior to the laboratory visit. At this point cytologic examination of smears of exudates or scrapings may no longer be helpful. To a limited extent, however, cytology is still useful in the diagnosis of some acute infections of the conjunctiva and cornea.

Smears taken during acute bacterial infection are likely to show numerous polymorphonuclear cells, together with the microorganism involved. If the organism possesses a characteristic morphology, it can be provisionally diagnosed, and time may be saved by using an optimal antibiotic before cultures provide the final identification. In cases where special media are indicated, such as in tuberculosis, the *Moraxella* group, or *Corynebacterium diphtheriae*, morphologic findings may serve to provide the laboratory with a clue toward the selection of special media for cultures. Fig. 4-16 illustrates a gram-positive coccus that was seen in a conjunctival scraping from a patient who proved to have conjunctivitis caused by *Staphylococcus aureus*. There was no evidence of phagocytosis. Such a scraping as this is helpful, since it almost certainly indicates a *Staphylococcus* infection and thus permits immediate

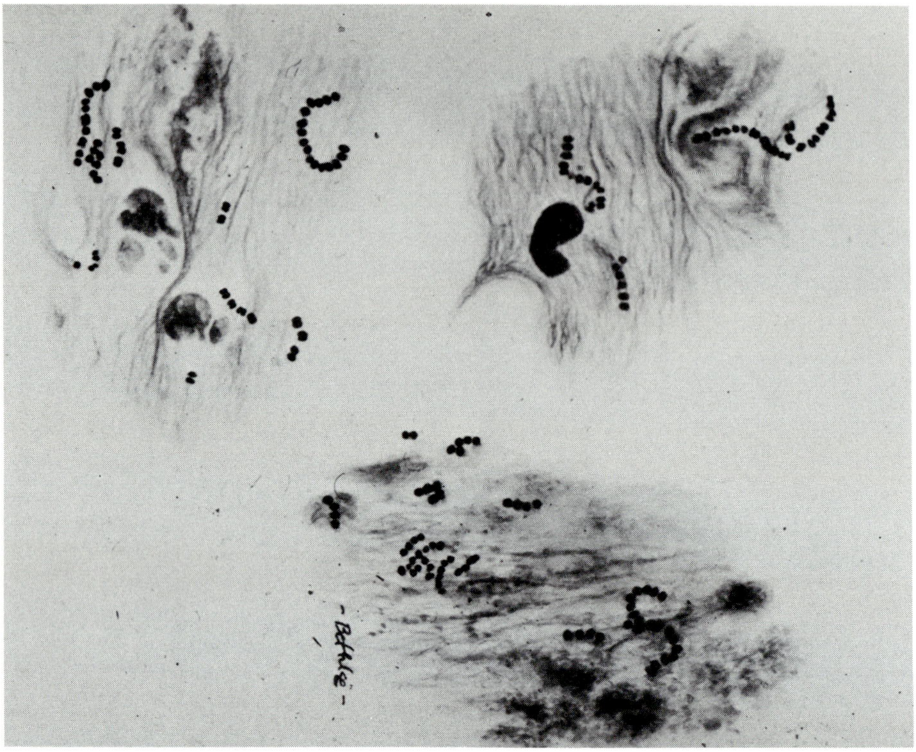

Fig. 4-17. Scraping from a membranous conjunctivitis caused by *Streptococcus hemolyticus*. (Gram stain.)

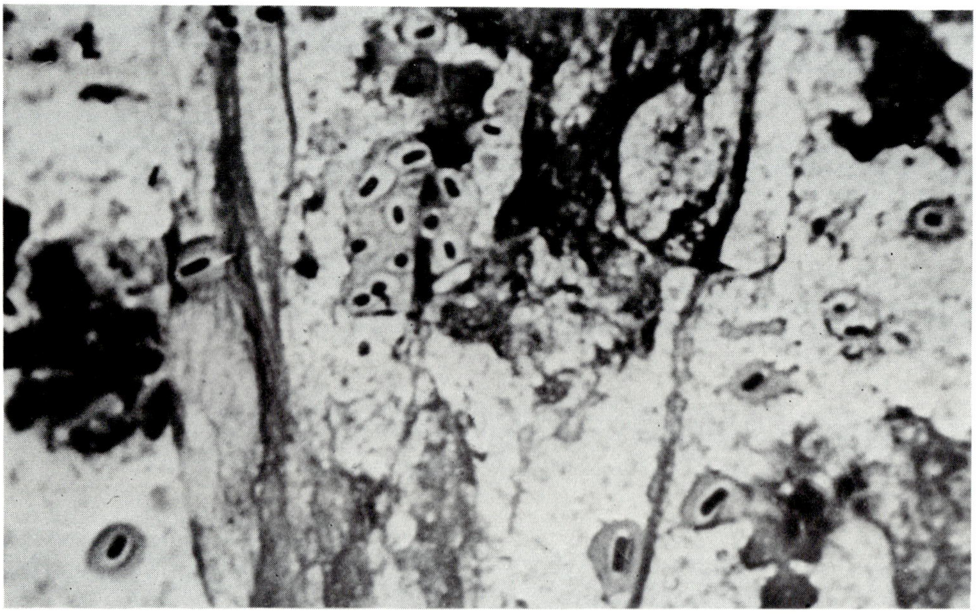

Fig. 4-18. Scraping from corneal ulcer. The encapsulated gram-negative rods proved to be *Klebsiella pneumoniae*. (Gram stain.)

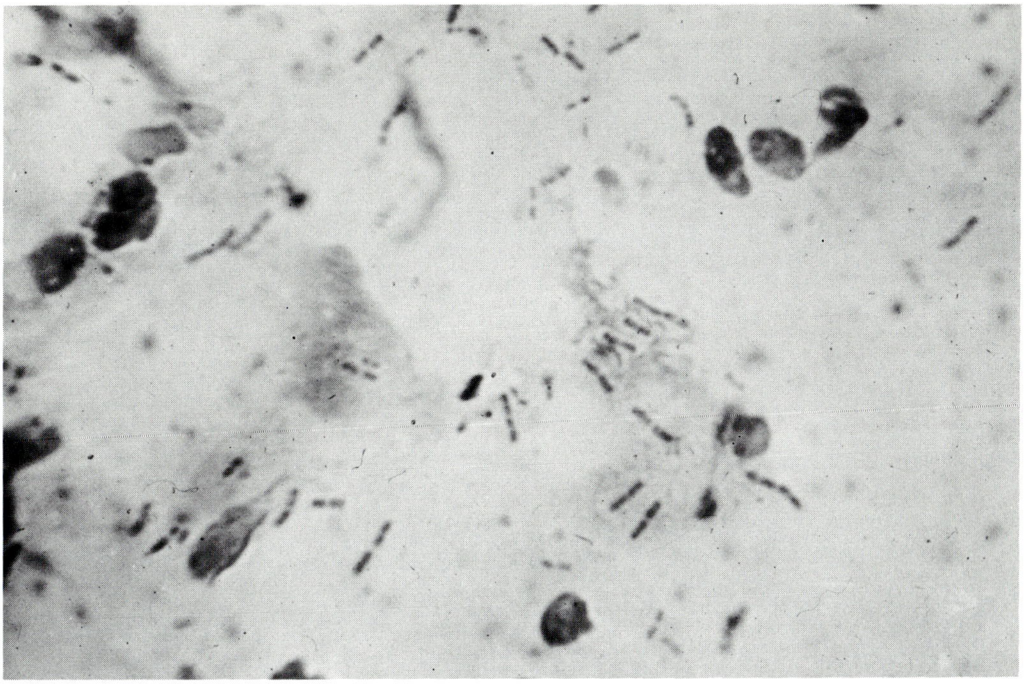

Fig. 4-19. Conjunctival scraping from a patient with angular conjunctivitis caused by the Morax-Axenfeld bacillus. (Gram stain.)

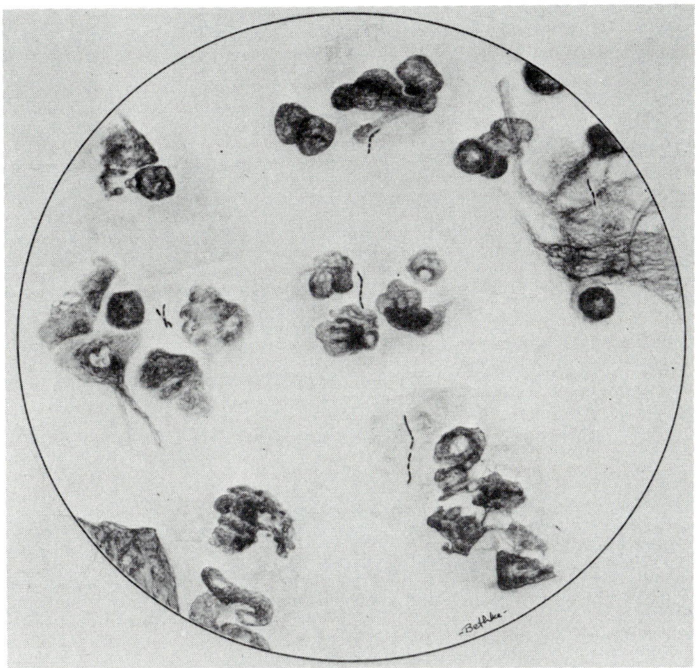

Fig. 4-20. Acid-fast bacilli in primary ocular tuberculosis. (Ziehl-Neelsen stain.) (From Bruce, G. M., and Locatcher-Khorazo, D.: Arch. Ophthal. **37**:375, 1947.)

treatment. Similarly, the presence of chains of gram-positive cocci suggests the probability of *Streptococcus hemolyticus* infection. Fig. 4-17 is a scraping from a membranous conjunctivitis caused by S. *hemolyticus* (see also Plate 1, *H* showing the eye from this patient). Similarly, the presence of gram-negative rods may suggest infection with an enteric pathogen. Fig. 4-18, a scraping from a corneal ulcer resulting from the encapsulated *Klebsiella pneumoniae,* is such an example. Antibiotic therapy should be started immediately, as gram-negative infections usually present the most serious therapeutic problems.

Not all gram-negative bacilli pathogenic for the eye are of enteric origin, for the diplobacillus of Petit (*Moraxella liquefaciens*), the Koch-Weeks bacillus (*Hemophilus aegypticus*), and the Morax-Axenfeld bacillus (*Moraxella lacunata*) are specific to the eye. Fig. 4-19 is a scraping from a patient with angular conjunctivitis caused by *Moraxella lacunata,* which shows the appearance of this gram-negative diplobacillus.

Primary tuberculosis of the eye is rare. Fig. 4-20 illustrates a smear of exudate from a tuberculous conjunctival ulcer; the smear has been stained by the Ziehl-Neelsen technique and shows scattered acid-fast bacilli (see Plate 2, *G,* showing the conjunctival ulcer from which the scraping was taken).

The examples of smears or scrapings from patients with acute bacterial infecions illustrate the variety of cellular response seen. It is evident that the cells are preponderantly polymorphonuclear cells but that some epithelial cells may be seen in the scrapings and occasionally a large mononuclear cell may be seen. The presence of the bacteria within or outside leukocytes can be of diagnostic value.

CHRONIC BACTERIAL INFECTIONS OF THE CONJUNCTIVA AND CORNEA

Chronic conjunctivitis is most frequently caused by staphylococci, members of the enteric groups of gram-negative bacilli, certain fungi, and occasionally a Vincent's infection. The cytology of chronic infections is characterized by a decrease in polymorphonuclear neutrophils and an increase in lymphocytes and large mononuclear cells. This cytology is not in itself pathognomonic of chronic infection nor does it make specific etiologic diagnosis, which depends upon the cultivation of the organism. However, there are a few important situations

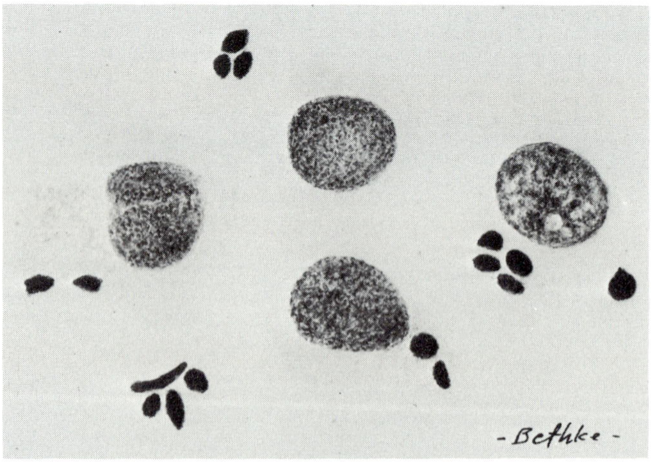

Fig. 4-21. A conjunctival scraping from a case of chronic conjunctivitis and meibomitis showing large gram-positive, oval, yeastlike organisms and a fragment of mycelium. This proved to be *Candida parapsilosis.*

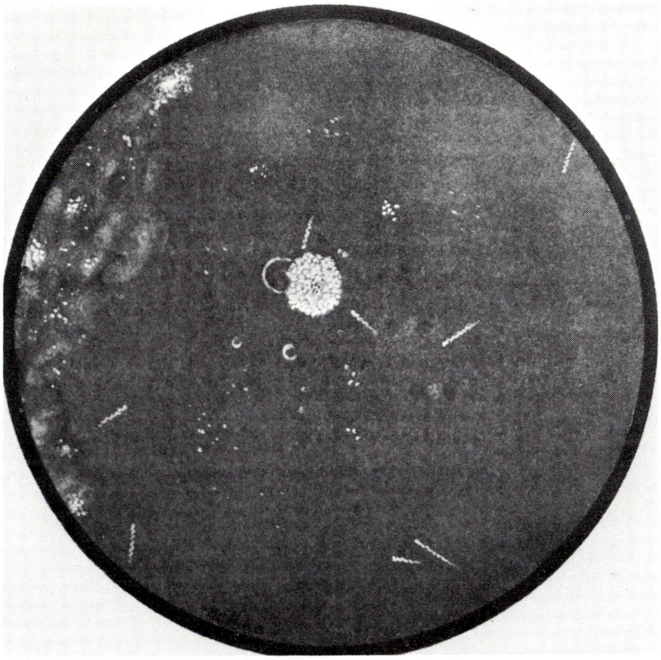

Fig. 4-22. A darkfield preparation of exudate from a patient with unilateral palpebral conjunctivitis with canalicular involvement caused by Vincent's infection. This field shows only the spirochetes. (From Burns, R. P., Macnie, J. P., Pfeiffer, R. L., and Locather-Khorazo, D.: Arch. Ophthal. **59**:236, 1958.)

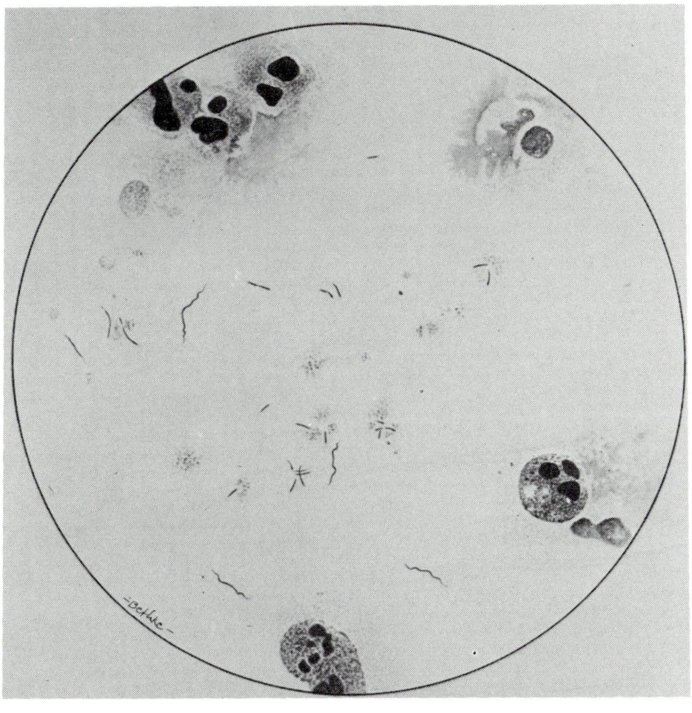

Fig. 4-23. A gentian violet stain of a smear from the same eye seen in Fig. 4-22. Fusiform bacilli as well as spirochetes can be observed. (From Burns, R. P., Macnie, J. P., Pfeiffer, R. L., and Locatcher-Khorazo, D.: Arch. Ophthal. **59**:236, 1958.)

where a provisional specific diagnosis is possible from the examination of smears. Fig. 4-21 shows a conjunctival scraping from a case of chronic conjunctivitis and meibomitis of 2 years duration. It proved to be caused by *Candida parapsilosis*. Large gram-positive yeastlike organisms lie free, and a fragment of mycelium is also present. These findings are diagnostic of a *Candida* infection. The same fungus was found in expressions of the meibomian glands. Smears for the recognition of mycotic infections are in general of great value. Certain rare chronic diseases of the eye may be diagnosed by such smears from scrapings. Fig. 4-22 is a picture of a darkfield fresh preparation showing spirochetes in exudate from a patient with unilateral follicular conjunctivitis and canaliculitis of 6 years duration, which proved to be caused by Vincent's infection. In Fig. 4-23, a gentian violet stain of a smear from the same case, fusiform bacilli as well as spirochetes may be identified. Since neither of these agents, which combine to produce Vincent's infection, are readily cultivated, the smear or fresh preparations examined by darkfield microscopy and the stained smear are of great diagnostic value.

CHLAMYDIA

Although acute and chronic chlamydial diseases can be identified best by cultural means, the presence of these agents causes the formation of cytoplasmic inclusion bodies, which may be recognized in scrapings. Plate 1, *E* shows a smear of a scraping from a case of acute trachoma in which two epithelial cells contain one and two small dark blue inclusions, respectively. The distribution of inclusion granules in epithelial cells follows a varied pattern that may be characterized by only a few scattered granules, or small clumps of granules, to massive deposits in the cytoplasm. These inclusion bodies are similar to those seen in inclusion conjunctivitis. They are difficult to find in chronic disease. Their reappearance indicates acute exacerbation. In contradistinction to viral infections, infections with *Chlamydia* produce an exudate rich in neutrophils and containing plasma cells (Fig. 4-14).[9,24]

VIRAL INFECTIONS

Conjunctival scrapings from patients with viral conjunctivitis show a variety of small and large mononuclear cells and lymphocytes. When no bacteria can be isolated to explain the conjunctivitis, it is assumed that it may be a chronic viral disease. Isolation of the virus is rare under such circumstances. The value of smears is largely that the character of the cells suggests the results of a previous viral infection. Fig. 4-13 illustrates the variety of cells that may be seen in chronic conjunctivitis free of bacteria. This scraping was obtained from a patient with chronic conjunctivitis whose past history and present bacteriologic status provided no explanation for the conjunctivitis, which therefore may have been of viral origin. No multinucleated cells were present, although such cells have been seen in about 170 cases of herpes simplex keratitis (Plate 1, *C*).

It is quite likely that the staining of scrapings with fluorescein-labeled antibodies specific to viruses known to cause viral infection may prove a useful adjunct in the diagnosis of some ocular viral diseases. Plate 1, *F* shows a scraping from the cornea of an 11-month-old child with acute keratoconjunctivitis; the scraping has been stained with fluorescein-labeled antibody to herpes simplex virus and was viewed in ultraviolet light. The viral antigen in the cell has bound the labeled antibody; and where this has occurred, blue-green color is seen and identifies the presence of the virus, thus confirming the presumptive clinical diagnosis.

NONINFECTIOUS INFLAMMATION OF THE EYE

In 1907 in India Herbert[10] examined ocular exudates in patients with spring catarrh; his diagnosis was largely based on the presence of eosinophils in the secretion. The greater the allergic reaction the higher the proportion of eosinophils found. It has since been learned that eosinophils may be observed in conjunctival epithelial scrapings as well as in smears of secretions. However, allergic inflammation of the eye, as in other areas of the body, can only be diagnosed with certainty when the specific allergen is found. This problem is discussed in Chapter 10.

Vernal conjunctivitis is the conjunctivitis attributed to an allergic response that was seen most frequently at the IOCPMC. This disease is characterized by a cobblestone type of follicular swelling, as is illustrated in Fig. 4-12. The scrapings contain epithelial cells, polymorphonuclear neutrophils, and eosinophils. This laboratory has examined ocular scrapings from 2,068 patients with allergic inflammation; 1,755 cases were diagnosed as vernal catarrh, 263 as hay fever, and 50 as allergic response to a variety of drugs or cosmetics. Neutrophils were present in all the eyes, eosinophils in 1,903, and basophils in only 74. In all 50 scrapings from patients with drug allergies no neutrophils were seen, and eosinophils were present only in the 16 cases caused by atropine. Other conditions in which eosinophils are sometimes found in the eye include ocular pemphigus, chronic trachoma, and chronic staphylococcus conjunctivitis.

Several factors may be responsible for keratinization of the epithelial cells of the eye: Sjögren's syndrome (keratoconjunctivitis sicca); nutritional disturbances, particularly vitamin A deficiency; exposure to radiation; age; or deficiency of lacrimal secretion, to mention some. The epithelium of both conjunctiva and cornea may be involved. The presence of keratinized cells should be considered abnormal when found in conjunctival or corneal scrapings, provided there is no contamination from the lid margins or caruncle. Numbers of goblet cells are found in keratoconjunctivitis sicca.

In mild degrees of vitamin A deficiency, keratinization of the epithelial cells is slight. A microscopic examination may indicate the possibility of deficiency in the early stages of vitamin A depletion. Clinical diagnosis includes three points: (1) wrinkling of the conjunctiva, (2) lack of luster, and (3) in some cases the development of Bitot's spots just outside the limbus. Bitot[5] in 1863 described these conjunctival spots, which are associated with night blindness (Fig. 4-24). These spots appear at the temporal limbus and are white, sharply defined, triangular patches; they are grossly visible and covered with a silver-gray foamlike substance, which is readily scraped off and which re-forms and may appear like

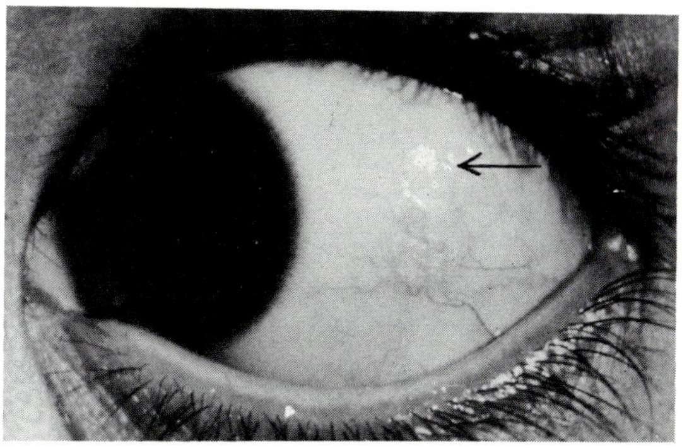

Fig. 4-24. Patient showing Bitot spots (arrow), small areas of keratinization. (Courtesy P. Thygeson.)

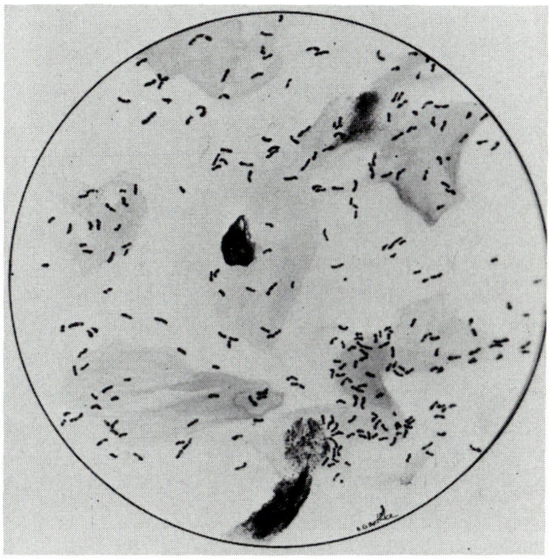

Fig. 4-25. Epithelial scrapling of conjunctiva of a patient with vitamin A deficiency. Note diphtheroids apparently growing on the dead cells. (From Thygeson, P.: Amer, J. Ophthal. **29**:1504, 1946.)

Table 4-2. Cytology observed in smears of exudates and scrapings in various ocular diseases

Disease	Cytology
None	Normal epithelial cells. Some may contain pseudoinclusion bodies or granules. A rare goblet cell.
Acute bacterial infections	Watery or mucopurulent discharge containing predominantly polymorphonuclear neutrophils. Bacteria may be identified.
Chlamydia infection	Cytoplasmic inclusion bodies in epithelial cells. Neutrophils, lymphocytes, plasma cells, macrophages.
Acute viral infection	Lymphocytes and large mononuclear cells. Some multinucleated epithelial cells.
Chronic bacterial, mycotic, and mycobacterial infections	Decrease in polymorphonuclear neutrophils and the appearance of some lymphocytes and large mononuclear cells. Fungi may be identified, also acid-fast bacilli.
Chronic infection of known or possible viral origin	Large mononuclear cells. Lymphocytes. Some multinucleated epithelial cells.
Allergies	Notable for numerous eosinophils and sometimes basophils.
Nutritional, physical, and chemical injuries, keratoconjunctivitis sicca, pemphigus	Squamous and/or keratinized epithelial cells, cicatrization. In vitamin A deficiency there may be numerous diphtheroids; in keratoconjunctivitis sicca, goblet cells and mucus; in pemphigus, occasional eosinophils.

plaques. They are more prevalent in children but may be present in adults. Fig. 4-25 shows scrapings from the bulbar conjunctiva of a patient with vitamin A deficiency. Note the epithelial cells covered with masses of diphtheroids. The relationship of Bitot's spots to vitamin A deficiency is under scrutiny.[15a,21a]

In several forms of trauma to the conjunctiva, such as allergic conjunctivitis, keratoconjunctivitis sicca, and vitamin A deficiency, the normal bacterial flora of the eye increases in volume, with the result that numbers of staphylococci and diphtheroids are seen in the scrapings.

A summary of the cellular changes found in ocular smears and scrapings in various types of inflammation is given in Table 4-2.

TECHNIQUE FOR PREPARING SMEARS FROM EXUDATES AND SCRAPINGS

Fig. 4-26 illustrates the tray of equipment needed for obtaining smears of exudates and scrapings from the conjunctiva, eyelid margin, and cornea. This tray is equipped with everything necessary to obtain the material at the bedside. If the patient is ambulatory, the scrapings are taken in the microbiology laboratory.

The three types of platinum spatulas employed for scrapings are standing to the left in front of the alcohol lamp and matches. The lamp is used to sterilize the spatula. Sterile gauze is in the jar in the shadow to the left. The spatula most frequently used is on the left; the "spade" in the center is sometimes helpful in recovering material from fungal infections and is preferred by some over the rounded spatula. The plastic bottle contains ophthaine 0.5%, for local anesthesia, and the glass holds the slips necessary for the laboratory records. Slides thoroughly cleaned with soap and water and alcohol are ready for use. Next to them in a glass test tube are small sterile swabs on toothpicks for recovering exudates. A wax pencil for writing on glass and a diamond glass-marking pencil, in the foreground next to two test tubes holding sterile cotton swabs in case of abundant amounts of exudate, are avail-

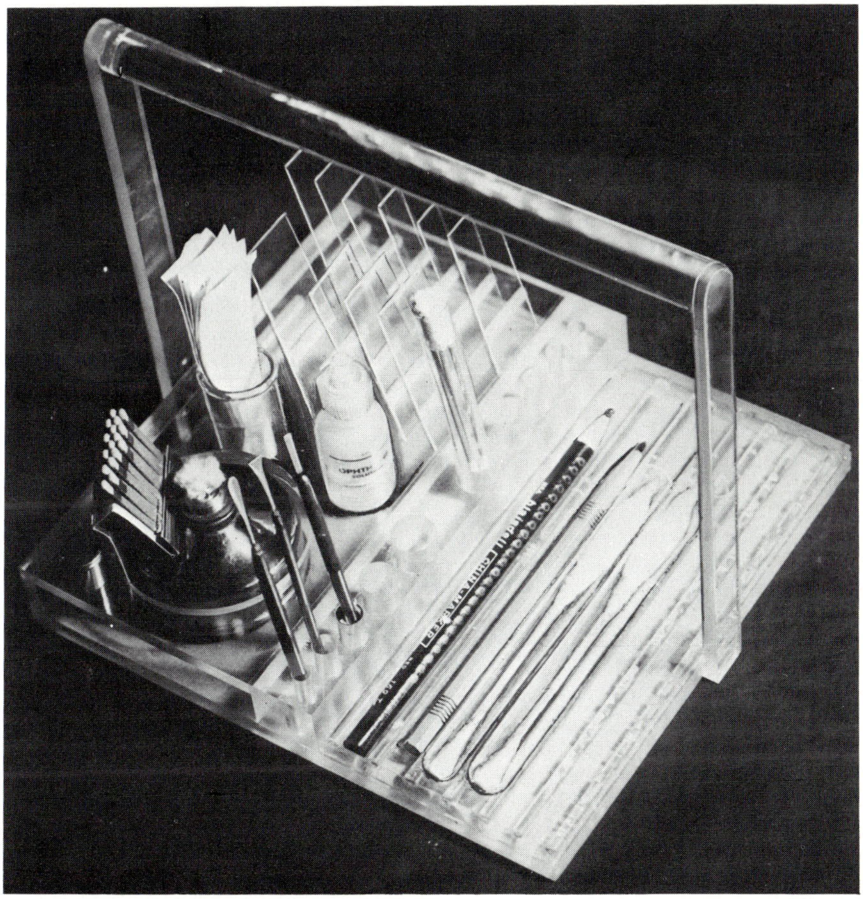

Fig. 4-26. Tray equipped for taking smears of exudates and scrapings from the eye.

able. The slides are marked with the diamond glass-marking pencil and carry the patient's name, the source of the material, such as OD, OS, C (for conjunctiva), K (for cornea), KU (for corneal ulcer), L (for lid), or any other information needed.

Fig. 4-27, *A* through *D*, illustrates the approach to taking ocular scrapings. The application of the material to the slide is most important. As indicated in Fig. 4-28, the spatula is gently rubbed over a small area of the slide. At least two slides are prepared. If the specimen is dry, a very small bit of water may be added to the slide to help spread the film more evenly. Much of the success for finding favorable fields for examination depends on obtaining a good distribution of the material without crushing the cells. In some instances, especially in suspected tuberculosis, after the smears are made the spatula may be placed in a few drops of broth. When the adhering material is loosened, the tube is put aside for centrifugation in case no acid-fast bacteria are found in the smears. The concentrated sediment from the centrifugate may be found positive for acid-fast bacilli. The slides containing the smears are returned to the rack to dry.

Usually a Gram stain is done immediately so that antibiotic therapy may be started if a presumptive diagnosis can be made.[7a] The Giemsa stain, a process that requires about 1¼ hours, is the stain of choice for histologic examination; and this stain, or some special stain indicated by the presumptive diagnosis, is used on the second

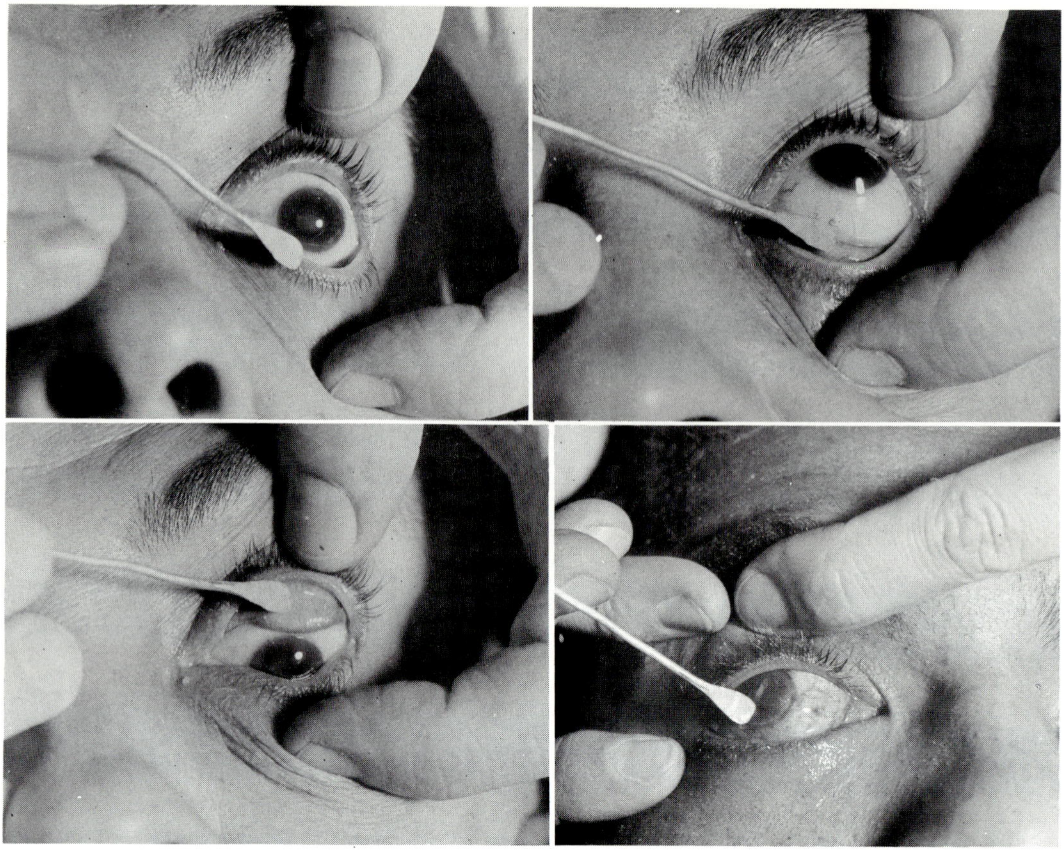

Fig. 4-27. **A,** Lid margin scraping; **B,** scrapings of the lower conjunctiva; **C,** scrapings of the upper conjunctiva; **D,** corneal scraping.

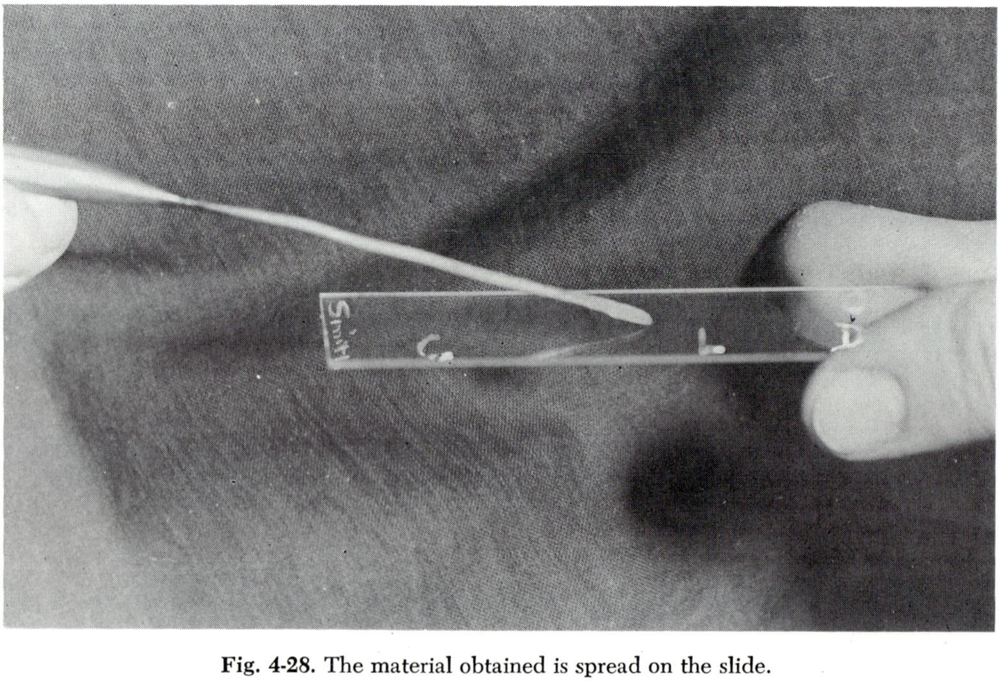

Fig. 4-28. The material obtained is spread on the slide.

slide. The Giemsa stain is made by fixing the slide in absolute methyl alcohol in a coplin jar for 5 minutes. The slide is then transferred to a jar containing freshly prepared Giemsa stain and placed in the incubator at 36° C for ½ to 1 hour. After passing through two changes of 95% alcohol, the slide is dried in the air and covered with emersion oil and a cover slip. The bacteria stain blue; the inclusions of trachoma or inclusion conjunctivitis appear deep blue; the eosinophils and their granules are pink; nuclear material and other miscellaneous granules are blue or green. In some laboratories Wright's stain is preferred.[7a]

SUMMARY

The examination of smears from exudates and scrapings offer the following diagnostic and therapeutic aids:

1. In the healthy eye only epithelial cells are found.
2. Acute infections of bacterial origin are characterized by numerous polymorphonuclear cells and often by the presence of the causative agent.
3. Although identification of the specific bacterium depends on its cultivation, this may be facilitated by preliminary inspection of the smear, after which special media may be selected.
4. Tentative recognition of the organism may indicate initiation of antibiotic therapy.
5. Trachoma or inclusion conjunctivitis can be diagnosed from the presence of epithelial cytoplasmic inclusion bodies.
6. The value of the smear from scrapings in acute viral infection lies in observing the lack of bacteria and the presence of lymphocytes.
7. The smears of scrapings obtained from cases of chronic trachoma or viral infection are often similar and show decreasing polymorphonuclear cells and increasing lymphocytes and monocytes.
8. Identification of fungal infection is possible.
9. Acid-fast rods, mycobacteria, can alert one to the possibility of tuberculosis.
10. Eosinophils are most frequently associated with an allergic disease.
11. Smears showing keratinized epithelial cells arise from a variety of physical and chemical injuries, malnutrition, cicatrization, and keratoconjunctivitis sicca.

It thus may be seen that the routine examination of smears from exudates and scrapings is well worth the extra time and care required, since diagnosis is often facilitated and therapy accelerated because of the information that such an examination yields.

REFERENCES

1. Agarwal, L. P., and Malhoutra, R. L.: Conjunctival smear cytology in xerosis, Ophthalmologica **130**:378, 1955.
2. Aubineau, E.: Chancre induré de la conjonctive, Ann. Oculist. **138**:16, 1907.
3. Axenfeld, T.: The bacteriology of the eye, translated by Angus MacNab, New York, 1908, William Wood and Co.
4. Barr, M. L., and Bertram, E. G.: A morphological distinction between neurons of the male and female, and the behavior of the nuclear satellite during accelerated nucleoprotein synthesis, Nature **163**:676, 1949.
5. Bitôt, P.: Sur une lesion conjonctivale non encore decrite coincidant avec l'hemeralopie, Gaz. Hebd. Med. Chir. **10**:284, 1863.

5a. Browning, S. H.: The value of the direct smear in the bacteriology of conjunctivitis, with analysis of a thousand cases, Ophthal. Rev. **31**:97, 1912.

6. De Azevedo, M. L.: Sex chromatin detection in epithelial cells of the conjunctiva, Ophthalmologica **142**:425, 1961.
7. De Azevedo, M. L.: Citologia ocular. Doctoral dissertation presented to the Faculty of Medicine at the University of São Paulo, São Paulo, 1962.

7a. Fedukowicz, H. B.: External infections of the eye, Des Moines, 1963, Meredith Corporation, p. 206.

8. Halberstaedter, L., and von Prowazek, S.: Zur Aetiologie des Trachoms, Deutsch. Med. Wschr. **33**:1285, 1907.
9. Hardy, D., Surman, P. G., and Howarth, W. H.: Cytologic survey of conjunctival smears

from aboriginal school children at Yalata, South Australia, Brit. J. Ophthal. **51**:54, 1967.
10. Herbert, H.: Clinical observations on spring catarrh, Brit. Med. J. **2**:1232, 1907.
11. Hirschberg, J., and Krause, F.: Zur Pathologie der ansteckenden Augenkrankheiten, Zbl. Augenheilk. **5**:270, 1881.
12. Hirschberg, J.: Wilhelm Werneck, Graefe-Saemisch Handbuch der Augenheilkunde **14**: 561, 1911.
13. Hogan, M. J., and Zimmerman, L. E.: Ophthalmic pathology: an atlas and textbook, ed. 2, Philadelphia, 1962, W. B. Saunders Co.
14. Howard, H.: Role of the epithelial cell in conjunctival and corneal infections, Amer. J. Ophthal. **7**:909, 1924.
15. Kamen, L.: Zur Aetiologie der epidemischen Bindehautentzündung, Zbl. Bakt. Parasit. Infekt. (Jena) **25**:449, 1899.
15a. Kimura, S. J., and Thygeson, P.: The cytology of external ocular disease, Amer. J. Ophthal. **39**:137, 1955.
16. Leber, T.: Keratomycosis aspergillina als Ursache von Hypopyonkeratitis, Graefes Arch. Ophth. **25**:285, 1879.
17. Lindner, K.: Über die Topographie der parasitären Bindehautkeime, Graefes Arch. Ophth. **105**:726, 1921.
18. Liotet, S., and Iris, L.: Étude analytique de la cytologie conjonctivale normale et pathologique, Arch. Ophtal. (Paris) **23**:143, 1963.
19. McKee, H. A.: A new method of making film preparations to demonstrate the presence of the gonococcus, Ophthal. Rec. **21**:4, 1912.
20. Moore, K. L., and Barr, M. L.: Smears from oral mucosa in the detection of chromosomal sex, Lancet **2**:57, 1955.
21. Norn, M. S.: Age variation in the frequency of lymphocytosis in the conjunctival fluid, Acta Ophthal. (Copenhagen) **40**:69, 1962.
21a. Paton, D., and McLaren, D. S.: Bitot spots, Amer. J. Ophthal. **50**:568, 1960.
22. Pedler, C., and Ashton, N.: Sex of nuclei in ocular tissues, Brit. J. Ophthal. **39**:362, 1955.
23. Schaudinn, F., and Hoffmann, E.: Vorläufiger Bericht über das Vorkommen von Spirochaeten in syphilitischen Krankheitsprodukten und bei Papillomen, Arbeiten, Aus Dem Kaiserlichen Gesundheitsamte **22**:527, 1905.
23a. Thygeson, P.: The cytology of conjunctival exudates, Amer. J. Ophthal. **29**:1499, 1946.
24. Thygeson, P.: The cytologic diagnosis of trachoma, Rev. Int. Trachome **32**:421, 1955.
25. Werneck, W.: Lettres au Docteur Florent Cunier: sur la structure de la conjonctive, Ann. Oculist. **14**:145, 241, 1845.

5

Bacterial infections of the eye

with **ELIZABETH H. GUTIERREZ**

During the period in which one of us (D. L.-K.) was in charge of the microbiology laboratory at the Institute of Ophthalmology, Columbia-Presbyterian Medical Center (IOCPMC), cultures from the eyes of some 40,000 patients were obtained. Records of findings have been kept in large ledgers, which, though somewhat reminiscent of a Dickens accounting house, have proved very valuable in that the clinical diagnosis and chart unit number accompany the detailed account of organisms seen in smears, isolated, identified, and checked for sensitivity to antibiotics. Through the years these readily available data have been assembled in secondary ledgers in various ways according to incidence of ocular disease, incidence of etiologic agents, relation to season, relation to known trauma or chemical treatment, incidence of infection per month and per year, and changing sensitivities of the microorganisms. Periodic cultures of normal eyes have been carried out in order to establish the ocular flora for comparison with that determined in disease and in relation to postoperative infections. Data for the normal flora are given in Chapter 2. Both eyes of every patient were cultured even when only one was involved. In this chapter, bacterial infections of the eye, as seen at the IOCPMC over a 30-year period, are discussed.

Neisser in 1879 was the first to describe a bacterial ocular pathogen, the gonococcus. A few years later, while studying the etiology of cholera in Egypt, Koch observed the second organism considered to be a primary pathogen of the eye. This organism was later isolated by Weeks and came to be known as the Koch-Weeks bacillus (*Hemophilus aegypticus*). In 1897 Morax isolated a diplobacillus from a case of subacute angular conjunctivitis. This bacterium, identified independently by Axenfeld, is now familiar as the Morax-Axenfeld diplobacillus, or *Moraxella lacunata.* A similar diplobacillus, *Moraxella liquefaciens,* described by Petit in 1898, causes serpiginous corneal ulcers. The experimental proof of the role of these organisms as agents of infection of the eye could not be established by transmission to animals, since they proved pathogenic only for man; but their etiologic relationship to ocular disease was demonstrated by experimental infection of the eyes of volunteers (Chapter 1). The flora of the normal eye contain bacteria that also may be found at times in ocular infections. These include *Staphylococcus aureus, Hemophilus influenzae,* and *Diplococcus pneumoniae,* among several others.

ACUTE CONJUNCTIVITIS

Acute conjunctivitis is the commonest type of infection seen at the IOCPMC. Table 5-1, covering the period 1938 to

Table 5-1. Etiologic agents in 8,068 patients with acute bacterial conjunctivitis: 1938-1968*

Etiologic agents	Premature babies (38)	Term babies (1,223)	Children to 18 years (3,062)	Adults (3,745)
Diplococcus pneumoniae	7	324	1,135	1,337
Hemophilus influenzae	3	136	1,032	1,148
Staphylococcus aureus	13	341	401	776
Neisseria gonorrhoeae	—	306	4	215
Streptococcus viridans	1	23	408	136
Hemophilus aegypticus	—	—	16	82
Hemolytic streptococci	2	7	12	20
Neisseria catarrhalis	—	5	18	16
Anhemolytic streptococci	1	—	—	6
Pseudomonas aeruginosa	7	—	2	—
Neisseria meningitidis	—	—	1	—
Proteus vulgaris	—	16	—	—
Escherichia coli	2	14	—	—
Diplococcus pneumoniae and *H. influenzae*	—	—	—	6
Diplococcus pneumoniae and *S. aureus*	—	25	—	—
Hemophilus influenzae and *S. aureus*	2	13	33	—
Streptococcus viridans and *S. aureus*	—	13	—	—
Hemolytic streptococci and *D. pneumoniae*	—	—	—	3

*Patients were premature or term babies, young children, and adults.

1968, presents data on 8,068 patients with acute bacterial conjunctivitis. These patients included premature babies, term babies, children to 18 years, and adults. In the 38 premature babies, *Staphylococcus aureus, Diplococcus pneumoniae,* and *Pseudomonas aeruginosa* accounted for 27 of the infections. The infections caused by *P. aeruginosa* were the most severe, and 4 of the children died of sepsis. This organism has proved to be difficult to control in patients of all ages. The pneumococci, *H. influenzae, S. aureus,* and *Neisseria gonorrhoeae* topped the list of agents causing acute conjunctivitis in the newborn. In 735 of these 1,223 babies the conjunctivitis developed before they left the hospital. Pneumococci, *H. influenzae,* and *S. aureus* also were agents of acute conjunctivitis in children to 18 years of age. *Streptococcus viridans* as well played a major role in the conjunctivitis of this group. *D. pneumoniae, H. influenzae,* and *S. aureus* each proved to be of major importance in acute conjunctivitis of the adult. Plate 1, *G* illustrates an acute bulbar conjunctivitis in an adult; the conjunctivitis was caused by *S. aureus.* Although *S. aureus* is a common inhabitant of the eye, the other two bacteria are only rarely found in the normal eye. There were 1,077 cases of acute conjunctivitis in adults in which no pathogenic bacterium was found.

Two hundred and seventeen cases of membranous or pseudomembranous conjunctivitis not included in Table 5-1 are presented in Table 5-2. Since such cases present a distinctive lesion, it was of interest to compare the etiologic agents producing this type of conjunctivitis with those of other cases. The single organisms producing membranous conjunctivitis most often were *Staphylococcus aureus* and *Streptococcus hemolyticus,* neither of which headed the list of organisms causing conjunctivitis reported in Table 5-1. Plate 1, *H* illustrates a streptococcal membranous conjunctivitis; Plate 1, *I* shows membranous conjunctivitis caused by *Corynebacterium diphtheriae.*

Table 5-3 indicates the sites of conjunctival lesions caused by some of the more important eye pathogens, and the nature of the exudates. From this table it may be

Table 5-2. Etiologic agents in 217 patients of all ages with membranous or pseudomembranous conjunctivitis: 1938-1968

Etiologic agents	Membranous conjunctivitis (163)	Pseudomembranous conjunctivitis (54)
Diplococcus pneumoniae	9	6
Staphylococcus aureus	47	27
Streptococcus viridans	6	2
Hemolytic streptococci	39	4
Escherichia coli	4	1
Hemophilus influenzae	8	2
Corynebacterium diphtheriae	4	3
Diplococcus pneumoniae and *S. aureus*	11	2
Hemolytic streptococci and *S. aureus*	12	1
Streptococcus viridans and *S. aureus*	5	3
Hemophilus influenzae and *S. aureus*	1	1
Escherichia coli and *S. aureus*	1	1
Staphylococcus aureus and *Neisseria catarrhalis*	10	1
Staphylococcus aureus and diphtheroids	6	—

seen that some bacteria are epithelial parasites and that in at least two instances (infection with the gonococcus or the pneumococcus) epithelial scrapings may give an early diagnosis.

CHRONIC CONJUNCTIVITIS

The diagnosis of chronic conjunctivitis, usually a low-grade infection of long duration, is made primarily by the attending physician. The determination of the etiologic agent is difficult because of several factors; perhaps the most important is that the patient has often been treated with antibiotics before the bacteriologic examination has been made. Other conditions, such as allergic reactions, eyestrain, or exposure to irritants, may introduce a nonbacterial factor that causes the appearance of infection. Furthermore, the fact that S. *aureus* and sometimes other potential pathogens are present in the normal conjunctiva makes difficult the evaluation of the relationship of these organisms to chronic infection. In spite of these hazards, the findings in the bacteriology laboratory were felt to justify the identification of the etiologic agent of chronic conjunctivitis in 562 children and 9,147 adults. The criteria applied were: (1) the organism must be present alone or in combination with another pathogen; (2) the organism must be present in large numbers; and (3) the use of antibiotics to free the eye of the pathogens must be associated with improvement in the conjunctivitis. In 4,857 instances the etiologic agent was undetermined. Cultures were sterile in 43 cases.

The bacterial agents causing chronic conjunctivitis in children and in adults are presented in Table 5-4. It may be seen that the mixed infections predominate in children. S. *aureus* alone or in association with *H. influenzae, D. pneumoniae,* or *S. viridans* accounted for 82% of the infections. *Escherichia coli* or paracolon bacilli caused another 10% of the cases. The majority (6,273) of cases of chronic conjunctivitis in adults were the result of infection with S. *aureus* only. The following combinations of organisms—*D. pneumoniae* with *H. influenzae* or S. *aureus; S. viridans* with *H. influenzae,* S. *aureus,* or *E. coli; Proteus vulgaris* with gram-positive cocci; and *E. coli* in association with paracolon bacilli and S. *aureus*—accounted for another 2,256

Table 5-3. Causative agents, sites of lesions, and nature of exudate in some types of conjunctivitis

Bacterium	Relationship to conjunctival epithelium	Site of conjunctival involvement	Character of exudate
Neisseria gonorrhoeae	Ephithelial parasite; found early in epithelial scraping	Bulbar conjunctiva; may involve entire conjunctiva	Early stage, serosanguineous discharge; later, profuse mucopurulent discharge with intracellular cocci
Neisseria catarrhalis	Perhaps an epithelial parasite	Affects whole conjunctiva	Sparse to profuse mucopurulent discharge with intracellular cocci
Hemophilus aegypticus	Epithelial parasite	Bulbar conjunctiva	Profuse mucopurulent discharge with numerous bacilli
Hemophilus influenzae	Epithelial parasite but may penetrate the epithelium to slight extent only	Bulbar conjunctiva	Thin, watery, or flocculent discharge with numerous bacilli
Diplobacillus of Petit (*Moraxella liquefaciens*)	Not an epithelial parasite	Usually invades whole conjunctiva	Fibrinous; absence of polymorphonuclear neutrophils
Diplobacillus of Morax-Axenfeld (*Moraxella lacunata*)	Secretes proteinase destructive of epithelium; tears protect most of eyes, however	Invades transitional epithelium near inner and outer angles of eyelid	Mild purulent discharge containing diplobacilli, adheres to lashes, especially near angles
Gram-negative bacilli*	Not epithelial parasites	Usually invade whole conjunctiva	Mild purulent discharge containing bacilli
Diplococcus pneumoniae	Epithelial parasite	Bulbar conjunctiva	Mucopurulent or serous; numerous organisms in epithelial scraping
Streptococci	Not epithelial parasites	Affect whole conjunctiva; exotoxin from virulent strains may rupture epithelium, give rise to membranous conjunctivitis	Catarrhal, rarely purulent
Staphylococcus aureus	Not an epithelial parasite	Proliferates on the surface of ocular membrane; inflammation results from liberation and diffusion of toxic products into the tissues	Thin, occasionally mucopurulent; generally scanty number of cocci
Corynebacterium diphtheriae	Epithelial parasite	Bulbar conjunctiva invaded only in severe cases; usually membranous; tarsal and retrotarsal folds affected	Yellow-glairy sticks to eyelashes; bacilli usually present
Francisella tularensis	Epithelium thickened; granulomatous reaction	Usually unilateral; small discrete ulcers more frequent on the lower than upper lid; bulbar conjunctiva rarely involved	Little if any exudate; diagnosis by culture difficult; animal inoculation and serologic tests used

**Escherichia coli*, *Proteus* group, *Aerobacter aerogenes*, *Klebsiella pneumoniae*, paracolon bacilli, and *Pseudomonas aeruginosa*.

Table 5-4. Etiologic agents in chronic bacterial conjunctivitis in 9,709 patients: 1938-1968

Etiologic agents	Children to 18 years (562)	Adults (9,147)
Staphylococcus aureus	60	6,273
Pseudomonas aeruginosa	2	28
Proteus group*	21	124
Escherichia coli or paracolon bacilli	60	90
Diplobacillus of Morax-Axenfeld (*Moraxella lacunata*)	9	76
Diplobacillus of Petit (*Moraxella liquefaciens*)	8	13
Klebsiella group†	5	30
Alcaligenes faecalis	—	4
Diplococcus pneumoniae with *Hemophilus influenzae* or *Staphylococcus aureus*	187	450
Streptococcus hemolyticus with *Hemophilus influenzae, Streptococcus viridans,* or *Staphylococcus aureus*	7	15
Anhemolytic streptococci with *Staphylococcus aureus*	—	3
Streptococcus viridans with *Hemophilus influenzae, Staphylococcus aureus,* or *Escherichia coli*	161	234
Klebsiella group with *Pseudomonas aeruginosa, Staphylococcus aureus, Proteus* group, or *Streptococcus viridans*	16	62
Proteus vulgaris and gram-positive cocci‡	—	913
Escherichia coli and paracolon bacilli with *Staphylococcus aureus*	—	659
Alcaligenes faecalis and *Staphylococcus aureus*	—	6
Pseudomonas aeruginosa with *Streptococcus viridans* or *Staphylococcus aureus*	—	20
Neisseria catarrhalis or *Herellea* species with *Staphylococcus aureus*	23	136
Nocardia species	—	7
Fusiform bacilli, *Treponema macrodentium,* and *Treponema microdentium*	—	4
Mycobacterium boris	3	—

**Proteus vularis, P. morgani, P. mirabilis,* and *P. rettgeri.*
†*Klebsiella pneumoniae* and *K. ozenae.*
‡The spreading *Proteus* organisms obliterate the colonial form of the cocci, preventing more precise diagnosis.

infections. Thus, when the etiologic agents in chronic conjunctivitis in children are compared with those seen in adults, considerable variation in the incidence of the various pathogens is apparent.

When the findings in acute conjunctivitis (Table 5-1) are compared with those in chronic conjunctivitis (Table 5-4), some marked differences between the incidence of the bacteria causing these two diseases are evident. *D. pneumoniae, H. influenzae,* and *S. viridans* may be as prominent as the staphylococci in initiating acute conjunctivitis.

Table 5-5 presents some of the findings in the four cases of chronic follicular conjunctivitis resulting from fusospirochetal or fusiform bacilli infection.[3] Figs. 4-22 and 4-23 illustrate the appearance of a dark-field preparation and a gentian violet stain of a scraping from the lesion of the second patient. The follicular conjunctivitis seen at the time the patient came to the IOCPMC is shown in Fig. 5-1.

Bacteriologic examination of the 1,077 cases of acute conjunctivitis and the 4,857 cases of chronic conjunctivitis in which no bacterial agent was thought responsible for

Table 5-5. Four cases of fusospirochetal or fusiform bacillus follicular conjunctivitis

Patient no.	Age	Sex	Clinical findings	Direct examination of purulent exudate	Isolation
1 (1935)	20	F	"Cold" OD for 2 weeks; purulent discharge; congestion and thickening of palpebral conjunctiva; few enlarged follicles in lower cul-de-sac; cornea clear; lacrimal sac not involved; left eye normal	Darkfield examination of secretion; few spirochetes; fusiform bacilli	Fusiform bacilli
2 (1938)	44	M	6 years' duration; follicular conjunctivitis of right eye and stasis of lacrimal canal; expression and irrigation of lacrimal canaliculi	Darkfield examination of secretion; spirochetes and fusiform bacilli	Fusiform bacilli Spirochetes
3 (1944)	51	F	History of tearing, redness, and stickiness of left eye for 1 year; severe papillary purulent conjunctivitis; no involvement of cornea; canaliculi dilated, curetted, and irrigated; rapid improvement	Darkfield examination; only fusiform bacilli seen	Fusiform bacilli
4 (1956)	28	F	16 months; redness, tearing, discharge of right eye; irrigation of painful canaliculi; follicular conjunctivitis	Darkfield examination; only fusiform bacilli seen	Fusiform bacilli

Data from Burns, R. P., Macnie, J. P., Pfeiffer, R. L., and Locatcher-Khorazo, D.: Unilateral conjunctivitis and canaliculitis due to fusospirochetal infection, Arch. Ophthal. **59**:235, 1958; and Dunnington, J. H., and Khorazo, D.: Conjunctivitis due to fusospirochetal infection, Arch. Ophthal. **16**:252, 1936.

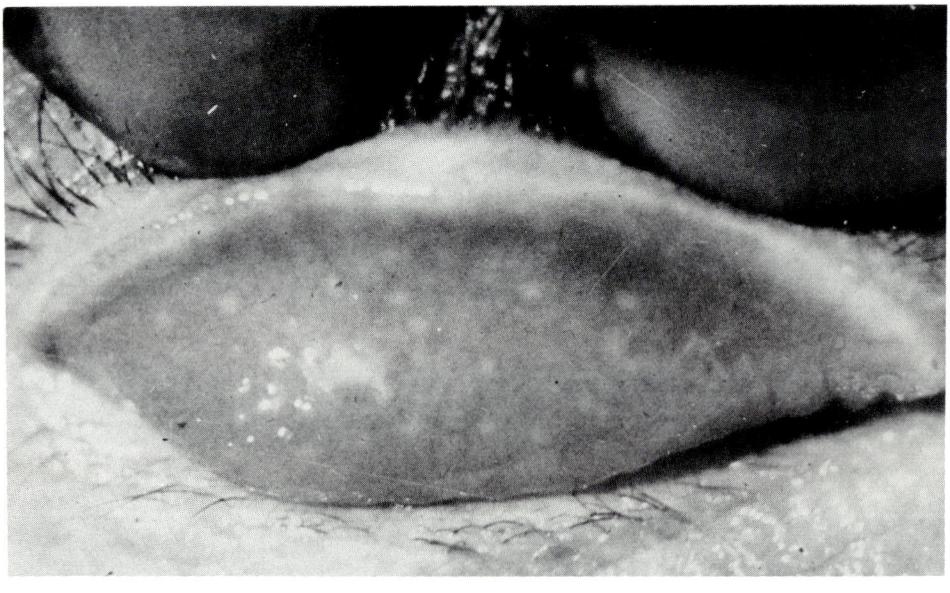

Fig. 5-1. Chronic unilateral follicular conjunctivitis caused by fusospirochetal infection. (From Burns, R. P., Macnie, J. P., Pfeiffer, R. L., and Locatcher-Khorazo, D.: Arch. Ophthal. **59**:236, 1958.)

Table 5-6. Etiologic agents in corneal ulcers in 3,535 patients: 1938-1968

Etiologic agents	Number
Diplococcus pneumoniae	1,233
Staphylococcus aureus	1,755*
Streptococcus viridans	15
Hemolytic streptococci	4
Pseudomonas aeruginosa	194
Proteus vulgaris	30
Escherichia coli	18
Paracolon bacilli	33
Diplobacillus of Petit (*Moraxella liquefaciens*)	77
Klebsiella pneumoniae	11
Nocardia species	1
Nocardia asteroides	1
Streptomyces species	1
Diplococcus pneumoniae and *S. aureus*	72
Hemolytic streptococci and *S. aureus*	17
Hemophilus influenzae and *S. aureus*	6
Pseudomonas aeruginosa and *S. aureus*	5
Pseudomonas aeruginosa and *K. pneumoniae*	1
Escherichia coli and *S. aureus*	61

*212 of these were marginal corneal ulcers.

the conjunctivitis yielded only *S. albus* or *S. aureus* in combination with diphtheroids. Forty-three of the cases had sterile cultures, a finding that is attributed to prior treatment with antibiotics. Many of these cases, on the basis of cytology, were probably of viral origin; some were allergic in nature. However, about half gave no evidence of these conditions. (See Chapter 4 on evaluation of scrapings.)

CORNEAL ULCERS

The bacterial agents isolated in 3,535 cases of corneal infections are listed in Table 5-6, which covers the period 1938 to 1968. The data indicate that *S. aureus* and *D. pneumoniae* are by far the most frequent causes of such infections, and if combined they account for 86% of the total. Plate 2, *A* illustrates a serpiginous corneal ulcer caused by the pneumococcus. *P. aeruginosa* occupies third place in these infections and accounts for 194 cases. Since *P. aeruginosa* usually is not pathogenic or when it does cause infection is often associated with trauma, the charts of the 194

Table 5-7. Type of injury causing 296 cases of bacterial infection of the cornea in adults: 1938-1968

Etiologic agents	Type of lesion	Number	Types of corneal injury
Pseudomonas aeruginosa	Corneal epithelium absent centrally	1	Struck by a piece of sandstone
	Corneal abrasion	1	Scratch with a newspaper
	Corneal ulcer	85	Incomplete removal of foreign bodies
	Hypopyon ulcer	1	While drilling struck by particles
	Corneal abscess	1	Instillation of contaminated drops
	Corneal ulcer	10	Instillation of contaminated drops
	Central corneal ulcer	1	Explosion of refrigerator, ammonium splashed on face
	Corneal exposure	1	Dryness, exophthalmos
Staphylococcus aureus	Corneal abrasion	57	Struck with shrubbery, finger, fingernails, fork; cut with glass, foreign particles; rust embedded in cornea; burns with lime and alkali
	Hypopyon ulcer	2	Injury with venetian blind; cinder removed by druggist
	Corneal ulcer	61	Injury with foreign particles
	Corneal aerosion	12	Foreign particles
Diplococcus pneumoniae	Corneal ulcer	1	Patient attacked and hit
		62	Injury with foreign particles

patients with corneal ulcers caused by pseudomonas were examined for history of trauma. The same procedure was carried out on records of some corneal ulcers caused by other bacteria. The results of this study are recorded in Table 5-7. This table shows that 102 patients with *P. aeruginosa* infections had a history of preceding trauma. Incomplete removal of foreign bodies preceded 85 of the infections.

P. aeruginosa may produce a most devastating infection of the eye and is also a difficult organism to treat with antibiotics. Within 24 to 48 hours it can produce a rapidly spreading ulcer with central necrosis. The infection should be considered of primary importance; and if the organism is suspected on the basis of the clinical picture and the presence of gram-negative bacilli, treatment should be initiated immediately. Plate 2, *B* illustrates such a rapidly progressing infection following removal of a foreign body.

Traumas of similar origin were present in the histories of 132 patients with corneal ulcers caused by S. *aureus* and in 63 patients with pneumococcal ulcers. Plate 2, *C* illustrates a marginal staphylococcal ulcer. Other types of predisposing injury in corneal ulcers have been described by Allen.[1] Although *Moraxella liquefaciens* (Diplobacillus of Petit) was among the first specific pathogens to be identified, it is one of the rarer causes of corneal ulcer seen in this country. Plate 2, *D* shows a corneal ulcer caused by *M. liquefaciens.*

The etiologic agents in 922 cases of corneal ulcers were not determined. One hundred and nine of these cases had sterile cultures, presumably because of antibiotic treatment prior to admission to the hospital. From the remaining eyes only staphylococci and diphtheroids were grown, and these organisms did not seem to be related to the cause of the lesion. It may be assumed that in some instances a virus was the etiologic agent, whereas in others prior antibiotic treatment had already removed the causative agent.

An attempt was made to determine if the strains of S. *aureus* causing either acute or chronic conjunctivitis or corneal ulcer were different from those strains carried by the patient in uninfected areas of the body. In order to carry out these studies, phage typing of staphylococci was performed. Many staphylococci are susceptible to lysis by one or more of 24 phages (viruses) that infect this bacterium. Such lysis is readily determined; and because of the multiple combinations of phages causing lysis of a specific type of staphylococcus, the organism is marked, making it possible to achieve accurate identification of a given strain. Cultures were taken from neighboring tissues as well as from the lesion in order to determine if the same staphylococcus was present in those noninfected tissues. Twenty-eight strains from the eyes of patients with acute conjunctivitis were phage typed; and strains isolated from the nose, throat, or hands, or in one case from an infected leg of the same patient, were also typed. The pattern of phage lysis (type) was the same for the staphylococci obtained from the infected and noninfected areas. Further studies on the normal disposition of typed S. *aureus* have shown that individuals usually carry the same type for many months.

Studies were carried out in the case of 35 patients who had chronic conjunctivitis. The results obtained were entirely comparable to those observed in cases of acute conjunctivitis. In addition, 31 cases of corneal ulcer yielded staphylococci that fell among the same types as were seen in the preceding two studies.[5,6]

Two other organisms, the pneumococcus and *H. influenzae,* causing conjunctivitis or corneal ulcers, were also typed in an effort to determine if a unique member of the group was responsible for these ocular infections. One hundred and twelve strains of *D. pneumoniae* isolated from acute conjunctivitis in children were typable; 62 belonged to type 1. In 236 adults with typable pneumococcal conjunctivitis, types 1, 2, and 3 accounted for 155 of the infections. Other types were found scattered among

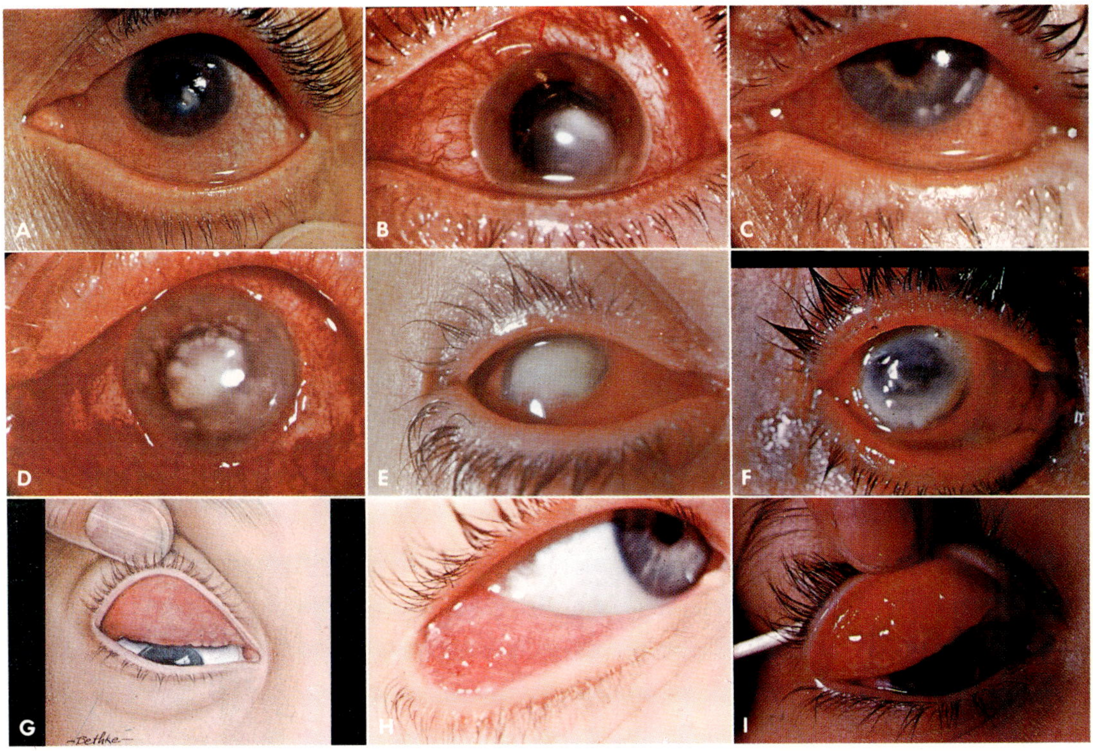

Plate 2. A, Serpiginous corneal ulcer caused by *Diplococcus pneumoniae.* **B,** Corneal ulcer caused by *Pseudomonas aeruginosa.* **C,** Marginal corneal ulcer with blepharitis caused by *Staphylococcus aureus.* **D,** Corneal ulcer caused by *Moraxella liquefaciens.* **E,** Endophthalmitis caused by *Staphylococcus aureus.* **F,** Endophthalmitis caused by *Proteus vulgaris.* **G,** Primary tuberculosis of the tarsal conjunctiva in a 9-year-old child. Note at about the middle of the upper tarsal conjunctiva a shallow, indolent ulcer, 4 × 5 mm in size with fairly well-defined reddish margin and a gray sloughing base. (See also Fig. 4-20.) **H,** Primary tuberculoma of conjunctiva in a 10-year-old boy. **I,** Papillary hypertrophy of the right upper lid with small areas of ulceration in an 11½-year-old girl with primary tuberculosis of the conjunctiva. (**B** and **D** courtesy Dr. R. W. Darrell; **G** from Bruce, G. M., and Locatcher-Khorazo, D.: Arch. Ophthal. **37**:376, 1947; **H** from DeVoe, A. G., and Locatcher-Khorazo, D.: Trans. Amer. Ophthal. Soc. **62**:205, 1964; **I** from Chandler, A. C., Jr., and Locatcher-Khorazo, D.: Arch. Ophthal. **71**:203, 1964.)

the remaining cases. Five hundred and eighty-six strains of *D. pneumoniae* isolated from corneal ulcers were also typed. Types 1, 2, and 3 accounted for 473 of the infections, and various types were found in the remainder. The distribution of types in the infected eye, exclusive of types 1 and 2, was not strikingly different from that which might be found in the normal throat.

Virulent *H. influenzae* may also be typed serologically, but the organisms isolated from conjunctivitis and corneal ulcers caused by this bacterium were with one exception not typable. It is concluded from the attempt to determine specific strains in infection that these three microorganisms, the staphylococcus, *D. pneumoniae,* and *H. influenzae,* show no specific strain causing conjunctivitis or corneal ulcer.

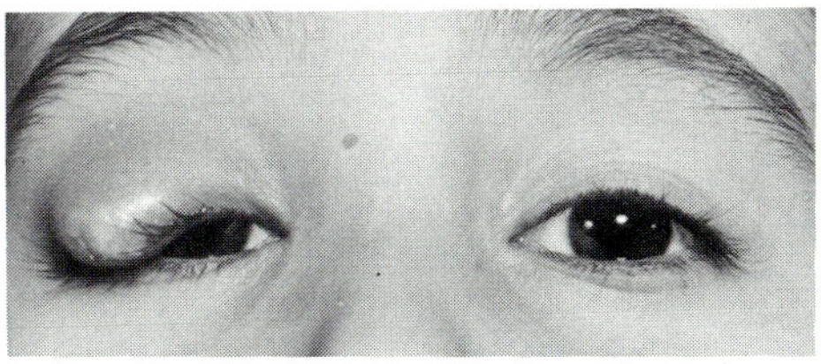

Fig. 5-2. Abscess, caused by *Staphylococcus aureus,* of right upper lid.

INFECTIONS OF THE EYELID

In the period of our studies (1938 to 1968) 8,486 patients with various bacterial infections of the eyelids were seen. The findings from these eyes are listed in Table 5-8 under six categories, which represent the clinical diagnoses. *Staphylococcus aureus* (Fig. 5-2) alone or in combination with other individual pathogens accounted for over 81% of the infections seen in all the groups. It was somewhat unexpected to find that almost all of the other infections

Table 5-8. Bacterial agents in 8,486 patients with various infections of the eyelids: 1938-1968

Microorganisms isolated	Eyelid abscess (228)	Hordeolum (230)	Meibomitis (325)	Acute and chronic chalazion (384)	Blepharitis (1,637)	Blepharoconjunctivitis (5,682)
Staphylococcus aureus	193	224	146	292	1,029	2,614
Streptococcus viridans	7	—	11	13	12	231
Diplobacillus of Morax-Axenfeld (*Moraxella lacunata*)	—	—	4	—	29	224
Escherichia coli	3	1	14	6	26	223
Klebsiella pneumoniae	1	—	44	—	29	213
Proteus vulgaris	—	—	11	5	16	160
Pseudomonas aeruginosa	—	2	8	1	15	146
Diplobacillus of Petit (*Moraxella liquefaciens*)	—	—	5	3	12	36
Diplococcus pneumoniae	7	—	6	11	29	26
Hemophilus influenzae	—	—	—	—	3	1
Hemolytic streptococci	3	—	4	3	3	—
Diplococcus pneumoniae and hemolytic *S. aureus*	7	2	16	9	20	275
Streptococcus viridans and *S. aureus*	3	—	7	10	226	215
Klebsiella pneumoniae and *S. aureus*	—	1	14	10	58	324
Proteus vulgaris and *S. aureus*	1	—	16	6	25	467
Escherichia coli or paracolon bacilli and *S. aureus*	—	—	6	6	49	363
Pseudomonas aeruginosa and *S. aureus*	—	—	11	4	46	136
Hemophilus influenzae and *S. aureus*	—	—	2	5	7	12
Hemolytic streptococci and *S. aureus*	3	—	—	—	3	16

were caused by one or another of 10 organisms, which, with the exception of *Streptococcus viridans,* are rarely found on the skin adjacent to the eye, or in the normal eye. In an additional 357 patients the etiologic agent was not determined.

INFECTIONS OF THE LACRIMAL SAC AND CANALICULI

Dacryocystitis is a common acute or chronic disease, most often unilateral, which is almost always secondary to obstruction of the nasal lacrimal ducts. Table 5-9 describes the results of cultures of 891 cases of dacryocystitis or lacrimal duct obstruction resulting from bacterial infection. The 551 cases carrying the diagnosis of acute and chronic dacryocystitis showed a preponderance of infections by *S. aureus,* with a scattering of cases involving the other 12 pathogens. Fig. 5-3 illustrates a staphylococcal dacryocystitis with draining abscess.

The three categories of lacrimal canaliculus disease showed a scattering of infectious agents, except for the 287 cases diagnosed lacrimal obstruction, 216 of which were caused by *Nocardia* species (Fig. 5-4). Three of the four cases of fusospirochetal or fusiform bacillus infection listed with the chronic conjunctivitis cases in Table 5-4 also had involvement of the lacrimal canals and might have been placed in Table 5-9 under the heading "lacrimal conjunctivitis." The findings from these patients are briefly summarized in Table 5-5.

Table 5-9. Etiologic agents in 891 patients with bacterial infections of the lacrimal apparatus: 1938-1968

Microorganisms isolated	Acute and chronic dacryocystitis (551)	Lacrimal obstruction (287)	Lacrimal abscess (25)	Lacrimal conjunctivitis (28)
D. pneumoniae (types 1, 3, 4, 6, 10)	43	12	3	1
Staphylococcus aureus (with or without diphtheroids)	282	17	3	12
Streptococcus viridans	4	1	1	1
Hemolytic streptococci	22	2	1	1
Pseudomonas aeruginosa	9	2	1	1
Proteus vulgaris	9	14	1	—
Escherichia coli	5	2	1	1
Klebsiella pneumoniae	15	4	4	1
Diplobacillus of Morax-Axenfeld (*Moraxella lacunata*)	5	1	—	—
Hemophilus influenzae	3	—	—	—
Corynebacterium diphtheriae (non–toxin producing)	—	1	—	—
Nocardia species	—	216	—	7
Streptomyces species	—	4	—	—
Diplococcus pneumoniae and *S. aureus*	68	—	—	—
Hemolytic steptococci and *S. aureus*	24	1	1	—
Streptococcus viridans and *S. aureus*	18	2	2	1
Klebsiella pneumoniae and *S. aureus*	25	2	1	1
Escherichia coli and *S. aureus*	13	3	3	1
Escherichia coli and pneumococci	1	1	1	—
Pseudomonas aeruginosa, Staphylococcus aureus, and *Streptococcus viridans*	3	1	1	—
Diplobacillus of Morax-Axenfeld and *S. aureus*	2	1	1	—

There were no failures to obtain a definitive etiologic diagnosis in the lacrimal area of the eye.

INFECTIONS OF THE SOCKET

Infection of the socket was seen in 987 patients; in all but two cases the causative agent was a bacterium. The two exceptions were infections caused by fungi (Chapter 13). S. *aureus* accounted for more than one third of the cases, with *Pseudomonas* and *Proteus* groups holding second and third place (Table 5-10). The bacterial flora in infections of the socket is similar to that found elsewhere in the eyes.

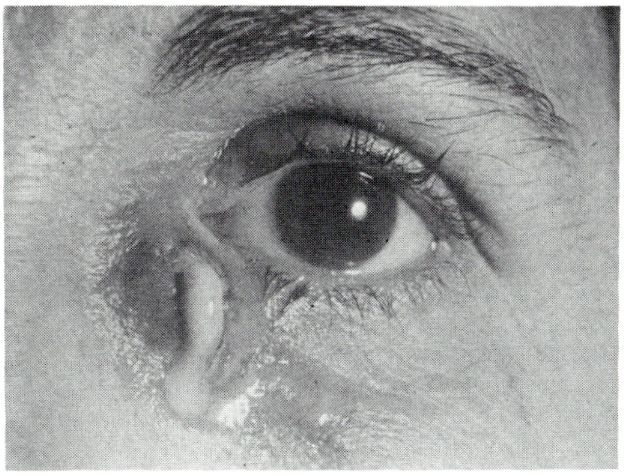

Fig. 5-3. Staphylococcal dacryocystitis with draining abscess.

ORBITAL CELLULITIS

From 1944 to 1968 cultures were obtained from 1,004 patients with a diagnosis of orbital cellulitis (Table 5-11). In 950 instances S. *aureus* was the causative agent, and in another 34 patients the staphylococcus in association with streptococci or pneumococci were isolated. Only infections of the eyelid show a somewhat comparable preponderance of staphylococcal infection.

ENDOPHTHALMITIS

Table 5-12 presents data from cases of endophthalmitis in which the etiologic agent was determined in the years 1945 to 1968. This represents only a portion of the

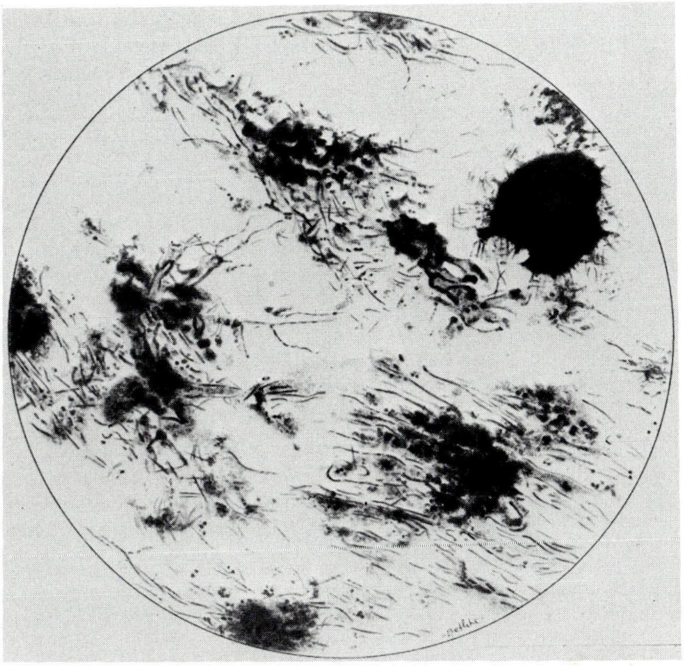

Fig. 5-4. Smear of expression from canaliculus of patient with lacrimal obstruction caused by *Nocardia* species. This bacterium was formerly classified as a fungus because of the branching filamentouslike appearance seen in the illustration.

Table 5-10. Bacterial infection of the socket in 987 patients: 1938-1968

Microorganisms isolated	Number	Percent positive
Staphylococcus aureus	351	35.5
Pseudomonas aeruginosa	112	11.3
Proteus group*	83	8.4
Escherichia coli	40	4.5
Diplococcus pneumoniae	37	3.7
Streptococcus viridans	25	2.5
Klebsiella pneumoniae	16	1.6
Hemolytic streptococci	5	0.51
Diplobacillus of Petit (*Moraxella liquefaciens*)	4	0.45
Diplococcus pneumoniae and *S. aureus*	69	6.9
Proteus vulgaris and gram-positive cocci†	52	5.2
Paracolon bacilli and *S. aureus*	44	4.4
Klebsiella pneumoniae and *S. aureus*	34	3.4
Pseudomonas aeruginosa and *S. aureus*	34	3.4
Streptococcus viridans and *S. aureus*	28	2.8
Hemophilus influenzae, S. aureus, and *D. pneumoniae*	16	1.6
Hemolytic streptococci and *S. aureus*	16	1.6
Beta-hemolytic streptococci and *D. pneumoniae*	10	1.1
S. aureus and *Neisseria catarrhalis*	7	0.7
S. aureus and *N. sicca*	2	0.22
Diplobacillus of Petit and *S. aureus*	2	0.22

**Proteus vulgaris*—62; *Proteus mirabilis*—21.
†The spreading *Proteus vulgaris* obliterates the colonial form of the organism, preventing more precise diagnosis.

patients with this clinical diagnosis, since bacteriologic examination was not made in some instances. The largest series of cultures were from eyes with postoperative infections, and here the staphylococcus was the most important pathogen.

SUCCESSFUL CULTIVATION OF OCULAR FLORA

The eye offers two special problems to challenge the skill of the microbiologist. The first of these is the extremely small amount of material available in many instances for culture. This amount may limit the number of inoculations of different, specialized media.[2] The small amount of material also puts pressure on the ophthalmologist or technician who takes the culture to return it to the laboratory promptly to prevent drying. The ideal condition is to have the patient come to the laboratory. The second problem that faces the microbiologist is related to the various flora that may cause infection of the eye. When a specimen comes to the routine microbiology laboratory in a general hospital, the accompanying slip states the source of the culture—sputum, throat, gastric lavage, stool, or abscess, for example. The selection of media for primary isolation is dictated by this information. By contrast, one may find in the eye almost any one of the upper respiratory tract, enteral canal, or skin inhabitants in addition to some bac-

Table 5-11. Bacterial agents in orbital cellulitis in 1,004 patients of all ages: 1944-1968

Microorganisms isolated	Number
Staphylococcus aureus	950
Diplococcus pneumoniae	8
Hemolytic streptococci	7
Pseudomonas aeruginosa	2
Proteus vulgaris	2
Anhemolytic streptococci	1
Streptococcus viridans and *S. aureus*	16
Hemolytic streptococci and *S. aureus*	13
Diplococcus pneumoniae and *S. aureus*	5

Table 5-12. Endophthalmitis—causative agents and preceeding injury in 105 patients: 1945-1968

Microorganisms isolated	Corneal ulcer	Surgery*	Trauma	Endogenous
Neisseria gonorrhoeae	1	—	—	—
Clostridium perfringens	—	—	1	—
Staphylococcus aureus	12	51†	4	2
Pseudomonas aeruginosa	5	1	—	3
Proteus vulgaris	2	3	1	—
Diplococcus pneumoniae (types 3, 8, 9, 14, 17, 21)	2	4	—	—
Streptococcus viridans	—	3	—	1
Hemolytic streptococci	—	1	—	—
Escherichia coli	—	1	3	1
Pseudomonas aeruginosa and *S. aureus*	—	1	—	—
Bacillus subtilis	—	—	1	—
Alcaligenes faecalis	—	—	—	1

*Thirty-five of these infections were "late" infections.
†In 13 of these cases the aqueous humor provided material for culture. This source was frequently the best for obtaining the etiologic agent in endophthalmitis.

teria peculiar to the eye. Judgment as to the handling of the culture has to be made promptly on a minimum amount of data. The microbiologist may receive considerable help from examination of smears of scrapings if these are available. Often the clinical judgment of the ophthalmologist is of great assistance. Each case is a "special" problem, and the success achieved in the laboratory often depends on cooperation from the ophthalmologist.

The prompt determination of the sensitivity of a pathogen to antibiotics is one of the most important functions of the laboratory. To isolate individual bacteria and determine their sensitivity in pure culture is routinely done. With a fast-moving infection, however, the minimum of 48 hours that this process requires may be highly damaging to the eye. Therefore, when severe inflammation is present, two extra plates are streaked at once and the entire spectrum of antibiotics is tested. Although the plates contain a mixture of organisms, it is rare to meet a situation in which at least one of the antibiotics has failed to inhibit all growth. This information, obtained overnight, is sometimes very helpful to the handling of the infection.

The sensitivity of S. *aureus* to the various antibiotics in common use at the IOCPMC was tabulated by month and by year. The strains of staphylococci found in this patient population showed a surprisingly constant seasonal and yearly pattern of sensitivity. The Institute has been free of problems associated with the spread of resistant, virulent organisms. Spot data analyzed from the sensitivity test on the other eye pathogens showed a similar stability among these organisms. The stability may be because of the fact that most of the hospital population are well except for the specific eye problem. Furthermore, the period of hospitalization is usually only a few days. Many of the cultures received came from the physicians' private offices and the clinic, where the infection could be handled on an outpatient basis. The variation in sensitivities of various strains within a species, however, makes the determination of the sensitivities of each strain still essential. If the patient fails to respond to treatment, frequent reculturing of the lesion and retesting of sensitivity is important.

Sensitivity of Staph

REFERENCES

1. Allen, H. F.: Current status of prevention, diagnosis and management of bacterial corneal ulcers, Ann. Ophthal. 3:235, 1971.

2. Burns, R. P.: Laboratory methods in diagnosis of eye infection. In Infectious diseases of the conjunctiva and cornea, Symposium of the New Orleans Academy of Ophthalmology, St. Louis, 1963, The C. V. Mosby Co.
3. Burns, R. P., Macnie, J. P., Pfeiffer, R. L., and Locatcher-Khorazo, D.: Unilateral conjunctivitis and canaliculitis due to fusospirochetal infection, Arch. Ophthal. **59**:235, 1958.
4. Dunnington, J. H., and Khorazo, D.: Conjunctivitis due to fusospirochetal infection, Arch. Ophthal. **16**:252, 1936.
5. Locatcher-Khorazo, D., and Gutierrez, E.: Bacteriophage typing of Staphylococcus aureus: a study of normal, infected eyes and environment, Arch. Ophthal. **63**:774, 1960.
6. Locatcher-Khorazo, D., Sullivan, N., and Gutierrez, E.: Staphylococcus aureus isolated from normal and infected eyes, phage types and sensitivity to antibacterial agents, Arch. Ophthal. **77**:370, 1967.

6

Postoperative infections of the eye

with **ELIZABETH H. GUTIERREZ**

Ocular surgery usually can be done at a selected time when the eye shows no evidence of infection. The operations considered in this chapter were for cataract extraction, muscle correction, repair of detached retinas, and treatment of glaucoma. The literature contains many references to infections that follow such surgery.[2,4,5,9,20] It is practically impossible to maintain sterility in the eye for any length of time, open as it is to the air and to the contiguous nose and skin. *Staphylococcus aureus,* a potential pathogen, is frequently found in the healthy eye (Chapter 2); and other, perhaps more virulent, organisms are sometimes present.[1a,19a] In the preantibiotic era, a semblance of sterility was achieved by the instillation of protein silver; with the advent of antibiotics the eye may be rendered apparently bacteria free for short periods of time.[6,12,18] Nevertheless, the area is one where some postoperative infections may be unavoidable.

Infections following cataract surgery at the Institute of Ophthalmology, Columbia-Presbyterian Medical Center (IOCPMC) from 1938 through 1955 have been reported. From 1938 to 1944, 2,508 cataract operations were performed on patients whose eyes had been cultured prior to surgery.[6] There were 11 cases of endophthalmitis caused by S. *aureus,* all occurring in the group of 529 patients who were carrying this organism. This was a 2% incidence of endophthalmitis in patients harboring this pathogen. There were no infections in the 1,706 patients who were not carrying S. *aureus.* In the last few years of this study 104 patients carrying S. *aureus* were given preoperative treatment with sodium sulfathiazole or penicillin ointments until the conjunctivas were free of the pathogens. Since no infection developed, treatment consisting of 5 local applications of antibiotics given over a 24-hour period prior to operation were performed routinely, starting with the year 1944. The antibiotics employed during the succeeding years have varied with the development of new agents and with the results of routine sensitivity tests.[13]

From 1945 to 1955[13] there were a total of 7,662 cataract extractions from patients who had preoperative antibiotic treatment, although not all patients had preoperative cultures taken (Table 6-1). In 567 patients, operation was deferred for supplementary treatment, since it was found that pathogens were not always eliminated by the routine preoperative application of antibiotics for 24 hours. There was a total of 6 cases of endophthalmitis, 5 of which occurred in a group of 3,854 patients in whom no preoperative cultures were taken. No postoperative infections were present in 2,263 patients known to be free of S. *aureus.* There was one infection among a group of 978 patients known to carry the

Table 6-1. Postoperative endophthalmitis following 7,662 operations for cataract extraction:* 1945-1955

Number of operations	Preoperative cultures	Postoperative endophthalmitis	Causative organisms
3,854	Not available	4	*Staphylococcus aureus*
		1	*Escherichia coli*
2,263	*Staphylococcus aureus* absent	None	
978	*Staphylococcus aureus* present	1	*Staphylococcus aureus* and *Pseudomonas aeruginosa*
567†	*Staphylococcus aureus* (507) *Escherichia coli* and *Proteus vulgaris* (60)	None	

*All patients received 24-hour preoperative antibiotic treatment.
†Operations deferred for supplementary local antibiotic treatment until the eye was free of potential pathogens.

Table 6-2. Incidence of postoperative infections in 15,278 patients with 24 hours of routine applications of antibiotics preceding cataract surgery: 1955-1968

Number of operations	Preoperative culture	Postoperative infection		Causative agent
13,319	Not done	Endophthalmitis	(15)	*Staphylococcus aureus*
		Conjunctivitis	(2)	
		Abscessed conjunctiva	(1)	
		Chalazion	(1)	
		Endophthalmitis	(2)	*Streptococcus viridans*
		Conjunctivitis	(1)	*Streptococcus viridans* and *S. aureus*
1,065	*Staphylococcus albus*	None		
726	*Staphylococcus aureus*	Endophthalmitis	(1)	*Staphylococcus aureus*
		Conjunctivitis	(1)	
28	*Proteus* group	Endophthalmitis	(1)	*Proteus vulgaris*
4	*Escherichia coli*	None		
136	*Diplococcus pneumoniae* *Streptococcus viridans* *Klebsiella pneumoniae* *Neisseria catarrhalis* with *S. aureus*	None		

staphylococcus; the infection was mixed, caused by S. *aureus* and *Pseudomonas aeruginosa.* No infection followed surgery among the 567 patients carrying pathogenic organisms whose operations were deferred until the eyes were free of pathogens.

Table 6-2 summarizes the incidence of infections following cataract surgery in the period 1955 to 1968 in 15,278 patients receiving 24 hours of routine prophylactic treatment with antibiotics (4 to 5 local applications in a 24-hour period). In 13,319 patients who had no preoperative cultures

Table 6-3. Pathogens found prior to local antibiotic treatment in 2,419 patients awaiting cataract extraction: 1943-1968*

Number of patients	Microorganisms isolated preoperatively	Treatment used
34	*Staphylococcus aureus*	Sulfathiazole
4	*Diplococcus pneumoniae*	
2	*Streptococcus hemolyticus*	
72	*Staphylococcus aureus*	Penicillin
147	*Staphylococcus aureus*	Combination of penicillin and streptomycin
2	*Hemophilus influenzae* and *S. aureus*	
57	*Staphylococcus aureus*	Terramycin
912	*Staphylococcus aureus*	Chloramphenicol
18	*Diplococcus pneumoniae*	
6	*Streptococcus viridans*	
3	*Streptococcus hemolyticus*	
20	*Diplococcus pneumoniae* and *S. aureus*	
4	*Hemophilus influenzae* and *S. aureus*	
683	*Staphylococcus aureus*	Erythromycin
3	*Pseudomonas aeruginosa*	Polymyxin
149	*Proteus* group	Chloramphenicol
108	*Escherichia coli*	
32	*Klebsiella pneumoniae*	Colymycin
113	*Proteus* group and *S. aureus*	Furacin
38	*Escherichia coli* and *S. aureus*	Neomycin
12	*Klebsiella pneumoniae* and *S. aureus*	Tetracyclines

*Operation deferred until pathogens were eliminated; no postoperative infections occurred.

taken, there were 15 cases of endophthalmitis caused by S. *aureus* and 2 caused by *Streptococcus viridans*. In the 1,065 patients who had preoperative cultures taken and who were found to carry only S. *albus*, no infections occurred. In the 726 patients whose cultures were positive for S. *aureus* there was one case of endophthalmitis. One case of endophthalmitis caused by *Proteus vulgaris* was present in 1 patient out of 28 who had carried *Proteus* organisms at preoperative culture time. There were another 136 patients carrying other potential pathogens, but no postoperative infection was noted.

Table 6-3 is a summary of the results obtained in a total of 2,419 patients who were seen from 1943 to 1968. On the basis of preoperative culture, these patients were found to carry potential pathogens, and they were treated with the various antibiotics listed until the eyes gave negative cultures (in 2 to 7 days). There were no postoperative infections in this group. These figures support the concept that the bacterial flora of the preoperative eye may be an important source of postoperative infection. The importance of S. *aureus* that many patients carried is emphasized by the observation that in the period 1938 to 1968, 5,034 patients who did not carry S. *aureus* in their preoperative cultures also did not have any postoperative infection. Adding the 5,034 patients free of S. *aureus* to the 2,419 in whom antibiotics were used to eliminate S. *aureus* gives a total of 7,453 cataract extractions performed in the absence of S. *aureus* and without a single postoperative infection.

The patient can be shown how to carry out preoperative antibiotic treatment at home, thus saving unnecessary days of stay in the hospital. S. *aureus* is usually eliminated in 2 to 3 days; but the gram-negative organisms—the *Proteus* group, *Klebsiella pneumoniae, Escherichia coli,* and *Pseudomonas aeruginosa*—may persist for as long as 7 days. The period of time required is determined in part by the care the patient takes. Since adjacent areas usually carry the same type of S. *aureus,* the patient is given instructions to wash his hands and face with a good disinfectant soap.

Other less serious infections have occurred following intraocular surgery. Conjunctivitis complicated recovery from cataract surgery in 32 patients in the period 1938 to 1968. In 28 instances the causative agent was S. *aureus,* in 4 *Proteus vulgaris.* S. *aureus* was also responsible for one case each of corneal ulcer, abscess of the conjunctiva, stitch abscess, infected bleb on the conjunctiva, and chalazion.

Surgery involving eye muscle, detached retina, or glaucoma was followed by postoperative infection in some instances. Table 6-4 presents the findings in 20,966 patients operated on at the IOCPMC from 1950 to 1968. Although preoperative cultures were very seldom taken, preoperative local anti-

Table 6-4. Incidence of postoperative infections in 20,966 patients following ocular surgery: 1950-1968

Number of operations	Types of operations	Postoperative complications	Causative agents*
12,263	Muscle surgery	Orbital cellulitis (11)	*Staphylococcus aureus*
		Conjunctivitis (38)	
		Sloughing ulcer on conjunctiva (1)	
		Stitch abscess (1)	
		Subconjunctival abscess (1)	
		Suppurative wound infection along with fascia lata suspension LUL (1)	
		Corneal ulcer (ptosis; Motais procedure) (1)	*Klebsiella pneumoniae*
		Conjunctivitis (1)	*Diplococcus pneumoniae* and *S. aureus*
		Conjunctivitis (1)	*Hemophilus influenzae* and *S. aureus*
4,912	Retinal detachment	Endophthalmitis (1)	*Pseudomonas aeruginosa*
		Conjunctivitis (3)	*Staphylococcus aureus*
		Orbital cellulitis (2)	
		Endophthalmitis (4)	
		Corneal ring abscess (1)	
		Infected surgical wounds (22)	
		Infected silicone sponge (2)	
		Infected suture site (3)	
		Cloudy vitreous (1)	
		Infected surgical wound (1)	*Escherichia coli*
3,791	Glaucoma	Endophthalmitis (2)	*Staphylococcus aureus*
		Corneal infiltration (1)	
		Infected blebs (2)	
		Endophthalmitis (1)	*Proteus vulgaris*
		Endophthalmitis (1)	*Diplococcus pneumoniae* Type 17

*The nonoperated eye, nose, face, and hand carried the same microorganisms as the infected eye.

biotic treatment was usually employed in cases of detached retina and in a few cases of glaucoma. Among the 12,263 patients undergoing muscle surgery there were 38 instances of conjunctivitis, 1 conjunctival ulcer, 1 abscess, 11 cases of cellulitis, and 1 suppurative wound infection, all caused by S. *aureus*. A corneal ulcer was the result of

Table 6-5. Susceptibility to bacteriophage lysis of strains of *Staphylococcus aureus* causing infection following cataract extraction compared with susceptibility of staphylococci isolated prior to surgery: 1957-1962

		Lysed by phage types			
		Preoperative cultures	Postoperative cultures		
Case number	Type of infection	Both eyes	Operated eye	Nonoperated eye	Other sources
1	Endophthalmitis	7, 53, 42B, 81	7, 53, 42B, 81	7, 53, 42B, 81*	
2	Endophthalmitis	53, 75, VA4	53, 75, VA4,	53, 75, VA4*	
3	Endophthalmitis	3B, 3C, 55	3B, 3C, 55	3B, 3C, 55*	Nose, 3B, 3C, 55*
4	Endophthalmitis	52, 80, 81	52, 80, 81	52, 80, 81*	Nose, 52, 80, 81*
5	Endophthalmitis	52, 80, 42B, 81	52, 80, 42B, 81	52, 80, 42B, 81*	Nose, face, skin, 52, 80, 42B, 81*
6	Endophthalmitis	52A, 79	52A, 79	52A, 79*	Nose, face, skin, 52A, 79*
7	Endophthalmitis	Nontypable	Nontypable	Nontypable*	Nose, nontypable*
8	Endophthalmitis	No culture	Nontypable	Nontypable*	
9	Endophthalmitis	No culture	52A, 79	52A, 79	Nose, 52A, 79
10	Endophthalmitis	No culture	52, 52A, 80	52, 52A, 80	Nose, 52, 52A, 80
11	Endophthalmitis	No culture	80, 53	80, 53	Nose, skin, 80, 53
12	Endophthalmitis	No culture	80, 53, VA4	80, 53, VA4	Nose, 80, 53, VA4
13	Endophthalmitis	No culture	52, 52A, 80, 42B, 81	52, 52A, 80, 42B, 81	Nose, 52, 52A, 80, 42B, 81
14-19	Endophthalmitis	No culture	Nontypable	Nontypable	Nose, nontypable
20	Endophthalmitis	No culture	Nontypable	29	Nose, 29; hand, skin, nontypable
21	Endophthalmitis	No culture	29, 52A, VA4	29, 52A, VA4	Nose, 29, 52A, VA4; hand, nontypable
22	Endophthalmitis	No culture	52, 52A, 80	52, 52A, 80	Nose, 52, 52A, 80
23	Conjunctivitis	52, 80	52, 80	52, 80*	Nose, 52, 80*
24	Abscess of conjunctiva	No culture	52, 80, 42B, 81	52, 80, 42B, 81	Nose, skin, air of patient's room, 52, 80, 42B, 81
25	Chalazion	No culture	47, 54, VA4	47, 54, VA4	Nose, 47, 54, VA4
26	Bleb on conjunctiva	No culture	80, 81	80, 81	Nose, 80, 81

*These cultures from the face and other sources were taken after operation.

K. pneumoniae infection, and *S. aureus* with the pneumococcus or *H. influenzae* caused conjunctivitis in two instances. Of 4,912 cases of detached retina only 40 were followed by infection. One case of endophthalmitis was caused by *Pseudonomas aeruginosa,* whereas 3 cases of conjunctivitis, a ring abscess of the cornea, 2 cases of cellulitis, and 4 cases of endopthalmitis were caused by *S. aureus.* Twenty-two infections of the wound were caused by *S. aureus* and one by *Escherichia coli.* Seven infections followed the 3,791 glaucoma operations; 2 cases of endophthalmitis, 1 corneal infiltration, and 2 infected blebs were caused by *S. aureus.* One case of endophthalmitis was produced by *Proteus vulgaris* and another by *Diplococcus pneumoniae* type 17.

Twenty-six strains of *S. aureus* isolated from cases of endophthalmitis or other infections following cataract surgery were phage typed. In 8 of the patients, preoperative isolates of the staphylococcus were also typed, as described in Chapter 5, p. 70. The purpose of this study was to determine if the patient carried the same type of staphylococcus in the eye prior to surgery as the type causing the infection. Table 6-5 shows that in 9 instances where preoperative strains were typed, the same strain was found to cause the postoperative infection. The same strain was present in the noninfected eye in 25 of the 26 patients, and the same strain causing the infection was also present in the nose and on the skin of the hands and face.

Plate 2, *E* and *F* illustrates postoperative endophthalmitis caused by *S. aureus* and *P. vulgaris,* respectively.

Others have reported postoperative infections, some or all of which may have been caused by exogenous sources of contamination. Winkler and Cason[20] have described a series of 11 cases of endophthalmitis that occurred following cataract extractions, 10 of which were caused by gram-negative bacilli (either *Aerobacter aerogenes, Pseudomonas aeruginosa,* or *Proteus vulgaris*) and one caused by *S. aureus.* In 4 of these 11 cases the infection was considered to be endogenous, since the causative organism was cultured preoperatively. In two other cases the possibility of an endogenous infection existed. Three cases probably were related to contamination of cotton pledgets used on the day of the operation. Custodis[4a] has reported a similar epidemic of infections involving 9 cases of iritis with hypopyon and 3 with less severe infection of the iris, all occurring within 3 days of the operation and traced to a solution of pilocarpine contaminated with *E. coli.*

It is important to examine factors that may contribute to the invasion by the bacteria present in the normal eye. One series of observations may have some bearing on this problem. The temperature of the eye is less than that of the internal organs of the body[1,19] and hence is lower than the optimal temperature for growth of the potential pathogens normally present in the eye. In 1954 cultures from the eyes of 15 patients were taken prior to a variety of operations and again 24 hours following operation. The results are presented in Table 6-6. During the 24-hour period the eye had been bandaged and probably had maintained a temperature nearer to that optimal for growth of the potentially pathogenic bacteria that were present. From Table 6-6 it can be seen that the colonies of the various microorganisms found preoperatively were considerably fewer than those found after 24 hours. Furthermore, in 12 instances an additional species of microorganisms was seen on the postoperative culture plate. This suggests that a bandage promotes conditions favorable for the multiplication of bacteria; and though this does not prove that bandaging would contribute to the development of infection, it suggests this possibility. This point of view may also gain some support from the latent period preceding the onset of postoperative infection; this period has varied from 2 to 7 days, with the peak incidence of infection occurring on the fourth day. Linhart[11] has reported an increase in bacterial colony

Table 6-6. Effect of surgical dressing on ocular flora in conjunctiva

Case number	Clinical diagnosis	Preoperative culture	Second culture 24 hours after surgery
1	Absolute glaucoma	15 colonies *S. aureus*, 12 colonies pneumococcus type 3, diphtheroids	Numerous *S. aureus*, pneumococci type 3, diphtheroids
2	Glaucoma	81 colonies diphtheroids	18 colonies *S. aureus*, diphtheroids
3	Pterygium	1 colony *S. aureus*, diphtheroids	Numerous *S. aureus*, diphtheroids
4	Extirpation of sac	23 colonies *S. albus*, diphtheroids	Numerous *S. albus*, diphtheroids, 13 colonies *S. aureus*
5	Esotropia	36 colonies *S. albus*	Numerous *S. albus*, *S. aureus*
6	Esotropia	3 colonies *S. aureus*	Numerous *S. albus*, *S. aureus*
7	Esotropia	7 colonies *S. aureus*	Numerous *S. aureus*, 6 colonies *S. albus*
8	Esotropia	1 colony *S. aureus*, diphtheroids	Numerous *S. aureus*, 14 colonies *S. albus*, diphtheroids
9	Esotropia	1 colony *S. aureus*	Numerous *S. aureus*, *S. albus*, diphtheroids
10	Congenital ptosis	45 colonies *S. albus*	Numerous *S. albus*, 27 colonies *S. aureus*
11	Paralysis of lateral rectus	42 colonies *S. albus*	Numerous *S. albus*, 10 colonies *S. aureus*
12	Esotropia	16 colonies *S. albus*	Numerous *S. albus*, *S. aureus*
13	Exotropia	22 colonies *S. albus*, diphtheroids	Numerous *S. albus*, 12 colonies *S. aureus*, diphtheroids
14	Exotropia	17 colonies *S. albus*	Numerous *S. albus*, 5 colonies *S. aureus*, diphtheroids
15	Congenital ptosis	2 colonies *S. albus*	Numerous *S. albus*, 44 colonies *S. aureus*

counts in patients with normal conjunctivas who wore an eye patch for 2 days.

Another factor that may influence the occurrence of infections following cataract extraction is the nature of the operation. At the IOCPMC since 1938 there have been 13,524 operations involving intracapsular extraction of the lens, 16 of which were followed by endophthalmitis, an incidence of 0.12%. In the same period there were 3,119 cases of extracapsular lens extraction, followed in 11 instances by endophthalmitis, an incidence of 0.35%. It would seem from these figures that endophthalmitis may be less likely to occur following intracapsular extractions. The added hazard of extracapsular extraction is also suggested by some other reported results.[2,5]

Culturing of the air from the operating room[14] and the routine monitoring of the sterility of instruments, dressings, solutions, and other objects that might come in contact with the patient's eye during surgery have failed to incriminate these objects as possible exogenous sources for the infections seen at the IOCPMC. In this respect the Institute of Ophthalmology at the Columbia-Presbyterian Medical Center has so far been fortunate.

Hughes and Owens[8] have stated that in a series of 2,086 operations performed without prophylactic antibiotic treatment, purulent endophthalmitis occurred in 21 patients. Staphylococci, streptococci, pneumococci, or *E. coli* were isolated from cultures of secretions in the lower cul de sac. These investigators believed that the sources of infection were "(1) obstruction of the lacrimal duct with resulting low grade chronic dacryocystitis; (2) inadequately treated chronic conjunctivitis; (3) sudden onset of an acute infection of the upper respiratory tract . . . ; (4) abscess around corneal scleral sutures . . . , and (5) undetermined causes." After they employed prophylactic measures with prolonged treatment, only 2 cases of postoperative endophthalmitis resulted out of a total of 1,200 cataract extractions. Maumenee and Michler[15] have emphasized the possible role of microorganisms carried on the skin as a source of postoperative infection. They recommend the topical application of antiseptics. Boyd, Maumenee, and McLean[3] recommend thorough bacteriologic studies of the lid and conjunctiva preoperatively, if the eye is inflamed, followed by adequate treatment prior to surgery. They use a subconjunctival injection of penicillin following surgery. Pearlman[16] also reports favorably on this type of prophylactic antibiotic treatment. Callahan[4] in a series of 1,653 cataract extractions lost 5 eyes with endophthalmitis. He believed that delaying the operation for adequate antibiotic treatment had reduced the number of infections in his series and might prevent future cases of endophthalmitis as more specific antibiotics were developed. Liehn and Schlagenhauff[10] reviewed 1,000 cases of cataract extraction in which 2 eyes were lost, one because of a mixed infection with pneumococci and a paracolon bacillus, the other from *E. coli* infection. They employed penicillin prophylactically.

Fine and Zimmerman[7] have collected the literature on mycotic infections of the eye and have reported the results of examination of eyes sent to the Registry of Ophthalmic Pathology. They employed stains appropriate for identifying fungi in the deep tissues. They found histologic evidence of fungal infection in 13 cases, 4 with a history of trauma and 9 following cataract extraction. These authors probably were in the position of receiving highly selected material in which the etiologic agent had not been identified. Fungi causing disease have not been cultured from postoperative infections in our experience, although expert assistance has been provided from the mycology laboratory.

Leopold and Apt,[9] and Theodore,[16a] and Theodore, Littman, and Almeda[17] have summarized the literature on fungal infections of the eye and have discussed the therapy in ocular infections in general. Chapter 13 describes the role of fungi in ocular infections.

REFERENCES

1. Adler, F. H.: Physiology of the eye: clinical application, ed. 3, St. Louis, 1959, The C. V. Mosby Co., p. 45.
1a. Allansmith, M. R., Anderson, R. P., and Butterworth, M.: The meaning of preoperative cultures in ophthalmology, Trans. Amer. Acad. Ophthal. Otolaryng. **73**:683, 1969.
2. Allen, H. F., and Mangiaracine, A. B.: Bacterial endophthalmitis after cataract extraction, Arch. Ophthal. **72**:454, 1964.
3. Boyd, B. F., Maumenee, A. E., and McLean, J. M.: Advances in cataract surgery, Highlights Ophthal. **3**:243, 1960.
4. Callahan, A.: Effect of sulfonamides and antibiotics on panophthalmitis complicating cataract extraction, Arch. Ophthal. **49**:212, 1953.
4a. Custodis, E.: Beitrag zur intraokularen Infektion nach Staroperationen, Klin. Mbl. Augenheilk. **133**:632, 1958.
5. Dellaporta, A., Riemer, F., and Harmuth, E.: Eine vergleichende Untersuchung über die Infektionshäufigkeit nach Kataraktoperation in den Jahren 1936, 1941, 1946 und 1948 mit Berucksichtigung der Penicillinbehandlung, Klin. Mbl. Augenheilk. **115**:369, 1949.
6. Dunnington, J. H., and Locatcher-Khorazo, D.: Value of cultures before operation for cataract, Arch. Ophthal. **34**:215, 1945.
7. Fine, B. S., and Zimmerman, L. E.: Exogenous intraocular fungus infections with particular reference to complications of intraocular surgery, Amer. J. Ophthal. **48**:151, 1959.
8. Hughes, W. F., and Owens, W. C.: Postoperative complications of cataract extraction, Arch. Ophthal. **38**:577, 1947.
9. Leopold, I. H., and Apt, L.: Postoperative intraocular infections, Amer. J. Ophthal. **50**: 1225, 1960.
10. Liehn, R., and Schlagenhauff, K.: 1000 intrakapsuläre Starextraktionen, ihre Ergehnisse und Komplikationen, Wien. Klin. Wschr. **64**: 988, 1952.
11. Linhart, R. W.: The effect of the eye patch on organisms of the conjunctival sac, Amer. J. Ophthal. **33**:1280, 1950.

12. Locatcher-Khorazo, D.: The effect on the ocular bacterial flora of local treatment with Chloromycetin (chloramphenical), Terramycin, or penicillin-streptomycin ophthalmic ointment in preoperative cataract cases and miscellaneous infections, Amer. J. Ophthal. **36**:475, 1953.
13. Locatcher-Khorazo, D., and Gutierrez, E.: Eye infections following cataract extraction with special reference to the role of Staphylococcus aureus, Amer. J. Ophthal. **41**:981, 1956.
14. Locatcher-Khorazo, D., and Gutierrez, E.: Bacteriophage typing of Staphylococcus aureus: a study of normal, infected eyes and environment, Arch. Ophthal. **63**:774, 1960.
15. Maumenee, A. E., and Michler, R. C.: Sterility of the operative field after ocular surgery, Trans. Pacif. Coast Otoophthal. Soc. **32**:172, 1951.
16. Pearlman, M. D.: Prophylactic subconjunctival penicillin and streptomycin after cataract extraction, Arch. Ophthal. **55**:516, 1956.
16a. Theodore, F. H.: Bacterial endophthalmitis after cataract surgery, Intern. Ophthal. Clin. **4**:839, 1964.
17. Theodore, F. H., Littman, M. L., and Almeda, E.: The diagnosis and management of fungus endophthalmitis following cataract extraction, Arch. Ophthal. **66**:163, 1961.
18. Thompson, R., Isaacs, M. L., and Khorazo, D.: A laboratory study of some antiseptics with reference to ocular application, Amer. J. Ophthal. **20**:1087, 1937.
19. Thygeson, P.: Ocular bacteriology, The Lancaster Course in Ophthalmology, The Ophthalmological Study Council, Division of Summer and Special Programs, Colby College, Waterville, Maine, p. 3.
19a. Whiston, G. J.: Review of postoperative endophalmitis, Montreal General Hospital—1955-1964, Canad. J. Ophthal. **2**:63, 1967.
20. Winkler, C. H., Jr., and Cason, L.: Bacteriology of the eye, role of gram-negative bacilli in infections following cataract extraction, Arch. Ophthal. **51**:200, 1954.

7

Aseptic technique in ophthalmology

HENRY F. ALLEN

Aseptic technique in hospital and office practice is a systematized, continuing effort to prevent infection by eliminating pathogenic microorganisms from the patient's environment. It is directed by the chief of service through his representative and must be supported by every member of the staff. It is of direct concern to the hospital administrator. It is above all a team effort, demanding the intelligent participation of all hospital and clinic personnel.

Aseptic technique can be no stronger than its weakest component. An error on the part of one individual can break the chain of asepsis. The duty of the ophthalmologist is to educate, to organize, and to inspire with the desire for perfection the members of his team. Only when discipline becomes second nature and any break in technique is detected instantly can it be said that the system is functioning as it should. Only by striving for the ideal of no infections can the incidence of infection be reduced to a minimum.

Foundations of asepsis

The basis for aseptic procedure rests on fundamentals relating to the communicability, virulence, and destruction of microbes and the resistance or susceptibility of tissues. These foundations are established in microbiology, epidemiology, and general surgery; specialized considerations determine their application to ophthalmology. Bacteriologic concepts include thermal death times of various groups and species of organisms, the relative sterilizing efficiency of moist and dry heat, and the ability of certain species to multiply in unpreserved solutions. Epidemiologic methods reveal modes of transfer and vectors of disease. Surgical principles stress operating room procedure and discipline, hemostasis, and respect for tissues. When infections occur, violation of basic principles should always be suspected. When claims for a new method or compound are at variance with existing knowledge of similar procedures and substances, acceptance should follow only after careful experimental and clinical evaluation of these claims.

Susceptibility of ocular tissues

Whereas other tissues can usually deal successfully with smaller or larger numbers of pathogenic bacteria, the cornea, lens, and vitreous being avascular are by nature especially vulnerable to attack by pathogens and even by organisms that are relatively nonpathogenic for vascular structures. The latter, though invaded, may emerge functionally unimpaired after elimination of infection by normal defense mechanisms with or without the help of specific therapy. But since transparency is

Modified from Allen, H. F.: Aseptic technique in ophthalmology, Trans. Amer. Ophthal. Soc. **57**:377-472, 1959.

synonymous with function in the cornea, lens, and vitreous, and since repair of damaged neural elements can occur to no significant degree in the retina, the development of an infectious process in the eye may lead to irreversible disability in spite of prompt and ultimately effective treatment. In intraocular infections there is literally no substitute for prevention.

Misconceptions and pitfalls

All ophthalmologists wish to prevent infection and presumably believe that they are taking all possible steps to do so. However, available evidence shows the need for wider understanding of the principles and practices on which aseptic eye surgery must be based. This evidence consists of: (1) continued occurrence of postoperative infections, both reported and unreported; (2) breaks in technique apparent to the casual observer in operating rooms and clinics; (3) use of preparations and devices, which not only are inefficient antiseptics, disinfectants, and sterilizers but may actually serve as vehicles of the very infections they are intended to prevent; and (4) the false sense of security generated in the minds of ophthalmic surgeons by the absence of infection from a series of intraocular operations. In some cases the absence of infection must be attributed more to the fact that infectious agents do not readily establish themselves in the eye than to the perfection of the technique employed. Only the busiest ophthalmic surgeons can cite a series large enough to have statistical significance. When postoperative infection strikes, it does so without warning. It may involve the eyes of several patients at once, and it usually destroys useful vision in the eyes it touches. For these reasons every avenue of exogenous infection must be considered and every means employed to block these routes and to eliminate organisms at their source.

Prophylactic antibiotics

Antibiotics may supplement but can never substitute for careful aseptic technique. In the brief history of these drugs, the development of bacterial resistance and of human hypersensitivity have refuted their infallibility against organisms and their innocuousness to patients. Antibiotic-resistant staphylococci and such refractory genera as *Proteus* and *Pseudomonas* forbid complacency. No antibiotic administered by any route can prevent infection resulting from irrigation of the anterior chamber with a pure culture of organisms in an aqueous solution. Anaphylactic deaths and other severe reactions make one consider the risk of sensitizing patients to future injections or of provoking a reaction in a previously sensitized patient. Before administering the antibiotics for prophylactic purposes, the surgeon must weigh their advantages against their hazards for each individual patient.

Responsibility for asepsis

The responsibility for aseptic technique, as for other aspects of patient care and protection, belongs to the physician who treats the patient. The surgeon who operates in ignorance of conditions and procedures in his hospital cannot shift responsibility to higher authority or impute negligence to subordinate personnel. Personal responsibility carries both the right and the obligation to investigate and to correct or insist in writing upon correction of deficiencies. Rigid self-discipline must precede criticism of infractions on the part of others.

In hospitals where ophthalmology is not a separate service, the ophthalmic chief must be prepared to educate the chief of surgery in the specific requirements of aseptic eye surgery. The hospital administrator, the chief of the nursing service, and the hospital pharmacist must be oriented in the same direction.

The initial institution of seemingly adequate precautions is not sufficient in itself. Many factors operate to inactivate or to infiltrate the barriers erected against bacteria. Periodic checks must, therefore, be carried out to ensure the continued effectiveness of current practices. Cultures of air, instruments, and supplies from the autoclave should be performed at regular intervals. Methods of conducting sterility surveys are outlined in this chapter.

THE DEVELOPMENT OF ANTISEPTIC AND ASEPTIC TECHNIQUE IN GENERAL AND OPHTHALMIC SURGERY

Concepts of infection before 1850

The history of aseptic technique began with the discovery of microorganisms and of methods for their destruction. Before the modern era, the value of dry heat (stoving) for rendering innocuous the fomites of scarlatina and smallpox was demonstrated by William Henry in 1831. It remained for Koch and Wolfhuegel[28] fifty years later to work out thermal death times of anhydrous spores. A device designed by a French physicist in 1679 and known as "Papin's Digester" was the precursor of the modern autoclave. Pasteur employed steam under pressure at 120° C for sterilization. Redard[41] demonstrated that this was an effective means of killing spores.

During the first half of the nineteenth century, postoperative suppuration and methods for its prevention received but scant mention in the ophthalmic literature. Infection was considered to be endogenous and therefore unavoidable in a certain percentage of cases. Travers[47] believed that the degree of inflammation following cataract extraction depended upon "bodily habit." He recommended cupping, purging, and an abstemious life; but his treatise contains no reference to cleanliness or to the care of instruments.

Ophthalmic surgery in the preantiseptic era, 1850-1875

The invention of the ophthalmoscope by von Helmholtz at midcentury marked the beginning of modern ophthalmology. A few years later the techniques of Albrecht von Graefe gave to intraocular surgery its first major advance since the introduction of cataract extraction through a corneal incision over 100 years before.

All of this preceded proof of the germ theory of disease by several years. The members of the First International Congress of Ophthalmology, meeting at Brussels in 1857, could scarcely have dreamed that 3 years later Pasteur would awaken the world to the science of bacteriology with his *Mémoire sur la fermentation alcoolique.* The rest of the third quarter-century would pass before Lister's contributions to antiseptic surgery would find their modified expression in the ophthalmic field.

Describing conditions as they were in the preantiseptic period, Ernst Fuchs[19] noted that when he started as an aspirant at the clinic of the University of Vienna in 1873, von Arlt "taught us to wipe Daviel's spoon between our lips before putting it into the eye, in order that it be moistened and made slippery." It is surprising that the incidence of cataract wound infection was only 8% to 10% under those circumstances. Following iridectomy, infections of the wound were exceptional. Fuchs attributed this difference to the role of free lens material in providing a good culture medium for bacteria. This it undoubtedly does. Kinoshita has observed *Pseudomonas* contamination of lens homogenates at 4° C.

The following year Fuchs was sent on detached service to Billroth's general surgical clinic. By a stroke of good fortune, Lister himself came to demonstrate his methods to Billroth over a period of several weeks, and personally assisted Fuchs during his stay. When Fuchs returned in 1876 to become an assistant in von Arlt's clinic, he applied antiseptic techniques to preparation of the operative field and to sterilization of instruments and supplies. By this time others were beginning to follow the new trend, and it was possible for the first time to visualize the beginning of the end of septic complications in intraocular surgery.

The antiseptic era, 1876-1886

The arrival of the new era was signalized in the ophthalmic literature in 1878 by Alfred Graefe's paper, "Antiseptic Wound-Treatment in Cataract Extraction."[20] Before his adoption of antiseptic measures, Graefe reported a minimum loss of 4% of eyes operated for cataract extraction, with an upper limit of 10% and an average loss of 5% to 6%. He succeeded in reducing these figures to the loss of 2 eyes in 114 consecutive operations by adoption of a modified Listerian routine.

Graefe's figures, both in regard to the preantiseptic incidence of intraocular infection and to reduction of this incidence by antiseptic techniques, were confirmed by a larger series reported by Horner[23] 3 years later. Both Graefe and Fuchs mentioned specifically that the carbolic acid spray, used as an integral part of the Listerian regimen during operations elsewhere in the body, was too irritating to patient and surgeon to permit its use in ocular surgery.

Beginnings of asepsis

In ophthalmology also, the trend changed from carbolic acid to bichloride of mercury. Landolt and Hirschberg were operators meticulous in their attention to details of asepsis and antisepsis. The former cleansed the lids and irrigated the conjunctival sac before and during operation with bichloride of mercury 1:5,000. The latter, with the Prussian passion for discipline, made every visitor wash his hands with soap, soak them in bichloride of mercury, and don a white robe before witnessing an operation. Hirschberg also subjected all his dressings, bandages, solutions, and instruments to high degrees of heat in containers specially made for the purpose. Like Landolt, he insisted on the most careful cleansing of the eye and the ocular adnexa before operation. Millikin[35] noted that pain could be avoided by making up bichloride of mercury with 4% cocaine solution, but stated that hyperemia of the conjunctiva was considerable as a result of the irrigation.

By the turn of the century all the basic principles of asepsis as we know them today had been clearly set forth, and few if any significant advances have been made since that time in this area. That infections have occurred and continue to occur can usually be explained by the failure to observe one or more of these principles.

THE PROBLEM OF OCULAR INFECTION

Etiology of ocular infections

Bacterial infections that follow elective intraocular surgery are almost always caused by a member species of one of two groups of vegetative organisms. The gram-positive cocci are most often represented by *Staphylococcus aureus,* less often by pneumococci, and more rarely by hemolytic streptococci. Among the gram-negative rods, *Pseudomonas aeruginosa,* the bacillus pyocyaneus, is the chief offender, followed by *Aerobacter aerogenes, Proteus* species, and coliform bacilli. Although spore-forming organisms are seldom identified in postoperative infections, they are often found in operating rooms and must always be taken into account. Mixed infection by *Proteus* organisms and *Bacillus subtilis* has followed retinal detachment surgery.

Postoperative intraocular fungus infections are not so rare as was formerly believed. Fine and Zimmerman[18] in 1959 reported 13 new exogenous cases of which 9 followed intraocular surgery. In 8 of these the operation was a cataract extraction. A latent period of days, weeks, or months after surgery preceded development of the clinical picture of plastic iridocyclitis with anterior endophthalmitis.

The globe is resistant to inward extension of external infection from the conjunctiva and orbital tissues. Trephine blebs and filtering cicatrices form an exception to this rule. They are particularly susceptible to pneumococcal infection.

In some cases of presumed bacterial endophthalmitis, the offending organism is never recovered. This failure may result from failure to tap the anterior chamber or from faulty culture techniques. Unless a blood culture is positive, a surgeon has no justification for attributing the cause of infection to endogenous sources. The recovery of a pathogenic organism from the conjunctival sac by no means establishes its origin. By the time endophthalmitis has developed, many of the possible sources of infection are no longer available for analysis. Since treatment is usually ineffective, the best hope lies in prevention of infection. The keys to prevention are anticipation and vigilance.

Epidemiology of ocular infections

History records many mechanisms for transmission of ocular disease. These range from the use of urine as an eyewash to the role of insects in carrying bacteria from eye to eye. Mother-to-child transmission is observed prenatally in gonorrheal ophthalmia and inclusion blennorrhea; postnatally, in herpes simplex and trachoma. Insect vectors are responsible for ocular filariasis and onchocerciasis. Swimming pools have been indicted in outbreaks of adenovirus infection and inclusion blennorrhea of adults. Animal hosts have been identified in cat scratch disease, tularemia, and others. Ingestion of infected meat may lead to trichinosis; of raw milk, to brucellosis and tuberculosis.

The most ironic methods of transfer are those mediated by medical personnel. Outbreaks of *Pseudomonas* infection from contaminated solutions and transmission of epidemic keratoconjunctivitis by infected tonometers, ophthalmoscopes, and unwashed fingers furnish the most common examples of iatrogenic spread of ocular disease. Ophthalmologists, among other physicians, can transmit serum hepatitis by breaking the skin with a knife or needle bearing this virus. Strict precautions are necessary if the eye physician is to avoid becoming a vector of disease.

Education of the public and of professional colleagues in the prevention of ocular infection is essential. In many cases, socioeconomic factors place the prevention of a given disease in the province of the public health officer. Where personal hygiene and individual precautions play a part, it is the ophthalmologist's duty to instruct his patient in the steps necessary for the protection of himself and others.

Incidence of postoperative infection

During the modern era of ophthalmic surgery, comprising approximately the past 100 years, statistics of the incidence of surgical infections have been derived almost entirely from cataract operations. The incidence of infection in intraocular procedures of all types is probably lower than that reported for cataract surgery, since it is generally admitted that the hazard of infection is less in simple iridectomy and other operations for glaucoma.

Figures such as those cited in Table 7-1 are necessarily derived from larger clinics. A series of fewer than a thousand operations has little statistical significance. Apart from large series, numerous cases of infection occur, which are never reported in the literature.

Incidence of infection is influenced by operative technique. Prolonged operating time, multiple entries into the anterior chamber, and excessive manipulation of the wound invite infection. Blood clots, traumatized tissues, and lens cortex are all good culture media. The infection rate is greater after extracapsular extraction than when the lens is delivered intact. There may also be a greater risk of postoperative infection in eyes of which the fellow eye has been operated during the same hospital admission. Patients may unconsciously rub the unoperated eye during the period intervening between the two operations. Topical antibiotics should be used in both eyes after operating on the first eye.

Table 7-1. Endophthalmitis after cataract extraction

Period	Rate per 1,000
Before 1875	40-100
1875-1900	10-20
1900-1950	11-12
1950-1970	1-2

Sources of ocular infection

Since it is not always possible to trace the origin of a given infection, all potential sources of contamination must be considered. Close attention must be paid to solutions and instruments that come into contact with intraocular tissues. Serious outbreaks of infection have been traced to preparations employed for their supposed antiseptic properties.

The main categories or sources of infection that must be considered in planning a system of aseptic technique are:

1. Solutions and medications
   - Saline for irrigation
   - Collyria
   - Ointments
   - Instrument disinfectants
   - Skin antiseptics
   - Injectables
2. Tissues
   - Skin of hands
   - Skin of operative field
   - Lid margins and lashes
   - Conjunctival sac
   - Lacrimal sac
   - Nasal mucosa
   - Corneal grafts
   - Vitreous implants
   - Fellow eyes
3. Objects and materials
   - Surgical instruments
   - Optical instruments
   - Tonometers
   - Magnets
   - Hypodermic needles, blood lancets
   - Drapes, dressings, masks and gowns
   - Rubber gloves, bulbs, droppers
   - Glass syringes, bottles, irrigating tips
   - Plastic tubing, sheeting, retractors
   - Contact lenses
   - Orbital implants
   - Intraocular lenses
   - Sutures
4. Airborne contaminants
   - Respiratory origin
   - Surface origin—skin, clothing
   - Ventilating system

These categories are separately considered in subsequent sections of this chapter.

DEFINITION OF TERMS

The following definitions reflect current usage.

STERILIZATION. Sterilization is the use of any process, physical or chemical, that destroys all forms of life. The concept of sterilization is absolute and permits no exceptions. It implies the destruction of all types of microorganisms. Since boiling water and most antiseptics will not destroy resistant bacterial spores, to refer to such agents as sterilizers is incorrect. Under the terms of this definition, sterilization can be achieved for practical purposes only with inanimate objects and restricted spaces. Living tissues may or may not be sterile; if unsterile, they can seldom be sterilized without being themselves destroyed, as is true for skin. A completely sterile environment can be achieved only under experimental conditions. In surgery, the effort to achieve sterility of environment can be considered successful if all potential pathogens have been eliminated from the operative field.

The suffix "-cide" is used to indicate an agent that will destroy that form of microorganism to the name of which it is appended. A sporicide is likely to be a complete sterilizer, since certain bacterial spores are the most resistant of organisms. On the other hand, germicides and bactericides are not necessarily sporicidal or virucidal and will therefore not be sterilizers if spores or viruses are present. The use of the term "cold sterilization" as commonly employed is a misnomer, since the processes usually designated by this term are not lethal to resistant spores.

DISINFECTION. Disinfection refers to killing of pathogenic agents by chemical or physical means directly applied. In the accepted sense, disinfection does not necessarily include the killing of resistant spores or the destruction of viruses. Certain disinfectants may have a sporicidal or virucidal effect; this is usually specified on the label. The term disinfectant is commonly used with substances applied to inanimate objects. Degerming the skin is accomplished with the help of antiseptics rather than disinfectants.

ANTISEPTIC. Antiseptics are substances that prevent or arrest growth or action of microorganisms, either by inhibiting their activity or by destroying them, especially agents applied to living tissue. Although we commonly think of antiseptics as germicides, the term originally implied only the ability to arrest putrefaction. In the modern sense of the word, antiseptic implies merely a bacteriostatic effect. Ability to kill spores or viruses is not implied by the term antiseptic. Bactericidal properties may rest with one or another antiseptic substance, depending on the conditions under which it is used. The first antiseptic in general surgery was carbolic acid, used by Lister as a 5% or 2½% solution.

SANITIZATION. Sanitization refers to reduction of the number of bacterial contaminants to safe levels as judged by public health requirements. This term is applied chiefly to the cleansing of utensils for eating and drinking. The standards implied are neither precise enough nor rigid enough for application to surgical procedures, especially in ophthalmology.

CORRECT USE OF TERMS. Certain of the above terms may have more than one meaning, and these meanings may overlap. Ambiguity can be avoided by specifying the circumstances and the microbiologic agents against which a given process is to be used and by limiting the term sterilization to those circumstances under which all forms of life are destroyed.

RESISTANCE OF ORGANISMS

Natural versus acquired or induced resistance

The ability of microorganisms to withstand exposure to adverse environmental influences is a subject of great complexity and of infinite variations. Its interest, both theoretical and practical, has been heightened by the development of chemotherapeutic and antibiotic agents. The appearance of acquired resistance, through processes of selection and of induced resistance (through mutation) is of obvious significance. However, the range in which such adaptation can occur is so limited as to be of little or no practical importance for purposes of surgical sterilization. The problem, therefore, lies not so much in the discovery of new means of killing organisms as in selecting and adapting agents of proved effectiveness on the basis of their suitability to the practical problems at hand. For this reason, only a brief résumé of the natural resistance of groups and species is pertinent to the present discussion.

Environmental factors

The principal physical agencies to which organisms may be subjected include heat, light, ionizing radiations, dessication, and supersonic vibrations. The range of chemical compounds employed against bacteria is almost unlimited. In every case the resistance of a given species or strain is influenced by the environmental conditions prevailing at the time of exposure to the particular agency. The most important of these conditions are the presence of moisture, the presence of organic matter, and the pH of solutions.

Within the range of ordinary environmental factors, microorganisms vary greatly in their ability to survive exposure to the various physical and chemical agents that may be applied to them. The most significant difference exists between the resistance of bacterial spores and that of all other microbial forms.

Spore-forming bacteria

Two bacterial genera, the aerobic bacilli and the anaerobic clostridia, have the property of forming endospores. Spores presumably represent a resting stage in the bacterial life cycle. Formation of spores is *sporulation; germination* signifies their return to the vegetative phase upon incubation in a nutrient medium.

Bacterial spores are the most resistant form of life, and it is believed that any process capable of killing resistant spores will result in the destruction of all other organisms as well. The resistance of spores extends to most types of physical and chemical agents and forms the basis of differentiation between absolute and relative methods of sterilization. Most spores are known to withstand boiling, ultraviolet light, and a wide range of chemicals that are lethal to other forms of microorganisms. Spores can survive indefinitely in solutions of disinfectants that kill vegetative bacteria in a matter of minutes. The differential between spores and vegetative forms of the same species is much smaller for gaseous sterilants.

Spore-forming species in the vegetative phase have no greater resistance than species that exist only in that phase.

Failure to use inocula or test strips rich in spore content can lead to false conclusions in evaluating sterilizing procedures.

Vegetative bacteria and fungi

The differences in resistance among non–spore-forming species are of less practical importance. The spores of fungi, though far less resistant than those of bacteria, are somewhat more resistant than vegetative forms. Bacteria and fungi in the vegetative phase are destroyed in 1 hour or less by boiling, by heating in the anhydrous state, and by many disinfectants. Certain species, such as the staphylococci, are more resistant than others, such as the neisseriae. For example, *N. gonorrhoeae,* an unusually delicate species, succumbs to 41.5° C in a few minutes; many strains of staphylococci withstand 60° C for 1 hour.

Most vegetative bacteria die out when dried, but tubercle bacilli have been found viable in dry dust after many weeks. Gram-negative organisms are seldom found in dust, although they occur occasionally in samples of room air.

Other differences between gram-positive and gram-negative species include the greater susceptibility of the former to penicillin and the cationic detergents.

Viruses

Although viruses can multiply only in the presence of living cells, most viruses can survive for a while in their absence. This property can readily be tested with viruses that can be propagated in tissue culture or in animal hosts. One of the more delicate viruses is that of herpes simplex. This agent is readily inactivated by heat (56° C for ½ hour) and by storage at room temperature. The latter result is the effect partly of oxidation and partly of phosphatase activity. Protection against both mechanisms is afforded by reducing agents such as cysteine and glutathione.

The resistance of adenoviruses to ether suggests that cleaning of tonometers with ether alone may not prevent transmission of epidemic keratoconjunctivitis. Although there is some evidence that swimming pools may be an epidemiologic factor in the spread of pharyngoconjunctival fever, it is probable that adenovirus type 3 in purified suspension is destroyed by 0.4-0.6 ppm residual chlorine.

The ability of inclusion blennorrhea virus (*Chlamydia oculogenitale*) to survive in swimming pools and to resist Credé prophylaxis with 1% silver nitrate suggests that the chlamydiae are either resistant to chemicals or protected from chemical action, possibly by the carbohydrate matrix that they possess.

Viruses that proliferate only in a human host present obvious difficulties to anyone wishing to test their resistance to heat and chemicals. In the case of serum hepatitis virus, studies with human volunteers have shown that this agent is killed by boiling for 15 minutes and by steeping at 60° C for 10 hours, but may survive for 1 hour or more at 60° C. The same virus has apparently remained infective after prolonged exposure to 0.2% tricresol. The practical importance of these data is apparent in relation to the sterilization of needles and sharp instruments.

PRINCIPLES OF STERILIZATION

Methods that kill all forms of microorganisms, including resistant spores, are always to be preferred to methods that merely kill certain species under certain conditions. Spore-forming species are constantly present in the environment and can never be discounted as a potential hazard. The sporicidal requirement provides a margin of safety over and above the minimum circumstances necessary for the destruction of vegetative forms. Because the eye may respond to infection in all-or-none fashion, acceptance of methods less than infallible is equivalent to playing "ophthalmic roulette."

The theory and practice of sterilizing processes are fully described in standard texts. The following paragraphs are intended only to provide a convenient summary. Ophthalmologists desiring fuller treatment of the subject are referred to source material.[4,32,38,50]

Requirements common to all methods

PROCESSING. The first requirement for sterilization is that the material must actually be subjected to the sterilizing process. Obvious though this may seem, instances of infection have occurred through the use of objects erroneously believed to have been processed. This accident can be avoided. Unsterile packages should never be stored in the sterilizing room or in a place where they can be picked up in the mistaken belief that they have already been sterilized. Sterile packages must be clearly labelled with heat-sensitive adhesive tape. Other types of thermal controls that indicate that a certain temperature has been maintained for a given period of time, may be used. None of these thermal controls is infallible, but they are useful adjuncts.

INCOMPLETE STERILIZATION. Next in disastrous effect to complete omission of the sterilizing procedure, and of far more frequent occurrence, is faulty or incomplete execution of the prescribed routine. Haste, impatience, ignorance, fatigue, and carelessness are the components of the human element, a factor that must be considered by every surgeon who does not, as indeed he cannot, personally supervise every step in the sterilization of every object used in the course of an operation. Indoctrination, training, and frequent checks on sterility are the only means of reducing such errors to a minimum.

TIME FACTOR. Time is essential to any sterilizing process. The critical time interval is that during which the object to be sterilized is actually exposed to the sterilizing agent, whether this be a certain degree of heat, a certain concentration of vapor, or a chemical in solution. Additional time must be allowed for penetration of the package and permeation of all parts of the object or material. Large packages and instruments require a longer time than small ones. The time required for objects to reach the sterilizing temperature is in addition to that required for sterilization.

CLEANING. Mechanical cleaning is necessary, not merely for esthetic reasons, but because the sterilizing action of heat, moisture, and chemicals is prevented or seriously delayed by the presence of organic residues. Few eye surgeons insist upon cleaning their own instruments with the aid of special illumination and of magnification. This practice should recommend itself to any surgeon who has found bits of tissue adherent to the teeth of forceps or to the points of diathermy electrodes. Whenever possible, instruments should be taken apart for cleaning. Joints should be worked back and forth in a detergent solution, and a stiff brush is essential for getting into crevices. Drying is important to prevent corrosion and because bacteria can proliferate wherever moisture is present. Ultrasonic cleaning is an important advance.

PACKAGING. The manner of wrapping must permit delivery without contamination of the contents. The material used for packaging must be permeable by the sterilizing agent. Cloth wrappings are suitable for steam sterilization, as are certain types of paper. Plastics are usually waterproof but may be permeable by certain gases. However, if they are permeable by the sterilizing gas but impermeable by air, the gas concentration attained within the package may be below that required for sterilization, for the simple reason that air connot be exhausted from the package. Glass and metal containers are suitable only for aqueous solutions or for materials that are to be subjected to dry heat.

Packages that are not to be used immediately after sterilization must be stored in such a way as to prevent contamination and should be resterilized after a long period of storage under certain conditions. Moisture or wetting is to be avoided at all costs, and any package that is not absolutely waterproof is considered to be contaminated if it has been in contact with liquid. Dry, imperviously wrapped packages may remain sterile for indefinitely long periods.

STERILIZING METHODS

Steam under pressure

Correctly performed, exposure of objects to saturated steam under pressure in the autoclave is the most rapid and dependable means of complete sterilization for practical use. For sterilization to occur, all objects in the autoclave must be exposed in their entirety to the action of saturated steam at the sterilizing temperature (121° C or higher). Moisture, heat, and time are essential; pressures achieved in the autoclave have no sterilizing action per se.

Saturated steam is water vapor at the maximum pressure and density for a given temperature. Because of Dalton's law of partial pressures, this situation cannot exist if another gas is present. If air has not been completely removed, steam will not be saturated, no matter what the pressure. At a given pressure, the maximum temperature for steam cannot be reached if air is present. Since air and steam do not mix readily, objects in contact with air are insulated from both heat and moisture. A film of oil or grease is also an effective means of shielding bacteria from the action of moisture. Since air is heavier than steam, modern autoclaves are evacuated through an opening at the bottom of the chamber, and the thermometer element is located at this point. In this way the sterilizing temperature is not recorded until all of the air has been exhausted from the chamber. Loading of packages, containers, and of the autoclave itself must be such that no air can be trapped by gravity at any point in the autoclave.

In the presence of saturated steam, temperature at equilibrium is a function of pressure. Ordinary autoclaves operate at 15 pounds per square inch (psi) and 121° C; high-speed autoclaves achieve 132° C at 27 psi. These temperatures kill resistant spores in minutes by moist heat; when moisture is absent, the same temperatures require almost the same number of hours to kill the same type of spores. Once the sterilizing temperature has been reached, exposure for 10 min at 121° C is considered sufficient to kill the spores of pathogenic bacteria. Solutions in containers are no exception to the time requirement. It takes longer to sterilize 1,500 ml of saline in a flask than 500 ml, just as it takes longer to boil a large volume of water than a smaller one.

Personnel entrusted with the responsibility of sterilizing instruments and other supplies must be thoroughly trained in the principles and use of the autoclave. The foregoing brief discussion is intended only as a review of principles with which all surgeons should be thoroughly familiar. Technical details of operation of the autoclave and its maintenance are available in manuals provided by the manufacturer. Periodic checks by professional maintenance men are advisable.

Dry heat (hot air)

Exposure to hot air in a gas or electric oven is the time-honored method of sterilizing glassware for bacteriologic purposes. This rigid test in daily use is sufficient indication of the efficacy of the process, but conditions of time and temperature must be met in all cases. Although dry heat is a dependable means of killing spores, it is far less efficient for this purpose than is saturated steam. Therefore, both a higher temperature and a much longer period of exposure are required for the sterilizing temperature to be reached at the interior of a package; 20 to 30 minutes are required for a cataract knife in a manufacturer's cardboard box to reach 140° C in a preheated oven. Much more time is needed for dry heat to penetrate a bulky package wrapped in several layers of insulating material.

When time is available, dry heat has clear advantages for sterilization of objects that are damaged by or impermeable by moisture and even of those that are not. The time can be shortened by the use of higher temperatures for glassware or metals.

Because of the poor heat-conducting properties of air, close attention must be paid to ensure that free circulation of air can occur through all parts of the loaded oven. Overloading or crowding is almost certain to mean that gross differences in temperature will exist in different parts of the oven.

The simplest hot air sterilizer is the electrically heated gravity-type oven, which depends upon circulation of air by thermal convection. Several such ovens are on the market for sterilization of small instruments used in ocular, aural, and dental surgery. Since these ovens are small and carry loads that normally permit free circulation of air through the entire chamber, they are usually reliable. Nevertheless, their accuracy should always be checked with the thermometer and their efficiency verified by the use of packaged dried spores as controls.

Larger ovens may be of the gravity-convection type or may include a turboblower to provide forced circulation of air. The latter type is greatly to be preferred when the load includes numerous packaged instruments, as it usually does in the surgical unit of a busy hospital.

Gaseous sterilization

A field of expanding potential is the use of gaseous agents for sterilization of materials and objects that would be damaged by ordinary methods of heat sterilization.

An ideal gaseous sterilant would be: (1) noncorrosive, (2) harmless to materials, (3) penetrative, (4) easily removed by aeration, (5) rapid in action, (6) of low toxicity to humans and animals, (7) nonflammable and nonexplosive, (8) convenient to store, (9) easy to handle, (10) readily available commercially, (11) inexpensive, and (12) bactericidal, sporicidal, virucidal, and fungicidal at ordinary atmospheric conditions.

Formaldehyde vapor has limited usefulness because of its corrosiveness to aluminum and other metals, its tendency to polymerize on surfaces, and the resulting difficulty of removing the compound following treatment of objects and spaces. Like formalin solution, it finds little application in ophthalmic sterilization.

Ethylene oxide combines sporicidal effect with penetration into packages, some liquids, and certain plastics. Although flammable, it can be handled in small quantities as the pure liquid and in larger volumes in combination with relatively inert gases, such as carbon dioxide and freon. Its effect is greatest in the range of moderate humidity, rather than at extremes of dryness and moisture. In hospital and surgical use its greatest application lies in sterilization of blankets and of plastics. It can also be used for sterilization of ophthalmic instruments, ampoules, plastic prosthesis and implants, and other items that would be damaged by heat or excessive moisture. Experience with ethylene oxide indicates the need for continual spore controls.

Flaming

Organisms subjected to the open flame are killed by charring. In bacteriology, flaming the mouths of test tubes containing culture media is a time-honored procedure. In ophthalmology, platinum wire loops and spatulas are sterilized by flaming before cultures or scrapings are taken from the conjunctiva and cornea. Flaming is an effective method of sterilizing stainless steel tonometers, but electronic tonometers cannot be flamed without incurring permanent damage.

Ionizing radiations

Although x-rays, beta rays, and gamma radiation have sterilizing properties, beams of high-voltage accelerated electrons (cathode rays) have proved to be the most practical for processing applications. Bacterial spores, yeasts, molds, and vegetative spores, in order of decreasing resistance, can be destroyed under conditions similar to those that may be used for practical sterilization of objects of limited thickness.

Miscellaneous methods

Under certain circumstances numerous agencies other than those listed above may prove destructive to living matter. Ultraviolet light, ultrasonic vibrations, strong acids and alkalies, boiling water, formaldehyde, and various other physical and chemical means may prove lethal to organisms if they are allowed to act under optimal conditions for a long enough time. Most of them, unfortunately, have limitations that render them unsuitable for surgical sterilization, or at least impractical by comparison with the more reliable methods just described.

DISINFECTANTS

Although we have noted that sterilization is, properly speaking, an absolute concept, it is possible, under certain circumstances, to achieve sterility by agencies other than those discussed above. The conditions and circumstances under which these methods may be effective sterilizers must be clearly defined. Since these circumstances usually exclude the presence of bacterial spores, the application of these methods for surgical purposes is limited. Only when it is impracticable to apply one of the absolute methods can the use of a method of relative effectiveness be justified. So rare are these occasions in ophthalmology that there is hardly any indication for using one of the latter methods. Nevertheless, antiseptics and disinfectants have a place in environmental sanitation and may be valuable when they are used with full realization of their limitations.

With the exception of strong denaturants unsuitable for clinical purposes, most chemicals are not sporicidal. Many, however, are bactericidal and qualify as disinfectants. Newer standards for the evaluation of germicides show a trend away from the historic but limited concept of the "phenol coefficient" and stress the importance of "use-dilution" tests and of evaluating compounds under circumstances paralleling as closely as possible those under which they are to be used.

Quaternary ammonium compounds

The quaternary ammonium derivatives, often referred to as cationic wetting agents or cationic detergents, have been extensively employed as instrument disinfectants, skin antiseptics, and preservatives for ophthalmic solutions. The quaternaries, or quats, as they are sometimes called, include several hundred compounds. The terms benzalkonium chloride and benzethonium chloride are often applied to some of the mixed alkyl quaternary ammonium derivatives. Ophthalmologists will more readily recognize such familiar trade names as Zephiran, Ceepryn, Phemerol, and Roccal.

Although cationic detergents are effective germicides in vitro against certain vegetative organisms, especially gram-positive cocci, their germicidal effectiveness is greatly reduced in the presence of organic matter. Moreover, they suffer from other serious limitations that restrict their usefulness: (1) lack of uniform sporicidal effect, (2) lack of uniform bactericidal effect, (3) possibility of contamination by pseudomonas, (4) reduction of efficiency by inorganic cations that may be present in tap water, (5) inactivation by soap and other anions, (6) incompatibility with a large number of other compounds, (7) toxicity to corneal endothelium and epithelium, (8) ability to bind bacteria to the skin, and (9) adsorption to skin, glass, rubber, and gauze.

The fact that the quaternaries in aqueous solution may carry pseudomonas renders them unsuitable for routine use in ophthalmology. Not only are the quaternaries less effective than other methods for the purposes for which they are employed in ophthalmic practice, but also their use has been attended by deleterious and even disastrous results.

Synthetic phenolic compounds

Environmental sanitation is aided by the residual surface disinfectant action of such compounds as orthophenylphenol incorporated in solution with other appropriate constituents. The low volatility of these compounds makes it possible to heat them to temperatures close to boiling without any objectionable odor. At such temperatures they kill resistant spores that are otherwise destroyed neither by boiling in plain water for several hours nor by the same compounds acting at room temperature. Although no direct application of this effect to ophthalmic surgery is immediately apparent, the usefulness of these compounds in hospital hygiene is considered in a later section.

Summary

Disinfectants must be evaluated under the conditions for which they are to be used. They are never to be used for sterilization when more reliable methods are practicable.

SOLUTIONS AND MEDICATIONS

Role of medications in ocular infections

The ability of tap water, distilled water, and aqueous solutions of many different substances to support bacterial multiplication has often led to ocular infections.

Through fear of admitting legal liability, hospitals and individual physicians are reluctant to publish details of infections traceable to contaminated solutions that were or may have been used in affected eyes. Most ophthalmologists have either first- or second-hand knowledge of one or more eyes that have been lost in this way. Instances of contaminated solutions, reported[5] and unreported, are too numerous to mention. Such incidents, in addition to the occasional cases reported in the literature, make it clear that a hazard exists whenever an aqueous solution of any description is instilled into an eye. Even solutions of antibiotics may become contaminated with organisms that lie outside their range of effectiveness.

The following examples are cited to prove this point:

1. Postoperative infection occurred in five eyes subjected to intraocular surgery during a single morning on a large eye service. All five eyes were lost from endophthalmitis. *Pseudomonas* organisms were recovered in pure culture from the five eyes and from undiluted, previously unopened stock bottles of benzalkonium chloride 1:1,000 and from the more dilute solutions that were used for preoperative preparation of the skin of these patients.
2. Postoperative infection occurred in six eyes subjected to intraocular surgery on two successive days in a large eye hospital. All six eyes were lost from endophthalmitis. *Pseudomonas aeruginosa* was recovered in pure culture from the six eyes and from a large demijohn used to fill 1,500 ml flasks with saline. After autoclaving, one flask was used to fill trays and basins for three operations. Among these were the containers for anterior chamber irrigant. Although none of the flasks available for culturing at the time infection was discovered was found to be contaminated, it was postulated that two or more flasks used for the six operations had escaped processing in the autoclave.
3. Postoperative infection occurred in three eyes subjected to intraocular surgery in a large general hospital. All these eyes were lost from endophthalmitis. *Pseudomonas* organisms were recovered from these eyes and from a solution of a cationic detergent in which cataract knives used on these cases were immersed. It was said that bronchoscopic instruments had been immersed in the same solution.
4. Following removal of embedded corneal foreign bodies in a large industrial eye dispensary, pseudomonas corneal ulcers developed in five eyes. Four eyes lost useful vision. *Pseudomonas* organisms in pure culture were recovered from previously unopened stock bottles of a proprietary sulfonamide solution that had been instilled into these eyes for an intended prophylactic effect.

In analyzing this series of clinical disasters we note that in three of the four instances the contaminated solution had been employed because of its supposed antibacterial effect. In one case the offending substance was used as a skin antiseptic; in another, as an instrument disinfectant; and in the third, as a chemoprophylactic agent. The causative agent of all these infections was the organism that is at once the most common contaminant of aqueous solutions and the most lethal in its effect upon the eye, *Pseudomonas* or *Bacillus pyocyaneus.* This omnipresent organism grows within a temperature range of 4° to 42° C and can reproduce in the presence of little or no nutritional substrate. It thrives in the anterior chamber and spreads rapidly through the corneal stroma, where it often forms a series of concentric ring abscesses. Other ocular pathogens often found in solutions are S. *aureus* and members of the coliform group.

Credit for arousing interest in this problem and for bringing it to the attention of the authorities belongs chiefly to Theodore and Feinstein.[45] Since 1953 the Federal Food, Drug and Cosmetic Act has been interpreted as requiring manufacturers of eye medicaments to prepare sterile solutions fortified with adequate preservatives. This requirement does not yet apply to eye ointments or to ophthalmic medications compounded and dispensed by local pharmacies or hospital pharmacies. It therefore behooves every ophthalmologist to familiarize himself with the principles of asepsis as they apply to ophthalmic medications.

Saline solutions

Aqueous solutions of sodium chloride are used in ophthalmology for irrigation of the anterior chamber, corneoconjunctival irrigation, wound irrigation, filling of gonioscopy lenses, and for intravenous infusion. Saline for any of these purposes is to be considered as a pharmaceutical in the strictest sense. Commercial saline is suitable for all.

SALINE FOR INTRAOCULAR SURGERY. The most dangerous solutions in ophthalmology are those of saline used to irrigate the anterior chamber at surgery or the conjunctival sac in the presence of an epithelial defect in the cornea. Contamination of such a solution means introduction of a pure or mixed bacterial culture into the interior of the eye or into the defenseless corneal tissues. In either event, loss of the eye is the most probable result. For this reason the principle of sterilization in the final container must be rigidly applied, and the container may be opened when, and only when, the operation is ready to begin.

Immediately before operation, the circulating nurse removes the cap from a 500 ml flask of saline, taking care not to contaminate the sterile lip of the container. The pernicious practice of pouring away a small quantity should be avoided, because the few drops of solution that run down the outside of the flask can run back again after being contaminated. The requisite number of sterile receptacles placed close together can be filled at a single pouring without repeated inversion of the flask. The flask is then emptied and permanently discarded. Under no circumstances should any fluid remaining in the bottle be used in another operation.

SALINE FOR CORNEOCONJUNCTIVAL IRRIGATION. Although the intact corneal epithelium is normally resistant to pseudomonas, broken epithelium and the stroma are not. Strict asepsis must be observed in all cases of corneal foreign body or abrasion. Many such eyes have been lost from unnecessary instillation of contaminated drops when otherwise healing would have been uneventful if no medication had been used. Examples of this have been cited above.

The same rigid criteria governing the use of saline in the anterior chamber must be applied when the corneal epithelium is broken. Even in the case of preserved solutions there is no substitute for the unit-dose preparation that has been sterilized in the final container. Every patient who requires irrigation of the conjunctival sac is entitled to a sterile solution. If an epithelial break is suspected, a previously unopened unit should always be used.

Individual disposable 15 ml bottles of 1.4% sterile sodium chloride are used in the clinics and wards of the Massachusetts Eye and Ear Infirmary. These bottles are handled aseptically and are used to moisten sterile cotton balls or fluorescein strips. Opened units remaining at the end of a clinic session are discarded. Bedside units are recapped after each use and are discarded when empty or when the patient is discharged.

Silicone bulb syringes used for irrigation are prepared in the central supply room as follows. The unsterile bulb is rinsed with distilled water, of which a little is purposely left in the syringe. It is then autoclaved and is ready for use. Failure to leave some fluid in the interior may mean that only the outside will be sterilized by steam at 121° C, the inside receiving only a substerilizing exposure to dry heat.

SALINE FOR GONIOSCOPY AND CONTACT LENSES. Since corneal abrasions can occur during gonioscopy and in fitting contact lenses, the principles governing the use of solutions for intraocular procedures should always apply.

SALINE FOR POSTOPERATIVE DRESSINGS. Saline is often used for swabbing the encrusted lid margins of operated eyes each time a dressing is changed. Wet swabbing increases the patient's comfort by relief of itching. Individual units are employed and a single container should never be used for more than one patient.

Collyria

The following principles apply to the manufacture and use of solutions of drugs commonly used in ophthalmic practice: (1) preparation under sterile conditions, (2) sterilization in the final container, (3) preservation against bacteria and fungi, (4) handling with aseptic technique, and (5) testing for sterility at intervals when open.

PREPARATION OF STERILE COLLYRIA. The compounding of collyria, formerly done by the local pharmacist, has fallen into the province of the wholesale manufacturer. This means that it has come under the jurisdiction of the Food and Drug Administration. Manufacturers have acquired the knowledge and the equipment necessary to produce sterile medications. Sterility is usually achieved by bacterial filtration of prepared solutions, which are then aseptically distributed into sterile containers. Filtration will not remove most viruses, but the likelihood of viral contamination is very slight.

The ophthalmologist is responsible for the sterility of the solutions he uses. For solutions to be used by patients it is better to specify commercially manufactured preparations or to dispense medications of known sterility than to run the risk that a contaminated solution might be dispensed by a local pharmacy. Collyria used in the operating room should be freshly opened.

STERILIZATION IN THE FINAL CONTAINER. As long as a given solution is sterile, the manner in which its sterility was achieved is immaterial. Sterilization in the final container offers a guarantee of sterility and should be employed whenever there is doubt about the manner of preparation. It usually requires autoclaving in sealed glass or metal containers and the observation of certain other requirements.

PRESERVATION OF COLLYRIA. Once the seal is broken, both the screwcap vial and the plastic dispensing bottle are subject to contamination by bacteria, fungi, and viruses. Bacteria and fungi can be inhibited by a suitable preservative.

A suitable preservative must be bacteristatic, fungistatic, effective in the presence of other substances, innocuous to the corneal endothelium and other tissues, compatible with other ingredients, chemically stable, and unlikely to sensitize patients when used over long periods of time. All of these properties must be maintained under conditions of actual use and especially within the pH range of maximum stability of alkaloids. The antibacterial powers of any preservative must be demonstrated against a representative number of strains of *Pseudomonas.*

Although many substances have been recommended and used as preservatives for collyria, only a few have been submitted to rigid testing of the above properties. These include benzalkonium chloride (Zephiran), chlorobutanol, phenylmercuric nitrate, phenylethyl alcohol, and a combination of polymyxin B sulfate with benzalkonium chloride.

The use of bactericidal preservatives must await the appearance of a single substance that is uniformly effective and that combines with its bactericidal effect the other properties desired in a preservative. Until such a drug becomes available, chlorobutanol 0.5% most nearly approaches the requirements for the ideal preservative, provided that its use is combined with careful handling.

Like other preservatives, chlorobutanol has certain disadvantages. It evaporates slowly from aqueous solutions. This effect can be minimized by the use of small, tightly stoppered containers. These are desirable in any event to prevent concentration of active ingredients by evaporation of water. Sealers inserted in plastic screwcaps should always be of rubber, never of cardboard.

Although chlorobutanol does not have a rapidly bactericidal effect, experimentally contaminated solutions containing chlorobutanol 0.5% almost invariably are free of vegetative forms at the end of 24 hours. In comparative studies the bacteristatic effect of chlorobutanol is superior to that of phenylethyl alcohol, benzalkonium chloride, and phenylmercuric nitrate in the strengths commonly used for preservation.

Finally, the case of fluorescein solutions is special. All authors agree upon the ineffectiveness of attempts to preserve this medication against contamination by *Pseudomonas* organisms. The use of sterile fluorescein papers, first suggested by Kimura,[26] is the standard method for staining the cornea in the presence of an epithelial break.

Handling of collyria. Contamination of sterile collyria can be avoided in the first place by careful technique in handling. Although viruses do not multiply in solutions, viral contamination of collyria can occur and virus particles can survive in them. In one instance 42 cases of epidemic keratoconjunctivitis were attributed to a single bottle of tetracaine hydrochloride. Another accident that has often occurred is contamination of one drug by another introduced by a dropper. Atropine contamination can produce acute angle-closure glaucoma through accidental dilatation of a pupil. For these reasons every solution that may be administered to more than one patient should be protected from microbial and pharmacologic contamination by the interposition of a sterile intermediary dropper, which enters the solution once and only once before being discarded.

In the Eye Clinic of the Massachusetts Eye and Ear Infirmary, autoclaved glass droppers are used once and discarded. Droppers do not need to be individually wrapped provided they are carefully handled and used in solutions containing an effective preservative.

Polyethylene "squeeze" bottles are convenient for use by patients and are less subject to contamination of their contents than the old-style dropper bottles. The contents must be preserved against bacterial contamination, which can be introduced by aspiration of the last drop after contamination of the dropper tip. Because ordinary polyethylene is pervious to chlorobutanol, some other preservative must be used. In the hands of the ophthalmologist and of properly trained nurses, contamination of the delivery tip by contact with conjunctival or skin surfaces can be avoided. If such contact occurs, the vial should be discarded. In the hands of careless or untrained personnel, contamination of the tips is almost certain to occur and to be ignored or overlooked. The contaminated tip can then convey infection to other patients. Sterile disposable droppers provide a greater safeguard in clinic practice where close supervision of personnel administering drops to large numbers of patients is not feasible.

Recent progress has been made in the development of unit-dose containers. They are, however, expensive.

Sterility testing of collyria. Since no preservative offers a complete guarantee of sterility after the seal is broken, periodic surveys of collyria in use should be carried out. Details of this procedure will be discussed in the section on sterility testing.

Ophthalmic ointments

Preparation and sterilization of ointments. The problem of ensuring sterility of ointments has not yet been satisfactorily solved in all cases. With certain exceptions, ointments are not marketed with the implication that they are sterile or have been sterilized. Contaminants have been found in eye ointments when they have been looked for. Fortunately, these are usually nonpathogenic bacteria and fungi.[9,10,48]

Heat sterilization of ointments in the tube is not practical for several reasons. Most commercial ointments are prepared by grinding the dry alkaloid powder into a petrolatum base in a milling machine. An alternative method is to dissolve the free alkaloid base in a fatty acid ester (such as polyethylene glycol 200 monostearate) that is freely miscible with petrolatum. In either case, heating the resulting anhydrous mixture to the required temperature of 140° C for 4 hours would result in layering of the suspension with consequent loss of uniform distribution of the active ingredient.

A compromise is reached by sterilizing the petrolatum base separately and adding the alkaloid to it. Heat sterilization of alkaloids is not always possible; for example, atropine base melts at 114° C. However, physostigmine salicylate and the sulfonamides will withstand 140° C.

HANDLING OF OINTMENTS. As in the case of collyria, a single tube of ointment should not pass from patient to patient without the interposition of a sterile intermediary. This may be a sterile glass rod or a sterile cotton swab.

SELECTION OF VEHICLE. The relative merits of prescribing a drug in aqueous solution or in an ointment base must always be considered. In general, ointments are indicated for treatment of conditions of the lids and lid margins. Certain disadvantages may attend their use in the conjunctival sac, namely: (1) greater risk of sensitization, (2) inhibition of epithelial regeneration by the ointment base, (3) retention of fat globules as foreign bodies under corneal epithelium, under the conjunctiva, or in the anterior chamber, (4) uncertain sterility, and (5) blurring of the cornea for ophthalmoscopy.

On the other hand, ointments prepared under sterile conditions offer less opportunity for bacterial proliferation following accidental contamination and adhere well to the lid margins.

Instrument disinfectants

Solutions of many chemicals used to disinfect instruments are dangerous for two reasons. First, they create a sense of security unwarranted by their antibacterial properties. Not only are most disinfectants not sporicidal, but their ability to kill vegetative bacteria is often contingent upon the absence of organic matter. In the second place, solutions of certain substances, especially the quaternary ammonium compounds, may themselves be contaminated with gram-negative bacteria.

The following solution is satisfactory for maintaining the sterility of instruments:

Ingredient	*Parts per 1,000 ml*
Isopropanol 99%	700.00
Roccal 50%	2.00
Triethanolamine	10.00
Potassium nitrite	1.00
Safranin O solution 2%	0.10
Water ad	1,000.00

This formula will kill most vegetative bacteria upon contact of 30 minutes or longer, but it is not sporicidal.

SKIN ANTISEPTICS. Like disinfectants, sulfonamides, and antibiotics, some skin antiseptics may be contaminated by the very bacteria they are intended to inhibit. A disastrous episode of this nature has been cited. Isopropanol 70% is satisfactory.

SUBSTANCES FOR INJECTION. Any of the injectables used in general medicine and surgery may be administered to ophthalmic patients. Some of the drugs used most commonly in ophthalmology are insulin, epinephrine, procaine, meperidine hydrochloride (Demerol), and aqueous or procaine penicillin. Most of these are prepared commercially and are fortified with one of several preservatives. Instances of contamination are rare.

Epinephrine for subconjunctival injection or other parenteral use can be obtained from a single dose unit such as the familiar 1 ml ampoule.

CONTACT LENS SOLUTIONS. Contact lens solutions have been found contaminated with *Pseudomonas* organisms. If a corneal abrasion occurs in the presence of a contaminated solution, the results can be extremely serious.

Case history. A 27-year-old language teacher had worn contact lenses for 2 years. One day she noted blurring of vision in the left eye. Examination showed a corneal ulcer from which *Pseudomonas* organisms was recovered. The same strain was present in the cassette equipped with sponge-rubber clips in which her contact lenses were stored in the presence of wetting solution. The ulcer was superficial and the strain was not highly virulent, but useful vision in the eye was lost.[19b]

Summary

The role of contaminated medications and irrigants in producing ocular infections of the most serious nature has been demonstrated. Because bacteria can multiply in unpreserved aqueous solutions, and because such solutions may contact the intraocular tissues or broken corneal epithelium, saline irrigants should be sterilized in the final container, dispensed on an individual basis, and discarded after a single use.

Collyria must be sterile, fortified with a suitable preservative and handled with aseptic precautions. Medications, whether collyria or ointments, which are to be used for more than one patient, should be administered by means of a sterile intermediary dropper or applicator.

Medications in use should be dated and checked for sterility at intervals. The use of unit-dose containers for operating rooms and accident rooms is recommended.

TISSUE CONTAMINANTS

Skin of hands

CUTANEOUS FLORA. The bacterial flora of normal human skin consists of transient and resident organisms. The transient population includes any organisms with which the individual has recently come in contact. They are the first to be removed by scrubbing. The resident bacteria maintain themselves by continuous reproduction on the skin, the birth rate being equal to the death rate unless it is altered by external influences. The superficial resident flora exists in the folds and crypts, the deep flora in the sweat glands, oil glands, and follicles of the skin. Nonpathogenic staphylococci form the bulk of the bacterial population, but pathogenic staphylococci and other pathogenic species may be found. Removal of the deep flora is never accomplished by scrubbing.

When an upper respiratory infection exists, the number of transient organisms and the relative proportion of pathogens on the skin are both markedly increased. Contamination of the skin with pathogenic transient organisms may result in the adaptation of these organisms to the skin, where they become part of the resident flora and may remain for weeks. For this reason the ophthalmic surgeon should protect his hands from contamination with pathogenic bacteria insofar as possible. The surgeon who operates on an infected patient should wear gloves not only for protection of the patient but also to prevent contamination of his own hands.

Because the normal skin is never sterile and cannot be made sterile, the wearing of sterile rubber gloves is recommended for all operators. But because rubber gloves may be torn or punctured during an operation, removal of dirt, grease, and bacteria must be carried out before an operation. The process of reducing the cutaneous flora has been designated *degerming* the skin. The most efficacious methods of accomplishing this object have been evaluated by surgical and skin bacteriologists.

DEGERMING THE SKIN. Rapid reduction of the cutaneous flora is accomplished in two stages: (1) mechanical removal of bacteria by scrubbing all accessible areas with a detergent and (2) killing the bacteria that remain on the skin by a skin antiseptic. A third process, (3) inhibition of the resident flora by a bacteriostatic substance deposited on the skin, is effective when it is allowed to act over a period of days. The principles underlying these processes should be understood by ophthalmic surgeons.

The effectiveness of mechanical cleansing of the skin depends upon (1) scrubbing in the presence of a surface-active compound, (2) friction, (3) time, and (4) hydrogen ion concentration (pH). The first two factors are self-explanatory. The time required is a function of these and of pH.

Surface-active agents include cationic, anionic, and nonionic compounds. There are hundreds of these compounds on the market, with more appearing yearly. The higher the alkalinity of any scrubbing process, the higher will be the negative charge on the cutaneous surface and on the bacteria.[6] Mechanical removal of bacteria is thus promoted by the mutual repulsion of similarly charged bodies. The alkaline detergents are therefore more efficient than the acid detergents.

Anionic detergents include soaps, sulfated alcohols and fatty acid esters, and sulfonated aliphatic and aromatic compounds. Soaps having a pH of 9.5 to 10.5 are the most alkaline and therefore the most efficient degerming agents in water of ordinary softness. The newer detergents, unlike soaps, are not precipitated by either acids or calcium and magnesium salts and therefore retain their cleansing properties in either acid solutions or hard waters.

Cationic surface-active agents are not effective for degerming the skin. They alter the electrostatic charge on the skin from negative to positive while leaving bacteria negatively charged. Bacteria thus temporarily bound to the skin by electrostatic attraction can be released by a subsequent alkaline rinse. These agents also lose some of their bactericidal power when in contact with the cutaneous surface. There have been instances of pseudomonas contamination of these agents resulting in loss of eyes. Thus, the quaternary ammonium compounds in aqueous solution are not only ineffective for purposes of degerming the skin but may even carry infection to the skin.

Killing of bacteria, other than spores, which remain on the skin after mechanical cleansing, is best accomplished by alcohol allowed to act for a sufficient time. Ethyl alcohol 70% is effective but is expensive and is subject to alteration in its concentration. Isopropyl alcohol is cheaper and is germicidal over a wide range of concentration. Iodine and its derivatives are not superior to isopropyl alcohol as skin antiseptics. The combination of mechanical scrubbing with soap and water followed by a 2-minute soak in 70% isopropyl alcohol renders the skin more nearly sterile than any other procedure for *rapid* degerming of the cutaneous surface.

Hexachlorophene leaves a bacteristatic film on the skin and lowers the bacterial population when it is used continually for washing. Added to soap it offers no advantage for *rapid* degerming of the skin.[7] Its value consists entirely in its cumulative effect over a period of time. For this reason, its addition to solutions of alcohol for soaking is recommended.

Fats are removed from the skin by emulsification during scrubbing with soap and water and by solution in alcohol. The skin feels dry when fat is thus removed. Cetyl alcohol added to the soaking solution provides a satisfactory substitute that leaves the skin soft and smooth without producing a greasy sensation. This emollient has the additional advantage of enabling the surgeon to don rubber gloves without the use of powder, thus eliminating objectionable talcs and starches from the operating room.

The above principles are applied in the following routine that has been used at the Massachusetts General Hospital and the Massachusetts Eye and Ear Infirmary since 1952.[8]

SURGICAL SCRUB ROUTINE

1. Wet hands and arms under running water and work up a lather with soap and brush.
2. Scrub each surface (fingers, hands, nails, arms to elbows) using three double strokes of the brush on each

surface. Rinse under running water (time—about 1 minute).

3. Clean nails with an orangewood stick.
4. Scrub each surface again with three double strokes of the brush (time—about 1 minute).
5. Rinse off soap completely and dry hands and arms with sterile towel.
6. Wet hands and arms thoroughly with the following solution:

Isopropyl alcohol (kills bacteria with 2 minutes of rubbing)	70.0 parts per 1,000 ml
Cetyl alcohol (substitutes for fats and oils of skin)	0.5 parts per 1,000 ml
Hexachlorophene (reduces resident flora when used daily)	0.1 parts per 1,000 ml
Water q.s. ad	100.0 parts per 1,000 ml

7. Rub hands and arms for a full 2 minutes, being sure that the skin is kept wet with alcohol solution the entire time. (This may be accomplished by continuous immersion, repeated immersion, or by repeated delivery of the solution from a dispenser.)
8. At the end of this 2-minute period, allow the hands and arms to dry by evaporation.

Recontamination of the hands can be avoided by wearing a separate pair of sterile gloves for preparation of the patient and injection of the local anesthetic. Alternatively, the surgeon may scrub his hands and the patient's skin with soap and water, administer the local anesthetic, and return to the alcohol soak for 1 minute before putting on his gown and gloves. Accidental contamination of the hands does not require repetition of the entire surgical scrub. The last bacteria to reach the skin are the first to be removed by soap or killed by an antiseptic.

The operative field

In ophthalmology the cutaneous operative field comprises the brow, the eyelids, and the anterior part of the temple and the cheek. Two stands of hair grow here, the eyebrow and the eyelashes.

The bacterial population of this area is comparable to the flora of other exposed areas of the body; that is, there is a preponderance of nonpathogenic staphylococci, but there may be pathogenic organisms among the transient and resident flora. Because skin pathogens adhering to instruments or sutures can be introduced into the eye, pathogens must be eliminated or reduced to a minimum.

Preparation of the operative field must be preceded by inspection to make sure that there are no traces of lid infection such as styes, furuncles, cellulitis, or impetigo. The bases of the lashes and the orifices of the meibomian glands should receive careful scrutiny for the presence of crusting and erythema.

Since it is impossible to study quantitatively the rate of removal of bacteria from a facial area, the principles of degerming derived from studies of hand scrubs must be applied. The scrub described for the hands is adapted, with minor modifications, to the skin of the operative field; that is, a scrub with sterile green soap solution is followed by a 70% isopropyl alcohol rub that should last a full 2 minutes. Cetyl alcohol is omitted; a few drops of eosin in the alcohol serve to indicate the area that has been prepared in this manner. The lids and lid margins are swabbed with alcohol on toothpick applicators, care being taken that the alcohol solution does not enter the conjunctival sac.

Proprietary cutaneous detergents are used in many hospitals for preparing the operative field. Because of their lower alkalinity, these are probably less effective in removing bacteria from the skin than are soaps. More serious are reports of severe keratitis resulting from prolonged contact of pHisoHex with the cornea. Browning and Lippas,[11] reporting two human cases and the results of animal experiments, identified the toxic agent as sodium octylphenoxyethoxyethyl ether sulfonate (Entsufon), an ingredient of pHisoderm and pHisoHex. Pure hexachlorophene 3%, present in pHisoHex, produced only mild stippling in a small percentage of animal eyes, whereas the sulfonated ether compound reproduced the epithelial denudation and deep stromal edema that characterized the clinical cases reported. Although both patients recovered full visual acuity after several weeks, the discomfort, disability, and the inevitable psychic trauma to patients should dictate extreme caution in the use of these agents in the vicinity of the eye.

Although shaving of hair is basic to skin preparation elsewhere on the body, shaving the eyebrow is not necessary provided scrub solutions are vigorously worked into the eyebrow and provided the brow is carefully walled off from the palpebral fissure during the operation itself.

Clipping of the lashes before intraocular surgery may do more harm than good. It is doubtful whether this practice is helpful in preventing infection. A solid-bladed speculum (Metscher) walls off the lid margins better than an open-bladed one.

The conjunctival sac

Pathogenic bacteria in the conjunctival secretions pose an obvious threat of infection at the time of intraocular surgery. Surveys of patients admitted for ocular surgery show that clinically healthy conjunctivas often harbor pathogens. Smith[42a] found pathogens in the eyes of 15% of 5,000 patients admitted to two London hospitals; only 3.5% of the 5,000 patients were classified as clinically "dirty." Cason and Winkler,[13] reporting conjunctival cultures from patients who showed no clinical evidence of an infectious process in either eye, found pathogens in 12%, including gram-negative rods in 5%. Khorazo and Thompson[25a] found S. *aureus* in 23% of 1,122 patients and other pathogens in an additional 11%. Dunnington and Locatcher-Khorazo[17] found pathogenic staphylococci preoperatively in 26% of 2,508 patients, alone or in combination with other pathogens. Postoperative endophthalmitis developed in 11 of the 529 patients in whom pathogenic staphylococci were found, but in none of 74 patients in whom other potential pathogens were cultured. Species that are pathogenic when introduced into the cornea or anterior chamber may thus be present in the conjunctival sac without producing symptoms or signs of conjunctivitis.

There is no infallible method for sterilizing the conjunctival sac preoperatively. Assuming that the lacrimal passages are patent, a suitable regimen is the use of drops containing chloramphenicol and polymyxin 4 times daily for 2 days before surgery, combined with erythromycin ointment to the conjunctiva and lids at bedtime.[3a]

The continued use of antibacterial medication in the conjunctival sac is desirable for at least the first week after operation, in view of the well-known effect of patching in creating an environment favorable for the proliferation of conjunctival bacteria.

The lacrimal sac

The lacrimal sac is of the greatest importance as a source of virulent organisms. Every well-trained eye surgeon is thoroughly imbued with the principle that reflux of mucopurulent material on pressure over the sac requires deferment of intraocular surgery until this focus of infection has been eradicated. In the absence of epiphora or of a mucocele, many surgeons prefer to proceed without irrigation or probing of the lacrimal passages than to take the chance of causing infection or edema by such manipulation. If epiphora is present with or without signs of infection, cultures should invariably be taken to determine the presence of pathogenic organisms before operating.

AIR HYGIENE FOR HOSPITALS

The role of airborne organisms in postoperative infections, like that of other environmental factors, is difficult to evaluate. Circulation of air in the operating room and loss of viability of most respiratory pathogens in air render futile retrospective attempts to recover an etiologic agent from the air by the time signs of endophthalmitis have appeared.

Coagulase-positive staphylococci are the most frequent cause of postoperative endophthalmitis and the pathogen most frequently recovered from air samples taken during eye operations. They are often recovered from the inside and outside surfaces of cloth masks worn by operating room personnel. Pneumococci and coliform bacilli, next in importance to staphylococci and pseudomonas in postoperative infections, may also be derived from the upper respiratory tract. Among rarer agents isolated from infected eyes, *Neisseria catarrhalis* has been cited by Givner[19a] as having a probable respiratory origin.

Early concepts and modern methods

The problem of organisms falling from the air upon open wounds became a concern of surgeons after Pasteur's demonstration of the role of airborne microorganisms in fermentation. Lister's techniques were directed primarily toward destroying airborne bacteria and isolating open wounds from them.

The introduction of the surgical mask by von Mikulicz in 1896 was perhaps the first attempt to check the dissemination of respiratory contaminants at their source. Twelve years later, at least one American eye surgeon felt that the use of the mask as a mouth protector was extreme and that its principal use in eye surgery was to control the surgeon's beard!

During the 1930's there was a reawakening of interest in the infection-producing role of airborne bacteria in general surgery. Renewed attention was directed toward their control by improved masking, ultraviolet irradiation of circulating air, and the use of germicidal aerosols and mists.

In recent years, mechanical ventilation by air of controlled temperature and humidity has been installed in most operating suites. The source of ventilation and the method of humidity control can have a profound influence on the number and species of organisms discharged from supply ducts. Aerosols of pathogenic bacteria can be generated in concentrations that could never be reached in ordinary atmospheric air and blown into spaces, such as operating rooms, where they can do the greatest damage. At the same time, great advances have been made in freeing air of particulate matter, chiefly through the development of filtering media of high efficiency against atmospheric dust and even smaller particles. Familiarity with the properties of these media can avoid inefficient, unnecessarily elaborate, and expensive installations.

Origin, nature, and fate of airborne contaminants

Microorganisms enter rooms in two principal ways. Some are carried in with atmospheric dust by currents of air. They include bacteria, spores, and molds in the dry state.

Other contaminants are carried in by personnel in their respiratory secretions, on the skin, on their clothing and shoes, or in bedclothes. They are liberated from these sources by activity on the part of the individuals concerned. The concentration of air contaminants derived from human sources is proportional to the following factors: (1) duration of occupancy, (2) number of occupants, (3) activity of occupants, that is, movements and forced expirations, (4) carriers of pathogenic organisms, and (5) intensity of growth from respiratory tracts of carriers. Of all these factors, it appears that the activity of individuals is the most important. Relatively few bacteria are liberated by people sitting quietly without speaking, whereas talking, laughing, coughing, and bustling about result in the liberation of many organisms from the mouth, skin, clothing, and bedding.

These organisms are distributed in air in three forms: (1) attached to dust particles, (2) in droplets, and (3) as droplet nuclei. A single particle may contain one or more bacteria. Dust particles vary greatly in size. Those larger than 10 μ settle at the rate of 1 to 2 ft per minute in still air; those smaller than 1 μ remain suspended for indefinite periods. Droplets evaporate at a rate proportional to their size and to the temperature and relative humidity of the environmental air. Large droplets are usually projected for several feet and fall to the ground before evaporating. Droplets of 10 μ diameter are propelled for shorter distances and evaporate almost instantaneously to form droplet nuclei. These lie almost entirely within the range of 1.34 to 2.68 μ diameter and settle at an average rate of 0.04 ft per minute in still air. Under ordinary conditions they remain in continuous suspension because of thermal and mechanical air currents.

The ultimate fate of airborne organisms depends upon environmental conditions. Spores remain viable indefinitely. Molds and fungi of various species are common airborne contaminants. On the other hand, *Pseudomonas* and other gram-negative species are seldom found in air samples.

Pathogenic bacteria do not multiply in ordinary room air or upon dry surfaces. However, certain bacteria can and do reproduce on moist surfaces, particularly if nutrient substances happen to be present. The rate of bacterial multiplication depends upon the growth requirements of the species involved and the extent to which these requirements are met under existing circumstances.

When the palpebral fissure is open, airborne particles impinge upon the cornea and the exposed conjunctiva just as they do upon other areas of the body's surface. Nonpathogenic gram-positive bacteria are usually destroyed by the lysozyme of the tears. Other organisms are mechanically removed by blinking and are washed away by the normal flow of tears. More rarely, airborne pathogens in droplets or spatters may establish themselves in the conjunctival sac. For example, the conjunctiva may be directly infected by meningococci expelled from the nasopharynx of a carrier or a case of meningitis. Adenovirus infections of the eye may be transmitted in the same manner.

Collection of data for periodic checks

RELEVANT DATA. Three items of information are required for periodic checks of conditions relevant to air contamination: (1) the temperature and relative humidity of the air in the operating rooms, (2) the direction and rate of flow of air currents in the surgical suite and the individual operating rooms, and (3) the bacterial count per unit volume of air and its breakdown into pathogenic and nonpathogenic species. The last of these is the most important, since it provides an index of total contamination in the environmental air.

TEMPERATURE AND RELATIVE HUMIDITY. The temperature and relative humidity are determined from readings of thermometers, psychrometers, and hygrometers. Variation of either of these factors within the limits found in operating rooms in the temperate zone probably has little effect upon bacterial contamination of room air or of surfaces in the operating room. Different species show marked differences in their rate of viability loss in relation to drying. Decay rates of gram-negative bacilli are faster than those of micrococci, corynebacteria, and mycobacteria.

AIR CURRENT TRACING. A simple, inexpensive indicator of air flow is the smoke from a cigarette. When a lighted cigarette is placed near the bottom of a closed door, it becomes apparent at once whether air is flowing into or out of the room at that point, and how fast it is moving. When it is held near the ceiling, the direction of air currents from a supply duct can be traced in the same manner. These currents indicate whether a positive or a negative pressure exists in the operating room relative to the corridor and to adjoining spaces, such as scrub rooms and anterooms for anesthesia. The same test can be applied to the operating suite as a whole by testing air currents at either end of the main corridor.

Quantitative measurement of air flow from duct outlets requires the use of flowmeters and anemometers. Such determinations are easily performed by air-conditioning engineers, who should make periodic checks and furnish pertinent data to the hospital.

COLLECTION OF AIRBORNE ORGANISMS. The simplest method for collection of organisms in air is the exposure of open petri dishes containing nutrient agar at strategic points in the operating room. The disadvantages of this method are: (1) only particles heavy enough to settle out by gravity will be collected, and (2) the volume of air sampled is unknown, a fact that prevents quantitative comparison of air samples. Nevertheless, the open plate technique, by permitting qualitative detection of pathogenic species, is better than nothing at all.

The problem of quantitative air sampling has stimulated the development of numerous ingenious devices too expensive for routine use.

COUNTS OF AIR CONTAMINANTS. In recording counts of organisms collected in the hospital it is essential to break down the total count into nonpathogens and pathogens. Under the former heading we include nonhemolytic staphylococci, species of sarcina, hay bacilli, and diphtheroids. These are usually of no interest, but their total count may be important as an index of air turbulence and human activity. When pathogens are found, the species should always be recorded. These often include *Staphylococcus aureus* and more rarely *Streptococcus hemolyticus, Diplococcus pneumoniae, Pseudomonas aeruginosa,* and other gram-negative rods. Because *Bacillus subtilis* and species of aspergilli may be pathogenic for the eye, notice should be taken if these occur with undue frequency in the operating room air.

Ventilation and air conditioning

Air entering the operating room suite should be free from dust and bacteria, controlled as to temperature and humidity, and supplied under slight positive pressure. Control of temperature and humidity is important for human comfort and efficiency as well as for minimizing explosion hazard from static electricity. Positive pressure is necessary in order to prevent entrance of unsterile air from uncontrolled sources. Under no circumstances should air be drawn into the operating suite from other parts of the hospital.

Achievement of these objectives is the problem of the ventilation engineer and the hospital architect. In existing hospitals the supply of air may or may not meet requirements. In hospitals under construction an opportunity for providing ideal conditions is present. The administration and the medical staff should understand the means of obtaining a properly cleaned and conditioned supply of air.

The intake for outside air should be located as far as possible above street level, preferably on the roof and always far removed from any exhaust outlets of other ventilating systems. Cold air must be warmed and sometimes humidified, while warm air must be cooled and sometimes dehumidified before delivery to the operating room. When the outside air is below 70° F, dehumidification is almost never necessary, because the relative humidity of heated air is automatically lowered by expansion.

Thomas,[45a] reviewing practical aspects of air conditioning in hospitals, recommends a central system of air conditioning to include the following features for operating and delivery rooms:

1. Winter humidification to reduce fire and explosion dangers of anesthetic gases
2. Summer cooling with some dehumidification to reduce fatigue and sweating
3. Eight to twelve changes of air per hour
4. A controlled temperature range of 72° to 80° F
5. A controlled relative humidity ranging from 50% to 60%
6. Proper filtering devices to remove particulate matter

Thomas takes issue with the Guide published by the American Society of Heating and Air Conditioning Engineers for requiring 100% outside air. He cites evidence suggesting that the use of 50% recirculated air presents no greater explosion hazard and is much more economical.

Air cleaning

Clean air is needed to maintain dilution of airborne contaminants derived from sources within the operating room; contaminated ventilating air would obviously compound the chances of infection. To ensure satisfactory performance over long periods, devices for delivering clean air should be simple, trouble free, and should require a minimum of maintenance. Recent developments in the field of air filtration permit realization of these objectives at reasonable installation and operating costs.[1]

DRY OR FIBROUS FILTERS. Dry filters are fabriclike media of wool felt, cotton batting, or thick mats composed of very fine glass fibers that may be bonded together by phenolic resins. By means of pleating, a great increase in effective filtering surface can be achieved. The more efficient of these filters may arrest up to 95% of ordinary atmospheric dust particles at a high rate of air flow and with a pressure drop across the filter bank usually less than 0.5 inch water gauge for a new filter. Examples of deep-bed glass fiber media are the American and Cambridge types.* Specifications of these media are available in manufacturers' brochures. They are composed of glass fibers averaging 0.8 to 3.0 μ diameter. Individual differences exist in the disposition of the medium (whether pocket, pleated, or expansion type) and in the manner of adaptation of the filter frame to the duct. Units presenting 4 sq ft superficial area provide an air flow of 1,000 cfm (superficial face velocity 250 fpm).

EFFICIENCY RATINGS OF AIR FILTERS. Although surgeons do not ordinarily carry out performance tests on air filters, an understanding of the basis for efficiency rating is important. A filter that is highly efficient against particles of 10 μ diameter may be extremely inefficient against particles of 1 μ diameter.

Deep-bed media are rated by the National Bureau of Standards (NBS) Discoloration Test using atmospheric dust as the test material; that is, against particles averaging 0.5 μ diameter. "Stain" efficiencies increase with the useful life of the filter as particles build up on the filter face. Efficiencies from 35% to 95% over the life of the different filters are achieved at the rated face velocity. The pressure drop for newly installed filters varies from 0.14 to 0.48 inches of water, depending upon the efficiency of the filter medium. Thus they combine high retention of particles with the advantages of lower initial and operating cost, easier and less expensive maintenance, and absolute freedom from shock and sparking hazards.

In order to conserve the efficiency of deep-bed media for fine (smaller than 5 μ diameter) particles, a viscous panel filter should be incorporated upstream from the former to screen out large particles and to postpone buildup of maximum allowable (dirty) pressure drop. The water gauge manometer should be inspected at regular intervals to prevent exceeding the maximum dirty drop.

Because no filter is better than the efficiency of its installation, this should be inspected for possible bypassing of the filter bed. A performance test should be carried out by the consultant, the manufacturer's representative, or the installing contractor to ascertain whether the completed assembly is functioning in a satisfactory manner. Faulty adaptation of the filter frame to the duct can reduce filtration by 50%. Under these circumstances, low manometer readings will give the erroneous impression that the pressure drop across the filter is below the maximum level permissible when actually the reverse may be the case.

A correctly installed, performance-tested bank of fibrous filters requires a minimum of maintenance. Its efficiency for fine particles increases with buildup of arrested dust at the filter face. A panel-protected filter bank may operate below the critical pressure drop for many months. Replacement of filter cartridges should be accom-

*American Air Filter Co., Louisville, Ky.; Cambridge Filter Corp., Syracuse, N. Y.

panied by careful vacuum cleaning of the duct.

Organisms liberated in the operating room

Sources of contamination. Most bacteria in operating rooms enter by ways other than ventilating air. Such bacteria are carried by: (1) particles containing bacteria and viruses freshly emitted from the respiratory tracts of the occupants as droplets or droplet nuclei; (2) particles of human origin arising from the skin, hair, and clothes of the occupants; (3) particles of nonhuman origin, including soil bacteria and spores, associated with clothes and bedding, and others similarly dispersed.

Particles in all three categories are continuously produced by activity of the occupants, and their concentration is continuously reduced by an adequate supply of bacteria-free ventilating air. Bacteria in the first category lose viability by decay. The resultant of the three forces of liberation, dilution, and decay determines the moment-to-moment concentration of airborne contaminants. Since the last two factors should be constant in suitably ventilated rooms, the main variable must be the rate of liberation of bacteria by the occupants. This factor is also the most difficult to control.

Respiratory contaminants. Most individuals expel very few bacteria in the course of quiet respiration. Forced expiration, as in talking, laughing, coughing, or sneezing, increases this number by expulsion at high speeds of droplets laden with bacteria. In the presence of an upper respiratory infection, the concentration of bacteria in secretions, the proportion of pathogens, and the virulence of these pathogens are all increased.

The two most obvious means of controlling respiratory contamination of the air are the avoidance of talking and the exclusion of individuals with coughs and colds from the operating room. In most operating rooms these means are seldom utilized.

Masking technique. Cloth masks are inadequate and obsolete. Modern synthetic fibrous masks are effective filtering devices.

Air that escapes around a mask is unfiltered and carries its bacterial burden into the room air.

Masks should be worn in the operating room even when an operation is not in progress. Since bacteria can remain airborne in a viable state for many hours, failure to observe this precaution can liberate organisms that may eventually find their way into open wounds.

The cooperation of anesthesia personnel is essential in preventing unnecessary dissemination of organisms. Induction of general anesthesia in the operating room is attended by a rise in airborne bacteria recovered in samples. By the same token, extubation of a patient on the table after operation may give rise to a spasm of coughing that is productive of atomized tracheobronchial secretions.

Bacteria from skin and clothing. Particles in these categories can be partially controlled by requiring a change to laundered cotton clothing of all individuals entering the operating room, by minimizing the movements of such individuals, and by applying grease or cream to exposed skin surfaces of the face and neck.

Blankets and bedding. One of the richest sources of bacteria, including many pathogens, and one of the easiest to control, is the blanket that accompanies the patient from the ward to the operating room. Blankets are easily sampled by passing an inverted blood agar plate rapidly and firmly across a section of blanket resting on a hard flat surface. The action of the nap in springing back throws up many bacteria and provides an adequate sample as an index of contamination. Large numbers of pathogenic staphylococci and other organisms are found in bed blankets.

Because of the danger from static electricity, wool blankets are never sent with patients to the operating room. Instead, a sterile cotton "ether blanket" should be placed over the patient after he has been transferred to the litter on which he is to be wheeled to surgery. The number of bacteria that settle upon this blanket during transportation of the patient will be few in comparison with those that collect in wool blankets in use for but a short time. Blankets should never be stripped off a patient in the operating room either before or after an operation, as large numbers of bacteria are liberated by these procedures. Instead, a sterile sheet should be draped over the patient and allowed to hang down over the sides of the table as soon as it has been wheeled in.

Practical studies

Bacterial counts taken in empty operating rooms ventilated under positive pressure by air filtered through deep-bed glass fiber media at the rate of 8 to 12 air changes per hour show negligible initial contamination and rapid disappearance of organisms introduced as droplet nuclei by nebulization. During operations the concentration of airborne bacteria-bearing particles, as calculated from colony counts, may vary from 0.66 to 5.2 colonies per cubic foot of air. The pathogen most frequently recovered is S. *aureus*. When this species has been found in the air, it has usually been demonstrated on the inside or the outside surface of the mask of a member of the surgical team. When S. *aureus* has been isolated from the air, it has often been found on the instruments at the end of an operation. On the other hand, instruments have been found to carry this organism when it was not recovered from the air or from the surgeons' masks.

Summary

Air samples taken in operating rooms always contain nonpathogenic bacteria and occasionally pathogenic species. Wounds can become infected by airborne organisms. Periodic checks of the concentration and species of airborne bacteria should be made.

Inadequately cleaned ventilating air can carry bacteria into operating rooms. Suitable fibrous filters clean air supplied to operating rooms.

The principal sources of organisms in the operating room air are the skin, clothing, and upper respiratory tracts of the occupants. Simple precautions, together with adequate ventilation, are more important than elaborate efforts to destroy bacteria liberated into the air. Unnecessary talking and activity are to be avoided. Masking technique and discipline should be strict.

STERILIZATION OF SPECIFIC ITEMS

Stainless steel items

Stainless steel instruments of all types, including scissors, are most rapidly and efficiently sterilized in the autoclave at 121° C. The time-honored formula of "15 min at 15 lb" offers an adequate margin of safety provided timing is begun only after the sterilizing temperature has been registered by the thermometer in the exhaust line. Unless air has been entirely evacuated from the chamber, this temperature will never be reached.

A complete set of instruments for a cataract operation can be folded into a towel and sterilized in a shallow, rectangular stainless steel basin wrapped in two more towels. The entire sterile package is delivered to the sterile nurse or to the operative assistant after he has donned mask, gown, and gloves.

Individual instruments needed during an operation can be sterilized in 5 minutes at 132° in a small, high-pressure autoclave.

Stainless steel instruments can also be sterilized in the final package by dry heat when time permits. In addition to instruments, stainless steel basins, trays, and other components of the operating kit can be sterilized in the autoclave. An item frequently overlooked are the steel trays that fit on the Mayo stands used for skin preparation and for instruments. Even though these are covered with sterile towels, they almost always get wet and can become contaminated from an underlying unsterile tray. For this reason all trays used in our operating rooms are autoclaved in paper wrappers sealed with Steritape.

Cutting-edge instruments

Cataract knives, glaucoma knives, keratomes, trephine blades, and other keen-bladed instruments cannot be autoclaved without corrosion of their cutting edges. Because most disinfectants lack sporicidal properties, dry heat offers the best method for sterilizing these objects.

The following method has proved satisfactory. The carefully cleaned instrument is packed in the original manufacturer's cardboard box with a silica gel packet* to absorb incidental moisture. The box is inserted into a syringe envelope, which is open at one end. Over this is passed a larger envelope, of which the open end is folded down to the level of the closed end of the inner sleeve and sealed with a wire strip. The sealed package is labelled with the surgeon's name, the name of the instrument, and the date.

A load of instruments packaged in this manner is then carefully packed in the sterilizing oven, which is equipped with a turboblower and provided with a thermometer and a timing device. In the event of power failure, the timer will not record a complete cycle. To provide an ample margin of safety, a cycle of 6 hours at 140° C is employed. Spore controls are included weekly. Instruments are sterilized after use and are carefully stored so that they are ready for reuse whenever they are needed.

Several complete cataract sets can be processed overnight and thus can be ready for an early morning operation. No damage to cutting edges results from multiple exposures to sterilizing cycles at 140° C. However, the blades should always be wiped with water (not with saline) and dried after wiping. Rinsing in saline may cause pitting of blades in a short time.

Not only eye instruments but other sharp instruments used in ear and dental surgery can be sterilized in the oven. Hypodermic needles, syringes, and many other heat-stable items are suitable for sterilization by dry heat. A well-insulated oven with provision for forced circulation of air is a worthwhile investment for any hospital.

Dry heat sterilizes instruments without introducing toxic substances or contaminants by way of disinfectants carried on knife blades. Christy[15] found a high incidence of striate keratitis after cataract operations in which knife blades soaked in Zephiran were used. When this practice was discontinued, marked reduction in the incidence of striate keratitis was observed.

Rubber bulbs and droppers

Silicone bulb syringes and eye droppers are suitable for sterilization by autoclaving. Sterilization will be readily effected if these items are partly filled with water before autoclaving. Sterilization is not complete unless some water is aspirated into the bulb, because trapped air prevents the entrance of steam from the outside.

Bulb syringes are conveniently sterilized in individual paper envelopes. If glass droppers with rubber bulbs are to be sterilized in a screwcap jar, the jar should be laid flat and the cover left off during sterilization. Otherwise air retained in the jar will prevent attainment of sterilizing conditions.

Droppers and irrigating bulbs that are to be used in intraocular surgery should be filled with fluid and autoclaved together with instruments for the same operation. Because of the intimate nature of their contact with the intraocular tissues, these precautions cannot be too strongly emphasized.

Heat-sensitive items

Optical instruments, electric cords, polyethylene tubing, diathermy points, enucleation implants, plastic prostheses, intraocular acrylic lenses, contact lenses, and many other objects that are subject to damage by sterilizing temperatures must be sterilized by means other than moist or dry heat. Ethylene oxide is recommended.

*Dri-Pax Silica Gel Air Dryer, Davison Chemical Co., Baltimore, Md.

Table 7-2. Relative merits of steam and gas sterilization

	Steam	Ethylene oxide
Action	Protein denaturation	Alkylation of SH group
Penetration	Rapid	Very rapid
Efficiency	Complete	Complete
Time required	15 min or less	4-12 hours
Equipment	Autoclave	Large or small chamber
Technical snags	Air removal	Prevacuum, correct RH, temperature over 70° F
Danger	Very little	Explosion hazard of pure ETO
Hazard	Inadequate if air not all removed	Toxic residual effect if aeration inadequate
Indications	Steel, glass, cloth	Plastics, delicate instruments
Contraindications	Rustable edges, heat-sensitive items	Previously irradiated PVC

Adapted from Rendell-Baker, L., and Roberts, R. B.: Medical and Surgical Rev. fourth quarter, 1969.

Tonometers

Causation of bacterial keratitis from contact with a contaminated tonometer is a rare possibility that could be eliminated by sterilization of the instrument between patients. Tonometers have transmitted infections by the viruses of inclusion blennorrhea and epidemic keratoconjunctivitis. In mass screening surveys for glaucoma, an infected tonometer could give rise to an epidemic of adenovirus keratoconjunctivitis. To cause an epidemic disease through an attempt to diagnose an endemic one would be ironic indeed.

The principal difficulty in sterilizing tonometers of the Schiøtz type is that a film of lacrimal fluid is drawn up by capillarity between the barrel and the plunger of the instrument each time it is used. This film of moisture, which is inaccessible to ultraviolet radiations, preserves bacteria and viruses in a viable state, so that succeeding patients are infected during displacement of the plunger.

Flaming of stainless steel tonometers is harmless to the instrument and offers the best guarantee of true sterility. To avoid coagulation of protein in the bore, the bore should be swabbed after removal of the plunger. The plunger and footplate should then be flamed separately. Tonofilms may be used instead of flaming.

Electronic tonometers present a delicate problem in that they must not be subjected to heat or to certain chemicals. The minimum acceptable routine for sanitization of electronic tonometers should include removal of the plunger and thorough swabbing of it and the barrel with sterile distilled water, using sterile cotton swabs and sterile pipe cleaners held in well-washed fingers. Applanation tonometers can be swabbed with sterile distilled water.

Sterilization versus disinfection

There are few items used in ophthalmic practice that cannot be sterilized. With a little forethought, presterilized, properly protected instruments and materials can be kept on hand to meet ordinary requirements. Disposable blood lancets and hypodermic needles help to prevent serum hepatitis. Office autoclaves and hot air ovens are available for instruments that are not damaged by heat. For those that are, hospitals need a device for gaseous sterilization. When means of sterilization are at hand, mere sanitization cannot be justified.

HOSPITAL HYGIENE

Staff attitudes

If aseptic technique is to succeed, all personnel in the hospital must be convinced of the necessity for energetic participation in the practices and procedures necessary for reducing the numbers of bacteria in the environment and for preventing their transmission from patient to patient. For all personnel to become convinced of this, the surgical staff must believe in the validity of such elementary precautions as washing the hands between visits to patients, wearing masks over nose and mouth, minimizing conversation and refraining from laughter in the operating room, and carrying out approved practices. If surgeons flout aseptic technique, nurses and corpsmen will find little incentive to observe it themselves or to enforce discipline upon orderlies and attendants. Because of the law of averages, single infractions may not show any effect upon the infection rate, but when breaks in technique are multiplied by many instances and individuals, it is only a question of time before disaster strikes.

Role of the laboratory

The hospital bacteriologic laboratory that limits its activity to isolation, identification, and sensitivity testing of strains recovered from patients is fulfilling only part of its proper function. A physician member of the committee on hospital infections should be given responsibility for supervision of spot checks, bacteriologic controls, and sterilizing practices in the operating and central supply rooms. The extent to which such an individual participates in inspections, sterility surveys, and in the taking and reading of cultures will largely determine his effectiveness. In general hospitals, a member of the ophthalmic staff should concern himself with both the specialized and the broader aspects of aseptic technique and hospital hygiene. By so doing he can provide liaison between the laboratory and the professional staffs, gain experience as an infections control officer, and be instrumental in preventing infections that might otherwise occur.

Committee on hospital infections

Because of accreditation requirements, almost all hospitals have a committee on hospital infections. The hospital bacteriologist and pharmacist should be ex officio members of this committee, which should also have a representative from each of the special services, including ophthalmology. The functions of such committees have been described elsewhere.

Routine controls

A schedule should be set up for routine sterility control of all lots processed in the pharmacy and central supply room. Spore samples processed with each lot should be sent for sterility testing, and the entire lot should be released only upon receipt of the bacteriologist's report of negative cultures, which becomes part of the permanent record of that lot. Carriers bearing 500,000 or more spores and suitably protected by envelopes can be included with objects to be sterilized, and their contents should be cultured aerobically and anaerobically. A log or ledger of all such routine checks should be kept.

Sterility surveys

A comprehensive survey of all the items used during a single operation should be carried out at intervals. Even though the results cannot affect that particular operation, possible sources of contamination may be revealed, and a body of information will be accumulated that may point to some potential source of infection. At the same time, the resident and nursing staffs become more conscious of infection and acquire some knowledge of sterility surveys.

Such surveys are best performed by residents and nurses, working as a team. About 30 to 40 cultures are taken each time. The following materials are furnished by the bacteriologic laboratory: culture tubes of fluid medium in racks, sterile swabs, and blood agar plates.

The manner of conducting a survey is as follows. At the beginning of an operation bacterial sterility controls (resistant spores) are removed from the autoclave, and settling plates are set out. At the end of the operation all instruments that have been used are swabbed with sterile swabs, which are immediately inoculated into tubes of fluid medium. Miscellaneous small items, such as sponges, swabs, sutures, and glass droppers, are dropped into culture tubes without swabbing. Samples of all solutions used in the preparation of the patient and during the operation itself are inoculated into individual tubes of broth. These may include liquid soap, isopropanol, procaine, epinephrine, saline (extraocular and intraocular), and a random sampling of collyria and ointments, whether or not these were used during the operation. The inside surfaces of gloves and masks used by the operating team are cultured by pressing them flat against the surface of blood agar in petri dishes. The cultures are incubated at 37° C and read at the end of 24 and 48 hours. Disruption of operating room routine is minimal; if all preparations have been made beforehand, an entire survey can be taken in 10 to 15 minutes.

Bedding precautions

Every patient entering the hospital is entitled to a sterile blanket and an impermeable pillowcase and mattress cover. These precautions are as elementary as the accepted routine of clean sheets daily. Blankets, pillows, and mattresses are often a formidable reservoir of staphylococci, other bacteria, and fungi. Because of the rapid turnover of patients on busy surgical services, a large, automatic ethylene oxide sterilizer is essential for larger hospitals.

Environmental sanitation and dust control

The high bacterial content of dust removed from modern vacuum cleaners is evidence of their effectiveness in reducing environmental contamination. Used in combination, adequate ventilation, blanket sterilization, vacuum cleaning, and residual surface disinfection with orthophenylphenol offer a four-way approach to reducing the number of bacteria throughout a hospital.

SUMMARY

Although the incidence of preventable infection in ophthalmology has been greatly reduced, major outbreaks (each involving the loss of several eyes) and an undetermined number of isolated cases of postoperative endophthalmitis continue to occur. There are also localized epidemics of adenoviral keratoconjunctivitis. Most, if not all, of the surgical infections and many of the cases of virus infection are preventable by stricter precautions on the part of opthalmologists.

Unfortunately, the standards observed in clinics in this country and in others offer no guarantee that similar surgical disasters and medically mediated epidemics will not continue. Community droppers and dispensing bottles pass from eye to eye in many clinics. Stagnant solutions of unpreserved irrigants can be seen in private offices as well as in hospital wards and clinics. Although unopened collyria and stock solutions are now required to be sterile, the possibility that opened units may become contaminated during careless handling is ever present. Collyria and irrigants, antiseptics and disinfectants, and antibiotics and sulfonamides must all be regarded with the suspicion that they may be contaminated by *Pseudomonas* organisms. When that suspicion arises, it should be confirmed or dismissed by cultural methods. Only a new bottle should be used for an injured eye.

For operating rooms, we must continue to stress all details of aseptic technique, with particular emphasis upon the elimination of unnecessary conversation before, during, and after operation. Adequate ventilation by adequately cleaned air is essential. An environmental survey of 1 case every 6 months is recommended as the minimum essential in spot checking for incidental contaminants.

Probably the most important source of postoperative endophthalmitis is the indigenous flora of the patient's conjunctival sac and lids.[3,31] Elimination or suppression of this flora, according to our latest figures, is best accomplished by the preoperative instillation of drops containing chloramphenicol 0.5% and polymyxin B sulfate 0.1% four times daily, combined with the nightly application of erythromycin ointment 0.5% to the conjunctival sac and the lid margins.[3a] This regimen should be instituted 36 to 48 hours before scheduled surgery.

The three As of asepsis are:

Aseptic technique

Atraumatic surgery

Antibiotic prophylaxis

Assiduous application of these principles will minimize postoperative infection in ophthalmic surgery.

REFERENCES

1. Allen, H. F.: Air hygiene for hospitals: efficiency of fibrous filters against staphylococcic droplet nuclei and bacteria-bearing dust, J.A.M.A. **170**:261, 1959.
2. Allen, H. F.: Aseptic technique in ophthalmology, Trans. Amer. Ophthal. Soc. **57**:377, 1959.
3. Allen, H. F., and Mangiaracine, A. B.: Bacterial endophthalmitis after cataract extraction, Arch. Ophthal. **72**:454, 1964.

3a. Allen, H. F., and Mangiaracine, A. B.: Bacterial endophthalmitis after cataract extraction. II. Incidence in 36,000 consecutive operations with special reference to preoperative topical antibiotics, Trans. Amer. Acad. Ophthal. Otolarying. To be published.

4. Aseptic methods in the operating suite: a report to the Medical Research Council, Lancet **1**:709, April 13, 1968.
5. Ayliffe, G. A. J., Barry, D. R., Lowbury, E. J. L., Roper-Hall, M. J., and Walker, W. M.: Postoperative infections with Pseudomonas aeruginosa in an eye hospital, Lancet **1**:1113, 1966.
6. Blank, I. H., and Coolidge, M. H.: Degerming the cutaneous surface: I. Quarternary ammonium compounds, J. Invest. Derm. **15**:249, 1950.
7. Blank, I. H., and Coolidge, M. H.: Degerming the cutaneous surface: II. Hexachlorophene (G-11), J. Invest. Derm. **15**:257, 1950.
8. Blank, I. H., Coolidge, M. H., Soutter, L., and Rodkey, G. V.: A study of the surgical scrub, Surg. Gynec. Obstet. **91**:577, 1950.
9. Bowman, F. W.: Microbial contamination of antibiotic ophthalmic ointments, J. Pharm. Sci. **58**:277, 1969.
10. Bowman, F. W., and Holdowsky, S.: Sterility of antibiotic ophthalmic ointment, J. Amer. Pharm. Ass. **48**:95, 1959.
11. Browning, C. W., and Lippas, J.: pHisoHex keratitis, Arch. Ophthal. **53**:816, 1955.
12. Burns, R. P.: Postoperative infections in an ophthalmologic hospital, Amer. J. Ophthal. **48**:519, 1959.
13. Cason, L., and Winkler, C. H.: Bacteriology of the normal eye: normal flora, Arch. Ophthal. **51**:196, 1954.
14. Chalkley, T. H. F., and Schoch, D.: An evaluation of prophylactic subconjunctival antibiotic injection in cataract surgery, Amer. J. Ophthal. **64**:1084, 1967.
15. Christy, N. E.: Chemically caused striate keratitis, Amer. J. Ophthal. **45**:5, 1958.
16. Dreisler, K.: Sterilization of tonometers, Arch. Ophthal. **53**:860, 1955.
17. Dunnington, J., and Locatcher-Khorazo, D.: Value of cultures before operation for cataract, Arch. Ophthal. **34**:577, 1947.
18. Fine, B. S., and Zimmerman, L. E.: Exogenous intraocular fungus infections with particular reference to complications of intraocular surgery, Amer. J. Ophthal. **48**:151, 1959.
19. Fuchs, E.: Memories of Vienna clinics, Amer. J. Ophthal. **9**:605, 1926.

19a. Givner, I.: Neisseria catarrhalis endophthalmitis, Amer. J. Ophthal. **32**:5, 1949.

19b. Golden, B., Fingerman, L. H., and Allen, H. F.: Pseudomonas corneal ulcers in contact lens wearers, Arch. Ophthal. **85**:543, 1971.

20. Graefe, A.: Die antiseptische Wundbehandlung bei Star Extraction, Graefes Arch. Ophth. **24**:223, 1878.
21. Guyton, H. G., and Decker, H. M.: Respiratory protection provided by five new contagion masks, Appl. Microbiol. **11**:66, 1963.
22. Guyton, J. S., and Woods, A. C.: Oral use of sulfadiazine for cataract extractions, Amer. J. Ophthal. **26**:1278, 1943.
23. Horner, M.: La methode antiseptique dans la chirurgie oculaire, Ann. Oculist. **86**:56, 1881.
24. Hughes, W. F., Jr., and Owens, W. C.: Postoperative complications of cataract extraction, Arch. Ophthal. **38**:577, 1945.
25. Jennison, M. W., and Edgerton, H. E.: Droplet infection of air, Proc. Soc. Exp. Biol. Med. **43**:455, 1940.

25a. Khorazo, D., and Thompson, R.: The bacterial flora of the normal conjunctiva, Amer. J. Ophthal. **18**:1114, 1935.

26. Kimura, S. J.: Fluorescein paper: a simple means of insuring the use of sterile fluorescein, Amer. J. Ophthal. **34**:466, 1951.
27. King, J. H.: Contamination of eye medications: practical methods of prevention, Amer. J. Ophthal. **36**:1389, 1953.

28. Koch, R., and Wolfhuegel, G.: Disinfection by hot air, Mitt. a.d. Kgl. Gesundheitsamt **1**:301, 1881, translated by W. W. Cheyne in Recent essays on bacteria in relation to disease, London, 1886, New Syndenham Society.
29. Lawrence, C. A.: Surface-active quaternary ammonium compounds, New York, 1950, Academic Press, Inc.
30. Locatcher-Khorazo, D., and Gutierrez, E.: Eye infections following cataract extraction, Amer. J. Ophthal. **41**:981, 1956.
31. Locatcher-Khorazo, D., and Gutierrez, E.: Bacteriophage typing of Staphylococcus aureus, Arch. Ophthal. **63**:774, 1960.
32. Lowbury, E. J. L.: Contamination of cetrimide and other fluids by Ps. pyocyanea. Brit. J. Industr. Med. **8**:22, 1958.
33. Lowbury, E. J. L., and others: Control of infection in ophthalmic surgery, Proc. Roy. Soc. Med. **60**:349, 1967.
34. Maumenee, A. E., and Michler, R. C.: Sterility of the operative field after ocular surgery, Trans. Pacif. Coast Otoophthal. Soc. **32**:172, 1951.
35. Millikin, B. L.: Cleanliness in eye surgery, Amer. J. Ophthal. **7**:175, 1890.
36. Murphy, J. T., Allen, H. F., and Mangiaracine, A. B.: Preparation, sterilization and preservation of ophthalmic solutions, Arch. Ophthal. **53**:63, 1955.
37. Parker, W. R.: Senile cataract extraction: comparative study of results in 1,421 operations, Tr. Sect. Ophth. A.M.A. **26**:202, 1921.
38. Perkins, J. J.: Principles and methods of sterilization, Springfield, Ill., 1956, Charles C Thomas, Publisher.
39. Price, P. B.: Bacteriology of normal skin: a new quantitative test applied to the study of the bacterial flora and the disinfectant action of mechanical cleansing, J. Infect. Dis. **63**:301, 1938.
40. Proskauer, C.: Development of the rubber glove in surgery and gynecology, J. Hist. Med. **13**:373, 1958.
41. Redard, P.: Desinfection des instruments chirurgicaux et des objets de pansement, Rev. Chir. **8**:360, 1888.
42. Reddish, G. F., editor: Antiseptics, disinfectants, fungicides, and chemical and physical sterilization, ed. 2, Philadelphia, 1957, Lea and Febiger.
42a. Rendell-Baker, L., and Roberts, R. B.: Gas versus steam sterilization: when to use which, Medical and Surgical Rev. fourth quarter, 1969.
42b. Smith, C. H.: Bacteriology of the healthy conjunctiva, Brit. J. Ophthal. **38**:719, 1954.
43. Swan, K. C.: Reactivity of the ocular tissues to wetting agents, Amer. J. Ophthal. **27**:1118, 1940.
44. Theodore, F. H.: Contamination of eye solutions, Amer. J. Ophthal. **34**:1764, 1951.
45. Theodore, F. H., and Feinstein, R. R.: Practical suggestions for the preparation and maintenance of ophthalmic solutions, Amer. J. Ophthal. **35**:656, 1952.
45a. Thomas, G.: Air conditioning in hospitals, Anesth. Analg. (Cleveland) **36**:32, 1957.
46. Thygeson, P.: The epidemiology of epidemic keratoconjunctivitis, Amer. J. Ophthal. **32**:951, 1949.
47. Travers, B.: A synopsis of diseases of the eye, ed. 3, London, 1824, Longman, Hurst, Rees, Orme, Brown, and Green.
48. van der Wyk, R. W., and Granston, A. E.: A bacteriological study of ophthalmic ointments, J. Amer. Pharm. Ass. **47**:193, 1958.
49. Vaughan, D. G., Jr.: Contamination of fluorescein solutions with special reference to Pseudomonas aeruginosa, Amer. J. Ophthal. **39**:55, 1955.
50. Walter, C. W.: The aseptic treatment of wounds, New York, 1948, The Macmillan Co.

8

Ocular tuberculosis

Man probably has been subject to tuberculosis for as long as or longer than history is recorded. Fig. 8-1 shows the skeleton of an Egyptian priest of Amen dating back to 2500 BC; the skeleton exhibits evidence of Pott's disease.[33] While excavating in Grennelle, France, Pales discovered two neolithic skeletons, one showing a hip lesion probably caused by tuberculosis and the other showing tubercularlike lesions of the spine.[15] Bartels stated that a neolithic skeleton from Heidelberg exhibited Pott's disease. Gordon further records the observations of Moodie, who found Pott's disease in a Peruvian skeleton from prehistoric times. Moodie was of the opinion that tuberculosis was widespread among Peruvian Indians. Gordon[15] credits Antoine Maitre-Jan with being the first to describe what probably was a tuberculous lesion of the eye. As quoted by Veith,[36a] Pott stated that his disease was characterized in part by "tedious obstinate ophthalmy." Lloyd[23] in 1930 presented a chronologic bibliography covering the published references to tuberculosis of the eye to that date.

Only clinical data and histologic examination were available for making the diagnosis of tuberculosis until the latter part of the nineteenth century. Furthermore, until the discovery of the ophthalmoscope by von Helmholtz in 1851, observations on tuberculosis of the eye were limited to external examination. Jaeger in 1851 was the first to observe tubercles in the choroid.[15] The tuberculous origin of these lesions was established microscopically by Manz,[25] who reported the case in 1858 and two additional cases in 1866. Cohnheim demonstrated that the choroidal nodules were histologically identical with the tubercles elsewhere in the body.[15]

DISCOVERY OF MYCOBACTERIA

In 1882 Robert Koch[19] stained a bacillus in tuberculous tissue by means of alkaline methylene blue, using vesuvine as a counterstain. He was able to demonstrate the consistent presence of these bacilli in such lesions. He found that cultivation was difficult and that special media were required to grow the organism. By successful animal inoculation he showed that the organism was the causative agent of tuberculosis. It was Ehrlich who discovered the fundamental acid-fast property of mycobacteria by using solutions of nitric acid for decoloration. Both Koch and Klebs recognized bovine tuberculosis as infectious for man; and both believed that the two strains, the human and the bovine, were the same.[35] In 1898 Theobald Smith[34] differentiated *Mycobacterium hominis* from *Mycobacterium bovis*. This was a second important step in the control of tuberculosis, because *M. bovis*, which infects cattle and which is shed in the milk, was soon found to be an important pathogen for man and more particularly for children. Though the figures differ from country to country, through the 1930s *M. bovis* accounted for 50% to 100% of lupus vulgaris infections in children to the age of 16 in Great Britain, 74% to 85% of cervical gland infections, and about 80%

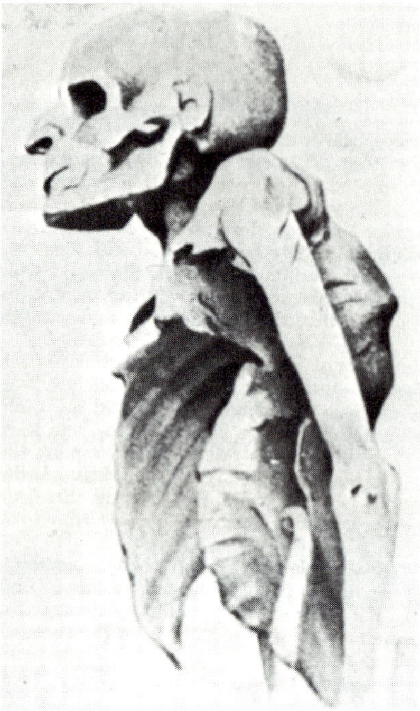

Fig. 8-1. Mummy of a priest of Amen (Twenty-first Dynasty) afflicted with Pott's disease. (From Gay, F.: Agents of disease and host resistance, Springfield, Ill., 1935, Charles C Thomas, Publisher, p. 958.)

of abdominal infections. The percentage of tuberculosis of the bone caused by *M. bovis* was variously reported as 18% to 60%.[35]

Today in many countries bovine tuberculosis is rare, as dairy herds are carefully screened for the disease and milk is pasteurized. The figures on the incidence of *M. bovis* in tubercular infections of the eye are unfortunately full of gaps because of the failure of many investigators to type the mycobacterium isolated from the eye. But from the data to be presented it appears that this pathogen has perhaps played a more important role in primary ocular infections than has *M. hominis*.

PRIMARY TUBERCULOSIS OF THE EYE

The occurrence of primary tuberculous infection of the eye is rare. At the Institute of Ophthalmology, Columbia-Presbyterian Medical Center (IOCPMC) from 1933 to 1970, among 163,948 patients examined only 3 cases of tuberculous infection of the conjunctiva that could be considered primary lesions were seen. In Table 8-1 reports

Table 8-1. Incidence of primary tuberculosis of the conjunctiva in various parts of the world*

Site of observations	Number of patients observed, incidence, or years covered	Number positive	Reported by
Baltimore Eye, Ear and Throat Charity Hospital, Baltimore, Maryland, USA	41,730	None	Bordley, 1902
Same	1870–1902	48	Bordley, 1902 (review of literature)
Guy's Hospital, London, England	1 in 3,200	29	Eyre and Durh, 1912
Finsen Institut, Copenhagen, Denmark	1909–1932	40	Blegvad, 1933; Lundsgaard, 1915
Seraphimer Hospital, Stockholm, Sweden	181,000 (1915–1934)	3	Samuelson, 1936
Oran, Algeria	60,000 (1936–1937)	2	Benalioua, 1938
Moscow Eye Clinic, Moscow, USSR	94,000	3	Ivanov, 1939
New York Eye and Ear Infirmary, New York, USA	30,000 per year for 20 years	None	Burchell, cited by Sitchevska and Sedan, 1947
Institute of Ophthalmology, Columbia-Presbyterian Medical Center, New York, USA	163,948 1933-1968	3	Bruce and Locatcher-Khorazo, 1947; Chandler and Locatcher-Khorazo, 1964; DeVoe and Locatcher-Khorazo, 1964

*This table presents only those studies containing information on frequency of disease. Individual case histories of primary tuberculosis of the eye are not included, except for Bordley's review.

from some other institutes of ophthalmology show equally small numbers of cases.

Primary tuberculous conjunctivitis occurs more often in children than in young adults and more frequently in females than in males. Such infection presumably is introduced into the eye by contaminated hands, fomites, or by exposure to dust or sputum particles containing tubercle bacilli. The patient sometimes mentions associated trauma. There is usually some fever with malaise; and the regional preauricular, submaxillary, and cervical lymph nodes become enlarged. This enlargement is in contrast to secondary infections of the eye, for in patients with some degree of immunity the adjacent lymphatic system is generally not grossly involved.

The first illustration of corneal tuberculosis is credited to Roy and Alvarez[28] (Fig. 8-2). The types of lesions produced in conjunctival tuberculosis are varied and are essentially the same as those listed by Sattler[30a,31] in 1874 and in 1891 and recorded by Duke-Elder.[12] Basically they are ulcerative or hyperplastic (nodular, hypertrophic, or polypoid). The *ulcerative* type is characterized by one or more small miliary ulcers, which may coalesce. They occur more often on the palpebral than on the bulbar conjunctiva. Tubercle bacilli may be recovered from the base of the ulcer. In severe cases the infection may spread to the cornea with pannus formation. Such lesions also may burrow through the thickness of the lid or penetrate the sclera. The *nodular* type shows the presence of small yellow or gray subconjunctival nodules, somewhat resem-

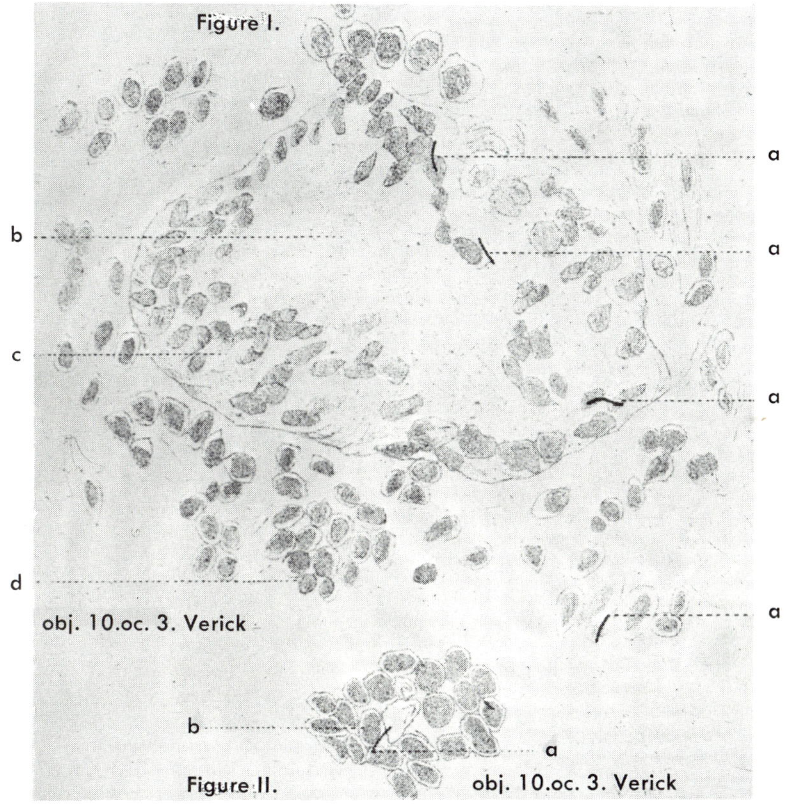

Fig. 8-2. A case of ulcerative tuberculosis of the cornea in a 4½-year-old girl. The corneal biopsy shown was taken about 8 months after the onset of symptoms. *a*, Tubercle bacilli; *b*, giant cell; *c*, numerous nuclei in a giant cell; *d*, round cells from infiltrated cornea. (From Roy, L., and Alvarez: Rev. Clin. Ocul. [Paris] **5**:187, 1885.)

bling granules of trachoma.[12] They tend to increase in size and become surrounded by follicles and granulation tissue. On histologic examination nodules prove to be miliary tubercles. The *hypertrophic* papillary type of conjunctival lesion is characterized by growth of granular tissue, usually developing from the fornices and associated with edema of the lids. In the fornices the granulations may become large, pedunculated, jellylike excrescences and may develop superficial ulcers. The *polypoid* type simulates a fibroma growing from the tarsal conjunctiva. On histologic examination a framework of connective tissue is found enclosing round cell infiltration with scattered giant cells containing tubercle bacilli. Bordley[4] reviewed the literature up to 1902 and assigned the cases to the categories described by Sattler.[31]

Table 8-2. Three cases of primary tuberculosis of the eye*

Special features of ocular disease	Other involvement	Course
Patient A: 9 years old, male September 1937: Painless swelling, right upper lid, for 9 days; shallow, indolent ulcer, upper tarsal conjunctiva; defined reddish margins; gray, sloughing base; surrounding follicles ulcerated; scraping from ulcer showed acid-fast bacilli, *M. bovis* cultured; positive tuberculin test; no history of previous exposure; x-ray films of chest, abdomen, and long bones negative[5]† (Plate 2, *G*)	Two enlarged preauricular lymph nodes, one ruptured, one incised at 5 months; tonsils removed in 4 years showed area of confluent tubercles	Treatment—irrigation with bland fluid; epithelium covered conjunctival lesion in 10 weeks; slow repair of lymph tissue; 9 years free of symptoms
Patient B: 10 years old, male March 1945: Painless swelling, lid of right eye, with mucous discharge; admitted in 2 months to another hospital; x-ray films of chest and abdomen negative; positive tuberculin test; biopsy of involved conjunctiva showed tuberculous lesions, acid-fast bacilli cultured; May 1945: admitted to the IOCPMC; yellowish granules on posterior surface of red and swollen right lid, also on bulbar conjunctiva near outer canthus; scraping and biopsy of swollen conjunctiva gave culture of *M. bovis*; histology typical of tuberculosis; intensive study gave no evidence of tuberculosis elsewhere except for local nodes[10] (Plate 2, *H*)	Concurrent with conjunctivitis, preauricular mass noted; submandibular gland enlarged 2 months later; preauricular node excised; tuberculous lesion	Conjunctivitis subsided over 6 month period; after 1½ years all lesions healed
Patient C: 11½ years old, female November 1961: Painless swelling, right upper lid; tearing "for a few days"; membranous tarsal conjunctivitis; scrapings negative for acid-fast organisms; in 2 weeks admitted to the IOCPMC; cobblestone papillae and small areas of ulceration; x-ray film of chest negative; positive tuberculin test; no known exposure to tuberculosis; 1 month later, scrapings and biopsy of conjunctiva showed acid-fast bacilli; *M. bovis* cultured; histologic examination of biopsy—tubercles, some with caseation, all with plasma cells, epithelioid cells, and Langhans' giant cells[6] (Plate 2, *I* and Fig. 8-3)	Concurrent with conjunctivitis, enlarged right preauricular node; subsequently mandibular node and right lateral glands of neck enlarged	PAS therapy started after biopsy; February 1962: conjunctival lesions healed; May 1962: submandibular and neck glands excised; 1963: patient doing well

*Patients seen at the IOCPMC.
†Superscript numbers refer to references at end of chapter.

Differential diagnosis of mycobacterial infection of the eye is usually difficult, since the lesion is variable and may simulate diseases such as Parinaud's syndrome, ophthalmia nodosa, trachoma, and others listed by Anhalt and his associates.[1] The difficult diagnostic situation is not helped by the infrequency with which tuberculous conjunctivitis is seen. The definitive diagnosis is made by identifying the mycobacterium.

In Table 8-2 three cases of primary tuberculosis of the conjunctiva seen at the IOCPMC are tabulated. Though the series is small, it represents several of the clinical and diagnostic features of this type of infection. All the patients were children under 12 years of age. The onset was insidious, since it was relatively painless. The patients did not present themselves for treatment until there was visible edema of the eyelid, and in each case the opinion was expressed that the condition had been present only a few days. But by the time the child had reached the ophthalmologist there was quite extensive involvement of the eye. Ulceration had taken place, and adjacent lymph nodes were enlarged. The mycobacterium was isolated, cultured, and typed in each instance. All three strains proved to be *M. bovis*. Even in the preantibiotic era the course of the disease under supportive treatment and surgical handling of the infected lymph nodes were satisfactory. The third patient received the usually highly effective general treatment with streptomycin and para-aminosalicylic acid (PAS).

It was quite unexpected to find that all three cases of primary tuberculosis of the eye seen at the IOCPMC were caused by *M. bovis*. This organism is most readily distinguished by its high pathogenicity for the rabbit, which is resistant to the human strain. A review of the literature has revealed a great sparsity of information about the type of tubercle bacillus found in primary lesions of the conjunctiva. Diagnosis was sometimes made only from acid-fast stains and histology. If the organism was grown and animal inoculation made, the

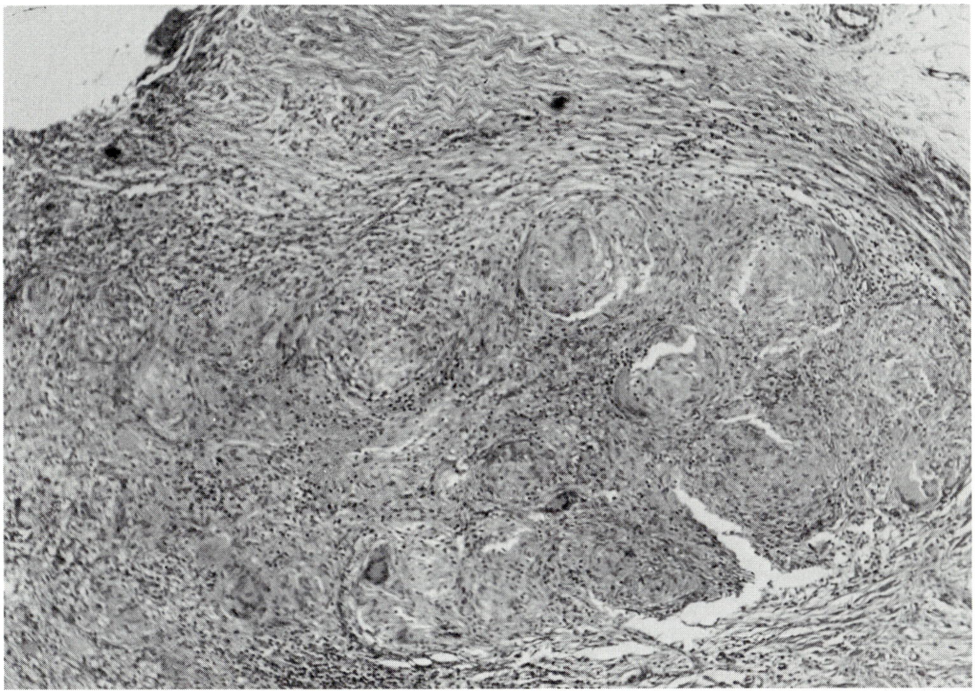

Fig. 8-3. Tubercles in conjunctival biopsy of lesion seen in Plate 2, *I*. Giant cells are evident. (From Chandler, A. C., Jr., and Locatcher-Khorazo, D.: Arch. Ophthal. 71:203, 1964.)

guinea pig was often the only animal tested. The guinea pig is equally susceptible to *M. hominis* and *M. bovis;* thus, such a test does not identify either. The following figures were obtained, however. Blegvad[3] reported 11 cases of primary tubercular conjunctivitis from the Finsen Institut; the mycobacteria were typed, and all were *M. bovis.* Samuelson[30] presented 3 cases of primary tuberculosis, one of which he was able to type. The infection was caused by *M. hominis.* Healy[16a] reported on 2 cases of primary tuberculosis of the conjunctiva, one of which was caused by *M. hominis* and one by *M. bovis.* Eadie[12a] reported 1 case caused by *M. hominis.* With the 3 cases from the IOCPMC, the totals are 15 cases caused by *M. bovis* and 3 by *M. hominis.* This data suggests that the eye of the child may be rather selectively susceptible to the bovine strain. More data on this point is needed.

SECONDARY TUBERCULOUS LESIONS OF THE EYE

Involvement of the eye, secondary to a primary tuberculous lesion elsewhere, may result from the manual introduction of the organism into the eye by the patient, extension of the disease from an adjoining area such as the skin or nasal passages in lupus vulgaris or the meninges in tuberculous meningitis, or from the dispersion of the bacteria via the bloodstream. In the latter situation any part of the eye may be infected (Table 8-3). The incidence of ocular involvement in a tuberculosis sanatorium, as reported by Donahue,[11] was 154 cases out of 10,524, or 1.4%, seen in the years 1940 to 1966.

Lupus vulgaris of the skin is thought to arise by direct inoculation of organisms into an abraded area. A subcutaneous tubercle is formed, which pushes to the surface. This is followed by proliferation of surrounding tubercles, leading to the formation of a lupus patch. When this occurs near the eye, the lids and the conjunctiva may become involved. The same type of evolution takes place in the mucous membranes of the conjunctiva. As in primary infections of the eye, the lesion is painless. The associated lupus tuberculosus of the skin indicates the correct diagnosis.

Miliary tuberculosis resulting from the spread of organisms through the bloodstream may seed tubercles in any part of the eye. Massaro and his co-workers[26] have

Table 8-3. Areas of the eye involved in tubercular infection

Orbit	Orbital abscess—extension from lacrimal gland or sinuses Periostitis—commonly involves tissues and bones of lateral orbital rim; painless red swelling
Lacrimal gland	Chronic dacryoadenitis
Eyelids	Primary lesions rare, but may be involved by extension from the skin
Conjunctiva	Conjunctivitis primary, or secondary to lesions elsewhere in the body
Cornea	Interstitial keratitis; deep (sclerosing) keratitis; corneal ulcer or abscess
Sclera	Proliferative ulcerative lesion; allergic exudative response
Iris	Iritis, a feature of tuberculous panuveitis
Ciliary body	Involved with iris and choroid in tuberculous panuveitis
Choroid	Infection most likely to occur with tuberculous meningitis or miliary tuberculosis, but may occur as only clinical manifestation of tuberculosis
Retina	Involved by contiguity with choroidal lesions; periphlebitis or exudative retinitis
Vitreous	Involved by retinal lesions (new blood vessels proliferate into vitreous with repeated hemorrhages)
Optic nerve	With tuberculous meningitis, optic neuritis not uncommon; also secondary to uveal and orbital lesions

recommended periodic mydriatic examination of the fundus of the eyes of patients with pulmonary tuberculosis. They describe 10 cases in which new choroidal tubercles were found, leading to the institution of therapy. According to Chapman and Whorton,[7] three fourths of 310 cases of acute generalized miliary tuberculosis, discovered at autopsy, had been missed clinically. Presumably a careful examination of the fundus would have corrected some of the missed diagnoses. This point has also been stressed by Olazábal.[27]

At the IOCPMC 2 cases of secondary ocular tuberculosis have been reported.[9,10] The first was in a 74-year-old man who in July 1962 became aware of pain and redness of the left eye. An "ulcer" of the sclera was cauterized elsewhere. In February 1963 the increasing ulceration of the sclera proximal to the limbus led to admission to another hospital where active pulmonary tuberculosis was diagnosed. Scrapings of the eye lesion did not show tubercle bacilli, nor were mycobacteria grown. Local treatment with steroids and atropine was given. In June 1963 the patient was admitted to the IOCPMC. At this time he was receiving PAS and isoniazid. A chest consultant considered the pulmonary condition clinically inactive. There was moderate edema of the lids and conjunctival injection of the left eye. The most striking finding was what appeared to be a large pigmented mass, 6 × 4 × 3 mm, herniating through a dehiscence in the sclera, which was absent except for a few remaining tags of tissue (Plate 3, *A*). Although long-term prognosis was poor, it appeared that an attempt should be made to repair the dehiscence. With the patient under general anesthesia, the conjunctiva was dissected free around the prolapsed uveal tissue. A large lamellar graft 15 × 20 mm was sutured into position. There were no unusual complications during the postoperative course. Acid-fast stains, cultures, and animal inoculation were made from conjunctival scrapings. Acid-fast bacilli were seen in the scrapings; cultures were positive; and guinea pig and rabbit inoculation identified the organism as *M. hominis*. The eye one year after the operation is shown in Fig. 8-4.

The second case was one of acute tuberculous panophthalmitis.[9] It is of particular interest because the primary lesion was discovered 40 years earlier in this 73-year-old man. The patient, first seen on February 4, 1966, had had pain and decreasing vision in the left eye during the previous 6 weeks. A diagnosis of granulomatous uveitis was made. Reactions to skin tests, including those using intermediate strength PPD,

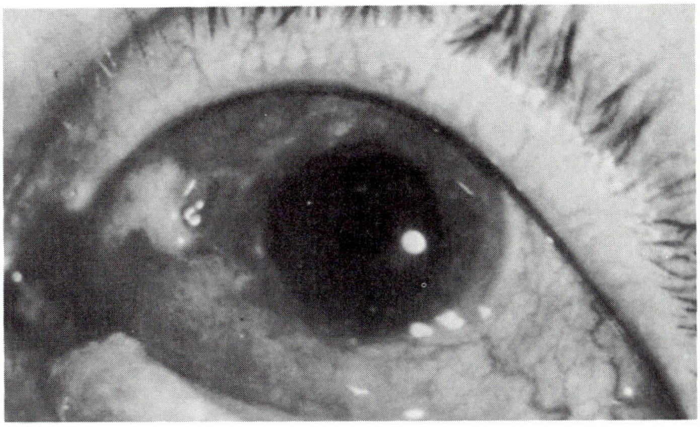

Fig. 8-4. Eye seen in Plate 3, *A* one year after operation. (From DeVoe, A. G., and Locatcher-Khorazo, D.: Trans. Amer. Ophthal. Soc. 62:209, 1964.)

Table 8-4. Ocular infections caused by atypical pathogenic mycobacteria

Lesion	History	Mycobacterium	Course	Reported by
Left eye, injection of cornea and sclera. Central corneal ulcer, 3 mm.	Piece of steel removed 5 months previously. Corneal ulcer treated with antibiotics and steroids for 3 months.	Scrapings negative for fungi. Sabouraud's agar, blood agar, thioglycollate broth, and Petragnani media inoculated. *M. fortuitum* isolated.	First treated with Chloromycetin, then amphotericin B until mycobacterium identified. Healed on streptomycin, followed by other antibiotics, in 3 months.	Turner and Stinson, 1965.
Right eye markedly injected and painful. Corneal ulcer, 2-3 mm, with margin of infiltrate two-thirds through cornea.	Piece of steel removed 6 months previously. Treatment with various antibiotics and steroids.	Cultures of scrapings for fungi and viruses. Diphtheroids cultured. Patient received lamellar corneal graft; from the removed corneal button *M. fortuitum* seen and identified.	Graft remained clear; one year later, right eye 20/50 + 2 vision, was painless, not injected.	Levenson and Harrison, 1966.
Right eye, limbal flush. Dense stromal corneal opacity 1 × 2 mm. Anterior chamber, trace of flare, 1+ cells.	Five weeks previously, struck by telephone cable in right eye. Minimal discomfort. No treatment.	Scrapings negative for fungi. Unclassified *Mycobacterium* group IV seen and isolated from corneal tissue on 21st hospital day.	Despite negative test reaction for fungi, antifungal treatment given, and lesion became worse. After organism identified, isoniazid, erythromycin, streptomycin therapy, later corticosteroids administered. Eye healed in 3 months.	Lauring, Wergeland, and Sack, 1969.
Necrotizing ulcer involving almost entire cornea, with hypopyon. (Patient seen in 1963.)	Eye believed to be end stage mycotic infection. Smear thought to show *Nocardia*. In 3 months eye had to be enucleated.	Culture of recovered organism identified as *M. fortuitum*. Thought to be nonpathogenic contaminant.	Enucleated eye diagnosed as having chronic keratitis. Six years later, after 2nd case, review of eye tissue showed many acid-fast bacilli.	Zimmerman, Turner, and McTigue, 1969.
Three weeks after keratoplasty, painful, inflamed eye. Antibiotics and steroids unsuccessful. Full-thickness graft after 4 months.	Continued inflammation. Patient transferred to Mt. Sinai Hospital, New York City.	Cultures taken prior to transfer identified as *M. fortuitum*. Keratectomy specimen, many acid-fast bacilli.	At Mt. Sinai Hospital, diagnosis of *M. fortuitum* confirmed. Mixed antibiotic treatment given. In 4 weeks lamellar graft sloughed, removed. No further deterioration.	Zimmerman, Turner, and McTigue, 1969. Wunsh, Boyle, Leopold, and Littman, 1969.

Table 8-4. Ocular infections caused by atypical pathogenic mycobacteria—cont'd

Lesion	History	Mycobacterium	Course	Reported by
Edema, scleral conjunctiva. Lower nasal quadrant of cornea, 4-5 mm epithelial defect.	Hit by piece of brick. Foreign body removed. After 6 weeks no improvement of persistent keratitis.	Gram-positive organism isolated, finally identified as *M. fortuitum*.	Initially treated as *Nocardia* infection. No improvement. When *M. fortuitum* recognized, PAS, isoniazid, and topical streptomycin treatment given.	Sexton, 1970.
Localized keratitis, outer one-third of left eye. Circle fibrin precipitate.	Foreign body acquired when using a grinder, removed some time previously from left eye.	Organism grown, *M. fortuitum*.	Same treatment as above successful.	

toxoplasmin, histoplasmin, blastomycin, and coccidioidin, were negative. The reaction to the test using brucellergen was "slightly positive." X-ray films of the chest showed fibrotic and fibrocalcific disease. Two weeks later exophthalmos of the left eye was noted. When the patient was admitted on February 27 for enucleation, the reaction to the tuberculin test was positive. The iris had become necrotic, and the corneal epithelium showed bullous elevation. Examination of the globe revealed a chorioretinal granuloma. There was necrosis of the overlying retina and inflammatory reaction in the vitreous. Areas of caseous necrosis were surrounded by lymphocytes, plasma cells, and giant cells. A large number of acid-fast bacilli were identified in the necrotic retina. The diagnosis was uveitis, scleritis, and orbital cellulitis specific to tuberculosis.

These two experiences with secondary tuberculosis of the eye seen at the IOCPMC give the extremes of ocular involvement; on the one hand, a localized and chronic lesion of conjunctiva and sclera; on the other, acute, rapidly progressing panophthalmitis. They illustrate the protein nature of pathology caused by *M. tuberculosis* and perhaps reinforce the plea of Massaro, Katz, and Sachs[26] for routine periodic examination of the fundus in cases of known tuberculosis.

ROLE OF ATYPICAL ACID-FAST BACTERIA IN OCULAR DISEASE

Several acid-fast bacteria have long been recognized as atypical mycobacteria.[14,18,20,29] They were formerly considered harmless saprophytes for man, although some were pathogenic for animals. Recent bacteriologic and clinical studies have shown that some of these mycobacteria may produce disease in man. The medical significance of these organisms and their classification may not yet be complete, but a tentative grouping offered by Runyon[29] in 1959 is currently widely accepted. Three of his four groups—I, III, and IV—contain bacteria that have caused human disease. One general infection caused by the Battey strain, group III has been reported to include infection of the orbit.[22a] Members of group IV have been reported in ocular disease. Table 8-4 summarizes data obtained from seven patients, six of whom had corneal ulcers from which *M. fortuitum*, a member of group IV, was isolated. An unclassified bacterium belonging to group IV was cultured from the corneal ulcer of the seventh patient.

The histories in each instance had some

common characteristics. The first of these was preceding trauma. Four patients had had foreign bodies removed from the cornea; one had been struck in the eye by a cable 3 to 5 months previously. Dr. Zimmerman's[38] first patient had come to him 6 years prior to the final infection with a lesion that resembled a crescentic laceration. Five years later the patient had an active dendritic ulcer. Two flare-ups with ulceration occurred at 4 month intervals. Eventually enucleation was necessary. Dr. Zimmerman's last patient developed intransigent inflammation 3 weeks after penetrating keratoplasty.

The second common characteristic of these infections was the failure to isolate immediately a recognized pathogenic organism. This led to treatment with a very wide spectrum of antibiotics and steroids. Four of the lesions were at one time suspected of being of fungal origin. Some of the difficulties of making an earlier bacteriologic identification of *M. fortuitum* in the patients reported in Table 8-4 probably were caused in some measure by the temperature for incubation, 36° C, and the use of Sabouraud's media, which is designed to favor only the growth of fungi. The cultural characteristics of *M. fortuitum* include rapid growth (2 to 5 days) on ordinary media and an optimum temperature for growth of about 25° C. The first culture obtained from Dr. Turner's[36] patient took 3 weeks to grow on Sabouraud's media, and the organisms were first identified as *Nocardia.* The first cultures from the patient of Dr. Levenson[22] (media not specified) grew diphtheroids. When the piece of cornea was cultured in thioglycollate broth and on blood agar, there was growth of a pleomorphic gram-positive rod resembling a diphtheroid. The Communicable Disease Center in Atlanta identified the organisms as *M. fortuitum.* Mycobacteria may resemble corynebacteria on Gram stain.

Dr. Lauring[21] had a similar experience. Organisms that grew on Sabouraud's media in 21 days were initially identified as *Nocardia.* Again the Communicable Disease Center, together with the National Jewish Hospital and Fitzsimons General Hospital in Denver, made the diagnosis of *Mycobacterium* group IV serotype II. Cultures from Dr. Zimmerman's first case were originally identified as *Nocardia* or *Actinomyces.* Again the Communicable Disease Center made the correct identification. *Nocardia* was also the original identification in Dr. Zimmerman's second case.

The histology of the lesions produced were similar and were reported as follows. Dr. Levenson reported "ulceration into the cornea stroma with a cellular infiltrate consisting of polymorphonuclear leukocytes and round cells in almost equal numbers and many slender pleomorphic bacilli with rounded ends . . . deep within the substantia propria." Dr. Lauring reported numerous bacilli in the corneal tissue and a stromal keratitis without abscess formation. The corneal tissue from Dr. Zimmerman's first patient showed a large area of corneal necrosis and inflammation with many typical beaded acid-fast bacilli present in the exudate. The iris temporally was densely infiltrated by lymphocytes and plasma cells. The keratectomy specimen from the second patient contained a deep ulcerated area with many polymorphonuclear leukocytes containing large numbers of acid-fast bacilli. In other areas of the eye additional similar microabscesses were seen.

The case histories of these 7 patients with infection caused by one of the group IV mycobacteria have been given in some detail because they pose an important differential diagnostic problem. These organisms are not sensitive to the drugs that are effective for the human and bovine strains of mycobacteria. Treatment of such cases requires knowledge of their specific sensitivities.

The question of the source of these bacteria is one that may also have some bearing on the origin of tuberculous infections of the eye. Chapman and Speight[8] have reported that of 458 samples of pasteurized milk sold in cartons, 2.8% contained mycobacteria, including *M. fortuitum* and others from group III. Harrington and Karlson[16] have raised the question as to whether the atypical mycobacteria as well as *M. tuberculosis* and *M. bovis* are always killed by pasteurization. They have shown that some of the atypical strains do survive this treatment. The 2 strains of *M. tuberculosis* and the 10 strains of *M. bovis* that they tested were killed by the treatment. This point becomes of special interest when the high incidence of bovine strains among the cases of primary tuberculosis of the eye is considered. Useful information would be obtained if possible sources of infection for all cases of primary ocular tuberculosis caused by the bovine strain were followed up.

Another practical diagnostic problem between infection by *M. hominis* or *M. bovis* and the atypical mycobacteria is the observation that there is crossing between tuberculins produced by *M. tuberculosis* and those derived from the atypical organisms.[9a] It may be that in some areas a large number of positive reactions to PPD are actually cross-reactions resulting from antibody response to atypical organisms. In evaluating the significance of a positive reaction to the tuberculin test one must thus realize that the positive reaction may not rule out one of the atypical mycobacteria as the causative agent of eye infection. Therefore such a reaction to the tuberculin test must not prevent looking for *M. fortuitum*.

SUMMARY

Primary tuberculosis of the eye that involves the cornea and conjunctiva is a rare disease today. It usually is unilateral only; the onset is insidious and painless; and, in contradistinction to mycotic infection, preceding trauma is often not mentioned. Lymph nodes contiguous to the involved eye become enlarged. Scrapings from the lesions usually will show acid-fast bacilli. In the 18 cases found where typing was carried out, 15 resulted from infection by *M. bovis*. The histology of the lesions is characteristic of typical tuberculous infection with infiltration of epithelioid cells and giant multinucleated cells, round cells, and scattered bacilli.

Secondary tuberculosis of the eye can be more difficult to diagnose when the lesions are not susceptible to direct culture and the primary disease is not recognized. Any or all parts of the eye may be involved. Sometimes the ophthalmologist may be the first to make the diagnosis of tuberculosis by seeing choroidal tubercles.

Differential diagnosis of infection caused by one of the atypical mycobacteria, notably *M. fortuitum*, may present an important problem because these latter organisms are not sensitive to the chemotherapeutic agents used for tuberculosis. The few infections with the atypical organisms so far reported have been associated with previous trauma and at one time in the course of determining the etiologic agent were considered as possibly caused by fungi. Biopsies of the lesions have proved most useful both for obtaining sufficient material to permit isolation and identification of the bacterium and for histologic evaluation. The lesions have shown many acid-fast organisms in fields filled with many polymorphonuclear neutrophils as well as mononuclear cells and no epithelioid or multinucleated giant cells.

REFERENCES

1. Anhalt, E. F., Zavell, S., Chang, G., and Bryon, M. H.: Conjunctival tuberculosis, Amer. J. Ophthal. **50**:265, 1960.
2. Benalioua: La primo-infection tuberculeuse de la conjonctive, Ann. Oculist. **175**:746, 1938.
3. Blegvad, O.: Fortgesetzte Untersuchungen über die Conjunctivaltuberkulose, Acta Ophthal. (Copenhagen) **14**:200, 1936.
4. Bordley, J.: Tuberculosis of the conjunctiva, Ophthal. Rec. **11**:368, 1902.
5. Bruce, G. M., and Locatcher-Khorazo, D.: Primary tuberculosis of the conjunctiva, Arch. Ophthal. **37**:375, 1947.
6. Chandler, A. C., Jr., and Locatcher-Khorazo, D.: Primary tuberculosis of the conjunctiva, Arch. Ophthal. **71**:202, 1964.
7. Chapman, C. B., and Whorton, C. M.: Acute generalized miliary tuberculosis in adults, New Eng. J. Med. **235**:239, 1946.
8. Chapman, J. S., and Speight, M.: Isolation of atypical mycobacteria from pasteurized milk, Amer. Rev. Resp. Dis. **98**:1052, 1968.

9. Darrell, R. W.: Acute tuberculous panophthalmitis, Arch. Ophthal. **78**:51, 1967.
9a. Davis, B. D., Dulbecco, R., Eisen, H. N., Ginsberg, H. S., and Wood, W. B., Jr.: Microbiology, New York, 1967, Harper and Row, Publishers, p. 863.
10. DeVoe, A. G., and Locatcher-Khorazo, D.: The external manifestations of ocular tuberculosis, Trans. Amer. Ophthal. Soc. **62**:203, 1964.
11. Donahue, H. C.: Ophthalmologic experience in a tuberculosis sanatorium, Amer. J. Ophthal. **64**:742, 1967.
12. Duke-Elder, S.: System of ophthalmology. Diseases of the outer eye, vol. 8, part 1, St. Louis, 1965, The C. V. Mosby Co., pp. 212-225.
12a. Eadie, S.: Primary tuberculosis of the conjunctiva treated with streptomycin and PAS, Brit. J. Ophthal. **38**:568, 1954.
13. Eyre, J. W. H., and Durh, M. S.: Tuberculosis of the conjunctiva, its etiology, pathology and diagnosis, Lancet **2**:1319, 1912.
14. Furguson, S. H., Prather, E. C., and Mayfield, C. L.: Clinically significant Mycobacteria, Southern Med. J. **63**:318, 1970.
15. Gordon, B. L.: Ocular and general tuberculosis, Hebrew Med. J. **2**:322, 1963.
16. Harrington, R., Jr., and Karlson, A. G.: Destruction of various kinds of Mycobacteria in milk by pasteurization, Appl. Microbiol. **13**:494, 1965.
16a. Healy, J. J.: Two cases of exogenous tuberculosis conjunctivitis displaying Parinaud's conjunctivo-adenitis syndrome, Trans. Ophthal. Soc. U. K. **66**:455, 1946.
17. Ivanov, N. K.: Tuberculosis of the conjunctiva, Vestn. Oftal. **14**(5):24, 1939.
18. Jawetz, E., Melnick, J. L., and Adelberg, E. A.: Review of medical microbiology, ed. 9, Los Altos, Calif., 1970, Lange Medical Publications, p. 186.
19. Koch, R.: Die Aetiologie der Tuberculose, Berl. Klin. Wschr. **19**:221, 1882.
20. Kubica, G. P., and Dye, W. E.: Laboratory methods for clinical and public health mycobacteriology, U. S. Department of Health, Education and Welfare Public Service, 1967.
21. Lauring, L. M., Wergeland, F. L., and Sack, G. E.: Anonymous mycobacterium keratitis, Amer. J. Ophthal. **67**:130, 1969.
22. Levenson, D. S., and Harrison, C. H.: Mycobacterium fortuitum corneal ulcer, Arch. Ophthal. **75**:189, 1966.
22a. Levine, R. A.: Infection of the orbit by an atypical mycobacterium, Arch. Ophthal. **82**:608, 1969.
23. Lloyd, R. I.: Tuberculosis of the conjunctiva, Amer. J. Ophthal. **13**:753, 1930.
24. Lundsgaard, K. K. K.: Die sogenanate primäre Konjunktivaltuberkulose und die Konjunktivaltuberkulose bei Lûpuspatienten, Klin. Mbl. Augenheilk. **55**:97, 1915.
25. Manz, W.: Tuberculose des Choriodea, Graefes Arch. Ophth. **4**:120, 1858.
26. Massaro, D., Katz, S., and Sachs, M.: Choroidal tubercles: a clue to hematogenous tuberculosis, Ann. Intern. Med. **60**:231, 1964.
27. Olazábal, F., Jr.: Choroidal tubercles: a neglected sign, J.A.M.A. **200**:374, 1967.
28. Roy, L., and Alvarez: Observation chinique de bacille de la tuberculose, dans la cornée, Rev. Clin. Ocul. (Paris) **5**:185, 1885.
29. Runyon, E. H.: Anonymous Mycobacteria in pulmonary disease, Med. Clin. N. Amer. **43**:273, 1959.
30. Samuelson, A.: Primary tuberculosis of the conjunctiva, Arch. Ophthal. **15**:975, 1936.
30a. Sattler, H.: Tubercular ulceration of the conjunctiva, J. Med. Sci. **68**:276, 1874.
31. Sattler, H.: Ueber die Behandlung de verschiedenen Formen der Conjunctivaltuberculose mit Tuberculin nebst experimentellen Untersuchungen über die Wirkung desselben, Ber. (21 Versammlung der) Ophth. Ges. **27**:33, 1891.
31a. Sexton, R. R.: Mycobacterium fortuitum infection of the cornea. In Polack, F. M.: Corneal and external diseases of the eye, Springfield, Ill., 1970, Charles C Thomas, Publisher, p. 25.
32. Sitchevska, O., and Sedam, M.: Primary tuberculosis of the conjunctiva, Arch. Ophthal. **30**:196, 1943.
33. Smith, G. E., and Dawson, W. R.: Egyptian mummies, New York, 1924, The Dial Press.
34. Smith, T.: A comparative study of bovine tubercle bacilli and of human bacilli from sputum, J. Exp. Med. **3**:451, 1898.
35. Steinbach, M. M.: Mycobacteria: the tubercle bacilli and tuberculosis. In Gay, F. P.: Agents of disease and host resistance, Springfield, Ill., 1935, Charles C Thomas, Publisher.
36. Turner, L., and Stinson, I.: Mycobacterium fortuitum as a cause of corneal ulcer, Amer. J. Ophthal. **60**:329, 1965.
36a. Veith, I.: This long disease, my life—postscript to "HE," Perspect. Biol. Med. **15**:110, 1971.
37. Wunsh, S. E., Boyle, G. L., Leopold, I., and Littman, M. L.: Mycobacterium fortuitum infection of corneal graft, Arch. Ophthal. **82**:602, 1969.
38. Zimmerman, L. E., Turner, L., and McTigue, J. W.: Mycobacterium fortuitum infection of the cornea: a report of two cases, Arch. Ophthal. **82**:596, 1969.

9

Ocular leprosy

JAMES H. ALLEN AND MARGARET BRAND

Leprosy is the oldest recorded disease of mankind.[26] In ancient cultures the visible features of the disease, its chronicity, and its incurability, coupled with lack of exact information on its mode of transmission, resulted in fear and superstition. From time to time many afflictions have been thought to be retribution for moral transgression, but leprosy has been unique in the intensity, ubiquity, and persistence of this superstition. In ancient India it was thought to be a curse of the gods. In China it was spoken of as "T'ien Ying," meaning "Retribution from Heaven."[29] The disease remains a great challenge to every branch of medicine, for in spite of the progress that medicine has made in general, leprosy presents many unsolved problems.

HISTORY

There has been much controversy regarding the origin of leprosy. Disease presumed to be leprosy was described in the Bible,[4,20] in the Susruth Samhita (India, approximately 600 BC), and in Chinese medical writings between 500 and 300 BC.[30] These writings infer much older awareness of the disease, although it is now agreed that a number of skin diseases and other afflictions were included. Nevertheless, fairly clear concepts of the disease seem to have emerged in the Middle East and the Orient by the second or third century before Christ. Pascha, quoted by Cochrane,[10] felt that the cradle of leprosy was ancient India, for sacred Sanskrit manuscripts mentioned leprosy. Pascha believed the disease spread from India to Egypt where conditions were favorable for its development. Baron,[6] in his recent publication *Man Against Germs*, stated: "Slowly the [leprosy] germs migrated to the West. They moved along the caravan routes through Persia, crossed the rivers Tigris and Euphrates, passed through mysterious Chaldea and sinful Babylon, traveled over the sands of the Syrian desert, over the Jordan through Canaan and the Wilderness of Shur into the Land of Goshen in ancient Egypt."* Thus the signs of leprosy became a part of the Old Testament, and they were described in Egyptian papyri written 5,000 years or more before the birth of Christ.

With the development of better communications and trade and of movements of armies and immigrants, the disease was introduced in various periods of time to every continent. As may be observed on the map (Fig. 9-1), the greatest incidence of leprosy now lies between the fortieth

*From the book *Man Against Germs* by A. L. Baron. Decorations by Doris Baron. Copyright © 1957 by A. L. Baron. Published by E. P. Dutton and Co., Inc. and used with their permission.

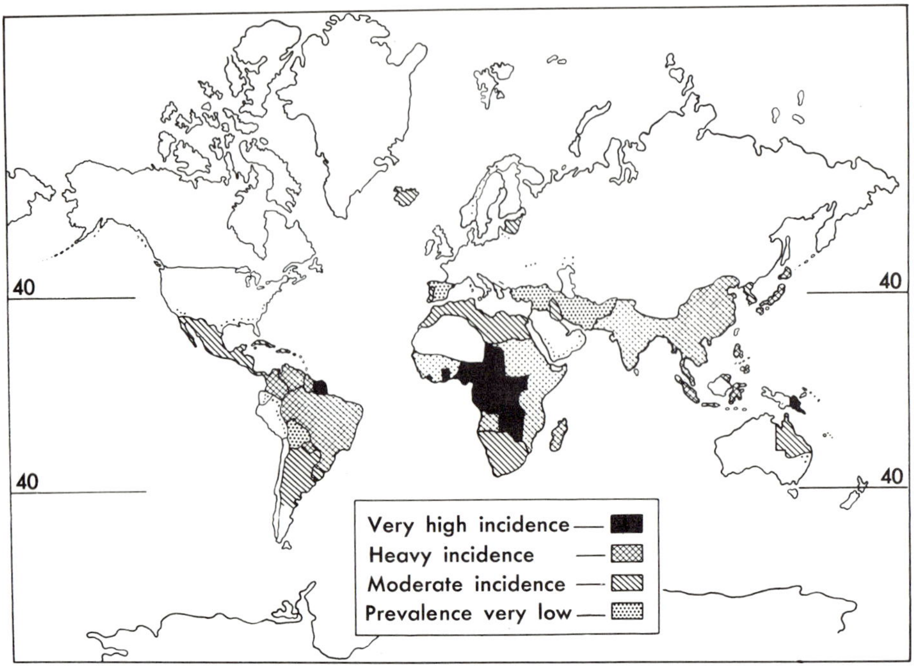

Fig. 9-1. Distribution of leprosy. (Adapted from Rogers, L., and Muir, E.: Leprosy, ed. 3, Baltimore, 1946, The Williams and Wilkins Co.)

parallels. Africa and Asia are the continents most affected. According to Holmes,[15] over 5,000,000 people are affected with leprosy throughout the world. A more accurate estimate probably is close to 10,000,000, and in the United States recent estimates vary from 5,000 to 10,000 cases. Apparently the disease was introduced into Mexico during the sixteenth century, and it is possible that leprosy spread into the part of this country that formerly belonged to Mexico. However, the earliest available reference to the disease within our present boundaries are to be found in Roman's *Concise Natural History of East and West Florida,* published in 1776. Therefore, leprosy has existed in the United States for more than 200 years, and it now is endemic in Florida, Louisiana, Texas, California, and Hawaii. It is interesting, as Cochrane[10] stated, that there is no evidence of leprosy among Eskimos.

The manner in which patients with leprosy were formerly treated, according to Badger,[4] "is not one of which we can be proud, generally they did not have a place to go. They were hounded from place to place, were isolated at the outskirts of the cities or in huts; in the woods . . . there were no institutions where they could go for treatment." Although a leprosarium had been established during the latter part of the nineteenth century in Louisiana, it was not until March 25, 1916, that Senator Ransdell presented a "Bill to Provide for the Care and Treatment of Persons afflicted with Leprosy and to Prevent the Spread of Leprosy in the United States" on a national scale. This bill became law, and in 1921 the National Leprosarium was established.

ETIOLOGY

Leprosy usually is prevalent in tropical and subtropical countries, and the incidence is greater in humid and moist countries where the rainfall is heavy. However, factors other than climate, such as poor personal hygiene and unsanitary and overcrowded living conditions, may be more important in accounting for the prevalence of the disease, for Iceland and Norway also have had large numbers of patients.

The causative agent of leprosy is an acid-fast bacillus that was originally observed by Hansen in 1873 to 1874 in Norway. Hansen[14] had seen this organism as early as 1868 in unstained scrapings of tissues from leprous lesions. When he used osmic acid for staining, he was able to demonstrate the bacilli clearly. Neisser[14] in 1879 also found the organisms in tissue sections, using fuchsin and gentian violet stains. All of Koch's postulates have not been fulfilled, since the organism cannot be cultivated nor can animals be infected;[31] however, the bacilli are considered the cause of leprosy because they are constantly present in the leprous lesions, in some instances in enormous numbers, and because there is a characteristic cellular reaction about them.

Hansen's bacillus belongs to the genus *Mycobacterium* and closely resembles the other pathogen in this genus. The organisms vary in size measuring from 1.5 to 8μ in length and 0.2 to 0.5μ in width. Some appear straight, some curved, some lie parallel to each other. Some stain solidly, but others show beading with bipolar staining. In the early stage of the disease, intracellular and extracellular masses of the bacilli adhere closely to each other, forming large bunches —"cigar bundles"—appearing in glomerations known as globi, which actually consist of tightly packed bacilli enclosed in capsular matter (Plate 3, *B*). The *Mycobacterium leprae* stains deeply and brilliantly with carbol fuchsin and resists decolorization. However, the results of the acid-fast stain may show unevenness, and some of the granular appearance may be explained on this basis. With metachromatic stains, beading and granules are observed.

Brieger[7] studied the structure *M. leprae* with the electron microscope. Since the tissues from which this material was obtained contained dead as well as living bacteria, he felt it was not possible to be certain of the appearance of a healthy organism. The bacilli rarely were found in the process of division, but some of them occasionally showed branching. In material from treated and untreated patients, the structure of the bacilli presented great variation. Many of the bacilli in sections of lepromatous nodules had lost their structure.

An interesting feature of *M. leprae* is that since its discovery, in spite of many attempts toward its propagation on a variety of artificial media, in tissue culture, in symbiosis with other organisms, and at varying temperatures, it still has never been grown. Also, attempts to transmit the disease to man[19] or to various animals with infected leprous material from human lesions have failed. However, Shepard[28] has shown that *M. leprae* can multiply to a limited extent in the footpads of mice but fail to exhibit gross signs of invasiveness. This has been confirmed by Rees[24] and by Janssens and Patlyn.[16]

The chief sites of infection are the skin, mucous membranes, and peripheral nerves. Clinical manifestations are a result of the lodgement and multiplication of the organisms in tissues and of the reaction by the host to such invasion. It is interesting that the human body has the capacity to harbor large numbers of the organisms for many years without ill effect. It may require months or years and additional stresses and strains before the resistance is broken and symptoms appear (Badger[5]). Therefore, it is not surprising that the exact incubation period in leprosy—the time interval before the infection causes disease in the individual—is not known and that it may be measured by years rather than by months or days. Rogers and Muir[26] cite Marchoux's case of a young surgeon who, while operating on a patient with leprosy, accidentally pricked his finger and developed leprosy some 8 or 9 years later. In contrast, Muir[20] observed leprosy in a 3-month-old child. Variable periods of incubation in leprosy have been recorded by a number of observers. Muir[20] considers that the average incubation period is about 3½ years and that the patient, if young, will be unable to remember the time of contact. The duration of the incubation period can be of great importance, since it may determine the source of the infection in an individual patient.

There still is uncertainty concerning transmission of Hansen's disease, although it is the oldest known infection. Prolonged and close association with someone known to have the disease is considered unwise, and yet minimal precautions seem to be adequate to prevent the infection. There is evidence that males are more susceptible than females; and in endemic areas, children and young adults are more susceptible to the infection than the middle-aged and elderly. This age difference in susceptibility is more striking in the case of leprosy than in the case of tuberculosis.

There is no simple technique to determine the presence of the leprosy bacillus in the body. The organisms may be found by acid-fast stains in large numbers in the nasal secretion even where there are no visible external signs of disease. Bacilli may be found in the dermal pulp scraped from shallow skin incisions or in material from ulcerations. Ulcerated nodules may discharge the organisms from the throat when one coughs and sneezes. The bacilli from the saliva may be swallowed and passed in the stools. Testicles, semen, and urine may contain them, as may the milk of the nursing mother. The bacilli may reach the sensory nerves from the skin or from the bloodstream. *M. leprae* may spread through the bloodstream to all parts of the body. The central nervous system is almost never invaded, perhaps because of the absence of Schwann cells, cells in which the bacilli frequently may be detected. In the severe type of leprosy the organisms are present in great numbers in the nose, mouth, skin, and upper respiratory passages and usually are increased when ulceration occurs, suggesting that the infection may occur by droplet transmission from the nose and the month as is common in tuberculosis; but, the actual pathways by which *M. leprae* enters and infects the various organs is not known.

Conclusive evidence that *M. leprae* can produce immunity is not yet available. Natural resistance to infection is present; and among different individuals exposed to infection, some acquire it, whereas others escape the disease. Rogers and Muir[26] were of the opinion that, as in tuberculosis, resistance to leprosy may be terminated by either massive or repeated infection, whereas slight infections may increase the resistance. The leprous individual may exhibit false-positive Wassermann, VDRL, and STS reactions, but reaction to the TPI test remains negative unless the patient also has syphilis. Similarly, reaction to the tuberculin test remains negative unless the individual has developed sensitivity to the tubercle bacillus. So far specific antibodies have not been demonstrated, nor is there evidence that *M. leprae* can produce general immunity. However, in 1919 Mitsuda discovered that intradermal injection of lepromin, a suspension of heat-killed *M. leprae* mixed with finely ground human skin, produced an intense inflammatory reaction, sometimes with ulceration, reaching a peak in about 3 weeks in patients with tuberculoid leprosy, but produced no visible reaction in patients with lepromatous leprosy. Later, Fernandez in 1940 reported that the late positive (Mitsuda) reaction usually was preceded by an early tuberculinlike response (Fernandez reaction) consisting of an area of erythema and edema at the site of injection 24 to 48 hours after injection. Although these tests are of no diagnostic value, experience has shown that reaction to the lepromin test is positive in individuals who have a strong biologic defense against leprosy and who develop tuberculoid or related forms of the disease.

Other immunologic studies[8] have shown that IgG, IgA, and IgM levels were significantly elevated in the sera of lepromatous patients, but serum levels in tuberculoid patients were not significantly different from control values. Serum levels of IgG and

IgA generally remained elevated even with prolonged therapy, whereas IgM levels tended to decline significantly with treatment in lepromatous leprosy. In reactional states in patients who had been treated for longer than 24 months, serum levels of IgA were unusually high.

Summary

It appears that since the discovery of *M. leprae,* the studies on leprosy have been hampered by the failure both to cultivate the bacilli and to transmit the disease to experimental animals. Very little is known about the incubation period or the mode of infection. *M. leprae* is able to live in tissues in enormous numbers for many years without producing overt disease.

CLINICAL TYPES OF LEPROSY

Clinically, leprosy may be classified as the lepromatous, tuberculoid, or dimorphous variety, although it may begin and exist for a time in an indeterminate type.

The *indeterminate* type consists of papules or pink or pale macules that have not developed sufficient character to permit differentiation into the usual varieties. The macule, usually single, commonly appears on the forehead as a circumscribed, nonelevated, hypopigmentation or hyperpigmentation exhibiting loss of sensation of cold, heat, and touch, usually in that order. The histologic appearance on biopsy of one of these lesions is that of small strands or groups of cells consisting of lymphocytes and macrophagic histiocytes with an occasional plasma cell, eosinophil, basophil, or polymorphonuclear leukocyte around the pilosebaceous system of the dermis and the nerve fibers and blood and lymph vessels, passing down toward the subcutis. Bacilli are few in number or may not be found. Reaction to the lepromin test may be weakly positive or negative. These lesions usually are precursors of tuberculoid or lepromatous leprosy but may develop into the dimorphous variety.

Lepromatous leprosy represents minimal resistance to the occurrence, multiplication, and dissemination of leprae bacilli, which are readily demonstrable individually or as

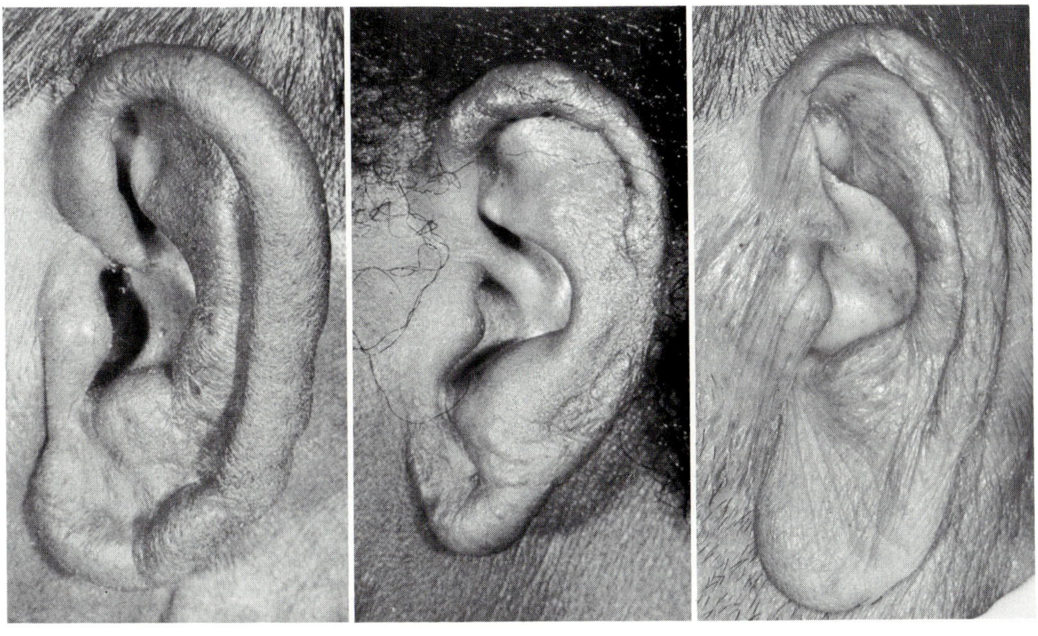

A B C

Fig. 9-2. Lepromatous nodules of the ear, **A**, **B**, and typical pendulous lobe, **C**.

A

B

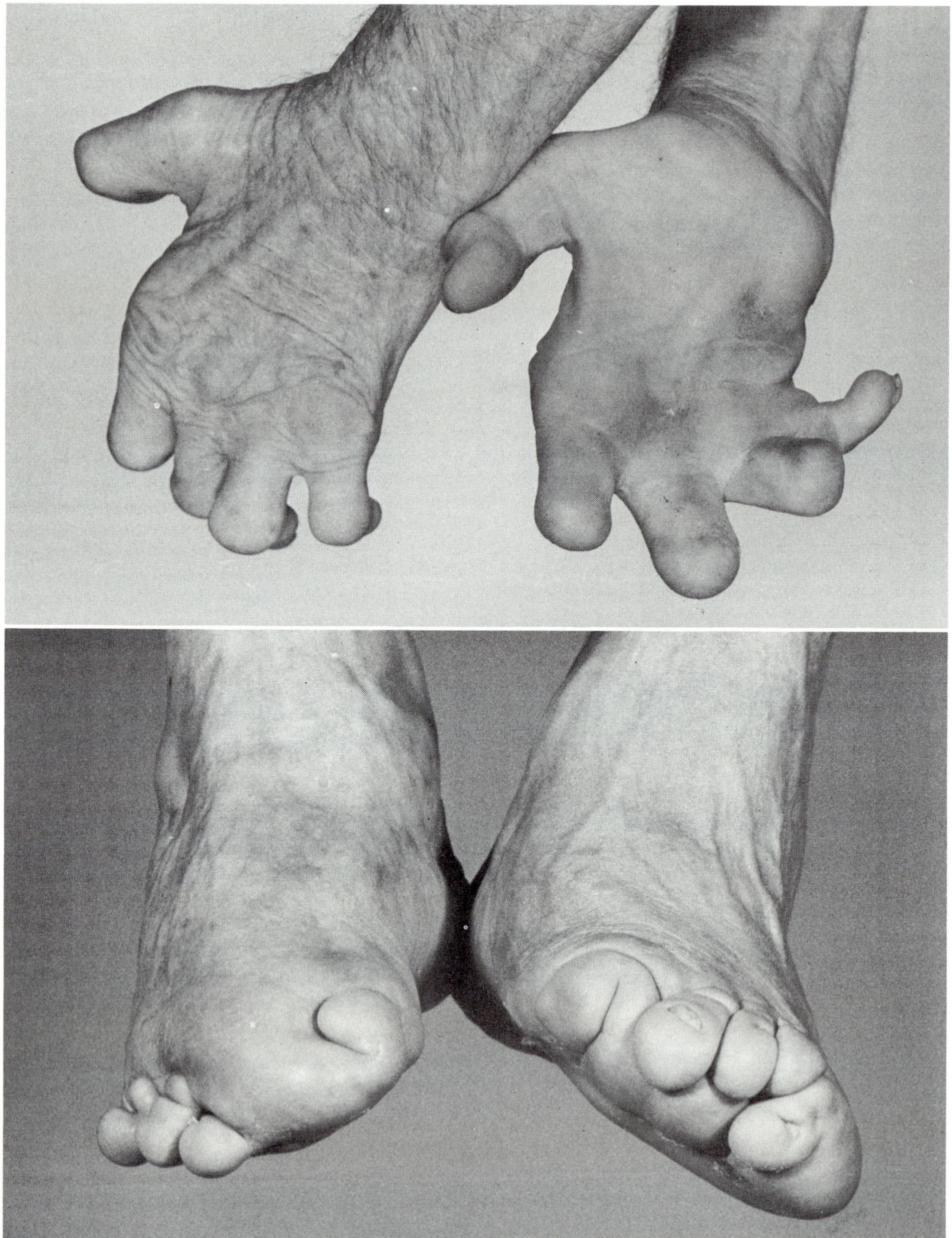

Fig. 9-3. Typical atrophic absorption of the distal phalanges.

globi in scrapings from skin and mucosa and in sections of lesions. Macular lesions of lepromatous leprosy begin as multiple, small, indistinctly marginated variations in the color of the skin and are symmetrically distributed over the whole body. They show no loss of sensation but become more erythematous and shiny in time. In some patients the macular lesions are so indefinite as to escape notice until infiltration of the skin occurs, producing either diffuse or nodular lepromatous lesions. The skin becomes infiltrated and thickened with exaggeration of the natural folds, which occasionally leads to the appearance of leonine facies. Infiltration around hair follicles causes loss of hair, especially of the brows, beginning in the outer halves. Cutaneous and subcutaneous nodules commonly develop on the brows, nose, chin, lobes and helices of the ears (Fig. 9-2), elbows buttocks, and knees. Infiltration of the mucosa also occurs especially in the nose where small punctate ulcers tend to develop especially on the septum, resulting in epistaxis. When it occurs, however, destruction of the nasal septum probably is secondary. The larynx occasionally is involved, reducing the voice to a whisper, and in some instances obstruction to respiration may require tracheotomy. Testicular involvement is followed by scarring and atrophy, but no serious involvement of the ovaries has been reported. Gynecomastia occurs frequently in older males. The bone marrow is invaded, and the distal phalanges undergo atrophic absorption (Fig. 9-3). Other lesions include rarefaction of bone and secondary osteitis, periosteitis, and osteomyelitis.

Microscopically, lepromatous leprosy is an extension of the cellular reaction described in the indeterminate stage. Groups and strands of lymphocytes and mononuclear cells are found around hair follicles, sweat glands, and sebaecous glands. The histiocytes are increased in numbers and have a foamy appearance because the pale-staining cytoplasm contains numerous vacuoles that contain leprosy bacilli. These cells are called foam cells, or lepra cells of Virchow. With time, some of these foam cells coalesce and form multinucleate giant foam cells with coalescense of the lipoid material, bacilli, and cellular debris to form globi. Later, large areas of dermis may be transformed into continuous masses of chronic inflammatory tissue with groups of mononuclear cells and plasma cells and containing large numbers of lepra cells packed with lepra bacilli. Bacilli also are found in the Schwann cells as well as in and between nerve fibers in this form of leprosy.

Tubercloid leprosy apparently represents high resistance to the occurrence, multiplication, and dissemination of the bacilli that are found with some difficulty in peripheral nerves and rarely in skin scrapings except during reactional states. The early lesion of the skin is a patch or macule with impaired sensation followed by hypopigmentation or erythema (Fig. 9-4). The typical tuberculoid lesion, or lepride, is raised and sharply marginated, with a pebbly surface, and extends by centrifugal spread, followed by atrophic changes and loss of sweating (Fig. 9-5). Basically, the lesion is an epithelioid cell reaction with giant cells of the Langhans type.

The central nervous system is not involved, but the peripheral nerves supplying the extremities are always affected in

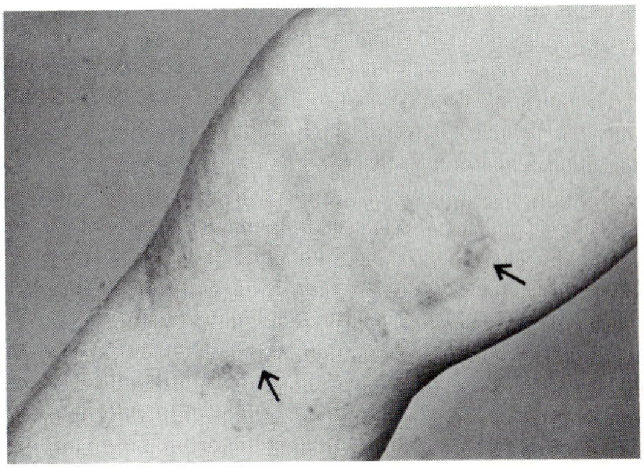

Fig. 9-4. Tuberculoid macule showing central hypopigmentation.

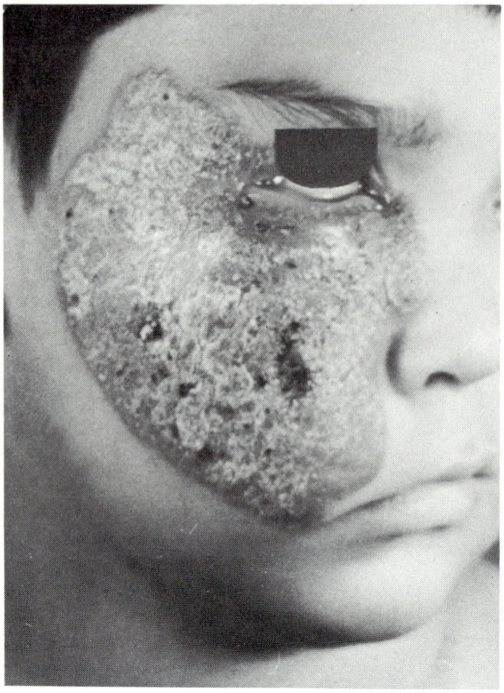

Fig. 9-5. Lepride showing typical pebbly surface and sharp margin.

advanced cases of both types of leprosy. The fine cutaneous nerves in the lesions are invaded, and ulnar, median, peroneal, posterior tibial, and auricular nerves often are enlarged and palpable. In lepromatous lesions the bacilli are in all parts of the nerve fibers and lepromas may develop within the nerve, whereas in the tuberculoid type an intense epithelioid reaction involves the nerve but bacilli are scarce. In either type, peripheral nerve involvement is followed frequently by atrophy and contracture of the muscles, associated with decalcification of the bones especially in the fingers and toes, the phalanges of which may be completely absorbed.

Polyneuritis occurs in both types but appears earlier and is more severe in tuberculoid leprosy. Numbness and tingling in an extremity may be the initial complaint.

The *dimorphous* variety has definite clinical and histologic characteristics of both lepromatous and tubercloid leprosy. The dimorphous macular lesion most commonly starts on the outer aspect of the thigh and is hypopigmented and anesthetic, with diffuse and ill-defined borders. Then for a few months or longer, multiple macular lesions appear in symmetrical distribution. Some are large with sharply defined edges; others are small with indistinct edges. The larger lesions have a dry surface with loss of light touch and thermal sensation, whereas the small ones show mixed features. The lesions are scattered symmetrically all over the body, some being larger with numerous smaller ones in between. They have indistinct borders, with the infiltration increasing centrally so that the most prominent part of the lesion is in the center, or in some cases in which healing has occurred centrally, the most prominent part is well within the spreading edge. This characteristic is in direct contrast to tuberculoid lesions, in which the edges are sharp and prominent. The superficial nerves are enlarged; the lepromin reaction is variable, being either negative or weakly positive; the histopathologic features also are mixed; however, there always is a free subepidermal zone. In some lesions the reaction, like that of tuberculoid leprosy, predominantly is lymphocytic, with epithelioid cells and giant cells frequently arranged in a focal manner. But in others that resemble lepromatous lesions the predominant cell is the macrophagic histiocyte, which develops into the foam cell of Virchow; but there are also some epithelioid cells and an occasional Langhans type of giant cell.

Reactions occur in the course of the disease and can be divided into two major categories: acute exacerbation and lepra reaction, or erythema nodosum leprosum.

Acute exacerbations may occur in any type of leprosy in preexisting lesions. The most prominent histologic feature common to all types of acute exacerbation is edema, but the other features vary with the variety of leprosy. In the lepromatous variety there often is an increase in bacterial activity along with extension of the preexisting clinical lesions. In some instances the exacerbation may represent a change from the indeterminate or dimorphous variety to the lepromatous or tuberculoid form of the disease. Generally, acute inflammatory cells are present, and even in the tuberculoid reaction there may be an increase in bacilli. But at times in pure tuberculoid leprosy there is an increase in edema in an epithelioid cell infiltrate but without bacilli. These reactions usually revert back to the more chronic phases of lepromatous or tuberculoid leprosy; however, the great danger from tuberculoid exacerbations is from increased nerve involvement and destruction.

The *lepra reaction* is an acute or subacute reaction that develops only in lepromatous leprosy and is thought by many to be a sensitization phenomenon of an allergic or anaphylactoid type to released components of the degenerated or dead bacilli. There usually are systemic symptoms as well as increased reaction in preexisting local lesions of the skin, eye, and other organs; however, the local reactions may develop where there has been no clinically apparent lesion. There are three specific lepra reactions; erythema nodosum leprosum, erythema multiforme, and erythema necroticans.

Erythema nodosum leprosum and erythema multiforme clinically resemble their like-named dermatologic counterparts but have distinctly different histologic characteristics. The reaction involves the mid and lower dermis, often extending into the subcutaneous tissue. A neutrophilic infiltrate is superimposed upon the usual lepromatous lesions. However, these cells tend to disintegrate in a few days as lymphocytes and plasma cells appear and increase in number. Vasculitis is frequent, and edema is a constant feature. Bacilli are decreased in number, especially the solid-staining forms, which may disappear completely. Fragmentation and disruption of elastic fibers and collagen in the dermis is frequent. In severe forms of the lepra reaction, a necrotizing vasculitis and fibrinoid degeneration of the vessel wall and perivascular tissues often is associated with dermal and epidermal necrosis and microabscess formation.

Erythema necroticans, or the Lucio phenomenon, is a special form of lepra reaction generally found in Central America and Mexico, in which patients without distinct skin lesions develop purple spots with scabbing on the extremities. Many of these lesions develop blisters and ulceration. In addition, they show a diffuse lepromatus infiltration of the skin, especially of the face and extremities. Histologically, there are two main types of lesions: one shows an intense neutrophilic and histiocytic infiltration into the dermis, with a severe, usually necrotizing, vasculitis of vessels larger than capillaries and of small arterioles; whereas in the more classical type there is dilation, necrosis, and thrombosis of capillaries and of larger vessels, especially in the lower dermis. In both of these severe forms the epidermis shows patches of depigmentation, degeneration, necrosis, and eventual sloughing. Numerous beaded bacilli may be found in the lesions.

OCULAR MANIFESTATIONS OF LEPROSY

Involvement of the eye rarely is a primary manifestation of leprosy; but few advanced cases, especially of lepromatous leprosy, fail to show some type of involvement of the eye or its adnexa. Ocular manifestations frequently occur in an insidious manner; therefore, Choyce[9] and Allen and Byers[2] have suggested that the eyes of patients with leprosy should be examined routinely. The relatively low incidence of ocular manifestations of infection reported in earlier studies might be because of the fact that observations of the eye were limited to gross examination. When slit-lamp biomicroscopy is applied, ocular involvements such as keratitis and iritis can be detected much earlier. Pillat[22] was the first to record the distinctive beading of corneal nerves viewed with the slit-lamp biomicroscope. Allen and Byers[2] advised the periodic repeated use of this instrument for the recognition of early corneal leprosy.

Elliot[12] made observations on the relationship of the usual time of appearance of clinical manifestations of ocular disease to the probable duration of the general disease. He concluded that the latent period varied for specific areas of the eye as much as 5 to 25 years or more. More recent observations tend to confirm the time ratio for ocular involvement in general, but these observations require modification of the details and also indicate that there may be considerable difference between the time of localization of bacilli in ocular tissues and the development of clinical signs of infection of those tissues.

Direct extension from infected adjacent skin was thought at one time to be the most common route by which the eye becomes infected with *M. leprae,* and it still may be a factor. Extension along the nerve fibers is considered the primary route of spread by some observers; however, the hematogenous route is probably the more important.

Whereas the diagnosis of the general disease is confirmed by skin biopsy, the diagnosis of ocular leprosy usually is based upon clinical findings. Skin scrapings from the lobes of the ear or from other sites, as well as biopsies of suspected lesions stained by Ziehl-Neelsen or Fite stains, may reveal acid-fast bacilli. In the lepromatous type of the disease, bacilli and globi are numerous, but in the tuberculoid type few or no bacilli may be found. Cultures and animal inoculation may be made in order to aid in differentiation from tubercle and other acid-fast bacilli. Failure to demonstrate the organisms in smears or scrapings and negative cultures do not exclude the diagnosis of leprosy. Numerous and repeated examinations are required in many patients. The techniques for the preparation of ocular scrapings and smears for examination in the laboratory are given in Chapter 4.

Large numbers of organisms may be present throughout the cornea (Plate 3, *B*). Although few changes are apparent, as Axenfeld[3] has stated, "The bacilli can spread in the lymph spaces of the cornea, where they are found in small masses between the lamellae; they often lie in small clusters cut off from the original point of entrance." Clusters of organisms under Bowman's membrane were reported by Meller.[3] Naar, as cited by Pillat,[22] was the first to make corneal scrapings. In one patient with keratitis punctata he failed to find bacilli in the corneal scrapings but did demonstrate them in smears from the conjunctiva, the nose, and the mouth. In three other patients the corneal scrapings were positive.

Pillat[22] made scrapings of corneal epithelium and of the mucous membrane of the nose, and obtained positive results. He observed that the keratitis punctata superficialis changed into uniform superficial pannus and later to interstitial keratitis. Pillat felt that "this indicates that a few leprosy bacilli in the cornea may produce miniature lepromas seen clinically as keratitis punctata superficialis. The bacilli may become destroyed, and the spot-shaped infiltrates may be absorbed. When, on the other hand, the number of bacilli is larger, the superficial infiltrates may flow together . . . and may even go into the depth of the cornea . . ." On the other hand, Pinkerton[23] has reported taking numerous scrapings from the cornea, where leukomatous spots were frequent, and found the bacilli only in a few cases. Scrapings from the lid margins frequently yield a larger number of the organisms. When diffuse infiltration of the conjunctiva occurs, a number of *M. leprae* are found. Excised nodules from the conjunctiva or lids contain a great number of *M. leprae* in the lepromatous type of the disease. Bacilli also have been found in the retina and choroid late in the course of ocular disease, but usually only in the anterior portions.

The incidence of ocular lesions of leprosy varies from approximately 15% of patients with tuberculoid leprosy to approximately 100% of patients with long-standing lepromatous leprosy. In addition, the character of the ocular involvement varies with the type of the general disease, although some ocular lesions are common to all types of leprosy.

In lepromatous leprosy one of the relatively early ocular involvements consists of thickening of the supraciliary ridges (Fig. 9-6, *A*) without evidence of inflammation. Eventually there is loss of hairs of the brows beginning laterally and progressing nasally (Fig. 9-7); but the swelling may persist for many months or even years without change or may progress with varying speed into the typical leproma of the brow (Fig. 9-8), forming a part of the so-called leonine facies of this form of leprosy. The granuloma of the brow (Fig. 9-6, *B*) may extend into the upper lid, or

A

B

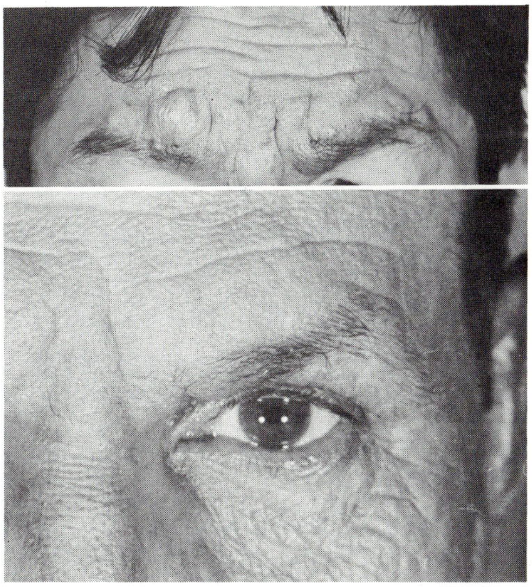

Fig. 9-6. A, Thickening of the superciliary ridges with early lepromatous nodule on the right side. **B,** Thickening of the brow with beginning loss of hairs in the outer portion.

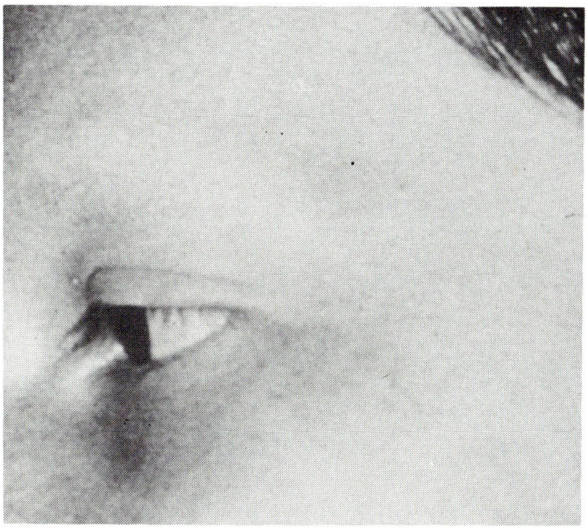

Fig. 9-7. Loss of eyebrows.

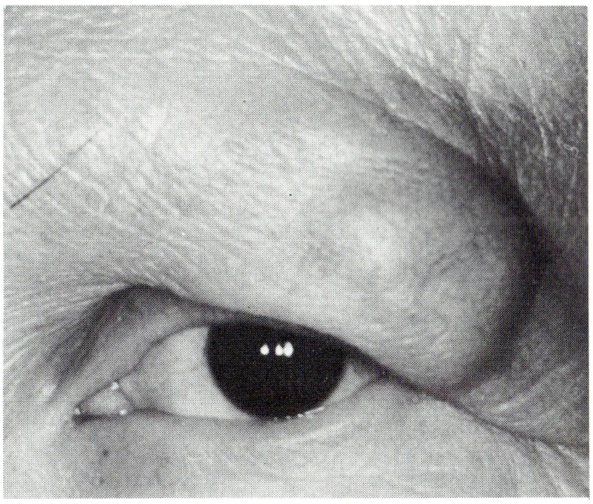

Fig. 9-8. Nodule in upper lid.

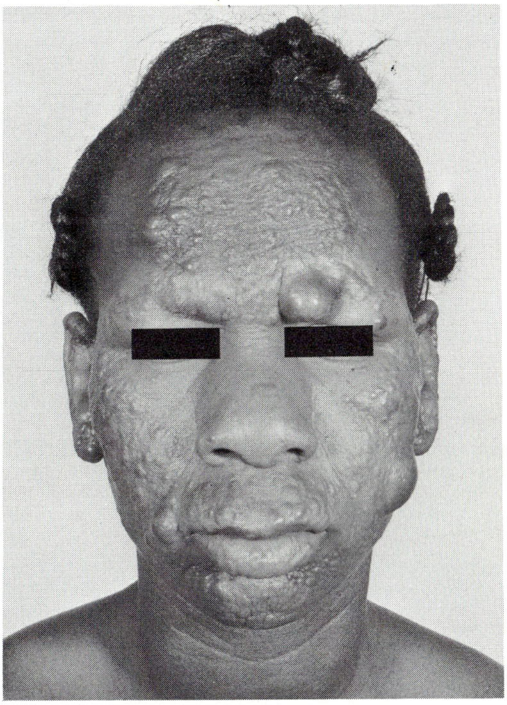

Fig. 9-9. Nodules of lid, brow, and face, showing typical distribution of early leonine character.

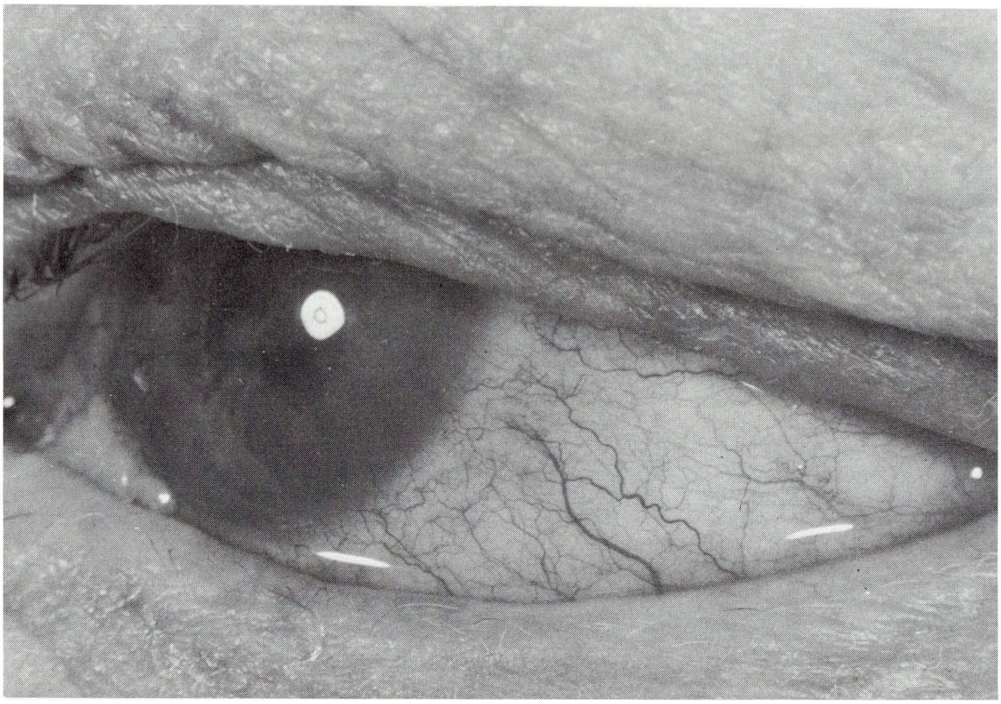

Fig. 9-10. Entropion of the upper lid.

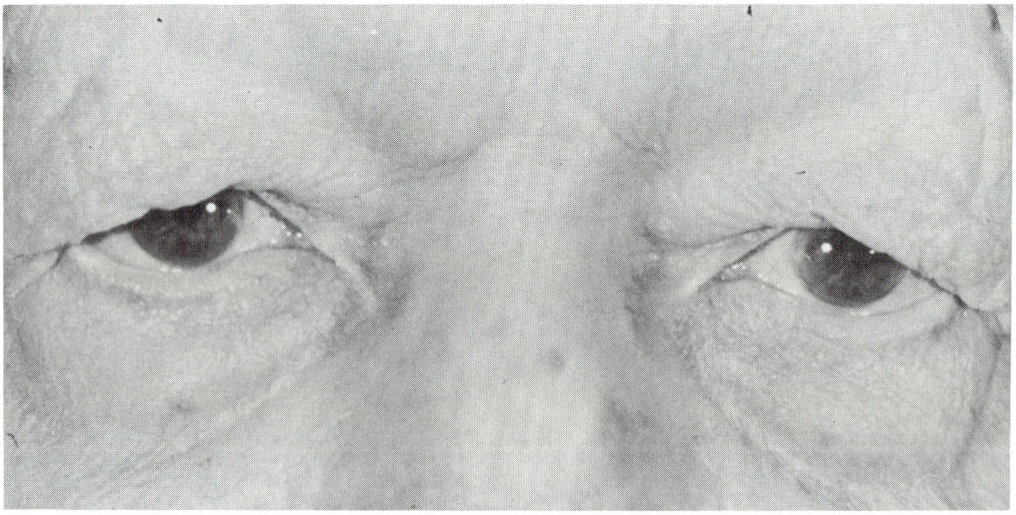

Fig. 9-11. Blepharochalasis.

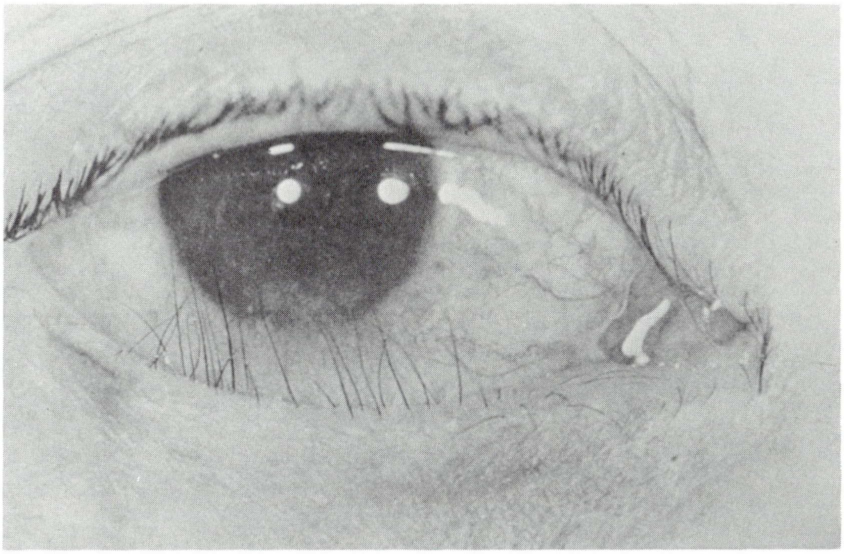

Fig. 9-12. Trichiasis. (From Holmes, W. J.: Geographic ophthalmology, Springfield, 1959, Charles C Thomas, Publisher.)

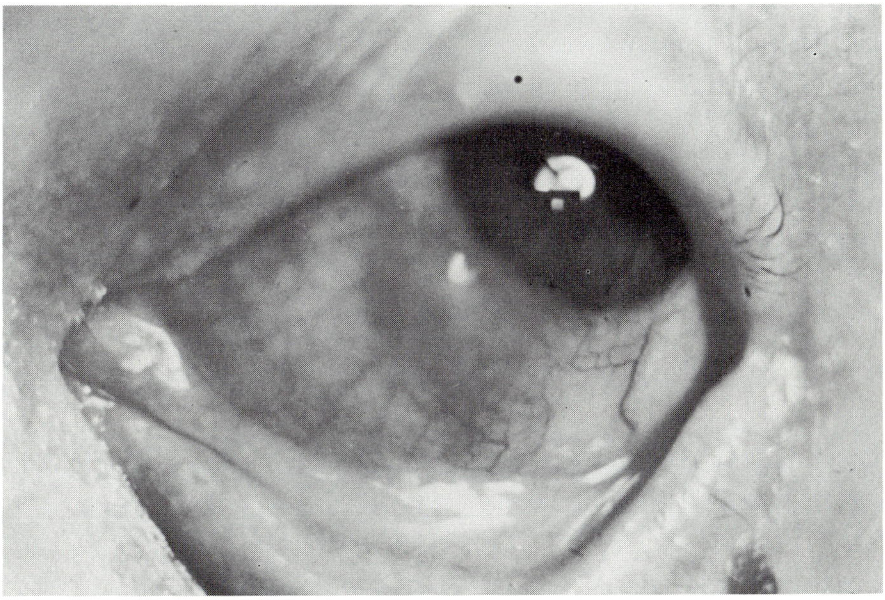

Fig. 9-13. Lepromatous nodular episcleritis.

occasionally small independent nodules may develop in the upper lid (Figs. 9-8 and 9-9), but practically never in the upper lid folds nor in the lower lid. During the inflammatory process, the tissues of the lid may become hypertrophic, or entropion may occur (Fig. 9-10). This may lead to corneal abrasions, then to spastic entropion of the lower lid. Later, after the lesions have resolved under systemic treatment, blepharochalasis may develop (Fig. 9-11). Frequently the ciliary margins of the lids are thickened, probably because of involvement of the follicles of the lashes, which results in loss of the lashes and occasionally in trichiasis (Fig. 9-12).

Conjunctivitis as such is not produced by *M. leprae,* even though the organisms may be found in variable numbers in the epithelial cells. Those patients who develop conjunctivitis do so because of coincidental superimposed infection.

Subconjunctival infiltrations occur especially around the limbus. These consist largely of chronic inflammatory cells in which miliary lepromata develop adjacent to the limbus. The infiltrations form a thin diffuse layer, which gradually disappears near the fornices. These lesions usually undergo remissions and exacerbations along with similar changes in other manifestations of the disease. However, miliary lepromata, once developed, tend to persist for long periods of time as pinpoint- to pinhead-sized, round, yellowish white, subconjunctival lesions. They are called pearls and are identical with pearls, or miliary lepromata, which occur in the cornea and other parts of the eye.

During acute reactions in the course of the disease or as the result of treatment, nodular episcleritis (Fig. 9-13) appears acutely and runs a subacute or chronic course, depending upon the course of the general reaction or the method of local treatment. Nodular episcleritis of leprosy is similar in its appearance to other types of episcleritis and in some instances, but not all, may be followed by local thinning of the sclera.

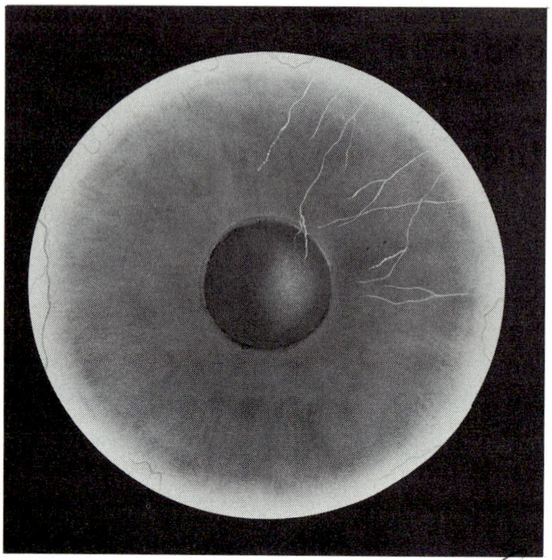

Fig. 9-14. Inflammatory opacification and beading of the corneal nerves.

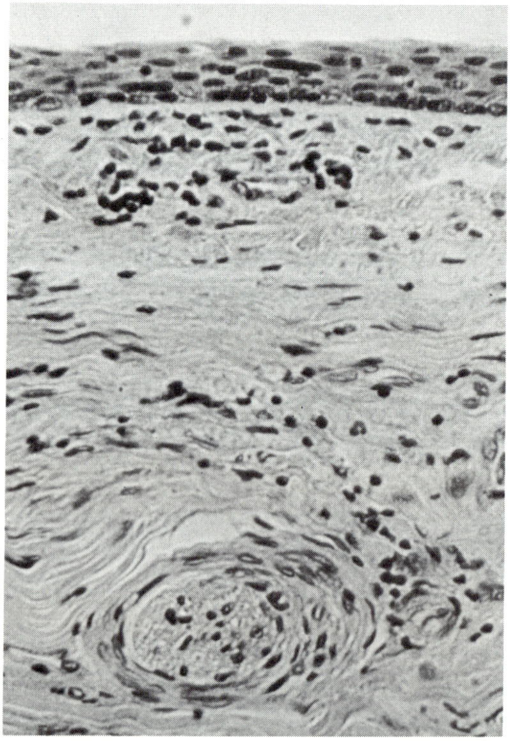

Fig. 9-15. Edema and infiltration of corneal nerve.

Japanese workers report that they have found leprosy bacilli in tears of 66% of patients without obvious ocular manifestations of the disease; however, clinical involvement of the lacrimal gland occurs only rarely.[11]

Nasolacrimal obstruction is frequent and secondary to nasal lesions of the disease, especially those producing periostitis and atrophy of the nasal bones. Secondary infection always ensues, as with any other type of nasolacrimal obstruction.

Initial clinical evidence of involvement of the globe may be inflammatory opacification of the corneal nerves (Fig. 9-14). It is a transitory asymptomatic phenomenon, visible only with magnification, which frequently first involves the nerves of the superior temporal quadrant; but several nerves in each or any quadrant may become involved atypically or in repeated episodes.

One or more, usually several, corneal nerves become swollen and opaque for a period of several weeks, then gradually become invisible again. The nerves become grayish white, fine, radial lines extending in from the limbus in the middle or deep stroma. The lines become branched after passing centrally for a short distance through the otherwise clear stroma, then gradually become finer and invisible at

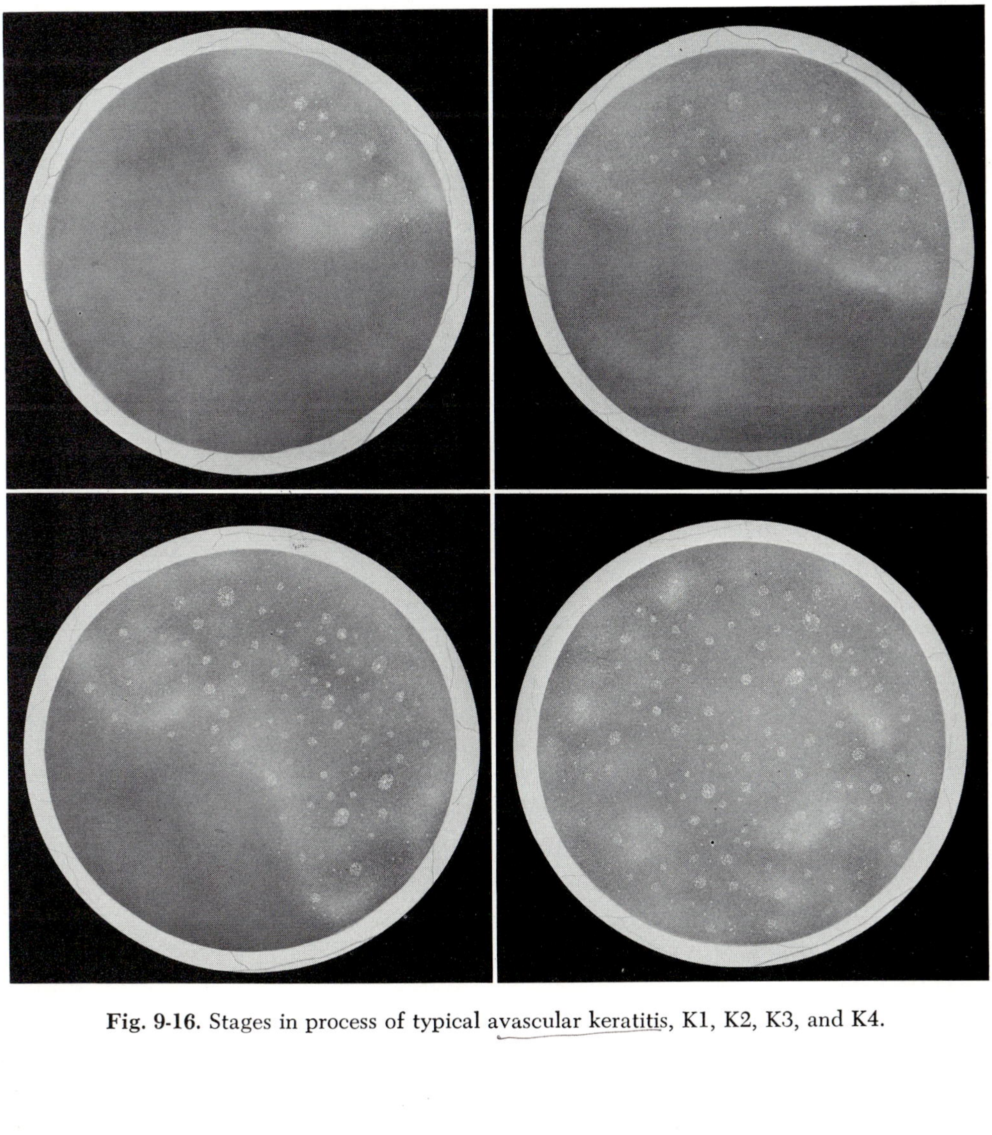

Fig. 9-16. Stages in process of typical avascular keratitis, K1, K2, K3, and K4.

variable distances from the limbus. Occasionally the opaque nerve may appear to have a sheath or sleeve around it for a short distance or have irregular swellings along its course. These changes are caused by edema of the nerves, with an accompanying infiltration of round cells and histiocytes in and around the nerves (Fig. 9-15). Bacilli may be found in Schwann cells, histiocytes, nerve fibers, and endoneural spaces.

The first corneal involvement that usually leaves permanent residual evidence of the infection is a superficial keratitis. The typical lesion begins as discrete patches of superficial thin, grayish white opacities, which appear first in the superior temporal quadrant, then coalesce, becoming confluent and diffuse, slowly spreading centrally and nasally, then downward into the inferior temporal quadrant, and finally into the inferior nasal quadrant (Fig. 9-16). Atypically, the lesion may begin in one of the other quadrants and spread to involve part or all of the cornea. Such atypical lesions may be initiated by trauma. Frequently in early stages the lesion is invisible except with magnification.

Upon biomicroscopic examination the early lesion is composed of a superficial thin, diffuse haze in Bowman's zone, with a variable number of punctate, chalky white opacities scattered through it. These chalky white opacities tend to develop in clusters composed of discrete, fine white opacities, producing a pathognomonic pattern of superficial stippling of the cornea. In some patients the keratitis, on gross examination, may seem to consist only of the diffuse haze, but even in these cases some very fine chalky deposits are seen on biomicroscopic examination. Either type of corneal involvement may spread slowly and continuously throughout the cornea, but in many patients the spread is interrupted by remissions that may occur after minimal corneal involvement or at any other stage.

As the active inflammation of the cornea subsides, the thin grayish white diffuse opacity may disappear or may persist, but the chalky white punctate opacities remain permanently. As the lesion persists, spreads, or recurs, some of the chalky white opacities increase in size and become visible, grossly measuring 0.25 to 0.5 mm in diameter. These are miliary lepromata and are sometimes called pearls. They are pathognomonic, do not disappear during remissions, and may become quite numerous.

The early and the most central opacities are superficial, lying in Bowman's zone; however, as the active lesion persists and spreads centrally and circumferentially,

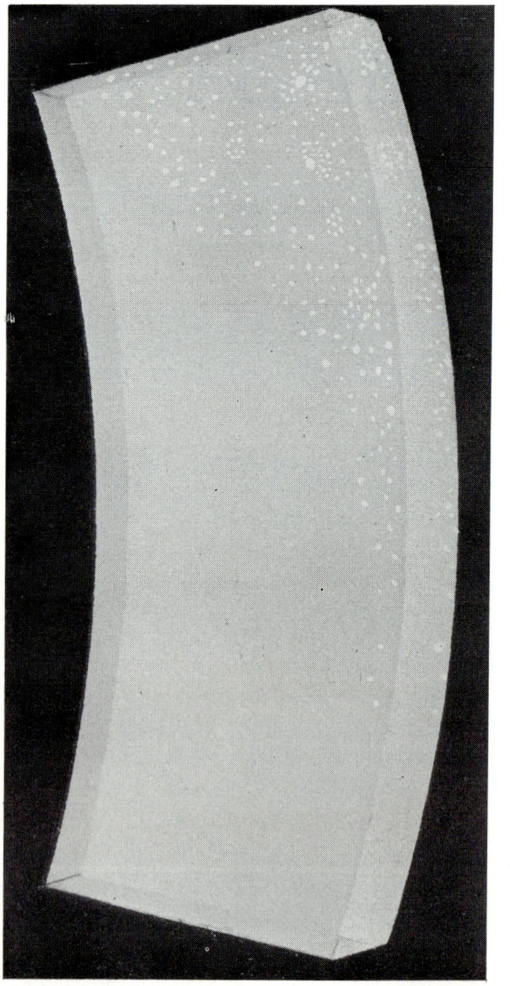

Fig. 9-17. Slit-lamp section of avascular keratitis in stage K3.

deeper layers become involved at the periphery of the cornea (Fig. 9-17). Thus the full thickness of the cornea tends to become involved first at the limbus and later centrally.

In some patients after an avascular keratitis has persisted for some time, or in some with repeated or severe attacks, superficial vessels of the limbus begin to extend into the cornea. Typically, the vascularization begins in the superior temporal quadrant, then involves the superior nasal quadrant, the inferior temporal quadrant, and finally the inferior nasal quadrant (Fig. 9-18). Vascularization of the cornea may become arrested at any stage, however. With severe or prolonged keratitis, the pannus may involve the whole surface of the cornea, but up to this point the avascular keratitis always is more extensive than the pannus. Atypical pannus formation may begin in any of the other quadrants and remain limited to that portion of the cornea or spread to involve any part or all of it.

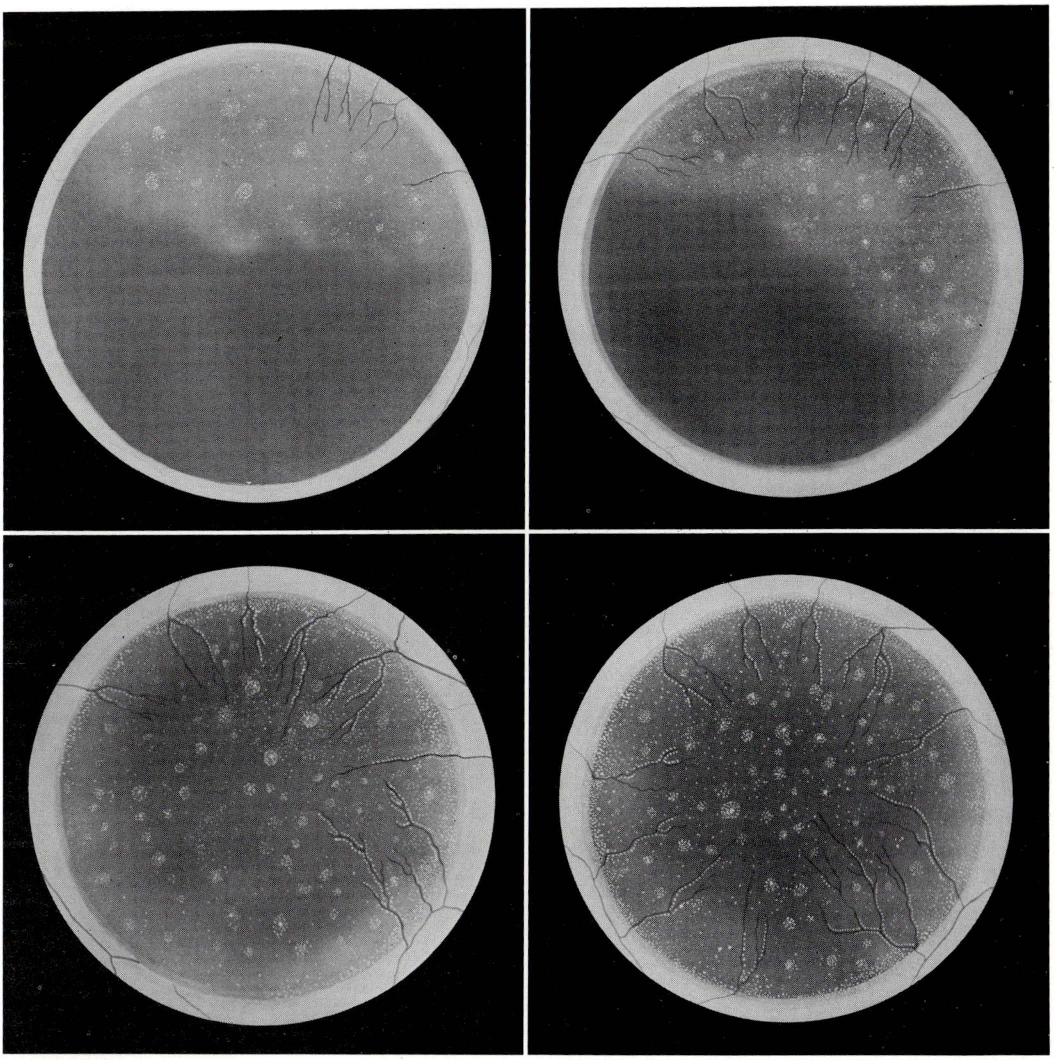

Fig. 9-18. Typical stages of pannus formation, which sometimes, but not always, follows avascular keratitis.

A

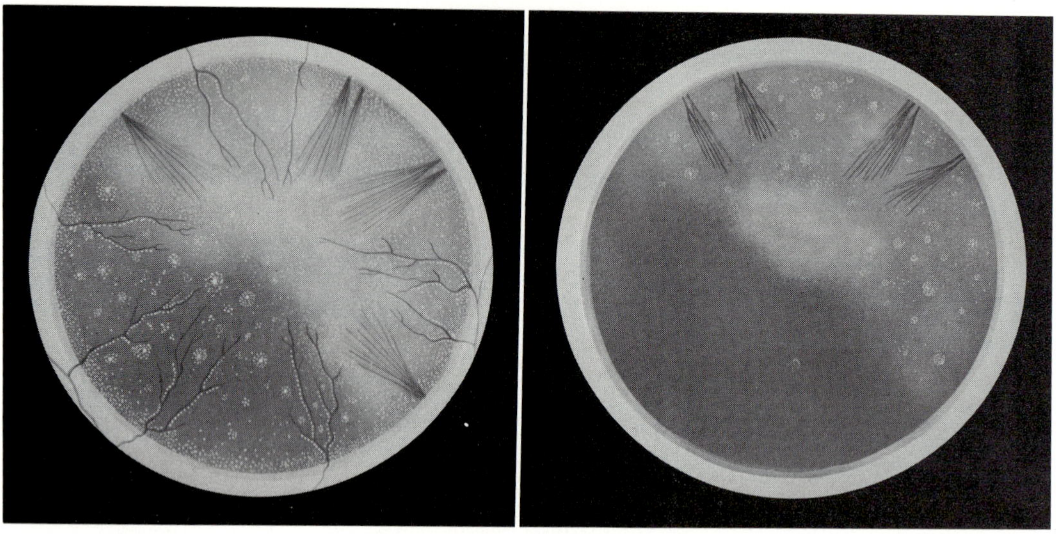

B

Fig. 9-19. A, Interstitial vascularization following pannus formation and avascular keratitis. **B,** Interstitial vascularization following avascular keratitis, but without pannus.

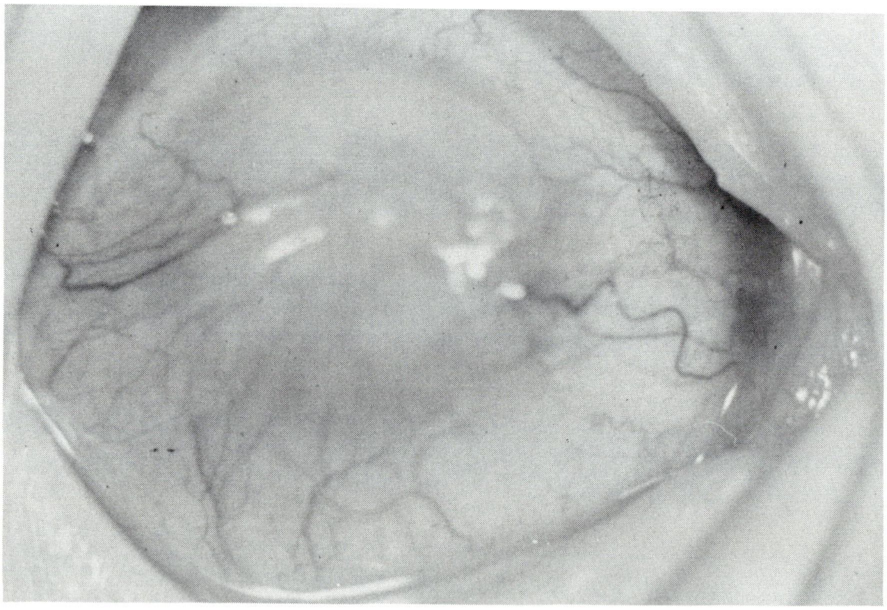

Fig. 9-20. Gross leproma of the cornea.

In a small proportion of patients deep or interstitial vascularization of the cornea may develop either in conjunction with superficial vascularization (pannus) or alone (Fig. 9-19). It develops as a consequence of prolonged deep infiltration and usually follows or accompanies pannus formation. In the typical case it begins in the superior temporal quadrant, eventually extending into other quadrants in the usual pattern of leprotic corneal spread. Not infrequently, however, deep vascularization may begin in the inferior temporal quadrant and extend from there. Interstitial

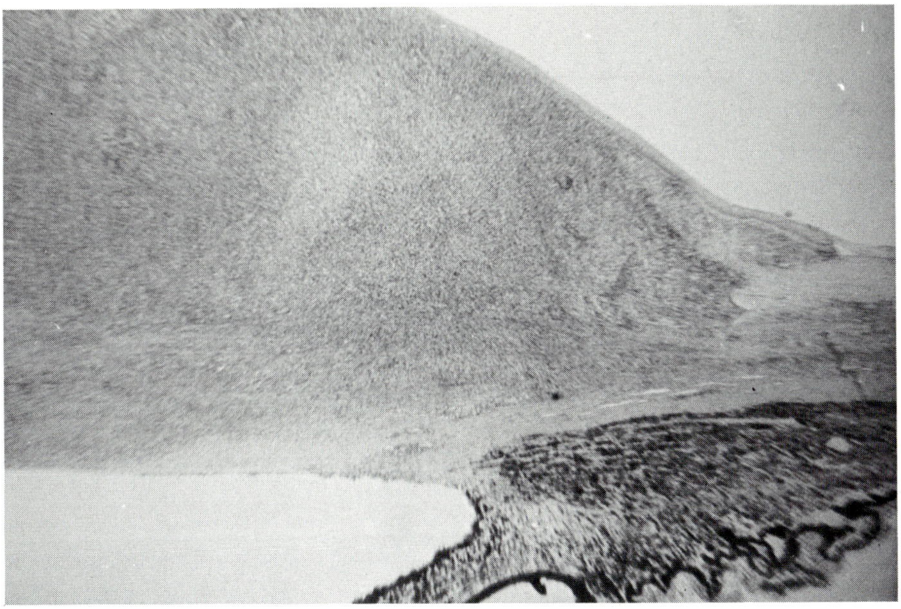

Fig. 9-21. Section of a gross leproma of the cornea.

leprotic keratitis without pannus formation occurs in some patients who have a severe granulomatous uveitis. In these patients a grayish opacity begins in the deep stroma at the limbus and extends centrally. Within the affected stroma between the newly developing vessels, there are small chalky white opacities that, once formed, usually remain, even though the inflammation may subside.

Gross lepromata occasionally develop at the limbus and involve the cornea (Fig. 9-20), or, more rarely, the involvement may be limited to the central part of the cornea. In some instances a corneal leproma resembles the fleshy type of pannus of trachoma, and in others it resembles an irregular lipoma. Pathologically, the lesions are typical lepromatous granulomas (Fig. 9-21) with both superficial and deep vessels surrounded by a heavy infiltration of lymphocytes and lepra cells, replacing practically all normal structures.

As a consequence of prolonged inflammation or repeated episodes of any of these types of corneal involvement, severe scarring ensues and under varying circumstances may undergo hyalinization or lipoid or calcium infiltration (Fig. 9-22).

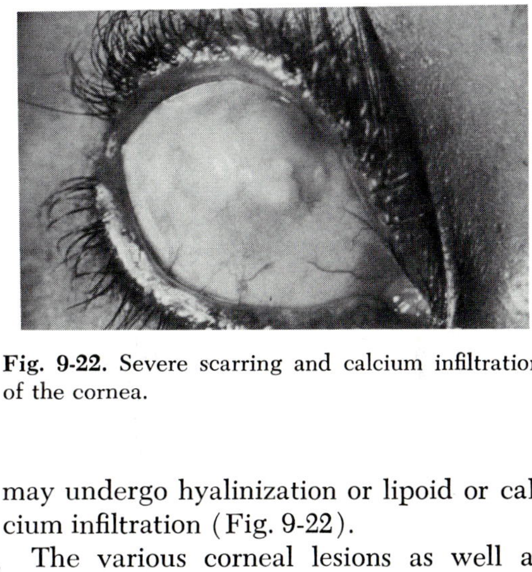

Fig. 9-22. Severe scarring and calcium infiltration of the cornea.

The various corneal lesions as well as other ocular lesions of leprosy are amazingly asymptomatic. The patient seldom is aware of corneal involvement until the lesion is well advanced, and even then he may complain only of a visual disturbance or slight circumcorneal congestion or rarely a mild photophobia. Frequently a superficial keratitis develops and subsides without the patient's knowledge. This apparently is the result of sensory nerve involvement and increases the danger of damage from relatively minor trauma.

Involvement of the iris and ciliary body occurs relatively early. Acid-fast bacilli probably are disseminated widely and localize simultaneously in the superficial or cooler tissues of the body, including the superficial tissue of the eye and adnexa as well as the anterior uvea. However, the organisms probably lie dormant or produce so little disturbance until they have increased tremendously in number that they fail to cause clinical signs for several years. Uveal involvement is limited to the iris, ciliary body, and occasionally the most anterior portion of the choroid. Organisms localize here, producing a mild subclinical inflammation consisting of an occasional lymphocyte and foam cell. After months or years, clinical signs appear in one of several forms: acute iritis, chronic iritis, nodular iritis, or chronic iritis with superimposed acute or subacute exacerbations.

An acute, subacute, or subclinical iritis always accompanies episodes of keratitis and some attacks of acute nodular episcleritis. The iritis is serous in type, characterized by an aqueous flare and fine floaters in the anterior chamber, with fine precipitates on the posterior surface of the cornea, but with relatively no symptoms. The inflammation usually has a slow onset with no gross evidence of the inflammation. In time, however, slight circumcorneal injection or mild photophobia occurs, and by this time posterior synechiae usually have begun to develop. Only by repeated periodic ocular examination with magnification may these lesions be found early. Occasionally an acute serous uveitis develops with moderate to intense circumcorneal injection, flare, and cells in the anterior chamber, but with negligible symptoms—the so-called red eye in patient terminology. The majority of these are recurrent episodes based upon an established and persistent mild or subclinical chronic anterior uveitis.

Chronic subclinical anterior uveitis probably exists in all leprosy patients from the time of the localization of organisms in the tissue and in some patients probably persists with only slight variation throughout the remainder of their lives. In others, mild, clinically apparent episodes alternate with subclinical periods; whereas in still other patients, nodular lesions (Fig. 9-23) develop in an episode of exacerbation of the iritis and persist as the acute

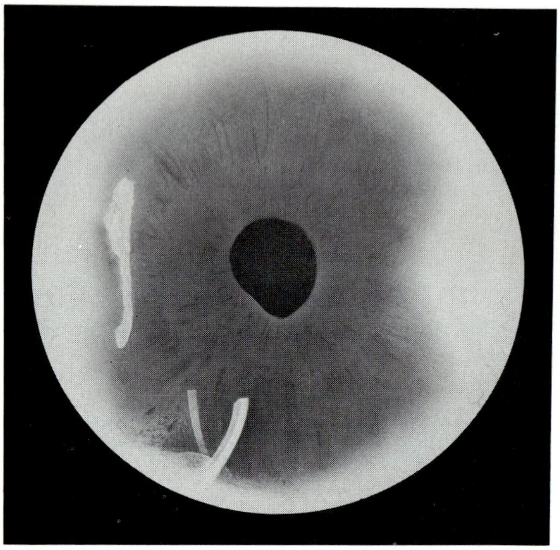

Fig. 9-23. Lepromatous nodular iritis showing nodule in the angle at 7 o'clock, as well as a pterygium and corneal scar.

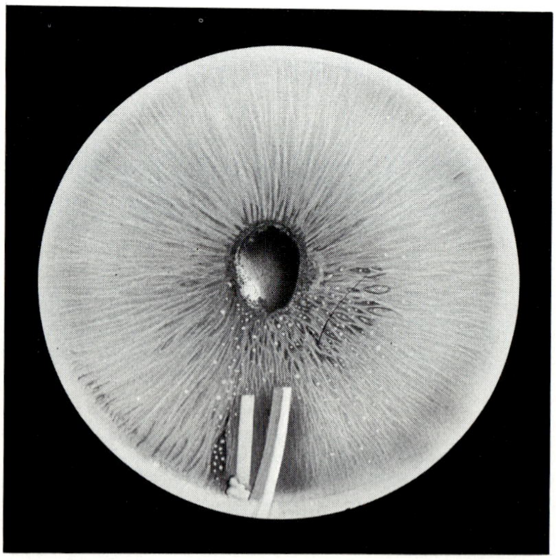

Fig. 9-24. Miliary lepromata, or pearls, of the iris, with a large conglomerate pearl in the angle at 6 o'clock.

serous lesions subside into a subclinical period. In other patients the nodules slowly and relentlessly extend, producing secondary glaucoma, cataract, and degeneration of the globe.

Miliary lepromata, or pearls of the iris (Fig. 9-24), develop as a result of the chronic inflammatory process. They develop in the stroma, usually in the pupillary portion of the iris, as the result of enlargement and fusion of lepra cells to produce giant lepra cells containing globi, which persist and eventually have calcium salts deposited in them. They continue to increase in size gradually and at other times coalesce with neighboring pearls to form a conglomerate pearl. As the pearls gradually increase in size, they appear to approach the surface of the iris, then protrude from the surface, and eventually they may break loose and migrate from place to place in the anterior chamber of the eye. Some "free" pearls have been followed for a number of years, and on the various examinations they were found in different locations on the surface of the iris or in the chamber angle. In a few instances the pearl could not be found in the anterior chamber but was found there again on later examinations. Thus "free" pearls may migrate into the posterior chamber and probably even farther.[1]

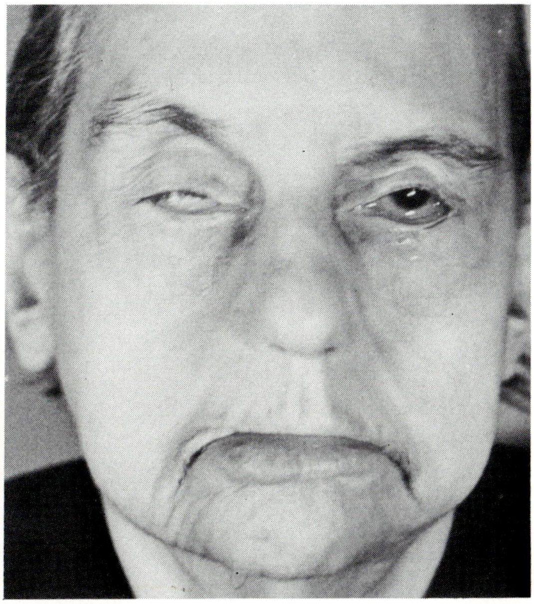

Fig. 9-25. Masklike facies in tuberculoid leprosy.

Complications of anterior uveal inflammation in leprosy include peripheral anterior synechiae from nodular iris or ciliary body lesions; posterior synechiae; occlusion and seclusion of the pupil; iris bombé; secondary glaucoma, both as the result of iris bombé and peripheral anterior synechiae as well as from angle obstruction from exudate in acute episodes of anterior uveitis; cyclitic membranes; cyclitic cataract; and atrophy and degeneration of the globe.

Tuberculoid leprosy, formerly designated as anesthetic leprosy, is characterized by much less frequent clinical involvement of the eyes, but the patient may have a smooth, masklike facies (Fig. 9-25). The skin of the face and lids frequently has areas of reduced sensation or anesthesia. This reduction or loss of sensation frequently includes the conjunctiva and cornea and is manifest by diminished blinking or even loss of the blinking reflex at times. Such patients may have foreign bodies lodged on their corneas without producing symptoms, and considerable damage may result.

In approximately 10% of tuberculoid cases paralysis of the facial nerve occurs. In some instances there may be slight to moderate recovery of function after several months, but as a rule the paralysis persists and atrophy of the affected muscles ensues. As a result, inadequate closure of the lids during the acute phase is followed by ectropion of the lower lid and in some instances by atrophy and vertical shortening of the lower lid in the chronic phase. Exposure keratitis (Fig. 9-26) frequently results and is more serious when there is associated corneal anesthesia, for it may lead to corneal ulceration, perforation, and even loss of the globe. In less severe forms of exposure keratitis, healing may be followed by infiltrative lesions, which resemble those seen in lepromatous patients. More rarely lesions

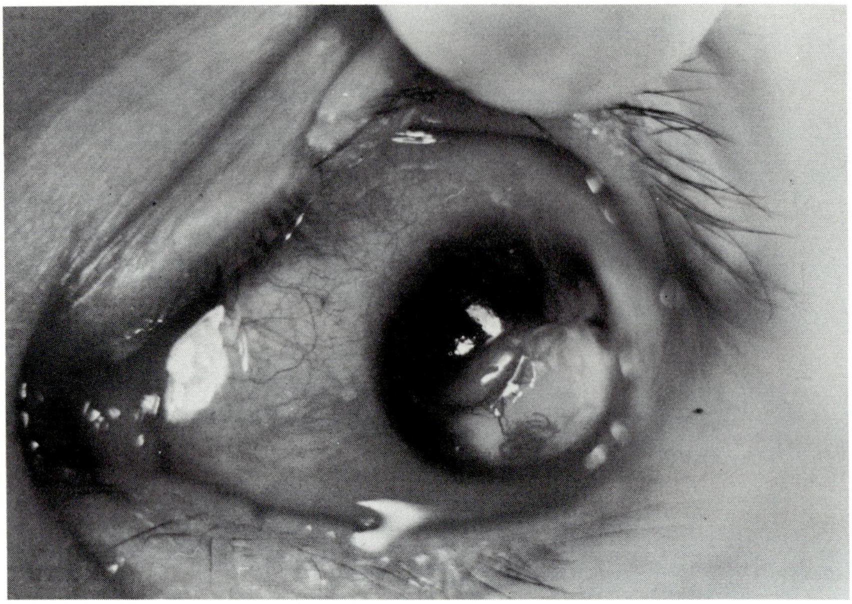

Fig. 9-26. Exposure keratitis.

identical with those seen in lepromatous leprosy also may be seen in the eyes of tuberculoid patients.

The posterior choroid probably is never involved other than by the passage of inflammatory cells in any type of leprosy until the eye begins to degenerate, and similarly there probably never is primary involvement of the retina or optic nerve. In a few instances pearls have been seen in the retina (Fig. 9-27). Although these undoubtedly are miliary lepromata, they probably represent "free" pearls that have migrated posteriorly because they always appear to be situated quite superficially in or on the retina and there is no visible associated inflammation of the retina (pearls always arise in an inflammatory infiltration in other parts of the eye). In one patient who has been observed periodically over a number of years there has been a decrease in the number of pearls visible in the retina, and in another the pearls have been observed in different positions at various times.

The eye and adnexa participate in the several types of general reactions. The lids participate in the skin reactions of acute exacerbations and in erythema nodosum reactions. The episclera may develop diffuse infiltrative lesions, nodular episcleritis, or lepromata. Corneal lesions increase and extend, and acute exacerbations of uveitis occur. Rarely the acute iritis may be accompanied by pseudohypopyon or hyphema.

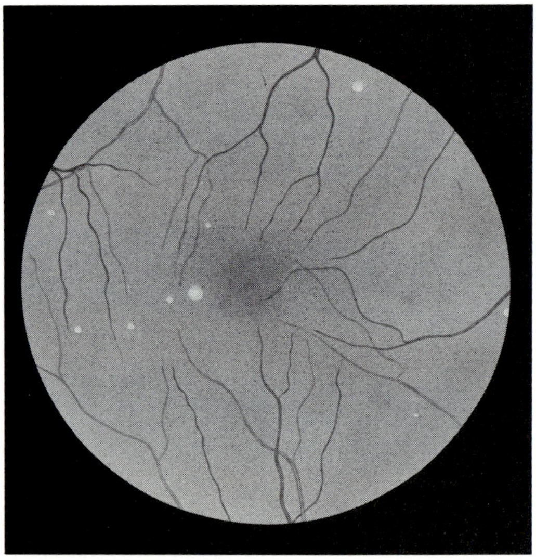

Fig. 9-27. Pearls of the retina.

A number of lesions have been described in patients with leprosy that also have been seen in patients with or without other disease. These include such things as central chorioretinoses, night blindness, uncomplicated senile cataracts, and pterygiums. Obviously, many of these are coincidental, for even though a patient has leprosy he still is subject to all the other ills and outrages of fortune that beset man. Thus the leprologist must bear this in mind in examining his patient and diagnosing the case.

THERAPY

Since the ocular lesions of leprosy are a part of a widely disseminated disease process, the basic treatment must be general treatment of the infectious process with special therapy for its local manifestations in the eye.

As a result of the report of the usefulness of glucosulfone (Promin) in 1943 by Faget and his associates,[13] the sulfones have become the basic form of therapy. The usual daily dosage of the various drugs is: glucosulfone, 1 to 5 gm intravenously; sulfoxone (Diasone), 0.3 to 0.6 gm orally; acetosulfone (Promacetin), 0.5 to 4 gm orally; and diaminodiphenylsulfone (Avlosulfon), 0.1 gm orally. However, these dosages are "maintenance doses," and it is prudent to start with smaller and less frequent doses, building up to a full dose in approximately 6 months in order to avoid exacerbations and early treatment reactions. In addition, the patient should be followed closely for toxic or side reactions.

The sulfones are not bactericidal against the leprosy bacillus, but they apparently inhibit multiplication of the organisms and thus assist the natural defenses of the host eventually to arrest the disease in a majority of patients.

Clofazimine (B663), a new drug, apparently is especially valuable in patients with organisms resistant to sulfones. The minimal effective dosage has not yet been determined, but it has been reported that 300 mg per day reduces the incidence of reactions of erythema nodosum leprosum. B663, however, has the objectionable feature, especially for light-colored patients, of causing a reddish black pigmentation of the skin.

Rifampicin also has recently been shown to have potential usefulness.[25] It appears that it may be bactericidal; however, more extensive studies will be necessary to permit adequate evaluation.

In erythema nodosum leprosum and related reactions, immunosuppressive agents, such as the steroids, phenylbutazone, and anthiomaline, have been used extensively. More recently thalidomide, which may be immunosuppressive, has been used successfully in preliminary trials. But its extent of usefulness remains to be determined.

Ocular lesions continue to develop in patients receiving sulfone therapy, especially during acute exacerbations and episodes of erythema nodosum leprosum; but it appears that the incidence and severity of ocular lesions may be decreasing, especially in those patients who have the benefit of therapy early in the disease and before the usual time of appearance of overt ocular lesions. Close observation and institution of local palliative and supplementary therapy seems to be improving the ocular prognosis in this disease.

Local application of heat under adequate control to prevent damage to anesthetic areas is helpful in all ocular inflammatory lesions of leprosy. In addition, mydriatics are especially important in placing the iris and ciliary body at rest and in preventing posterior synechiae and secondary glaucoma. When additional control of the inflammatory lesion is necessary, topical application of steroids is valuable and important; but their use must be controlled carefully to avoid the development of steroid glaucoma and cataract.

Traumatic lesions, secondary infectious processes, or other coincidental eye lesions are treated in the same manner as in patients without leprosy.

Elective intraocular surgery, such as cataract extraction, should never be done until the eyes have been quiescent for a minimum of 6 months, but otherwise should be done after the usual preparation and in the usual manner for that particular procedure. The usual postoperative routine should be observed.

Lid surgery for the correction of trichiasis, ectropion or entropion, lid lag, and paralysis of the orbicularis may be done when deemed necessary except during reactions. Healing usually is prompt and satisfactory. Lacrimal obstruction is corrected by extirpation of the sac rather than by dacryocystorhinostomy because of the nasal bone involvement.

Glaucoma should be controlled medically until ocular inflammation has been quiet for several months; but under these conditions, iridectomy and external filtering procedures may be done without undue complications.

Keratoplasty has been reported successfully accomplished by several surgeons but should not be done until after the inflammatory lesions of the eye have been controlled for at least 6 months.

CONCLUSION

In spite of years of research and enormous numbers of references on leprosy, the disease still remains a major medical problem. However, the conception of leprosy has changed with the years, as Wayson[31] has stated: "Instead of thinking of it as a disease of foul-smelling sores and grotesque facial mutilations, we shall consider it a communicable affection of protean manifestations, whose commencement may be acute or is so insidious many times that neither the patient nor his physician is aware of the presence of the infection." Great progress has been made in the humane attitude toward patients afflicted with Hansen's disease; leprosariums have been established; and finally, the use of sulfone drugs and cortisone has resulted in an improved prognosis. Choyce[9] reported regression with delay in ocular complications, but he also stated that no patient has yet had a "complete cure" of eye lesions. Nevertheless, blindness from leprosy can be a thing of the past if an early diagnosis is made and appropriate treatment undertaken. Furthermore, recently developed drugs hold additional promise for improved results.

REFERENCES

1. Allen, J. H.: The pathology of ocular leprosy, II. Miliary lepromas of the iris, Amer. J. Ophthal. **61**:987, 1966.
2. Allen, J. H., and Byers, J. L.: The pathology of ocular leprosy, I. Cornea, Arch. Ophthal. **64**:216, 1960.
3. Axenfeld, T.: The bacteriology of the eye, translated by Angus MacNab, New York, 1908, William Wood and Co., p. 344.
4. Badger, L. F.: History of leprosy in the United States, Ann. N. Y. Acad. Sci. **54**:6, 1951.
5. Badger, L. F.: Epidemiology. In Cochrane, R. G.: Leprosy in theory and practice, Bristol, 1959, John Wright and Sons, Ltd., p. 58.
6. Baron, A. L.: Man against germs, New York, 1957, E. P. Dutton and Co., Inc., p. 80.
7. Brieger, E. M.: The submicroscopial structure of the Mycobacterium leprae. In Cochrane, R. G.: Leprosy in theory and practice, Bristol, 1959, John Wright and Sons, Ltd., pp. 22-28.
8. Bullock, W. E.: Min-Fu Ho and Mei-Jan Chen: studies of immune mechanisms in leprosy, J. Lab. Clin. Med. **75**:863, 1970.
9. Choyce, D. P.: The eyes in leprosy. In Cochrane, R. G.: Leprosy in theory and practice, Bristol, 1959, John Wright and Sons, Ltd., pp. 160-170.
10. Cochrane, R. G.: The history of leprosy and its spread throughout the world. In Cochrane, R. G.: Leprosy in theory and practice, Bristol, 1959, John Wright and Sons, Ltd., p. 1.
11. Cochrane, R. G., and Sloan, T. B. M.: Tuberculoid leprosy affecting the palpebral portion of the lachrymal gland, Leprosy in India **12**:83, 1940.
12. Elliot, D.: An interpretation of the ocular manifestations of leprosy, Ann. N. Y. Acad. Sci. **54**:84, 1951.
13. Faget, G. H., Pogge, R. C., Johansen, F. A., Prejean, B. M., and Eccles, C. G.: Pormin treatment of leprosy: a progress report, Public Health Rep. **58**:17, 1943.
14. Gay, F. P., and others: Agents of disease and host resistance, Springfield, Ill., 1935, Charles C Thomas, Publisher, p. 1027.
15. Holmes, W. J.: Geographic ophthalmology, Springfield, Ill., 1959, Charles C Thomas, Publisher, p. 42.
16. Janssens, P. G., and Patlyn, S. R.: Experience with mouse inoculation of leprosy bacilli

originating from the Congo, Int. J. Leprosy **31**:522, 1963.
17. Kellersberger, E. R.: The social stigma of leprosy, Ann. N. Y. Acad. Sci. **54**:126, 1951.
18. Kirwan, E. W. O'G.: Ocular leprosy with reference to certain cases shown, Proc. Roy. Soc. Med. **48**:108, 1955.
19. McKinley, E. B.: The bacteriology of leprosy, Int. J. Leprosy **7**:1, 1939.
20. Muir, E.: Manual of leprosy, Baltimore, 1948, The Williams and Wilkins Co., pp. 3, 10.
21. Muir, E.: Relationship of leprosy to tuberculosis, Leprosy Rev. **28**:11, 1957.
22. Pillat, A.: Leprosy bacilli in the scrapings from the diseased cornea in a leper and comments on keratitis punctata superficialis leprosy, Arch. Ophthal. 3:306, 1930.
23. Pinkerton, F. J.: Leprosy of the eye: an analysis of the records of 512 cases of leprosy in the Hawaiian Islands, Arch. Ophthal. **56**:42, 1927.
24. Rees, R. J. W.: Limited multiplication of acid fast bacilli in footpads of mice inoculated with Mycobacterium leprae, Brit. J. Exp. Path. **45**:207, 1964.
25. Rees, R. J. W., Pearson, J. M. H., and Waters, M. F. R.: Experimental and clinical studies on Rifampicin in treatment of leprosy, Brit. Med. J. **1**:89, 1970.
26. Rogers, L., and Muir, E.: Leprosy, ed 3, Baltimore, 1946, The Williams and Wilkins Co.
27. Ruge, H. G. S., Fromm, G., Fuhner, F., and Guinto, R. S.: Serological findings in leprosy: an investigation into the specificity of various serological tests for syphilis, Bull. W.H.O. **23**:793, 1960.
28. Shepard, C. C.: The experimental disease that follows the injection of human leprosy bacilli into footpads of mice, J. Exp. Med. **112**:445, 1960.
29. Skinsnes, O. K.: Leprosy in society, I. Leprosy has appeared on the face, Leprosy Rev. **35**:21, 1964.
30. Skinsnes, O. K.: Leprosy in society, II. The pattern of concept and reaction to leprosy in oriental antiquity, Leprosy Rev. **35**:106, 1964.
31. Wayson, W. E.: Leprosy of the eye, ear, nose and throat, Laryngoscope **43**:991, 1933.

10

Allergy in relation to ophthalmology

FREDERICK H. THEODORE

In ophthalmology, perhaps more than in any other specialty, allergy has come to be accepted as a major etiologic mechanism. An increasing number of apparently unrelated ocular affections are now best explained on the basis of hypersensitivity. This is not surprising in view of the fact that the eye and its adnexa offer a unique opportunity to observe and study, both clinically and experimentally, all the fundamental allergic reactions to an extent not possible elsewhere in the body. Unfortunately, however, because ocular allergies often resemble inflammations of nonallergic origin, on many occasions allergy is not recognized when it is present, or it is erroneously diagnosed when it does not exist.

Most of the difficulties that arise in the recognition and classification of allergies, especially of the external eye, stem from the fact that allergy itself is not a single entity, but instead may assume a number of forms. If, however, the clinical manifestations of these allergies are correlated and classified in accordance with the various allergic mechanisms involved, many otherwise troublesome diagnostic problems are clarified.

GENERAL CONCEPTS OF ALLERGY

Allergy is considered a specifically altered capacity to react as judged from previous experience of the same individual or from experiences of other individuals of the same species. The term is generally used to denote acquired hypersensitivity, although tendencies to develop allergy are influenced by heredity. Atopy is the term used to designate allergy with a hereditary background, that is, with a familial history of allergy.

The concept of hypersensitivity on an immunologic basis is less than 70 years old, having first been introduced as anaphylaxis by Portier and Richet[24] in 1902. It was confirmed independently by Theobald Smith,[31] who noted the reaction with horse serum at just about the same time. The name allergy was coined by von Pirquet[45] in 1906 and has been used ever since because it is so neat an expression.

Allergens

Substances that can cause allergic states, and thereafter allergic reactions, are almost limitless. Besides foreign proteins, foods and digestive products, and nitrogenous materials as in pollens, the list includes chemicals, drugs, metals, and living or dead microorganisms (molds, yeast, fungi, bacteria, viruses, parasites, metabolites). Physical influences such as light, heat, and cold, as well as emotional factors, also cause allergic responses.

It is thus obvious that although some of these substances are true antigens, and others, such as pollens, show some degree of antigenicity, many are frankly not antigens in the usual sense. Many of these allergic excitants or allergens are believed to combine with proteins or some other substance of the host's tissues and to assume thereby the nature of an artificial antigen, thus causing allergic reactions.

The concept of allergy has until now been basically oriented on the assumption of an antigen-antibody relationship, an approach that has proved very useful but that has failed to explain many phenomena in the field of allergy. Thus even the allergist versed in immunology is often obliged to make diagnoses solely on a clinical basis. Vernal conjunctivitis, for example, the mechanism of which is still obscure, does not fit neatly into such a framework but seems to require a special chain of allergic circumstances and allergic responses for its occurrence. However, for clinical purposes it is convenient to divide allergic reactions into two types: (1) the immediate and (2) the delayed. Although the distinctions are not always clearcut and some overlapping occurs, this classification is of great value.

THE IMMEDIATE ALLERGIC RESPONSE. "Immediate" allergic responses occur shortly after application or absorption of the allergen, usually within a few minutes. Immediate reactions occur in asthma, hay fever, urticaria, unusual cases of drug sensitivity, and gastrointestinal disturbances, and are generally caused by serum or other proteins, danders, pollens, dusts, or foods. The reaction has the following characteristics:

1. Skin tests give a typical wheal in a few minutes.
2. A drop of the allergen in the eye is followed promptly by itching, tearing, redness, and chemosis.
3. Circulating antibodies, such as precipitins, are often demonstrable.
4. Passive transfer (Prausnitz-Küstner phenomenon) occurs.
5. Desensitization following the injection of minute quantities of antigen is often successful and results in the formation of "blocking antibody," which combines readily and specifically with the allergenic material and "neutralizes" it.
6. Histamine plays a dominant role in the production of the reaction.

THE DELAYED TYPE OF ALLERGIC RESPONSE. In the delayed type of allergic response, which is also known as the tuberculin or bacterial type, it is a matter of hours, often 24 to 48, before reaction occurs. Contact allergy, caused by drugs or chemicals, and bacterial allergy constitute the major clinical forms of delayed allergy.

In contradistinction to the immediate type of allergic response, the delayed type fails to show certain characteristics:

1. Circulating humoral antibodies are absent. The cells themselves are the seat of the antigen-specific reaction.
2. In most instances passive transfer cannot be produced.
3. Histamine does not appear to play a significant role in the reaction.

However, anaphylactic and immediate reactions, as well as passive transfer of serum, may occur at times with both chemical and microbial antigens, especially if the sensitization is intense.

Microbiallergic reactions

I have coined the term microbiallergic to describe reactions caused by microbial allergy.[41,42] It is now an established fact that many of the harmful effects that microorganisms can exert in the human body are manifestations of allergy. Beyond the direct toxic nature of microbial infection, allergy may convert a harmless protein product of bacterial disintegration into a violent and lethal poison. In ophthalmology such bacterial allergy, especially to staphylococcal products, is of great importance in diseases of the eyelids, conjunctiva, cornea, and sclera; hypersensitivity to products of the *Streptococcus* and the tubercle bacillus appear to play an important role in uveal diseases and in scleritis. Similar allergic reactions may result from fungal products and parasitic agents. Moreover, bacterial exotoxins may likewise incite microbiallergic reactions.

Bacterial allergy and bacterial immunity are entirely distinct and different processes.

Autogenous allergy

The concept of sensitization to antigens of one's own tissues, or autosensitization, long recognized by ophthalmologists in the causation of sympathetic ophthalmia and phacoanaphylactic uveitis, is now belatedly gaining generalized acceptance. Such diseases as acquired hemolytic anemia, thyroiditis, and certain forms of encephalitis may arise on this basis. There is evidence suggesting that the sensitization in rheumatic fever is not to the *Streptococcus* but is an autosensitivity induced by the streptococcal infection. A similar mechanism may be involved in the pathogenesis of glomerulonephritis. In ophthalmology, as will be noted later in this chapter, autogenous allergy may serve to explain many as yet incompletely elucidated reactions of apparently alergic nature.

ALLERGY OF THE CONJUNCTIVA

There could hardly be a better site in the body than the conjunctiva for the study of basic allergic reactions. The juxtaposition of readily accessible mucous membrane to the adjacent thin and delicate skin of the eyelids provides the opportunity for all types of allergic reactions to occur to an extent and with a frequency that do not exist elsewhere. Although the nasal mucosa is often the site of explosive airborne allergies, contact allergy is relatively rare. The reverse is true of the skin. Only in the conjunctiva are both of these forms of allergy, as well as reactions to microbial allergens, commonly encountered. Such allergic responses may result from local exposure to excitants or as part of a generalized hypersensitivity.

The outline below classifies the various types of conjunctival allergy that are encountered in clinical practice.

Allergy of the conjunctiva

A. Atopic conjunctivitis
  1. Atopic (familial history of allergy), rarely anaphylactic
  2. Immediate alergic response (in a few minutes) after contact
  3. Positive intradermal wheal test reaction in 15 to 30 minutes
  4. Causes: inhalants, such as pollens, dusts, fungi, animal epidermals
  5. Types
     a. Acute atopic conjunctivitis—major characteristics: chemosis, eosinophilia
     b. Chronic atopic conjunctivitis—major characteristics: itching, slight edema, eosinophilia

B. Microbiallergic conjunctivitis
  1. Atopy not essential
  2. Delayed allergic response
  3. Delayed positive intradermal test reaction (24 to 48 hours); immediate urticarial reaction may occur
  4. Causes products of microorganisms: bacteria, fungi, parasites, possibly viruses
     Major characteristics: irritation, burning, some follicles

C. Allergic dermatoconjunctivitis
  1. Atopy not essential
  2. Delayed allergic responses (24 to 48 hours)
  3. Positive patch test in 1 to 5 days
  4. Contact allergy to locally applied drugs or chemicals
     Major characteristics: eczema, eosinophilia

D. Vernal conjunctivitis

Atopic conjunctivitis

By the term atopic conjunctivitis we describe the conjunctival reaction occurring in atopy and in anaphylaxis. This is a clearcut antigen-antibody response and should not be confused with the conjunctivitis occurring in so-called atopic dermatitis, which is by no means a clearly distinguished entity. As the outline above indicates, atopic conjunctivitis is divided into acute and chronic varieties.

ACUTE ATOPIC CONJUNCTIVITIS. This type of hypersensitivity is characterized by a sudden or immediate hyperemia and edema. Marked chemosis of a glassy appearance, associated usually with a watery, but sometimes mucopurulent, discharge, occurs. It is the conjunctival prototype of the immediate type of allergic response and usually is caused by the airborne group of allergens: pollens (Fig. 10-1), animal danders and feathers, mold spores, dusts, insects, and scents. The conjunctival reaction is similar to the general inflammatory edema that involves the upper respiratory tract.

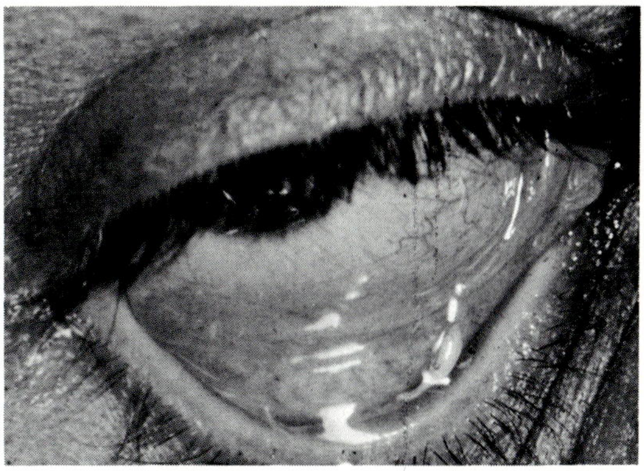

Fig. 10-1. Experimentally induced conjunctivitis in ragweed-sensitive hay fever patient. A small amount of pollen (still visible) was placed in lower conjunctival sac 7 minutes before picture was taken. (From Theodore, F. H., and Schlossman, A.: Ocular allergy, Baltimore, 1958, The Williams & Wilkins Co. © 1958, The Williams & Wilkins Co., Baltimore.)

A similar picture may occur in food allergies, such as egg and milk, but in that event the ocular reaction has only a minor role in a dramatic general systemic reaction. A familial history of allergy (atopy) is generally obtained.

As in the nasal symptoms of hay fever, the reaction may be so intense that a profuse mucopurulent discharge occurs. Itching and burning may be intolerable. Eosinophils often occur in abundance in the secretions. Vasoconstrictors, like epinephrine, phenylephrine, (Neo-Synephrine), and naphazoline (Privine), help control the reaction, which usually subsides rapidly once the excitant is removed.

Skin tests of the intradermal type give an immediate wheal response in most cases of this group. Ophthalmic tests, by means of the direct instillation of the suspected allergen in weak dilution, are generally not safe in these cases. Severe, and possibly permanent, ocular damage may result. Because of chemosis, early epidemic keratoconjunctivitis may be confused with acute allergic conjunctivitis. The virus infection, however, is differentiated by the presence of preauricular lymphadenopathy. In scrapings, mononuclear cells are found instead of eosinophils.

Chronic atopic conjunctivitis. In contradistinction to the often dramatic and generally severe reactions that occur in acute atopic conjunctivitis, the chronic form frequently shows little or no objective evidence of inflammation in comparison to the irritating subjective symptoms of itching, burning, photophobia, and dryness that are usually present. As a result, the patients often are considered psychoneurotic or else are thought to be suffering from chronic catarrhal conjunctivitis. Since the cultures from many patients with chronic conjunctivitis are found bacteriologically negative, it may be that a significant number of such so-called cases actually are overlooked forms of chronic atopic conjunctivitis. In fact, even when the ophthalmologist is alerted to the frequency of chronic atopic conjunctivitis, if he performs routine epithelial scrapings in cases of conjunctivitis, he is often surprised to find numerous eosinophils in cases that clinically did not appear allergic.

The conjunctiva often appears rather pale. A minor degree of conjunctival edema may be suggested by the somewhat juicy appearance of the conjunctiva, especially in the lower fornix in its temporal portion. Although the response is essentially papillary, follicles may appear in long-standing cases, especially where there is relatively little inflammatory reaction. In other patients, where a more subacute process occurs, there may be considerable injection, as well as slight chemosis. Corresponding to the grade of the reaction in general, there may be a slight watery discharge or a mucopurulent one. In either event, eosinophils are found in epithelial scrapings, always in diagnostic numbers, although less numerous than in acute atopic conjunctivitis.

Chronic atopic conjunctivitis is often known as simple allergic conjunctivitis.

The diagnosis of chronic atopic conjunctivitis is often difficult because the condition may resemble other forms of chronic conjunctivitis, in particular, microbiallergic conjunctivitis caused by *Staphylococcus* organisms. The differentiation of these two

Table 10-1. Differentiation of chronic types of allergic conjunctivitis

	Chronic atopic conjunctivitis	Microbiallergic conjunctivitis caused by *Staphylococcus* organisms
History	Familial allergy frequent Other associated allergies	Familial allergy infrequent No associated allergies
Allergens	Pollens, danders, inhalants, foods	Bacterial products, mainly *Staphyloccus* toxin
Allergic response	Immediate	Delayed
Symptoms	Burning, irritation, and often severe itching	Burning, irritation, and often marked dryness
Discharge	May be mucopurulent	Watery, no pus
Lid margins	Usually uninvolved	May be swollen; possible blepharitis
Conjunctiva	May appear same in both types Often little objectively noted Sometimes edematous	May appear same in both types Papillary, but scattered follicles may appear Dry, no chemosis
Cornea	Generally not involved	May have superficial punctate keratitis involving inferior portion of cornea
Epithelial scrapings	Eosinophiles almost always found sooner or later	No eosinophiles
Cultures	Normal flora	Toxin-producing staphylococci found, or normal flora
Intracutaneous *Staphylococcus* toxin or toxoid	Moderate delayed response	Marked delayed response, at least 3 × 3 cm, usually more; may have marked immediate response also; may get systemic reactions (arthritis)
Response to vasoconstrictors	Local use often affords considerable symptomatic relief	Generally no great relief
Response to antihistaminics	Oral use often affords marked symptomatic relief	Generally no relief at all
Response to cortisone	Local use usually affords marked symptomatic relief	Relief in some cases, but not the rule
Best treatment	Elimination of cause	*Staphylococcus* toxin or toxoid injections

From Theodore, F. H.: The classification and treatment of allergies of the conjunctiva, Amer. J. Ophthal. **36**:1698, 1953.

forms of chronic allergic conjunctivitis is shown in Table 10-1.

The conjunctivitis that occurs often does not permit any ready means of distinguishing between the two types, although there generally are slight differences. However, more important than the appearance of the conjunctiva itself are the history; the finding of the eosinophils; the response to certain avenues of therapy, such as local vasoconstrictors, steroids, and oral antihistamines; and, if possible, the elimination of the cause of the allergy. These clues afford the framework for differentiating chronic atopic conjunctivitis from other forms of chronic inflammation of the conjunctiva.

Microbiallergic conjunctivitis

Bacteria, fungi, and helminths appear to be capable of inciting microbiallergic conjunctivitis. The status in regard to viruses is not clear.

Bacteria. There is very little evidence that bacteria other than the *Staphylococcus* play an important role in the production of allergic conjunctivitis. Apparently a combination of two factors operates in the pathogenesis of this condition: (1) chronicity, with the opportunity for repeated reinfection, and (2) the formation of antigenic exotoxin or other sensitizing substances. Most bacteria that produce potent, but not necessarily allergic, exotoxins, such

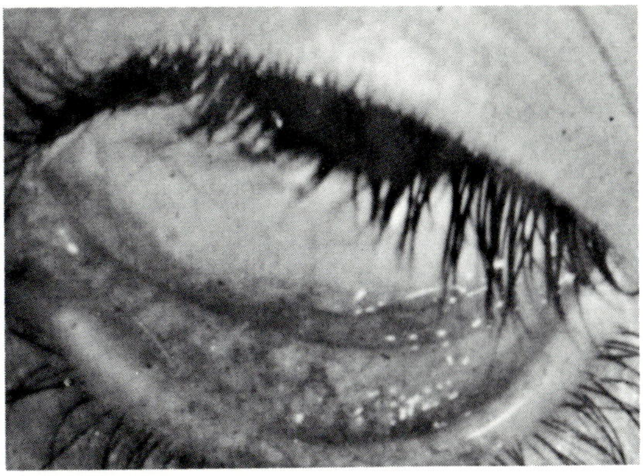

Fig. 10-2. Microbiallergic conjunctivitis caused by *Staphylococcus*. Quiescent stage, minor symptoms. Note follicles in lower lid. (From Theodore, F. H., and Schlossman, A.: Ocular allergy, Baltimore, The Williams & Wilkins Co. © 1958, The Williams & Wilkins Co., Baltimore.)

as the diphtheria and tetanus bacilli, cause acute processes. Only the *Staphylococcus* appears to fill both requirements in this respect. It must be emphasized that microbiallergic conjunctivitis may occur without the presence of or previous exposure to what we consider pathogenic organisms. Even nonpathogenic bacteria can bring about an allergic state in certain individuals. This fact would explain the occurrence of microbiallergic conjunctivitis where only so-called non-toxin-producing *Staphylococcus albus* is found. The appearance of allergic conjunctivitis caused by *Staphylococcus* is seen in Fig. 10-2.

Studies of bacteriophage typing of *Staphylococcus* organisms by Locatcher-Khorazo and Gutierrez[17] may offer, by inference, additional confirmation of the role of bacterial allergy in staphylococcal infections. Although many phage types were isolated by these authors from normal eyes, it was rare to find more than one strain in the eyes of any single individual, and the same phage type was present in the nose as well. Staphylococcal ocular infections, including unilateral postoperative infections, were caused by the same type that was present in the normal eye of the same individual. In eight postoperative infections the same phage type found before operation was responsible. Repeated ocular cultures showed that the same type of *Staphylococcus* persisted for months, even after antibiotic therapy.

Although others have reported microbiallergic conjunctivitis to streptococcal and gonococcal products, I have not encountered such instances.

In a detailed study of 60 instances of all forms of conjunctival allergy, other than those caused by contact allergy, investigated at the Fondation Rothschild in Paris, Morault[21] found that 7 cases resulted from bacterial allergy. According to Morault, the responsible organisms, which in some instances were multiple, were: *Pneumococcus,* 5 cases; *Streptococcus hemolyticus,* 5 cases; *Staphylococcus aureus,* 3 cases; *Streptococcus viridans,* 1 case; coliform bacillus, 1 case; and *Bacillus pyocyaneus,* 1 case.

Fungi. Allergic conjunctivitis caused by mold spores is not uncommon. Essentially an inhalant form of allergy, like pollen allergy, the allergic reactions these fungi arouse have many of the characteristics of the immediate atopic response. *Alternaria* and *Cladosporium,* as well as yeasts, have been responsible.

Other types of fungi, of more pathogenic character, cause allergy only after a primary infective focus has been established. Here the mechanism is of the delayed tuberculin type. The main ones of this group are the dermatophytes, such as *Trichophyton* and *Candida albicans (Monilia),* causing skin diseases. Thus, after a demonstrably infected primary dermatitis has occurred, id reactions may appear elsewhere. These id lesions reveal no fungi and disappear spontaneously when the original lesion is successfully treated. In the eye such allergic reactions occur mainly as eczematous lesions affecting the eyelids; only rarely is the conjunctiva involved.

Helminths. Conjunctival allergy to intestinal parasites has been produced experimentally. Laboratory workers in this field, especially those dissecting the parasites, may contact allergic conjunctivitis from finger-to-eye contact. Reactions similar to hay fever with conjunctivitis and asthma also occur. Slaughterhouse workers also develop similar symptoms, which disappear when such exposure no longer occurs. At least two instances of recurrent allergic conjunctivitis related to *Oxyuris* infestation have been recorded.

Allergic dermatoconjunctivitis

Contact allergy of the eyelids and conjunctiva constitutes by far the most common form of allergic reaction encountered in ophthalmic practice. It is generally caused by the local use of drugs; it can also be caused by cosmetics, articles of clothing, jewelry, animal or vegetable products, plastics, or chemicals used in industry. In those instances where the conjunctiva is the focal point of contact, as in the use of ophthalmic drugs, the allergic reaction generally begins as a conjunctivitis, soon involving the adjacent skin of the eyelids in a typical eczematous dermatitis. The particularly apt term allergic dermatoconjunctivitis has been applied to this clinical picture. When the eyelid skin is the site of the primary contact, conjunctival allergy plays little or no role in the manifestations, and an allergic eczematous dermatitis occurs without conjunctivitis. This form of reaction usually is the result of exposure to cosmetics, apparel, jewelry, metals, plants, or chemicals, and is the most frequent cause of acute ocular eczema. Although the allergic mechanism is basically the same, only allergic dematoconjunctivitis is discussed at this point; allergic eczematous dermatitis of the eyelids is discussed later in this chapter.

In contact allergy of the conjunctiva, the responsible agent almost always is an ophthalmic drug. Since the conjunctiva is usually the focal point of contact, the allergic reaction generally begins as a conjunctivitis but soon involves the adjacent skin, becoming a typical allergic dermatoconjunctivitis. The major diagnostic characteristics of this type of reaction, in the order of their appearance, are (1) severe itching of the eyes, (2) papillary conjunctivitis, (3) eczema of the skin of eyelids, and (4) conjunctival eosinophilia. If the conjunctivitis is caused by eye drops, the earliest signs of eczema may be at the canthi and on the lower lids; if ointments are the offending agents, the lid margins may first be involved. Although any ophthalmic drug may at times result in allergy in susceptible individuals, allergic dermatoconjunctivitis is usually encountered as a result of using one of the following important groups of medicaments: anesthetics, antibiotics, sulfonamides, mydriatic alkaloids, or mercurials. Moreover, even if the active drug itself is harmless, allergy may often result from other ingredients in ophthalmic vehicles, especially preservatives and ointment bases.

ALLERGENIC DRUGS. Many ophthalmic drugs are true sensitizers. On occasion probably every drug used in the treatment of the eyes has resulted in allergic dermatoconjunctivitis in some individual. In fact, there is probably no drug or chemical in existence that everyone can use with impunity. Although nonprotein substances are in themselves not primary antigens, it is believed that they form true antigens in the body by union with the host tissues. These relatively simple chemicals, known as haptens, combine with body proteins, forming conjugates that act as antigens. The hapten confers specifically on the conjugate; hence, the allergy is directed against the hapten and not against the protein. This process explains why the substitution of a drug that is chemically similar to one that previously caused sensitivity in a patient is dangerous. Thus, after allergy to one sulfonamide has developed, another sulfonamide is very likely to cause sensitivity. Benzamine and other chemicals with paralinked amino groups, as compared with ortho- and meta-attachments, are especially prone to cause contact allergies. Unfortunately, very many of the drugs we use fall into that category.

Local anesthetics. Apparently every local anesthetic that is used for instillation is a potential sensitizer and has been known to cause allergic conjunctivitis. Of the commonly used ones, those least likely to do so appear to be cocaine, phenacaine (Holocaine), and possibly piperocaine (Metycaine), tetracaine (Pontocaine), butacaine (Butyn), dibucaine (Nupercaine), and Larocaine are particularly likely to cause reactions and frequently are the causes of cases of conjunctivitis that get progressively worse despite treatment. Proparacaine (Ophthaine, Ophthetic) not only may cause a typical allergic dermatoconjunctivitis, but on occasion may incite a hyperallergenic corneal reaction of the greatest severity.

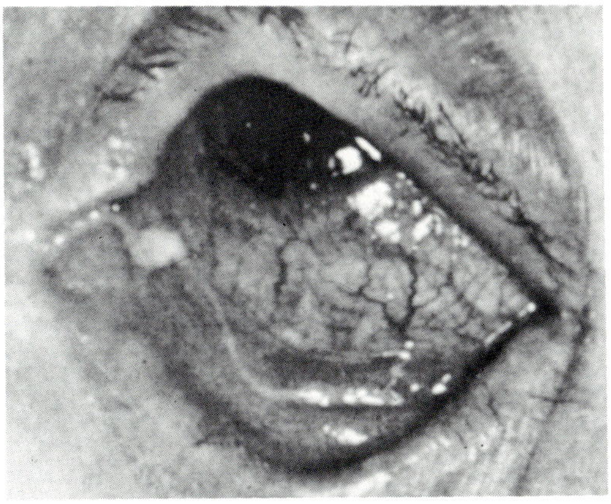

Fig. 10-3. Allergic dermatoconjunctivitis caused by hyoscine. (From Theodore, F. H., and Schlossman, A.: Ocular allergy, Baltimore, 1958, The Williams & Wilkins Co. © 1958, The Williams & Wilkins Co., Baltimore.)

Antibiotics. Penicillin is notorious for its sensitizing tendencies, especially in the ointment form. Streptomycin, bacitracin, the tetracyclines, chloramphenicol (Chloromycetin), erythromycin, and neomycin all may cause allergies. Neomycin is particularly important in this respect because it is used in combination with so many other antibiotics and corticosteroids.

Sulfonamides. All sulfonamides are prone to cause allergic reactions after prolonged topical use.

Mydriatic and miotic alkaloids. Allergy to atropine is a common occurrence, resulting in a typical allergic dermatoconjunctivitis with eczema, papillary conjunctivitis, and conjunctival eosinophilia. Both hyo-

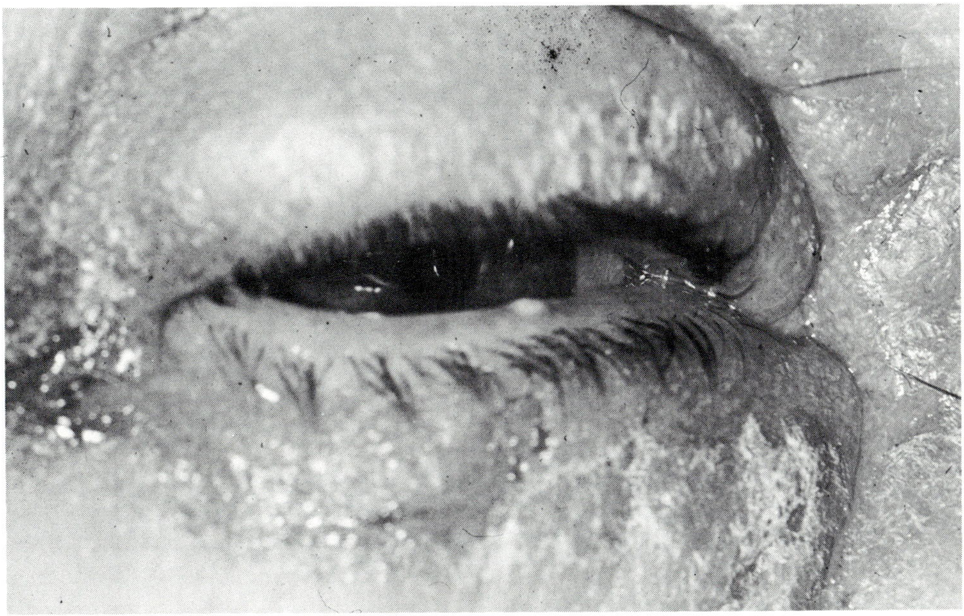

Fig. 10-4. Allergic dermatoconjunctivitis caused by eserine. Typical full-blown picture after using drops for several months. (From Theodore, F. H.: Trans. Amer. Acad. Ophthal. Otolaryng. **58**:708, 1954.)

scine and homatropine may also cause sensitivities (Fig. 10-3), but the eczematous component in these drugs is less evident. Atropine, however, sometimes causes follicular conjunctivitis without eosinophilia or dermatitis resulting from conjunctival irritation (see below).

The miotic alkaloids, on the other hand, are rarely sensitizers. The use of pilocarpine or eserine (physostigmine) only occasionally results in true allergic dermatoconjunctivitis (Fig. 10-4). Instead, the prolonged administration of these and other related synthetic miotics may produce follicular conjunctivitis, without eczema and eosinophilia, which appears to be caused by drug irritation, not by allergy. This will be elaborated upon later. Those very rare instances in which allergic dermatoconjunctivitis as well as follicles occur are explained by the fact that primary irritants may also be, or can become, sensitizers.

Other common ophthalmic drugs. Mercurials are well-recognized sensitizers, as are drugs ranging from dionin to boric acid, including zinc salts, silver protein (Argyrol), and naphazoline (Privine). Nitrofurazone (Furacin), quarternary ammonium compounds like benzalkonium (Zephiran), phenylephrine (Neo-Synephrine), and many others may also cause allergies. Even topical corticosteroids may cause an allergy. Idoxuridine may cause severe allergies, especially after prolonged use. Follicular irritation from use of this drug, involving the lower conjunctival sac, is a frequent occurrence.

Ophthalmic vehicles. Preservatives used in eye solutions may be the unsuspected cause of allergy.[43,44] This especially applies to the mercurials and to benzalkonium chloride. Ointment bases may cause allergies, usually to lanolin or petrolatum.

THE SYNDROME OF DRUG IRRITATION.[34,40] Although most cases of drug intolerance are caused by drug allergy, enough instances of drug irritation occur to make it an important differential consideration. The importance of the distinction between these two types of drug reaction lies in the fact that in drug irritations the use of the same drug may be continued if it is prepared in a manner that ensures no more irritation, whereas in allergies an entirely different drug must be substituted. Clinically, differentiation is generally simple.

Substances that come in contact with the skin and mucosa may be classified as (1) primary irritants and (2) cutaneous and mucosal sensitizers. Primary irritants cause an inflammation by direct action at the site of contact only, if allowed to act in sufficient intensity or quantity for a long enough time. Cutaneous and mucosal sensitizers usually cause no changes on first contact; but after about 5 to 7 days the entire skin, or the mucous membranes, will react specifically on further contact at the original site or elsewhere. These are the sensitizers that cause contact allergy.

Although some drugs are themselves primary irritants, and almost every drug may at times be irritating, conjunctivitis caused by irritation usually occurs following the prolonged use of preparations that are prone to deteriorate into irritating products if not prepared in a manner that will hinder or prevent this breakdown. This is particularly apt to occur with alkaloids but can also occur with the use of many chemicals, including antibiotics, especially neomycin, and, as stated above, idoxuridine.

The clinical picture of conjunctivitis resulting from drug irritation is that of a nonspecific watery inflammation of the conjunctiva in which, in contrast to allergic dermatoconjunctivitis, there is neither dermatitis of the eyelids nor conjunctival eosinophilia. In chronic cases, especially with the use of the alkaloids, follicular conjunctivitis may be the outstanding feature. The conjunctival involvement is less diffuse and less uniform than in allergy; often the area of most irritation, the lower lid and adjacent bulbar conjunctiva, bears the brunt of the involvement. Results of skin patch tests with these low-grade irritants are negative. In practice, it is important to know that such drugs as atropine usually cause allergies, but that on occasion irritation may occur because of formation of irritants like tropic acid and tropine.

The miotic alkaloids and the synthetic miotics cause irritations much more frequently than they do allergies. However, occasional allergies, especially to aromatic compounds like pilocarpine, eserine, neostigmine (Prostigmin), and Humorsol (demecarium bromide, a quaternary ammonium compound containing two neostigmine molecules), are encountered. Allergic reactions from isoflurophate (Floropryl) seem to be even rarer. The one allergic reaction I experienced with isoflurophate proved to be caused by the peanut oil vehicle. However, allergies must be expected from all miotic drugs if their use is sufficiently widespread.

The basis for the commonly encountered irritative, often follicular, conjunctivitis following the prolonged use of miotics appears to stem from their breakdown products, which are of course related to their chemical composition. All the aromatic miotics contain methyl ammonium radicals. Pilocarpine degrades to acetic acid, propionic acid, ammonia, and methylamine. Eserine forms rubeserine and methylamine through a rapid deterioration. Neostigmine appears to be more stable, but irritation occurs because of the formation of dimethylamine. Humorsol, a related drug (as noted above), appears to cause irritation by the same mechanism. Furtrethonium iodide (Furmethide) is another methyl ammonium agent with extremely marked irritating propensities, because of which the drug is no longer available.

Two aliphatic compounds, methacoline (Mecholyl) and carbachol (Doryl) also contain methyl ammonium radicals that apparently break down to methylamine or dimethylamine. There are two other aliphatic compounds that do not contain methyl ammonium radicals: isoflurophate and echothiophate (Phospholine iodide). Follicular reactions from isoflurophate are not rare. The drug degrades to hydrochloric acid and elemental fluorine. A phosphorus derivative of choline, echothiopate appears to decompose by hydrolysis to thiocholine and the diethyl ester of phosphoric acid and causes irritation possibly on this basis.

Although allergic reactions to epinephrine products used in glaucoma occur, follicular irritative reactions appear to be more common. This drug also contains a methylamine radical. Another particularly interesting phenomenon is the deposition of clumps of melanin pigment in the interior fornix after the use of epinephrine solutions, because of the "dopa" reaction. In contrast, I have encountered a number of allergic reactions to phenylephrine, another methyl ammonium compound, but no characteristic irritative follicular conjunctivitis. The absence of such irritation may lie in the fact that the drug is more stable and is used less frequently in the individual patient in such high concentrations.

Vernal conjunctivitis

Vernal conjunctivitis is a recurrent, bilateral, interstitial inflammation of the conjunctiva occurring in warm weather. Although the exact causation of the disease is unknown, it is included among allergies of the eye because the condition has so many allergic facets. The most likely hypothesis is that vernal conjunctivitis is a form of physical allergy and that it is the ocular reaction to the warm season of especially predisposed atopic individuals whose constitutions have been conditioned by a number of general organic factors.

Clinical aspects. Vernal conjunctivitis is a disease of warm climates. In the Mediterranean area an incidence of up to 2% of all patients examined in eye clinics has been reported; in New York City the probable figure is less than 1/10 of 1%. The condition almost always affects boys rather than girls, in a proportion of more than 3 to 1. After puberty the incidence is about equal in both sexes. It is a disease of childhood that usually occurs in those from 6 to 20 years of age. Colored races are particularly prone to the limbic form of the disease. In most patients a familial incidence usually occurs, with an allergic background being present more than half the time. In addition, over 50% of all patients with vernal conjunctivitis suffer from other types of allergic diseases of atopic nature, such as hay fever, asthma, atopic dermatitis, and allergies to foods, dust, and molds.

SYMPTOMS. The outstanding symptom of the disease is extreme itching. Photophobia is also a frequent complaint.

OBJECTIVE FINDINGS. Vernal conjunctivitis is a bilateral condition, occurring in two main forms: the palpebral and the limbal. In a significant percentage of patients a mixed type occurs in which both the conjunctiva and the corneal limbus show changes (Fig. 10-5). The palpebral form of vernal conjunctivitis is practically always limited to the tarsal conjunctiva of the upper lid where, in long-standing cases, large cobblestone vegetations appear. Involvement of the conjunctiva of the lower lid indicates extreme severity of the condition in that individual.

The disease is essentially proliferative, characterized by a marked and continuously increasing formation of hyalinized

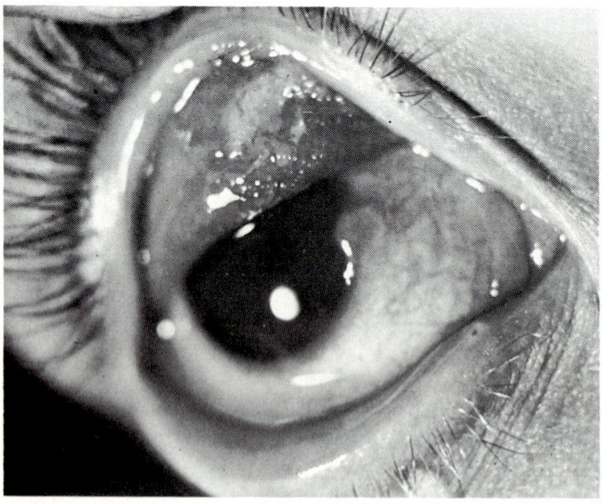

Fig. 10-5. Vernal conjunctivits. Mixed type, showing palpebral and limbal involvement with thin pseudomembrane. (Courtesy Clay-Adams Co. From Theodore, F. H., and Schlossman, A.: Ocular allergy, Baltimore, 1958, The Williams & Wilkins Co. © 1958, The Williams & Wilkins Co., Baltimore.)

connective tissue. This opaque tissue imparts a milky, bluish appearance to the conjunctiva by obscuring the capillaries, which normally give it a pink color. No matter of how many years' duration, in other forms of allergic conjunctivitis the capillary markings are never obliterated. Sometimes patients with subjectively very severe vernal conjunctivitis may show only slight conjunctival thickening and the presence of microscopic papillae containing central blood vessels ("blood points"). Usually, however, the proliferation progresses to the formation of the classical excrescences, which are hard, flat, large, polygonal papillae of varying size, with a predilection for the tarsus of the upper lid. In some countries vernal conjunctivitis, because of this predominant upper lid involvement, may be confused with trachoma. When one is in doubt, epithelial scrapings revealing conjunctival eosinophilia are helpful; however, the two conditions may coexist. Follicular conjunctivitis, despite its lower lid predilection, true follicular character, and preauricular adenopathy, is sometimes confused with vernal conjunctivitis.

The discharge that occurs in vernal conjunctivitis is of great diagnostic value. The tenacious, thick, "chewing-gum" pseudomembrane, which may be peeled off the conjunctiva without bleeding, is characteristic. Even if a membrane is not present, exposure of the everted lid, massage, or the heat of a camera light or slit lamp will result in its formation. The extremely alkaline secretion is notable for the masses of eosinophils or eosinophilic granules it contains.

The limbic proliferations of the bulbar type of vernal conjunctivitis may occur without any palpebral lesions. They appear as yellowish gray gelatinous elevations in the palpebral fissure zone. Trantas' spots are white points that sometimes cap the excrescences and are pathognomonic of vernal conjunctivitis. As differentiated from phlyctenules, vernal lesions do not stain with fluorescein. Furthermore, there is in general less inflammatory reaction than in phlyctenular keratoconjunctivitis. Conjunctival eosinophilia is a valuable differential in determining the diagnosis.

CORNEAL LESIONS. The most frequent and characteristic corneal lesion of vernal conjunctivitis is a superficial epithelial keratitis, requiring biomicroscopy for its recognition, located usually in the upper half of the cornea. The cornea looks white, as if flour had been blown over it, and stains in a punctate fashion. These lesions clear rapidly as the condition improves and thus offer an excellent index of the efficacy of treatment. Other types of corneal involvement occur much less commonly, some by direct extension of the limbal process, others being deeper and central, leaving serious opacities. Still others resemble dystrophies, such as pseudogerontoxon.

ETIOLOGY. On the basis of all the clinical characteristics of the disease and its clinical course, with exacerbations during warm weather and clearing in all but the most severe cases during the winter or in migration to a cold climate, it appears that vernal conjunctivitis is a form of physical allergy to the warm season.[46] This peculiar allergy occurs only in especially predisposed atopic individuals. The special factors that predispose these individuals may be endocrine, metabolic, allergic, and possibly infectious. In some way these factors all combine to condition atopic individuals so that the warm season acts as a trigger mechanism, setting off a sort of chain reaction precipitating the disease.

ALLERGY OF THE EYELIDS

The eyelid proper is often the site of allergic reactions. In fact, such allergies occur so commonly that they appear to constitute, at least statistically, the most important form of ocular allergy encountered in clinical practice. Because the eyelids represent a transitional structure consisting of the conjunctiva and the skin with the lid margin in between, allergies of both the conjunctiva and the eyelids often overlap and occur at the same time. The most important such combined allergic reaction, allergic dermatoconjunctivitis, has already been described. The outline below classifies all types of allergic reactions of the eyelids that are encountered.

Allergy of the eyelids

- A. Anaphylactic and atopic allergy (immediate reaction)
  - 1. Allergic edema (urticaria, angioneurotic edema, serum sickness): drugs, animal sera, insect bites
- B. Contact allergy (delayed reaction)
  - 1. Allergic dermatoconjunctivitis: drugs, chemicals
  - 2. Eczematous contact dermatitis: cosmetics, drugs, chemicals, apparel
- C. Microbial allergy (delayed reaction)
  - 1. Infectious eczematoid dermatitis
    - a. Bacterial: *Staphylococcus, Streptococcus*
    - b. Fungal: trichophytosis, moniliasis
  - 2. Infections of the lid margin (usually staphylococcal)
    - a. Blepharitis
    - b. Meibomitis
    - c. Hordeolum
    - d. Chalazion

Allergic edema of the eyelids

Anaphylactic and atopic allergic reactions of the eyelids manifest themselves basically as urticaria or angioneurotic edema. Such reactions may occur in serum sickness, from insect bites, from the ingestion of all types of foods and many drugs, and sometimes, although rarely, from inhalants and contactants. Even microbial allergens, particularly fungal products, may cause urticarial reactions about the eyelids. In addition, physical agents, such as cold or sunlight, may result in such urticaria.

Contact allergy of the eyelids

The skin of the eyelids is particularly susceptible to allergic inflammation for several special reasons.[35,36,38] First, its fine texture and extreme thinness readily permit minor traumatization and the penetration of noxious substances of all types. Second, because of their location, the eyelids are especially exposed to physical trauma (rubbing, heat, sun, wind, and ocular secretions) and to various drugs and chemicals applied elsewhere on the head and face.

Thus, although a facial cream or hair tonic is not directly applied to the eyelids, the eyelids may eventually prove to be the only site of the eczema, as even a minimal amount of the irritant, indirectly contacted by means of a pillowcase during sleep or from the fingers, is able to penetrate sufficiently here to cause the reaction, in contrast to its inability to penetrate the thicker and stronger skin where it was originally applied so generously. Similarly, the skin of the eyelids often reacts to bacterial products or ocular medicaments occurring in tears, which would be harmless elsewhere on the skin.

Contact allergy of the eyelids usually results from the use of cosmetics or ophthalmic drugs. Allergy to plants is, however, not uncommon. Less often articles of apparel, jewelry, metals, plastics, other chemicals, and animal or vegetable products, too numerous to mention, may cause a reaction. The relative importance of the various contactants causing allergic eczematous dermatitis is difficult to evaluate. However, it appears clear that cosmetics and drugs are the two major offenders. The dermatitis, which may be either unilateral or bilateral, occurs mostly in women, probably more because they use cosmetics so universally than because of any endocrine factor. There need be no previous history of familial or personal allergy. The diagnosis is based on a careful history, positive patch test reaction, and the ruling out of other major causes of eyelid eczema, namely primary ocular infection or generalized dermatoses. In addition, one must be certain that the contact dermatitis present is caused by allergy rather than by primary irritation. The highlight of therapy is to eliminate the sensitizing agent; the use of any other allergenic substance may seriously aggravate the condition.

The mechanism for the production of contact allergy has been fairly well established and has been described earlier in this chapter. The site of eczematous (contact type) allergic dermatitis appears to be strictly epidermal, not to be deeper in the

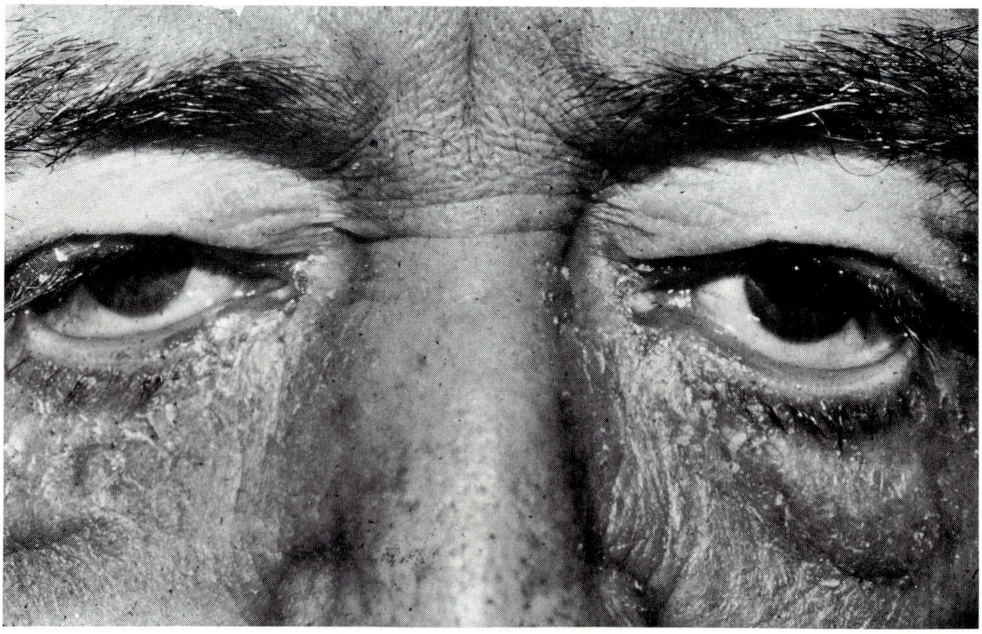

Fig. 10-6. Contact allergy to witch hazel applied to eyelids. The conjunctiva was uninvolved. (From Theodore, F. H., and Schlossman, A.: Ocular allergy, Baltimore, 1958, The Williams & Wilkins Co. © 1958, The Williams & Wilkins Co., Baltimore.)

skin. For this reason, in order to prove contact allergy, patch tests are necessary. Immediate-wheal testing by intradermal injections is not a correct diagnostic procedure here, because even the most superficial intracutaneous or scratch test carries the allergen through the epidermis into the cutis.

Ophthalmic medicaments. Most instances of this form of allergy begin in the conjunctiva, as it is generally the focal point of contact of the drug. However, certain medicaments that are directly applied to the skin of the eyelids do not cause conjunctivitis and might be briefly mentioned. These include antiseptics such as iodine, picric acid, mercurials, Zephiran, boric acid, and witch hazel (Fig. 10-6). Most of the time, however, ointments, especially those used to relieve itching or irritation of the eyelids, and particularly those containing anesthetics, antihistaminics, or even corticosteroids (Fig. 10-7), are the prime affectors. Reactions may occur from the use of all types of adhesive tapes.

Cosmetics. Cosmetics have been widely used for thousands of years, despite sporadic, unsuccessful attempts to outlaw the custom, such as the introduction of a bill in the British Parliament in the eighteenth century proposing to make the beguiling of men into matrimony by their use punishable as for witchcraft. So much is now known about the action of cosmetics on the skin, and the exclusion of harmful ingredients is so regulated by law, that the good accomplished by their use far outweighs the occasional harm that occurs. Actually, if we consider how universally cosmetics are used, the percentage incidence of allergies to them is extremely low.

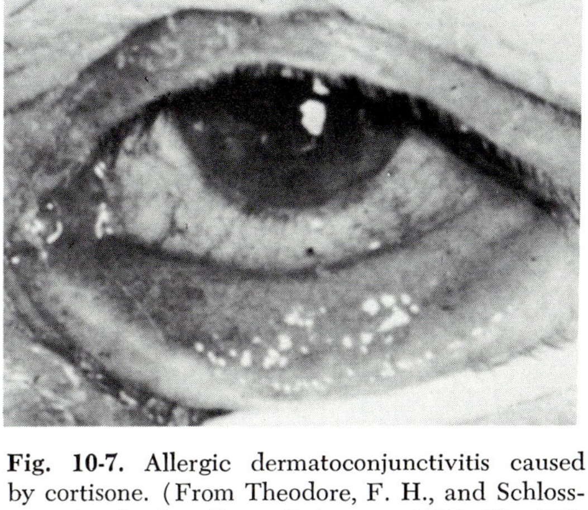

Fig. 10-7. Allergic dermatoconjunctivitis caused by cortisone. (From Theodore, F. H., and Schlossman, A.: Ocular allergy, Baltimore, 1958, The Williams & Wilkins Co. © 1958, The Williams & Wilkins Co., Baltimore.)

Unlike drug allergy, cosmetic allergy usually begins by involvement of the upper lid especially at the medial portion. Generally the conjunctiva is uninflamed and without eosinophilia. In the diagnosis of eyelid eczema caused by cosmetics it must be remembered that only the eyelids may react even if the allergenic substance was applied at a place remote to them. Careful history taking is essential; the use of leading questions often is important in opening avenues of thought otherwise dismissed by the patient as immaterial. Just because a cosmetic has been used previously without reaction for a long time does not mean it should be completely exonerated, because the manufacturer only now may have changed the formula or the method of production in some way. In diagnostic testing for cosmetic sensitivity it is better to apply the cosmetic in the way it is generally used instead of doing a patch test, because in normal use the uncovered cosmetic loses most of its substance by evaporation. Covering the cosmetic by a patch does not permit this evaporation and may give rise to false-positive reactions with cosmetics that are actually harmless when used in the ordinary manner.

Nowadays most allergies to cosmetics are caused by the perfumes used and by impurities in manufacture, as the hitherto most flagrant offenders have been eliminated. Sometimes, although the cosmetic itself is innocent, contamination of the containers may cause allergies. Allergies to a few important types of cosmetics are noted below.

Nail polish and nail lacquer. These used

to be extremely common but now occur less frequently. The offending ingredients are believed to be the synthetic resins, such as methacrylates, and possibly the dyes used.

Face powder. Face powders used to be sensitizers because of the orris root and the rice powder content. These ingredients are rarely used at present, having been replaced by titanium salts. Now any allergy to face powder is usually traced to perfumes and to impurities in manufacture and packaging.

Facial creams. Facial creams such as plain cold cream and vanishing creams are not often sensitizers. In both, the major offender is either lanolin or cocoa butter and almond oil. Emulsifying agents and perfumes should also be suspected.

Lipstick. Lipstick dermatitis is usually caused by the indelible dyes used.

Perfumes. The extremely complicated nature of perfumes makes such products especially liable to cause allergies. Their universal use, not only alone but to make other products more attractive, makes them a common cause of contact allergy.

Hair preparations. Hair dyes and rinses contain both sensitizers and toxic products. The most commonly used ingredient, paraphenylenediamine, may be both toxic and allergenic. Generally allergies occur from its use, but in susceptible persons serious toxic reactions may develop. Paraphenylenediamine is also the major sensitizer in allergy to furs. Metallic dyes may also cause allergies. Vegetable dyes are safer. Hair tonics and locations also contain sensitizing agents.

OTHER CAUSES OF CONTACT ALLERGY OF THE EYELIDS. These include wearing apparel, such as dyed fabrics, especially if the dyes tend to "bleed" or come out of the fabric easily, and laundering and dry-cleaning materials. Allergy to leather usually occurs because of the manufacturing process. Shoe polishes and shoe dyes may cause severe allergy. Furs may cause allergic dermatitis of the eyelids because of the dyes used in their manufacture. Allergy to jewelry is not uncommon, particularly to nickel, cobalt, platinum, copper, chromium, aluminum, and gold. Spectacle frames may cause allergies. Most reported cases are those caused by metallic (white gold) frames. Here the allergy is caused by the nickel content. Allergy to plastic eyeglass frames arise from sensitivities to the various chemicals used in the manufacturing process.

Infectious eczematoid dermatitis

Eczematoid dermatitis of the eyelids may arise on an allergic basis as a complication of bacterial, fungal, or other microorganismal infection present elsewhere.[37] This basically allergic response to infectants must not be confused with the numerous types of dermatitis resulting from direct invasion of the skin of the eyelids by many bacteria, viruses, and fungi. The latter are entirely distinct and not germane to the subject. Allergic reactions of the eyelids caused by bacteria generally are the result of neighboring infection of the adnexa, although rare syphilids and tuberculids need not follow this pattern. In fungal infections, however, the original focus may be far from the eye and entirely unrelated to it. In either event, the eczema appears to be in large measure a manifestation of microbial allergy. Although microbial dermatitis elsewhere on the body may result from a variety of infectants, including *Staphylococcus, Streptococcus,* and *Escherichia coli,* as far as the eyelids are concerned the important bacterium involved is the *Staphylococcus.* On rare occasions streptococci are responsible. Eyelid eczema caused by fungus sensitivity, an unusual occurrence to begin with, appears mainly as trichophytosis or moniliasis. All types of infectious eczematoid reactions appear prone to secondary contact type allergies, especially from medicaments. Since the reverse also happens—that is, the secondary infection of primarily allergic dermatitis—diagnostic problems may arise. About the eyelids, however, fewer such differential difficulties should occur, because the only type of infectious eczematoid reaction of practical importance encountered—staphylococcal eczema

—is generally associated with other ocular findings that afford valuable diagnostic clues.

Staphylococcal eczema of the eyelids

The importance of staphylococcal infections of the lid margin and conjunctiva as a major cause of eczema of the eyelids has not received the emphasis it deserves. Although dermatitis actually is a relatively infrequent complication of such common infections, recent experience indicates that the condition is the most frequent cause of chronic eyelid eczema that has been encountered; yet because its importance is not generally appreciated, it is often overlooked.

Many unrecognized, recurrent cases of

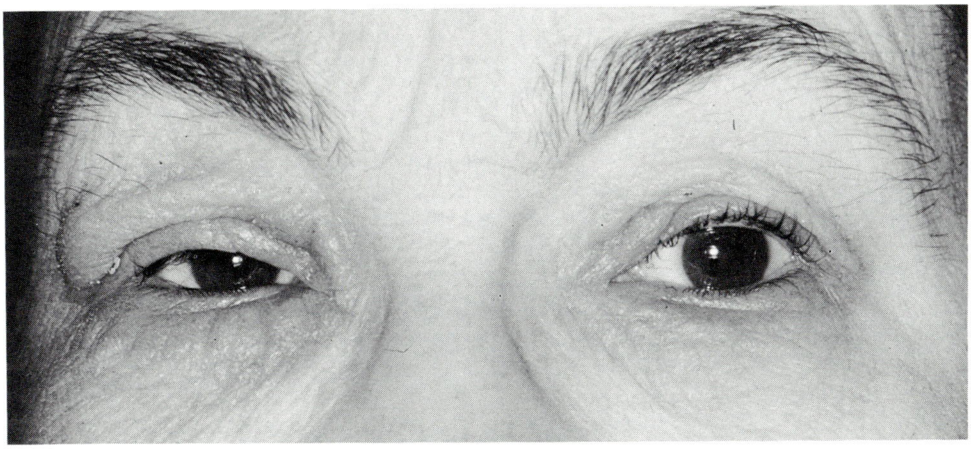

Fig. 10-8. Staphylococcal eczema of the eyelids. (From Theodore, F. H.: Trans. Amer. Acad. Ophthal. Otolaryng. **58**:708, 1954.)

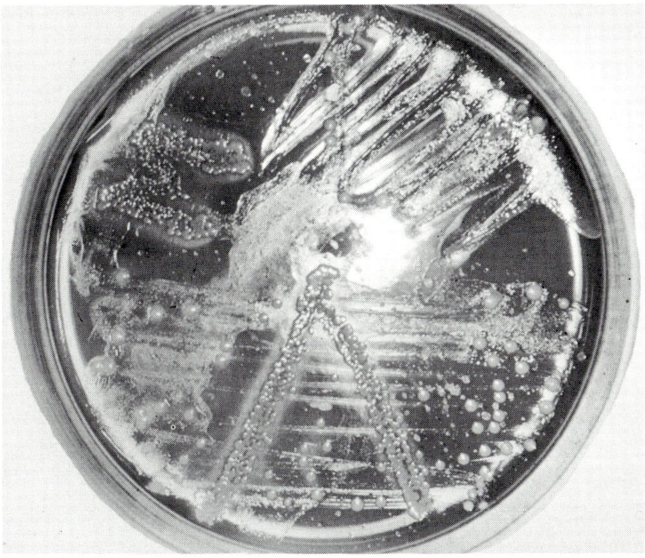

Fig. 10-9. Culture of conjunctiva and eyelids (patient seen in Fig. 10-8) revealing numerous colonies of pathogenic *Staphylococcus aureus;* growth in form of M (top left quadrant) was obtained from expressed meibomian secretion. (From Theodore, F. H.: Trans. Amer. Acad. Ophthal. Otolaryng. **58**:708, 1954.)

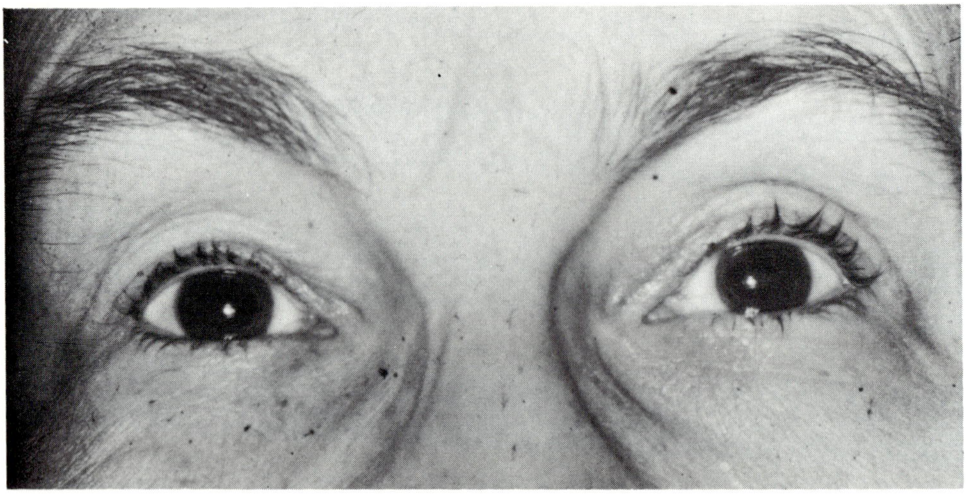

Fig. 10-10. Same patient as in Fig. 10-8. Complete cure of staphylococcal eczema. At this time bacterial cultures and skin tests were negative. (From Theodore, F. H., and Schlossman, A.: Ocular allergy, Baltimore, 1958, The Williams & Wilkins Co. © 1958, The Williams & Wilkins Co., Baltimore.)

staphylococcal eczema of the eyelids are treated unsuccessfully for years as instances of contact allergy. One cannot distinguish between the two conditions on the basis of the character of the dermatitis, as they look very much alike. What is required for the diagnosis and successful treatment of staphylococcal eczema is the demonstration that the focal point of the process is not the skin, but instead is the eye and its adnexa. When this is demonstrated and proper treatment instituted, the eczema, which is a secondary complication, gradually disappears. The key to the diagnosis is routine detailed ophthalmologic examination, both clinical and bacterial. This almost always will reveal the basis for the dermatitis, even if the primary focus is obscure, such as a minute abscess of a meibomian gland.

The following findings differentiate staphylococcal eczema of the eyelids from the allergic variety: (1) blepharitis, with scaling, and often ulcers of the eyelid margin; (2) meibomitis, either diffuse or focal; (3) superficial epithelial keratitis involving the inferior half of the cornea, readily seen on slit-lamp examination after staining with fluorescein, considered as pathognomonic of staphylococcal conjunctivitis; (4) strongly positive conjunctival and lid margin cultures, showing many toxin-producing staphylococci, often entirely out of numerical proportion to the objective clinical findings; and, (5) absence of eosinophils in epithelial scrapings, which instead usually reveal neutrophils and staphylococci, especially on the lid margins (Figs. 10-8, 10-9, and 10-10).

Lid margin affections

In long-standing blepharitis, meibomitis, recurrent hordeola, and recurrent chalazion, all conditions in which staphylococcal infection play an important role, secondary microbial allergy often supervenes. Desensitization therapy is an integral and often necessary part of the long-term treatment.

ALLERGY OF THE CORNEA

A large part of corneal disease is allergic in nature.[29] The cornea manifests all recognized forms of allergic reactions, including the atopic, microbial, and contact types. Furthermore, other diseases that occur in allergic individuals, such as atopic dermatitis and possibly rosacea, demonstrate corneal lesions.

It is interesting that some of the fundamental experimental work in ocular allergy was performed with the cornea as a shock organ. As early as 1909 Weekers[49] produced phlyctenules in rabbits sensitized to bovine tuberculosis. During the following 20 years this work was confirmed and expanded by many investigators. Wessely[51] in 1911 was a pioneer in demonstrating that the cornea is capable of reacting anaphylactically to produce parenchymatous keratitis. Thus two of the most important corneal diseases of that era, namely, interstitial keratitis and phlyctenular ophthalmia, were shown to have an allergic etiology. These pioneer investigations have been considerably extended by more modern studies, including the experimental induction of local selective tissue sensitivity of the cornea and the corneal limbus. Immune corneal rings have been produced experimentally by a number of investigators.[41]

The classification of corneal allergy

Similar to allergies of the conjunctiva, eyelids, and other parts of the eye, the various manifestations of corneal allergy can best be understood when they are considered on the basis of the allergic mechanism involved. In fact, this mechanistic approach has particular advantages in regard to the cornea, because different types of allergy may give relatively similar clinical pictures and because the type of reaction depends to a great extent on the degree of hypersensitivity, time of exposure, and other factors that alter the clinical picture. A classification of corneal allergy is presented in the following outline.

Allergy of the cornea

A. Atopic allergy (immediate reaction)
   1. Topical allergens: superficial keratitis (rarely ulceration)
   2. Generalized allergy: superficial and marginal keratitis (rarely deep)

B. Contact allergy (delayed reaction)
   1. Drugs: superficial keratitis, deep ulceration
   2. Other contactants: superficial keratitis, deep keratitis

C. Microbial allergy
   1. Lues, tubercle bacilli, other bacteria: interstitial keratitis
   2. Tubercle bacilli, staphylococci, other bacteria, coccidioides immitis, nematodes: phlyctenular ophthalmia
   3. Staphylococci, bacillary dysentery: marginal infiltrates and ring ulcers
   4. Herpes simplex virus: disciform edema of the corneal stroma
   5. Adenoviruses: subepithelial opacities
   6. Virus of trachoma: keratitis, opacities

D. Keratitis of possible allergic origin
   1. Vernal catarrh
   2. Keratitis associated with atopic dermatitis
   3. Rosacea keratitis
   4. Periarteritis nodosa

E. Allergic reactions in corneal transplants
   1. Interstitial keratitis

F. Autogenous reactions

Atopic reactions of the cornea

Atopic reactions of the cornea are most commonly caused by pollen allergy or by certain ingestants. They are chiefly superficial in nature, although occasionally deep keratitis does occur. Superficial keratitis resulting from atopy is much more common than the reports in the literature seem to indicate. Because of the mildness of atopic corneal reactions, most cases are not referred to the ophthalmologist. Others may be missed by allergists who have no experience in the use of the slit lamp. Also, many atopic reactions are self-limited or improve as a result of the treatment of the general atopy.

CORNEAL REACTIONS TO POLLENS AND DUSTS. Although the conjunctiva is commonly affected by hay fever, corneal involvement is much less frequent and occurs in more severe cases. It is generally confined to superficial keratitis with a few isolated areas that stain with fluorescein. I have also noted mild keratitis in conjunctival tests utilizing pollen extract. Such keratitis is often self-limited and responds readily to the same treatment as the conjunctivitis. This mild lesion presents no problem either diagnostically or therapeutically and should give little cause for concern. More severe reactions may occur from other pollens, such as corn and orris root. In severe generalized hypersensitivity to dusts the cornea may become involved.

Corneal reactions to ingestants. Corneal allergies caused by foods are generally more severe than those caused by inhalants. Although they may at times be superficial, they tend to involve the corneal stroma. Foods that have been incriminated include cottonseed meal, wheat, strawberries, cucumbers, cheese, Coca-Cola, egg white, chocolate, rye, and nuts.

In addition, corneal allergy has been reported from the internal use of a mixture containing caffeine, phenacetin, and antipyrine.

Contact allergy of the cornea

The cornea is often involved in contact allergies of the eye. Usually this is part of an allergic dermatoconjunctivitis, so that the involvement of these tissues points to the correct diagnosis. Since the cornea may show only mild superficial keratitis, its involvement may be easily overlooked when other parts of the eye have a more marked reaction. In some instances the lid and conjunctiva are slightly affected, but the keratitis is extremely severe. On occasion the superficial cornea may show a similar picture to that of atopic allergic keratitis, and differential diagnosis will then depend on history and elimination of the offending allergen.

However, many times the corneal involvement may dominate the scene. Severe contact keratitis may extend into the deeper layers of the cornea and may be accompanied by an iritic condition. Occasionally the process is essentially subepithelial, with no staining of the cornea.

The responsible allergens include a variety of ophthalmic medicaments, such as local anesthetics, mydriatic alkaloids, antibiotics, sulfonamides, mercurials, quaternary ammonium compounds, lanolin, coal tar dyes, orris root, and vegetable products.

Special emphasis in regard to possible severe hyperallergic reactions from the use of some of the newer and better local anesthetics such as proparacaine, and to a lesser degree from benoxinate (Dorsacaine), must be made. I have reported a number of instances of bilateral necrotizing epithelial reactions requiring hospitalization of the patient in some cases because of severe disability from pain and poor vision after the instillation of a single drop.[42] Fortunately, recovery was complete in these acute idiosyncrasies. However, the constant home use of such anesthetics for chronic eye complaints may cause severe deeper corneal allergies that may result in permanent disabilities and visual loss.

Microbiallergic keratitis

Allergic reactions of the cornea to products of bacteria, protozoa, fungi, and helminths and to other similar protein products give a wide variety of corneal lesions. It is interesting that certain bacteria are associated with certain specific corneal changes. The classical picture of interstitial keratitis is caused by the spirochete of syphilis, and phlyctenular keratoconjunctivitis is most commonly traceable to the products of the tubercle bacillus.

Interstitial keratitis. An allergic mechanism appears to offer the best explanation for the occurrence of the two major types of interstitial keratitis encountered clinically; namely, luetic and tuberculous. Evidence for an allergic etiology is based on: (1) the ineffectiveness of specific (antiluetic) therapy, (2) the effectiveness of corticosteroids and foreign protein therapy, (3) the rare onset of interstitial keratitis during the course of systemic arsenic therapy (Jarisch-Herxheimer reactions), and (4) experimental production by allergic techniques of lesions identical in essential details to syphilitic parenchymatous keratitis.

Phlyctenular keratoconjunctivitis. It is now generally accepted that phlyctenular keratoconjunctivitis is a manifestation of endogenous allergy to not only tuberculoprotein[32] but also other bacterial antigens, especially staphylococcal, and rarely to gonococcal and diplobacillary products. In-

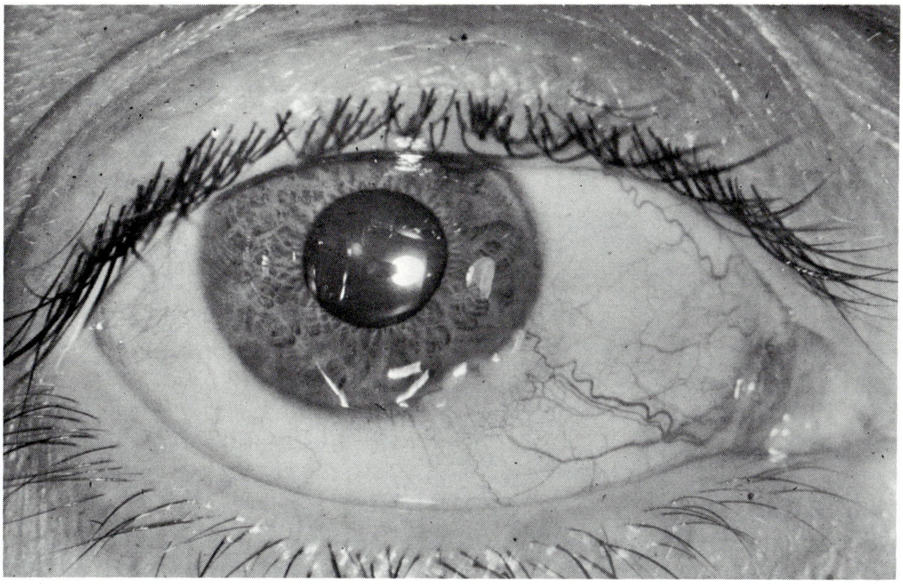

Fig. 10-11. Phlyctenular keratoconjunctivitis complicating ulcerative colitis. Excellent result with topical hydrocortisone. (From Theodore, F. H., and Schlossman, A.: Ocular allergy, Baltimore, 1958, The Williams & Wilkins Co. © 1958, The Williams & Wilkins Co., Baltimore.)

stances have been encountered in patients allergic to coccidioidin and in patients with leishmaniasis, trypanosomiasis, moniliasis, ascariasis, and helminthiasis. Phlyctenules have been produced experimentally by many allergic methods, using various antigens in appropriately sensitized animals. These include tuberculin, staphylococcal products, horse serum, and chemicals, which were instilled into the conjunctival sac. The dramatic response to corticosteroid therapy in all types of phlyctenulosis is further suggestive evidence of the allergic nature of the disease (Fig. 10-11).

MARGINAL ULCERS AND INFILTRATES. Simple marginal or catarrhal ulcers and infiltrates are probably the most common manifestations of corneal allergy. Although it has not been proved conclusively that marginal ulcers in bacterial conjunctivitis are allergic in nature, the weight of evidence favors an allergic etiology, especially as regards the *Staphylococcus;* here the antigen is probably the exotoxin of the bacterium. Marginal ulcers caused by other bacteria, such as the diplobacillus or the Koch-Weeks bacillus, may occur as a result of direct toxic action. In favor of an allergic etiology for such infiltrates and ulcers are the following findings:

1. Marginal ulcers rarely appear early in the course of conjunctivitis caused by staphylococci or diplobacilli. They occur commonly after the infection has been present for a period of time, often after repeated exacerbations.
2. Patients often show evidence of hypersensitivity to bacterial exotoxins through positive reactions to skin tests, or they may have foci of infection in sinuses and tonsils and other remote areas of the body. However, in some cases reactions to the skin tests are only slightly positive.
3. It is difficult to isolate bacteria from scrapings of marginal ulcers.
4. Thygeson[47] claims that he has never observed a catarrhal ulcer caused by the pneumococcus. This is probably because of the fact that no exotoxin has been demonstrated in association with pneumococci.
5. There are many similarities between marginal ulcers and phlyctenules,

which are universally conceded to be allergic manifestations.

6. Marginal ulcers have been observed in atopic and contact allergies, such as tetracaine sensitivity, as well as in vernal catarrh.
7. Marginal ulcers in general respond very well to corticosteroids.

RING ULCERS. Ring ulcers give the appearance of coalescing marginal ulcers but seem to have a different etiology, although they are allergic in nature. Systemic microbial allergy seems to play a role. I have encountered this condition in patients with ulcerative colitis; Thygeson has described it in bacillary dysentery.

DISCIFORM EDEMA OF THE CORNEAL STROMA. Edematous reactions of the cornea of disciform character may arise in the course of various types of keratitis, particularly herpetic, or may appear without any clearly demonstrable cause. The tendency has arisen to group all such instances of corneal edema under the term disciform keratitis. The disadvantage of considering all disciform stromal edema as one entity lies in the fact that, whereas in herpetic keratitis corticosteroids may be contraindicated, in other disciform lesions such therapy may be of value. Beneficial effects in these cases may result from the action of the corticosteroids on the possible allergic component.

Originally disciform keratitis was meant to describe a disklike opacity situated in the corneal stroma, which often assumed twice its usual thickness in the involved area and was associated with descemetitis. Usually the corneal epithelium was relatively intact, and staining with fluorescein revealed little or nothing. Most such cases were attributed to herpes simplex infection on the basis of exposure to viral infections (colds, herpes labialis), often in association with trauma, and it was hypothesized that the virus had somehow entered the stroma through the epithelium. Many times the so-called point of entrance could not be demonstrated. Such cases were of themselves very serious; resultant central opacities, after the edema of the cornea had subsidized, would reduce vision to the extent of industrial blindness. There seems no clearcut evidence, other than circumstantial, that the condition is always caused by herpes simplex. Sometimes herpes zoster and vaccinia seem causative. In still other instances the cause is not demonstrable.

The role of hypersensitivity in the causation of disciform keratitis has been accepted by many, although the evidence is partially hypothetical and inferential. Braley[4] has long been an important exponent of the allergic nature of disciform keratitis. Jones[16] has restated Braley's original concept in a graphic manner. He visualizes the corneal stroma as an immunologic blotter that absorbs antigens arising from virus proliferating in the epithelium. The subsequent arrival of antibody gives rise to a fixed tissue antigen-antibody union resulting in edema or even necrosis.

It has long been my opinion that there are two types of disciform keratitis: (1) the type without clinical evidence of herpetic keratitis and (2) the type occurring in association with demonstrable herpetic ulceration.[46] My hypothesis is that in the first (classical) variety the cause has not been demonstrated and may possibly be allergic in nature; in the second form, where a herpetic ulcer preexists, although allergy possibly operates in the production of the stromal edema, the infectious component of the process predominates in the stroma to the extent that corticosteroids should either not be used at all, or else with caution, concomitantly with idoxuridine. Fig. 10-12 illustrates an interesting example of herpes simplex keratitis in a successful graft.

ADENOVIRUS KERATITIS. A microbiallergic basis for the subepithelial capacities occurring in epidemic keratoconjunctivitis, caused by adenovirus type 8, appears to be a strong possibility. I have observed many patients in whom the opacities, which occur at a time when infectivity is over, clear dramatically with the use of topical steroids only to reappear when the medic-

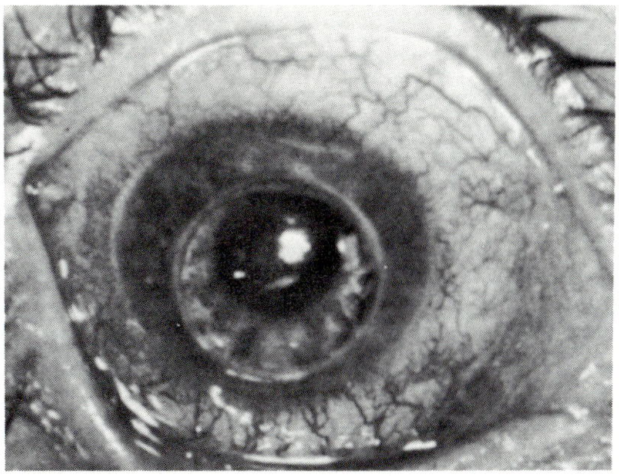

Fig. 10-12. Herpes simplex keratitis of a corneal graft. The patient had a successful keratoplasty performed 1½ years previously because of corneal opacification following disciform keratitis. The present herpetic infection is explained by the fact that the donor material assumes the susceptibilities and characteristics of recipient tissue. (From Theodore, F. H., and Schlossman, A.: Ocular allergy, Baltimore, 1958, The Williams & Wilkins Co. © 1958, The Williams & Wilkins Co., Baltimore.)

ament is discontinued.[41] Some of these patients receiving steroids show the recurrence of such opacities as much as two years after the original virus infection if the drug is stopped completely. For this reason, to avoid a form of steroid "addiction" in the patient, I do not advocate their use unless central opacities seriously bother the patient, either subjectively or visually.

Keratitis of possible allergic origin

VERNAL CATARRH. Except for the limbal proliferations, corneal lesions of vernal catarrh are an often overlooked feature of the disease. They may be divided into two groups: (1) those occurring as direct extension of the limbic and conjunctival disease and (2) those in which there is no such direct extension. In the first group are included crescentic, raised, fleshy processes and pannuslike formations. The lesions that do not arise from direct extension of the conjunctival process may be toxic or possibly nutritional in origin. The most important of these is superficial epithelial keratitis. Corneal ulcers and dystrophies may occur.[46]

KERATITIS ASSOCIATED WITH ATOPIC DERMATITIS. Corneal involvement of varying intensity may complicate chronic atopic dermatitis. According to Hogan,[15] the corneal affection may occur simultaneously with or follow repeated exacerbations of conjunctivitis. The superficial third of the periphery of the cornea is affected first. The corneal stroma near Bowman's membrane becomes clouded. The lesion gradually spreads deeper into the stroma, and after some time blood vessels push in from the limbus. The corneal epithelium covering the area of keratitis becomes edematous and shows minute punctate staining with fluorescein. In some instances the entire cornea becomes hazy and vascularized, with resultant diminished visual acuity.

Two other types of corneal lesion have been described in association with atopic dermatitis. Pillat[23] reported a case with superficial punctate keratitis. In rare instances keratoconus is associated with atopic dermatitis. Patients with this corneal condition manifest severe and extensive dermatitis with lichenification and pigmentation, severe bronchial asthma, and reactions to food and inhalant allergens. It is possible that by carefully studying such cases, ophthalmologists will gain better insight into the pathogenesis of keratoconus. Keratoconus is also a complication of vernal catarrh. Steroid therapy, both local and systemic, is the indicated form of treatment.

ROSACEA KERATITIS. The etiology of rosacea is obscure. Although a few observers maintain that it is an allergy, there is little definitive evidence to substantiate this theory.

KERATITIS IN PERIARTERITIS NODOSA. Keratitis has been described as a complication of periarteritis nodosa.

Allergic reactions in corneal transplants

It is probable that allergy plays a role in the clouding of corneal grafts, occurring from the tenth day to the sixth week after operation. Castroviejo[8] believes that this corneal opacification is the result of uveitis, an allergic response to foci of infection harbored in the nose or the throat. Maumenee,[18] on the other hand, showed experimentally that the recipient can become sensitized to donor material following corneal transplants, and he concluded that this allergic reaction is in large measure responsible for the clouding of grafts after the tenth day.

In a later paper Maumenee[19] stressed the importance of the homograft allergic reaction as the most important single cause of delayed opacification of the graft in an eye that has been properly selected for corneal transplantation. This reaction is characterized by progressive edema of the stroma of the graft, which eventually may become thickened and vascularized or may clear spontaneously if the reaction first occurs many months after transplantation. Evidence that this reaction is to a homograft may be summarized as follows: (1) the response is localized to the graft; (2) it occurs much more frequently in heavily vascularized than in avascular corneas; (3) a similar clouding can be experimentally produced in corneal grafts of rabbits by increasing the dose of homograft antigen by transplanting skin from the same donor to the recipient; (4) corneal stroma and endothelium are capable of eliciting the homograft reaction; and (5) penetrating autografts of the entire cornea in man do not develop a delayed opacification. It is reasonable to assume that the homograft reaction may also occur in lamellar transplants, although there is less evidence in this regard.

ALLERGY OF THE SCLERA

The widespread use of antiinfective agents and the control of syphilis and tuberculosis has resulted in the lessening importance of infection in the causation of scleritis. Thus, although scleritis in itself is a relatively infrequent disease, the percentage of scleral inflammations of probable allergic origin is very high—perhaps higher than in any other ocular structure. However, because the sclera, unlike the conjunctiva, cornea, and uvea, does not lend itself so readily to the experimental investigation of allergic phenomena, it has been largely ignored in this respect. We are therefore forced to depend chiefly on clinical observations for the evaluation of the various allergic mechanisms that appear to operate in the production of scleritis. These indicate, first, that allergy is indeed an important etiologic mechanism and, second, that many instances of scleritis are best explained on the basis of microbial allergy. The outline below offers a classification of allergic reactions of the sclera.

Allergy of the sclera

- A. Atopic allergy (immediate reaction)
    1. Inhalants: episcleritis
    2. Food allergy: episcleritis
- B. Microbial allergy (delayed reaction)
    1. *Streptococcus, Staphylococcus:* episcleritis, scleritis
    2. Tubercle bacillus: scleritis, sclerosing keratitis
    3. Other microorganisms: episcleritis, scleritis
- C. Collagen diseases (mechanism unknown)
    1. Gout, rheumatic fever, rheumatoid arthritis, periarteritis nodosa: scleritis, episcleritis

Atopic reactions

Most atopic allergic reactions causing scleritis arise from foods, generally fish, and especially seafood. Inhalant allergies are rare but may occur from ragweed.

Microbiallergic reactions

If we consider certain collagen diseases, such as rheumatoid arthritis, to result from bacterial (streptococcal) allergy, then it would be safe to say that most cases of scleritis have a microbiallergic origin. Clinical and confirmative laboratory experiences indicate that such allergy is in general evoked chiefly by three organisms: *Streptococcus, Staphylococcus,* and the tubercle bacillus. However, the well-known relationship between scleritis and what was originally considered the focus of infection, but which I prefer to call an antigenic focus, indicates that although these organisms dominate the picture, many others, such as enteric bacilli and perhaps even parasites, may be incriminated, although the evidence here is less clearcut.

Scleritis in collagen diseases

Gout, which has allergic facets, often is accompanied by scleritis. Scleritis likewise occurs in periarteritis nodosa, a collagen disease in which allergy appears to play an important role.

Tenonitis

Except for the rare instance of tenonitis arising from direct infection, such as that complicating trauma or extraocular muscle surgery, the obscure etiology of tenonitis appears best explained in certain instances on the basis of allergy. The rarity of the disease makes etiologic evaluation difficult. Its exudative character, its transient, recurrent, yet benign course, its association with collagen disease, its relationship and similarity to scleritis, and its response to corticosteroids and foreign protein therapy all suggest that an allergic component may play a role in its causation. However, we know of no known instance where tenonitis has arisen on the basis of atopy, such as food allergy. That microbial allergy may operate is suggested by its association with rheumatoid arthritis and infective antigenic foci. In this regard it is possible that the chemosis and other ocular findings in trichiniasis are caused by tenonitis arising secondary to muscle infestation, either as toxic or allergic response to products of trichinella.

ALLERGY OF THE UVEA

There is considerable evidence, based upon anatomic, experimental, and clinical data, that allergy plays an important role in the causation of endogenous uveitis.[11,41] Anatomically, the extremely vascular uvea offers a particularly favorable site for the concentration of proteins, antigens, and antibodies originating elsewhere in the body. Furthermore, it is known that local antibody formation can and does occur in the uvea itself. Since the uvea thus affords such an ideal shock organ for the study of allergic reactions, it is not surprising that investigators in the field of immunology have utilized this structure experimentally in the production of allergic reactions ever since the introduction of the concept of anaphylaxis. As a result, much of the basic knowledge of hypersensitivity in general stems from such experiments. Allergic uveitis has been induced in laboratory animals by means of horse, cat, and other foreign sera, egg albumin, various microbial products, and by tissue proteins, either alone or in combination with Freund's adjuvant (heat-killed tubercle bacilli in mineral oil).

These observations show that all forms of allergic mechanisms operate in the production of uveal inflammation. Work by Silverstein and Zimmerman[30] also confirms this. The authors indicate that endophthalmitis may be produced in the guinea pig by two distinct immunologic mechanisms: (1) delayed hypersensitivity and (2) antigen interaction with circulating antibody. By varying the method of sensitization, the route of administration, and the dose of antigen, the several immunologic mechanisms may be stimulated to produce ocular lesions. According to these authors, not only may acute nongranulomatous uveitis caused by a delayed hypersensitivity result from microbiallergic processes involving bacterial antigens, but it may also arise as a consequence of the tuberculin type of hypersensitivity to simple bland protein antigens, such as crystalline egg albumin or bovine serum albumin.

More recent contributions relating hypersensitivity to the etiology of uveitis, offering additional detailed evidence, include those by Aronson and his associates,[1] Böke,[3] Campinchi and his associates,[7] Coles,[9] Maumenee and Silverstein,[20] Remky,[27] Schlaegel,[28] Wittmer,[52] and Woods.[53]

The following classification is useful for understanding the clinical manifestations of uveal hypersensitivity.

Allergy of the uvea

A. Anaphylactic and atopic reactions: uveitis from sera, pollens, animal proteins, foods, drugs, angioneurotic edema
B. Microbiallergic reactions
   1. Nongranulomatous uveitis (allergy apparently the main factor): *Streptococcus, M. tuberculosis, Staphylococcus, Gonococcus, Pneumococcus*
   2. Granulomatous uveitis (allergy not primary factor but may alter the nature of the inflammatory response): tuberculosis, syphilis, toxoplasmosis, brucellosis, helminthiasis
   3. Viral uveitis: herpes simplex, herpes zoster, poxviruses, myxoviruses, arboviruses, others
   4. Mycotic uveitis: *Candida,* histoplasmosis
C. Autogeneous allergic reactions
   1. Sympathetic ophthalmia (allergy to autogenous uveal pigment)
   2. Endophthalmitis phacoanaphylactica (allergy to autogenous lens protein)

Atopic reactions

Anaphylactic and atopic reactions of the uvea, although rare, offer the best clinical corroboration of the fact that the uvea may participate in generalized allergic reactions. A prime example of this is uveitis complicating serum sickness, as originally described by Theodore and Lewson[45] and later described by others.[10] Other instances of atopic allergic uveitis may result from hypersensitivity to ragweed, house dust, cat dander, and other inhalants, and to foods. In this category allergy plays the primary role in the uveal inflammation.

Microbiallergic reactions

Although the terms anterior and posterior uveitis and panuveitis have much in their favor, the classification most widely used, that of nongranulomatous and granulomatous types, based on histopathologic studies, is a convenient tool. Microbiallergic reactions of the uvea may occur in both nongranulomatous and granulomatous uveitis. In the anterior nongranulomatous variety, where no direct bacterial infection can be demonstrated, allergy appears to be the primary factor. Even in those granulomatous form of uveitis where microorganisms can be demonstrated, a secondary microbial allergy often alters and aggravates the inflammatory state.

Although specific hypersensitivity to any of the bacteria listed in the outline may cause anterior nongranulomatous uveitis, allergy to *Streptococcus* organisms is most commonly implicated. However, studies have failed to establish a correlation between elevated antistreptolysin-O titers and uveitis. Furthermore, skin tests with bacterial vaccines may be nonspecific, and convincing proof of the value of desensitization in a disease as variable and unpredictable as uveitis is not yet at hand.

All types of tuberculous uveitis have allergic components. Anterior uveitis may occur as a manifestation of tubercle bacillus hypersensitivity in the absence of direct infection, just as it is known to occur in phlyctenular keratoconjunctivitis and scleritis. Even in actual tuberculous infection of the uvea, as in posterior granulomatous uveitis, a secondary allergic reaction may dominate the clinical picture. Exacerbations of uveitis following testing or therapy with tuberculin are known clinically. Moreover, it has been found that destruction of bacilli by means of chemotherapy can occasionally liberate sufficient antigen to cause a focal allergic response.

In ocular toxoplasmosis both local and systemic sensitization to the toxoplasma occurs at the time that the organism forms pseudocysts in the retina. Generalized sensitization is manifested by a positive dye titer. When years later pseudocysts rupture, the hypersensitive tissues react with the liberated organism to produce an allergic reaction clinically manifested as posterior uveitis.

Autogenous reactions

Long before the concept of autoallergy or sensitization of the host to his own tissues was utilized to explain certain systemic diseases, the ophthalmologist had recognized that two unique types of autogenous allergy occur in the eye; namely, phacoanaphylactic uveitis and sympathetic ophthalmia.

Phacoanaphylactic uveitis. Phacoanaphylactic uveitis occurs as the result of a severe allergic reaction in persons sensitized to lens protein, which has entered the anterior chamber as the result of surgery, trauma, or the altered permeability of the diseased lens capsule. Although endophthalmitis phacoanaphylactica clinically appears to be a definite allergic reaction, the fact that its experimental production in animals has required adjuvants besides lens protein, has led some investigators to believe that the mechanism is toxic rather than allergic. However, clinical experiences with the use of fish lens extract in the treatment of cataracts in human beings offers excellent experimental confirmation of two facts: (1) the allergic basis for endophthalmitis phacoanaphylactica and (2) the organ specificity, rather than species specificity, of allergy to lens protein. In three reports, uveitis was induced by repeated injections of fish lens protein and cured by intracapsular cataract extraction. [5,25,26]

Sympathetic uveitis. Analysis of what is known experimentally and clinically about sympathetic ophthalmia leads to the conclusion that the most acceptable pathogenesis of this entity is some form of hypersensitivity. The allergic reaction apparently requires special exciting factors, some of which are still unknown. However, uveal pigment appears to be the basic exciting antigen, as first shown by Elschnig in 1910. Woods[53] has demonstrated a specific antibody to uveal pigment in human beings after perforating ocular wounds, demonstrable on intradermal skin testing. Friedenwald,[14] utilizing histologic studies on the skin of persons who had received such intradermal injections of suspensions of uveal pigment, felt that the uveal pigment granules acted as a specific antigen and that the disease was primarily allergic in nature.

The concept that the allergic reaction resulting in sympathetic ophthalmia is somewhat more complicated, requiring special circumstances for its development, is suggested by recent work. Collins[12] found that in order to produce the picture in in guinea pigs it was necessary to employ Freund's adjuvant in addition to uveal pigment. Naquin,[22] however, was unable to duplicate this work. Blodi[2] recently analyzed a total of 170 eyes with sympathetic ophthalmia and found that 39, or about 23%, showed evidence of a phacoanaphylactic reaction. He felt that this association was higher than could be expected by chance coincidence and that their simultaneous occurrence lent additional weight to the concept of an allergic pathogenesis in sympathetic uveitis.

The concept of autoallergy, or allergy of the host to his own tissues, although still largely an experimental one, has other provocative applications in the field of uveitis. It has been found that in producing experimental allergic encephalitis, in which animals formed antibodies to their own central nervous system myelin following single injections of myelin extract, three quarters of the animals developed a nongranulomatous uveitis limited to the anterior segment.[6] Fernando,[13] injecting bovine albumin tagged with radioactive iodine into the vitreous of nonsensitized rabbits, found that an allergic uveitis developed on the basis of the original injection. No second, or "shocking," dose of antigen was necessary. His autoradiographs demonstrated that the antigen accumulated most intensely in the ciliary body and lens, structures rich in mucopolysaccharides. This association of antigen with tissue polysaccharide suggested to him the possible formation of a polysaccharide-antigen complex that resulted in autosensitization.

These and other experiments indicate that the mechanisms of uveal allergy are even more complex than previously presumed and that there are probably many avenues in which hypersensitivity operates in uveitis. Autoallergy may some day serve to explain many now obscure uveal reactions. Moreover, the hypothesis of autogenous hypersensitivity resulting from a microbial antigen may clarify much that is lacking for our full acceptance and understanding of microbiallergic uveitis.

ALLERGY OF THE RETINA AND OPTIC NERVE

The optic nerve and retina are frequently the site of reactions resulting from exposure to various types of noxious agents. Although most of such phenomena are obviously toxic in nature, often definite allergic manifestations appear to occur. In general, allergic reactions of the retina and optic nerve appear to follow the usual lines of allergy seen elsewhere. With the exception of contact allergy, which obviously cannot occur, anaphylactic, atopic, and microbiallergic reactions have been noted.

In evaluating reactions occurring in the retina and optic nerve, one must make a distinction between allergy and hyperreactivity, especially in regard to drugs. Everyone accepts the fact that when poisons are taken in large enough or toxic doses, tissue death will result. It is generally not realized, however, that in certain hyperreactive individuals minute amounts of the same drug may cause a similar reaction. It should be clear that this is not allergy, because the person so affected reacts in a manner only quantitatively different from that of the average person. For example, most persons will react to large doses of atropine taken internally, with the classic pharmacologic and toxic actions of the drug, such as vomiting, tachycardia, fever, and dilatation of the pupil. When, however, an individual reacts in the same manner with the same symptoms if we inject a very small amount of atropine, or reacts similarly after its local instillation into the eye, this is in a sense a toxic effect following a minute dose, or hyperreactivity. In other words, the only difference in the reaction here is a quantitative one as regards dosage. When, however, a person is allergic or hypersensitive to a drug, he responds with entirely different symptoms, which are essentially allergic in character. These are asthma, rhinitis, urticaria, skin eruptions, and other accepted allergic phenomena. These are not the pharmacologic effects of the drug. Moreover, when such reactions occur, they are the same no matter what particular drug the patient has used. Other examples of hyperreactivity that are important to the ophthalmologist occur in quinine amblyopia, reactions with minute amounts of nicotine, or following the use of atropine and cocaine. Marked ciliary spasms from extremely small amounts of pilocarpine and other miotics should also be noted.

Toxic and hyperreactive affections of the retina and optic nerve reveal little immediate objective evidence of tissue involvement, so that diagnosis depends on subjective findings, especially those of central vision and visual fields. In most instances of neuroretinal allergy, however, reactions are exudative and hemorrhagic, so that they are readily apparent on ophthalmoscopic examination. The only major exceptions appear to be those rare cases of retrobulbar neuritis arising on an allergic basis.

The outline below classifies all known instances of neuroretinal allergy.

Neuroretinal allergy

- A. Anaphylactic and atopic reactions
  1. Serum
  2. Food
  3. Pollen
  4. Drug
  5. Angioneurotic edema and urticaria
- B. Microbiallergic reactions
  1. Tuberculin
  2. Other organisms
- C. Other reactions of possible allergic origin
  1. Eye changes in periarteritis nodosa
  2. Central angiospastic retinopathy

Atopic reactions

Most instances of proved neuroretinal allergy have occurred in the course of serum sickness. Now that antisera are used less frequently, such occurrences are encountered far less often. Food allergy resulting in neuroretinitis has been reported to occur from peanuts, fish, chocolate, milk, eggs, and Coca-Cola. Pollens such as primrose and ragweed have been incriminated.

Sulfa drugs, penicillin, and procaine have been observed to give rise to allergic retinal reactions. Generalized angioedema caused by a variety of agents has resulted in retinal exudative lesions. Instances of retrobulbar neuritis occurring on the basis of atopic allergic reactions, usually caused by foods, have also been reported.

Microbiallergic reactions

Even though instances of microbiallergic neuroretinitis are rare, a number of rather convincing cases have been reported. Weizenblatt[50] has described such a reaction occurring on two occasions in a patient with marked cutaneous sensitivity to old tuberculin, 5 to 7 days after skin testing with this antigen. Other reports describe similar exudative retinitis from tuberculin injections and in trypanosomiasis.[46] Retrobulbar neuritis has resulted from prophylactic vaccination against rabies.

Other reactions of possible allergic origin

Periarteritis nodosa, a disease in which hypersensitivity mechanisms are believed to play an important role, often causes neuroretinal lesions. Central angiospastic retinopathy must also be included in this category.

Retinal detachment

Some rare instances of detachment of the retina occurring on an allergic basis have been reported. Unfortunately, in almost every instance only presumptive evidence was available to make such a diagnosis.

REFERENCES

1. Aronson, S. B., Gamble, C. N., Goodner, E. K., and O'Connor, G. R.: Clinical methods in uveitis, St. Louis, 1968, The C. V. Mosby Co.
2. Blodi, F. C.: Sympathetic uveitis as an allergic phenomenon, presented at the special program of the American Society of Ophthalmologic and Otorhinologic Allergy, October 19, 1958.
3. Böke, W.: Uveitis and allergy. In Remky, H., editor: The uveal tract and its endogenous inflammations, vol. 5, no. 3, Boston, 1965, Little, Brown and Co., pp. 755-788.
4. Braley, A. E.: Experimental herpes simplex, Amer. J. Ophthal. **35**:1737, 1952.
5. Breinin, G. M.: Danger of fish lens protein injection as treatment for cataract, J.A.M.A. **152**:698, 1953.
6. Bullington, S. J., and Waksman, B. H.: Uveitis in rabbits with experimental allergic encephalomyelitis, Arch. Ophthal. **59**:435, 1953.
7. Campinchi, R., Faure, J. P., Bloch-Michel, E., and Haut, J.: L'uvéite—phénomènes immunologiques et allergiques, Paris, 1970, Masson et Cie.
8. Castroviejo, R.: Ocular allergy, cornea and lens, Trans. Amer. Acad. Ophthal. Otolaryng. **54**:242, 1952.
9. Coles, R. S.: Uveitis. In Sorsby, A., editor: Modern ophthalmology, vol. 4, Washington, 1964, Butterworth's, p. 636.
10. Coles, R. S., and Shapiro, A.: L'uvéite biliterale anterieure compliquant la maladie du serum, Bull. Soc. Franc. Ophtal., pp. 67-70, 1971.
11. Coles, R. S., and Theodore, F. H.: Clinical aspects of uveal hypersensitivity, Arch. Ophthal. **62**:223, 1959.
12. Collins, R.: Further experimental studies on on sympathetic ophthalmia, Amer. J. Ophthal. **36**:150, 1952.
13. Fernando, A. N.: Immunological studies with I^{131} labeled antigen in experimental uveitis. Thesis presented at the New York University Post-Graduate Medical School, 1959.
14. Friedenwald, J. S.: Notes on allergic theory of sympathetic ophthalmia, Amer. J. Ophthal. **17**:1008, 1934.
15. Hogan, M. J.: Atopic keratoconjunctivitis, Amer. J. Ophthal. **36**:937, 1953.
16. Jones, R.: The management of ocular herpes, Trans. Ophthal. Soc. U.K. **79**:425, 1959.
17. Locatcher-Khorazo, D., and Gutierrez, E.: Bacteriophage typing of Staphylococcus aureus: a study of normal, infected eyes and environment, Arch. Ophthal. **63**:774, 1960.
18. Maumenee, A. E.: The influence of donor-recipient sensitization on corneal grafts, Amer. J. Ophthal. **34**:142, 1951.
19. Maumenee, A. E.: Biological responses to corneal homografts, Trans. Amer. Acad. Ophthal. Otolaryng. **64**:765, 1960.
20. Maumenee, A. E., and Silverstein, A. M.: Immunopathology of uveitis, Baltimore, 1964, The Williams and Wilkins Co.
21. Morault, S.: Enquète allergologique et traitement par desensibilisation spécifique dans les conjonctivites allergiques. Thesis presented for the degree of Doctor of Medicine to the Faculté de Médecine de Paris, July 6, 1959.
22. Naquin, H. A.: An unsuccessful attempt to

produce hypersensitivity to uveal tissue in guinea pigs, Amer. J. Ophthal. **39**:196, 1955.
23. Pillat, A.: Zur Mitteilung der Hornhaut beim Ekzem, Wien. Klin. Wschr. **50**:768, 1937.
24. Portier, P., and Richet, C.: De l'action anaphylactique de certains venins, Compt. Rend. Soc. Biol. **54**:170, 1902.
25. Posner, A.: Endophthalmitis phacoanaphylactica induced by injections of lens protein: notes on ophthalmology, Eye Ear Nose Throat Monthly **32**:42, 1953.
26. Posner, A.: Complications following injection of fish lens protein for cataract, J.A.M.A. **151**:317, 1953.
27. Remky, H.: Etiologic diagnosis of endogenous uveitis. In Remky, H., editor: The uveal tract and its endogenous inflammations, vol. 5, no. 3, Boston, 1965, Little, Brown and Co., pp. 789-822.
28. Schlaegel, T. F., Jr.: Essentials of uveitis, Boston, 1969, Little, Brown and Co.
29. Schlossman, A. X., and Theodore, F. H.: The classification of allergies of the cornea, Acta XVIII International Congress of Ophthalmology, Brussels, 1958, vol. 2, Brussels, 1959, Imprimerie Medicale et Scientifique, S. A., p. 1136.
30. Silverstein, A. M., and Zimmerman, L. E.: Immunologic endophthalmitis produced in the guinea pig by different pathogenic mechanisms, Amer. J. Ophthal. **48**:435, 1959.
31. Smith, T.: As cited by Chase, W. W.: The allergic state. In Dubos, R. J., editor: Bacterial and mycotic infections of man, Philadelphia, 1948, J. B. Lippincott Co., p. 113.
32. Sorsby, A. P.: The aetiology of phyctenular ophthalmia, Brit. J. Ophthal. **26**:159, 189, 1942.
33. Theodore, F. H.: The classification and treatment of allergies of the conjunctiva, Amer. J. Ophthal. **36**:1689, 1953.
34. Theodore, F. H.: Drug sensitivities and irritations of the conjunctiva, J.A.M.A. **151**:25, 1953.
35. Theodore, F. H.: Differentiation and treatment of eczemas of the eyelids, Trans. Amer. Acad. Ophthal. Otolaryng. **58**:708, 1954.
36. Theodore, F. H.: Ocular eczema: its classification and treatment, J. Mount Sinai Hosp. N.Y. **21**:255, 1955.
37. Theodore, F. H.: Staphylococcal eczema, Acta XVII International Congress of Ophthalmology, New York, 1954, vol. 2, Toronto, 1955, University of Toronto Press, p. 609.
38. Theodore, F. H.: Eczema of the eyelids, Ann. Allerg. **14**:484, 1956.
39. Theodore, F. H.: Bacterial allergy of the eye, Trans. Amer. Acad. Ophthal. Otolaryng. **65**:184, 1961.
40. Theodore, F. H.: Drug irritations from miotics, Eye Ear Nose Throat Monthly **42**:74, 1963.
41. Theodore, F. H.: Allergic keratitis. In King, J. H., and McTigue, J. W., editors: The Cornea World Congress, Washington, 1965, Butterworth's, p. 197.
42. Theodore, F. H.: Idiosyncratic reactions of the cornea from proparacaine, Eye Ear Nose Throat Monthly **47**:66, 1968.
43. Theodore, F. H., and Feinstein, R. R.: Practical suggestions for the preparation and maintenance of sterile ophthalmic solutions, Amer. J. Ophthal. **35**:656, 1952.
44. Theodore, F. H., and Feinstein, R. R.: Preparation and maintenance of sterile ophthalmic solutions, J.A.M.A. **152**:1631, 1953.
45. Theodore, F. H., and Lewson, A. C.: Bilateral iritis complicating serum sickness, Arch. Ophthal. **21**:82, 1939.
46. Theodore, F. H., and Schlossman, A.: Ocular allergy, Baltimore, 1958, The Williams and Wilkins Co.
47. Thygeson, P.: Marginal corneal infiltrates and ulcers, Trans. Amer. Acad. Ophthal. Otolaryng. **51**:198, 1946.
48. von Pirquet, C.: Allergie, Munchen. Med. Wschr. **53**:1457, 1906.
49. Weekers, L.: Nouvelle pathogénie des phlyctènes, Bull. Acad. Roy. Med. Belg. **23**:577, 1909.
50. Weizenblatt, S.: Allergic ocular reactions to tuberculin (bilateral cyclitis and neuroretinitis), Arch. Ophthal. **41**:436, 1949.
51. Wessely, K.: Ueber anaphylaktische Erscheinungen an der Hornhaut (experimentelle Erzeugung einer parenchymatoson Keratitis durch artfremdes Serum), Munchen. Med. Wschr. **59**:1713, 1911.
52. Witmer, R.: Klinik und Diagnostik der Uveitis in heuter Sicht, Klin. Mbl. Augenheilk. **138**:609, 1961.
53. Woods, A. C.: Endogenous inflammations of the uveal tract, Baltimore, 1961, The Williams and Wilkins Co.

11
Ocular toxoplasmosis

G. RICHARD O'CONNOR

Within the past 25 years *Toxoplasma gondii* has come to be considered one of the most important causes of retinochoroiditis. This intracellular protozoan parasite, measuring approximately 2.5 × 6.5 μ, belongs to the class Sporozoa; and as such it can be thought of as a "second cousin" to the more familiar malarial parasite.

The organism has two distinct morphological forms. In its invasive or proliferative form it is crescentic in shape (Fig. 11-1). The more sharply pointed end of this crescent presents a conoid or primitive mouth (Fig. 11-2) by means of which the organism presumably attaches itself to the host cell and invades it. *Toxoplasma* has a very distinctive type of movement in liquid media. Bringmann and Holz[4] believe that it achieves its gliding motion by periodic contraction of a network of fibrillary organelles (toxonemes) (Fig. 11-2), which originate from a ring at the base of the conoid and fan out into the cytoplasm. By electron microscopic studies Ludvik[26] has shown that the toxonemes extend only one fifth of the distance from the anterior (conoid) end of the organism to its posterior pole. There are, however, certain rodlike organelles that extend in a zig-zag fashion from one end of the organism to the other. Hogan and his co-workers[15] have confirmed the presence of rodlike contractile organelles, and they have also shown that the cell wall is made up of several discrete morphologic layers.

Until recently it was thought that the organism multiplied by simple binary (longitudinal) fission. Goldman and his associates[12] have shown, however, that the actual process of cell division is preceded by internal budding, or "endodyogeny." A pair of buds appears on the anterior surface of the parent nucleus in the earliest stages of reproduction. These buds then develop into the miniature conoids (anterior cones) of the daughter cells and seem to be the organizing influence for division of the cytoplasm (Fig. 11-3). The organism is not able to survive outside its host cell for more than a few hours and is totally unable to withstand certain elements of the external environment, such as heat, drying, or changes in osmotic concentration. For this reason the exact mode of its transmission from one host to another has always remained somewhat of a mystery.

A second, more resistant form of the organism has the appearance of a cyst. After invasion of the host cell, the organism may reproduce itself 25 to 100 times by repeated division (Fig. 11-4); however, the resulting daughter cells may remain inactive as a rounded mass within the host cell, (Fig. 11-5). A process of cyst formation may then take place in which the nucleus of the parasitized cell generally becomes pushed to one side. Until recently it was thought that the host cell membrane became thickened into a cyst wall. Because the host provided the material of the cyst

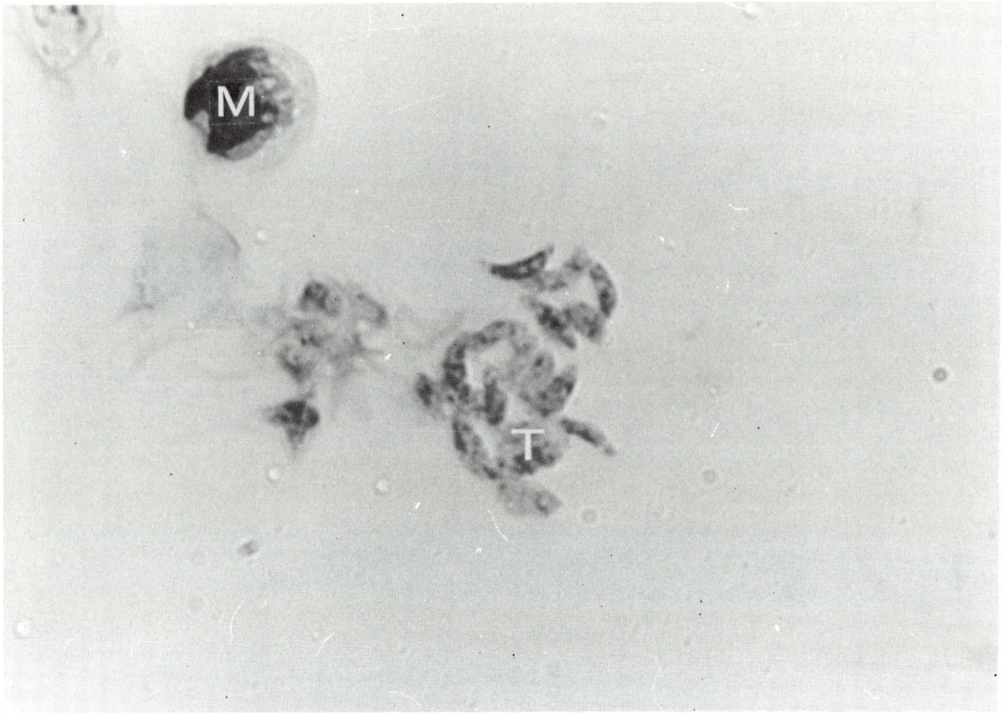

Fig. 11-1. *Toxoplasma* organisms in a Giemsa-stained smear of peritoneal exudate from an infected mouse. *M,* Macrophage; *T, Toxoplasma* organisms. (×1,000.)

wall, the cyst was generally called a pseudocyst. Hogan and his co-workers[16] believe that the preferred term is cyst, since the parasites themselves can be shown to contribute to the cyst wall. Whatever the fine points of this argument may be, the older term pseudocyst is still used by some authors; and since the work of some of these is quoted in this chapter, the reader will encounter both terms.

Although the cysts (Fig. 11-6) are nonchemotactic, they are prone to periodic rupture in the tissues. Frenkel and Jacobs[9] state that organisms liberated from the cysts are generally destroyed in the ensuing inflammatory reaction. If, however, the degree of immunity of the host has declined and a sufficient level of antibody is not available in the tissues at the site of rupture, the liberated organisms appear to be able to invade new cells and proliferate in them. It is apparently the recurrent multiplication of organisms in the retina that accounts for the chronic, progressively destructive nature of the infection.

Although only one species of *Toxoplasma* is known, many strains of widely differing virulence have been isolated. The classical RH strain, for example, has a high degree of virulence for man, mice, and rabbits. It is generally lethal to mice within 3 to 5 days after inoculation. Strain JQ, on the other hand, is relatively avirulent for mice and tends to produce chronic infections of long duration.

Much of what is now known about virulence has been provided by tissue-culture studies. The organism does not seem to be at all fastidious about the type of cell on which it grows. Chorioallantoic membranes of chick embryos have long been used as a culture medium. So, too, have HeLa cells, derived from human cervical carcinoma. Although it has long been thought that high degrees of virulence are correlated with both an increased proportion of cells in-

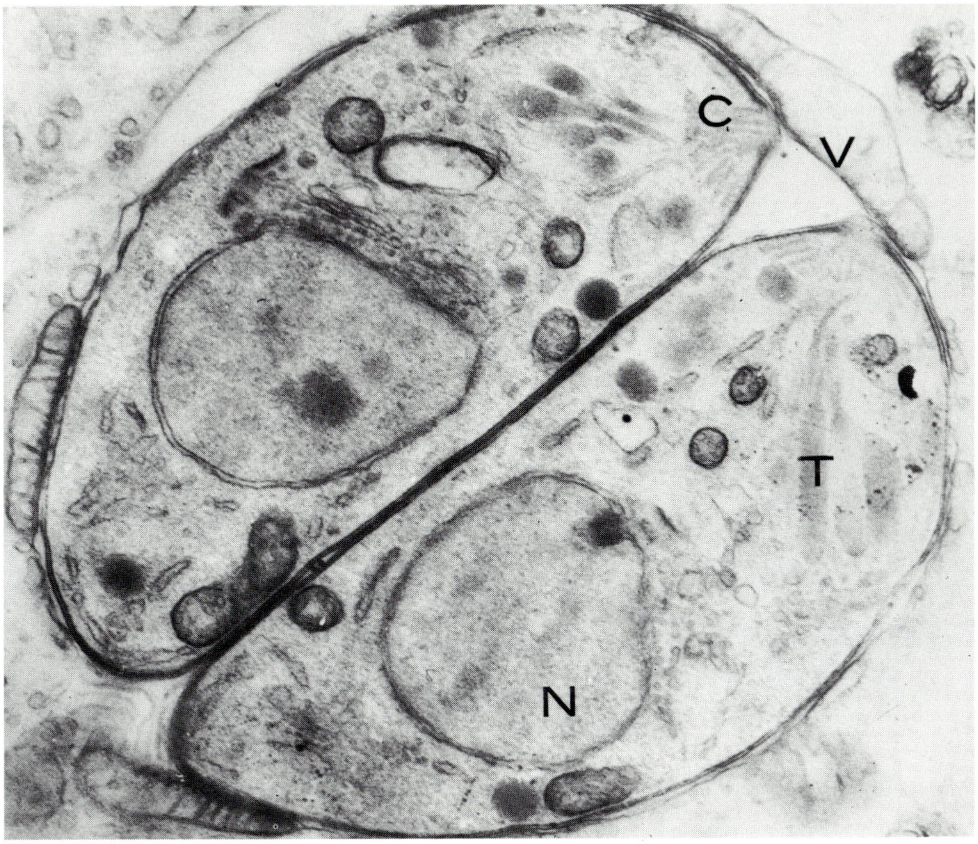

Fig. 11-2. An electron micrograph of two recently divided *Toxoplasma* organisms lying within a vacuole of host cell cystoplasm. *C,* Conoid; *V,* wall of cytoplasmic vacuole; *T,* toxoneme; *N,* nucleus. (×24,000.)

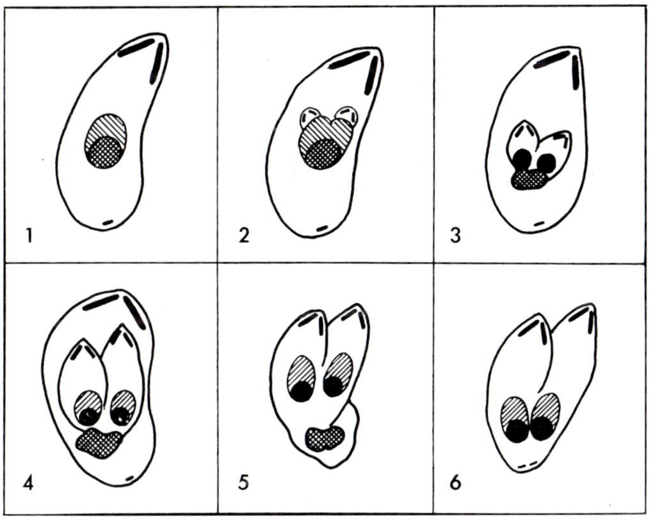

Fig. 11-3. Diagrammatic representation of division by internal budding (endodyogeny). Two polar bodies resembling the conoid of the parent cell appear at the anterior pole of the nucleus. Subsequent stages of division are apparently organized by them. (From Goldman, M., Carver, R. K., and Sulzer, A. J.: J. Parasit. **44:**161, 1958.)

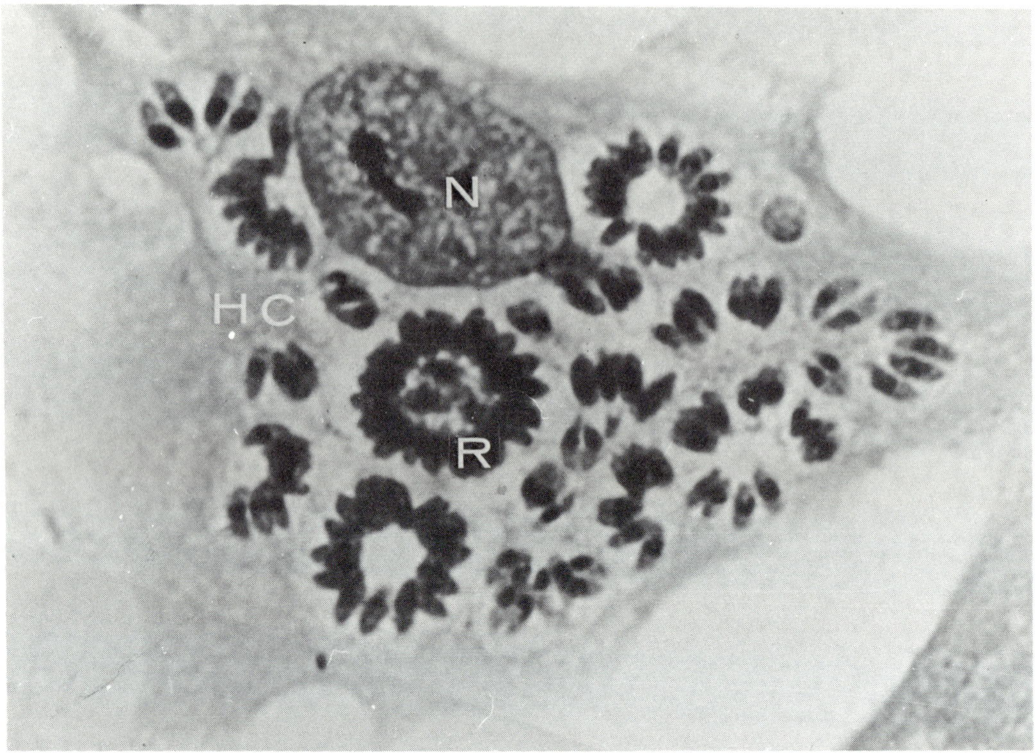

Fig. 11-4. *Toxoplasma* parasites multiplying in the cytoplasm of a HeLa cell (in tissue culture). *N,* Nucleus; *HC,* host cell; *R,* rosette. (×1,000.)

vaded and a more rapid multiplication of the organisms within the cells, the tissue-culture experiments of Hogan and his co-workers[16] and Kaufman and his associates[25] have left no doubt about this. Strains known to have a high degree of virulence in mouse infections have shown the same highly destructive effects on many types of cells in tissue culture. Strains of low virulence, on the other hand, produce much less cell destruction and have a tendency to produce terminal colonies in tissue-culture cells relatively soon after inoculation.

Toxoplasma is widely distributed among warm-blooded vertebrate hosts. Cats, dogs, pigeons, rodents, and many meat-yielding animals, such as hogs, have been shown to be infected. By and large, infected animals (including humans) do not appear to be sick, and the parasitic relationship between the organism and its host is a harmonious one. On the basis of serologic studies it appears that human populations in many areas of the world are infected. Some regions, such as Tahiti, have a very high rate of infection, whereas others, such as Iceland, have virtually none. Populations in high-altitude areas appear to be less infected than groups from tropical or sea-level areas.

Little is known about the transmission of the disease to man. Although the transplacental passage of the organisms from mother to child seems to be well established in the congenital form of the disease, the epidemiology of the adult, or acquired, form is poorly understood. It is known that cats, dogs, and rodents carry the organisms in their excreta and on their mucous membranes. Blood-sucking arthropods, such as ticks, may harbor the organism for short periods of time; and Jacobs[18] has demonstrated the persistence of viable toxoplasmas in the body louse *(Pediculus humanus)*

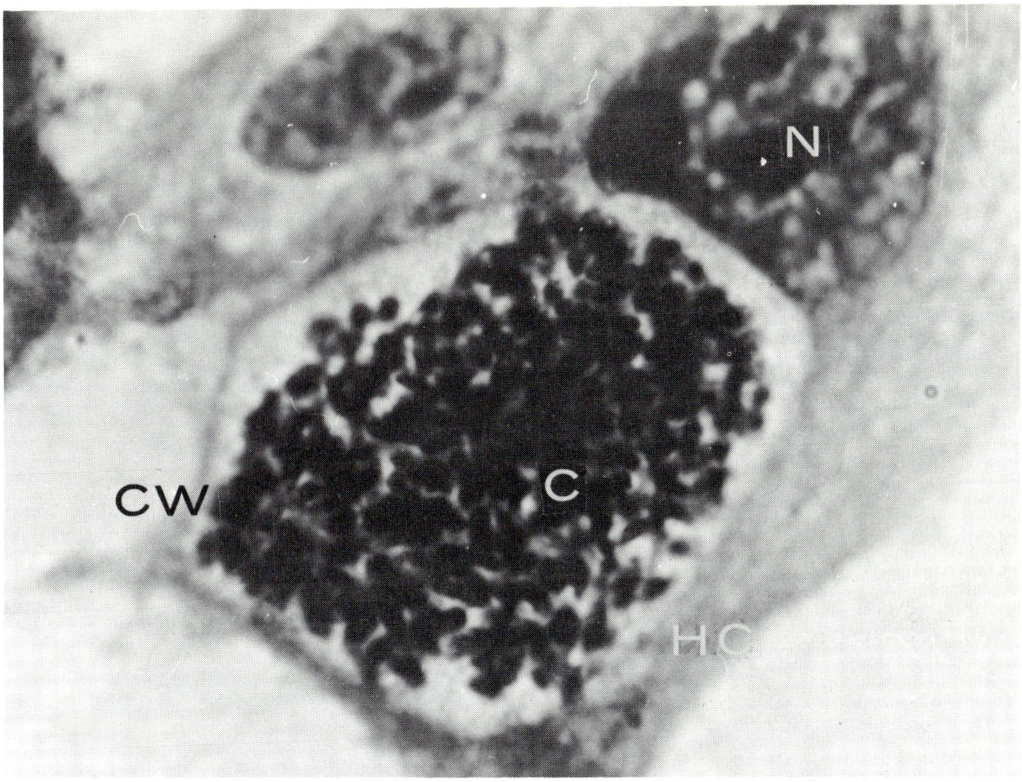

Fig. 11-5. Cyst formation in tissue culture. *N,* Nucleus; *C,* cyst; *HC,* host cell (retinoblastoma); *CW,* cyst wall. (×1,000.)

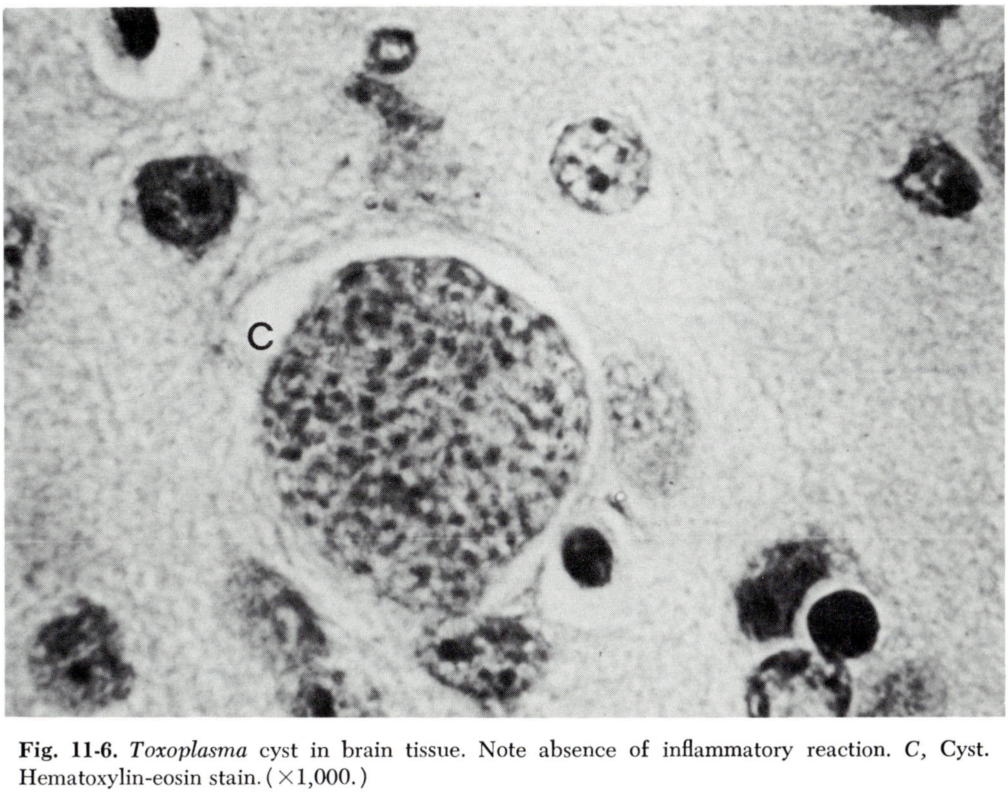

Fig. 11-6. *Toxoplasma* cyst in brain tissue. Note absence of inflammatory reaction. *C,* Cyst. Hematoxylin-eosin stain. (×1,000.)

for as long as 6 days. Jacobs, Woke, and Jones[23] also showed that the ingestion of infected flesh could cause infection in mice. It is quite possible that the same holds true for human beings, although there is still much uncertainty about the whole problem. Current work indicates that the oocysts of *Toxoplasma* may be shed in the feces of cats, and this may provide an important clue as to the transmission of the parasite to man.

Whatever the source of infection, it appears that the organisms multiply locally at the site of penetration and eventually spread by hematogenous dissemination to all parts of the body. Although the initial stages of the disease may be accompanied by remittent fevers, malaise, maculopapular rash, and myalgias, the chronic stages of the disease associated with pseudocyst formation are usually asymptomatic. Were it not for affections of the eye and central nervous system, many more cases of toxoplasmosis would undoubtedly go unnoticed.

HISTORY

Although the parasite was discovered by Nicolle and Manceaux[31] as early as 1909, its importance in human disease was not suspected until 1923, when the Czechoslovakian ophthalmologist Jankû[24] described intracellular parasites in sections of retina taken from eyes with so-called congenital coloboma of the macula. The organisms were not definitely identified as *Toxoplasma* at this time, nor were isolations of the parasite performed. In 1937 Wolf and Cowen[48] recovered *Toxoplasma* from the tissues of an infant who died of "encephalitozoic encephalomyelitis." It was recognized that this child had bilateral chorioretinitis, and the organisms were later identified in tissue sections; but living parasites were not recovered from the retinal tissues.

Wilder[46] in 1952 reported a series of 53 human eyes in which organisms with the morphologic characteristics of *T. gondii* were observed in tissue sections. Although severe necrotizing inflammatory reactions could be seen in the retina, choroid, ciliary body, iris, and sclera, the parasites themselves could be found *only* in the retina. This was a fundamental discovery, and it is the reason why the disease is more properly referred to as *retinochoroiditis* rather than chorioretinitis. As yet, however, the particular predilection of the organism for the retina itself has not been fully explained.

Conclusive proof that granulomatous retinochoroiditis could be caused by *Toxoplasma* was not obtained until the now classical work of Jacobs, Fair, and Bickerton[20] was published in 1954. These authors obtained a freshly enucleated eye removed from a 30-year-old white man who had suffered from recurrent retinochoroiditis for 8½ years. They divided the eye into two halves. One half was used for the preparation of routine histologic sections. The retina and uveal tissues from the other half were removed by dissection, ground in a mortar, and injected into mice, chick embryos, and various tissue cultures. After suitable periods of incubation, *Toxoplasma* organisms, identified by irrefutable morphologic and immunologic criteria, were obtained from all of the injected specimens. Cysts of *T. gondii* were seen on histopathologic sections of the remaining half of the eye. With the exception of the fact that the organism could not be grown on artificial media, Koch's postulates had, indeed, been fulfilled. A positive skin test for toxoplasmosis as well as a postoperative rise in the *Toxoplasma* dye test titer gave additional support to the diagnosis in this patient.

Hogan and his co-workers[17] reported a similar isolation from the eye of a 20-year-old white male in 1958. This patient had allegedly had macular choroiditis in his right eye since the age of 1½ years. The case was thought to represent congenital toxoplasmosis in which the organisms had persisted in the retina and perhaps elsewhere in the body for 20 years. Habegger[13] reported the isolation of *Toxoplasma* from the subretinal fluid of a patient who suffered an inflammatory detachment of the retina. Ansari and Minou[1] reported finding the organisms in a lesion of the conjunctiva. In the strictest sense, it is only in this type of observation, when the organisms are visualized in, and if possible, isolated from ocular tissues that an absolute diagnosis of ocular toxoplasmosis can be made.

DIAGNOSIS

Although the observations listed above leave little doubt that *Toxoplasma* is the causative agent of certain forms of ocular disease, the isolation of the organism can be achieved only rarely from tissues. From the practicing ophthalmologist's point of view, it cannot be looked upon as a practicable diagnostic method. From the patient's point of view, there is little to be gained from establishing the diagnosis on an enucleated eye. On the whole we are still forced to make the diagnosis on indirect evidence, and the greatest part of this is derived from serologic testing.

Various serologic methods are now available for the diagnosis of toxoplasmosis. Each is presented briefly from the point of view of its theoretical background, its advantages, and its disadvantages.

Neutralization test

The *Toxoplasma* neutralization test of Sabin and Ruchman[40] utilizes the principle that the serum of an immune patient will neutralize a given suspension of *Toxoplasma* organisms to the extent that the injection of a standardized mixture of serum and organisms fails to produce the usual necrotizing skin lesion in a rabbit. This test has been largely abandoned because neutralizing antibodies are heat labile and will not survive passage through the mail. They are destroyed by the usual procedures for serial dilution. In addition to these factors, they disappear relatively early in the disease and do not necessarily indicate active disease. At best, the test is cumbersome, expensive, and impractical to perform.

Complement-fixation test

A complement-fixation test for toxoplasmosis was described by Warren and Sabin[45] in 1942. The original antigen used for this purpose was a 10% suspension of infected rabbit brain in physiologic saline. Later an extract of *Toxoplasma*-infected chick chorioallantoic membrane was found to be more suitable, being less anticomplementary than the rabbit brain suspension. Complement-fixing antibodies were detected in monkeys about 2 weeks after infection, but they began to disappear at the end of 2 months. In one established case of acute toxoplasmosis in a human subject, complement-fixing antibodies did not appear until the thirty-second day of infection and disappeared within 3 months.[38] The usefulness of this test in studies of chronic disease was obviously limited; and this test, like its predecessor the neutralization test, has been largely abandoned. The test is used occasionally in determining whether the disease is in its earlier or more acute stages.

Toxoplasma dye test

The mainstay of our present diagnostic regimen is the Sabin-Feldman dye test, which was described by these two authors in 1948.[39] The test depends on the observation that the cytoplasm of living *Toxoplasma* organisms, when acted upon by a specific antibody in the presence of a complementlike "accessory factor," loses its affinity for methylene blue at pH 11. The titer refers to the highest original dilution of serum at which 50% of the extracellular *Toxoplasma* organisms lose their affinity for the dye. The reaction appears to result from minute breaks in the cell membrane of the organism and is related to the depolymerization of ribose nucleic acids within its cytoplasm. It is almost invariably accompanied by swelling of the parasite. Studies by Bringmann and Holz[3] and by Strannegård[43] on the ultramicroscopic morphology of the organism during the dye test procedure have shed some light on this subject.

As a rule dye test antibodies in titers of 1:256 to 1:4,000 develop within 10 to 20 days following infection and may remain at these high levels for 5 years or more without reinfection. It is rare indeed for a patient with an established *Toxoplasma* infection to become totally seronegative even after 5 or 10 years. Treatment with antimicrobial agents, such as pyrimethamine (Daraprim) and the sulfonamides, may be associated with a twofold to fourfold rise in titer during the first 2 weeks of therapy. It may be that this is associated with widespread necrosis of the organisms and the liberation of large amounts of antigen. In no case, however, is the patient rendered seronegative by treatment. It is assumed that the encysted forms of the organism are not reached by the antimicrobial agents. It may be that periodic breakdown of the cysts provides an antigenic stimulus adequate for the maintenance of dye test antibodies in low titer.

The dye test has been the basis for such studies as those of Hogan[14] and those of Jacobs and his associates,[22] in which attempts were made to correlate the incidence of granulomatous uveitis (chorioretinitis) with positive serum dye tests. There seems to be little doubt that patients with chorioretinitis show a higher incidence of positive dye tests than those with nongranulomatous anterior uveitis or control subjects selected at random. In evaluating these surveys, however, one must always be mindful of (1) the incidence of positive tests in the control population of the locality in which the survey is being conducted, (2) the mean age of the group being studied, and (3) the minimum titer that is thought to represent a positive test (such as 1:16 or 1:64). In the study of Jacobs, Cook, and Wilder,[19] for example, all of the 21 patients in whom toxoplasmic chorioretinitis was diagnosed histologically showed positive serum dye tests. In one case antibodies were present only in the undiluted sample, and in another case they were present at a titer of only 1:2. The ages ranged from 16 to 71 years. On the basis of Feldman's[8] population survey, 50% of the people in this age group might have been expected to show dye test antibodies anyway.

The incidence of low titers in some of the patients described by Jacobs, Cook, and Wilder[19] deserves some comment. It must be remembered that the eye is a relatively isolated organ and that retinal lesions have a relatively meager vascular supply. Therefore, as far as the production of circulating antibodies is concerned, the isolated retinal lesion must surely represent a minor antigenic stimulus. If the eye lesions were the only residue of chronic infection in a given patient, the low titer of circulating antibodies would be easy to understand. By the same token one cannot necessarily expect to find a rise in the titer of serum antibodies with each exacerbation of inflammatory disease in the retina. The point of all these observations is to emphasize the caution that must be taken in evaluating a single dye test result. The finding of dye test antibodies in the serum indicates nothing more or less than that the patient has been exposed to toxoplasmosis at some time in his life. Fourfold increases or decreases in titer (correlated with the appearance or disappearance of complement-fixing antibodies), a positive skin test, or symptomatic changes may give some indication of the activity of the disease; but single isolated blood tests are of use only when they are completely negative.

Hemagglutination test

In 1957 Jacobs and Lunde[21] described a hemagglutination test for antibodies to *Toxoplasma*. This test was based on Boyden's[2] observation that sheep erythrocytes treated with tannic acid could bind antigens to their surfaces. If these coated red cells were then suspended in a medium containing specific antibody, they could be agglutinated by the latter. The agglutination is not a gross clumping of cells as one might expect, but rather a fine network that is best demonstrated on a bowl-shaped glass surface. If antigen-coated cells are merely suspended in solution in a small glass tube to which no antibody has been added, they will sediment in such a way as to form a compact pellet or button on the bottom of the tube. If, on the other hand,

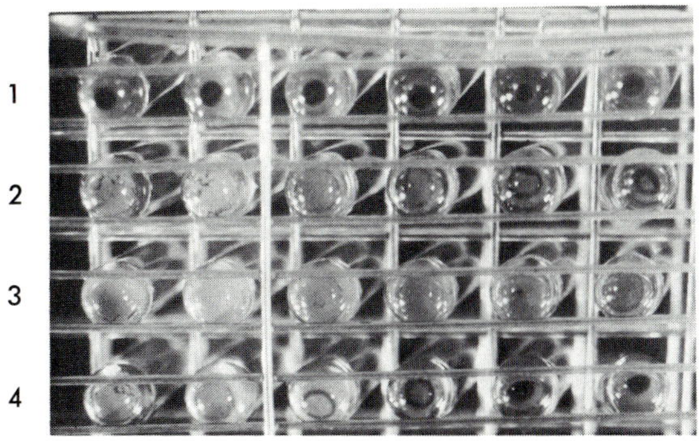

Fig. 11-7. The hemagglutination test for toxoplasmosis. Typical appearance of the tubes as seen from the botton. Fourfold dilutions of each serum are arranged in horizontal rows. Serum 1, negative; serum 2, positive, 1:1,024; serum 3, positive, 1:16,384; serum 4, positive, 1:256.

they have been mixed with specific antibody before they are allowed to settle, the sedimentation pattern is quite different. The cells will be spread out in an even, fine reticulum over the entire bottom of the tube (Fig. 11-7). As the antibody is progressively diluted, the agglutination observed is correspondingly less, and intermediate patterns represented by rings or discs are noted instead. In this way the agglutination patterns have been graded from "4+," represented by a fine network spread over the entire bottom of the tube, to "0," represented by the compact button. A "2+" reaction, represented by a diffuse ring in the bottom of the tube, is taken as the endpoint for titer determination.

The test is now performed in many laboratories throughout the United States and Europe. It is not a foolproof test, in that numerous small factors, such as the cleanliness of the glassware, the shape of the bottom of the hemagglutination tube, and the age of the normal rabbit serum used as a stabilizing medium, may all play a significant role in the readings obtained. For this reason one should take particular note of procedural details and variations from the original Jacobs-Lunde test when evaluating the results of a given laboratory.

Maloney and Kaufman[29] have developed a procedure for using formalin-fixed human type O cells in the *Toxoplasma* hemagglutination test, and Park[35] has published a method for preserving alcohol–formalin-fixed sheep cells in the lyophilized state. The advantages of these methods are obvious. If stable, antigen-coated erythrocytes can be prepared in large lots and preserved indefinitely, the normal variations in titer that are observed when a standard serum is tested against two different lots of freshly sensitized cells can be eliminated.

The use of preserved cells also makes it possible for small laboratories in outlying communities to test for hemagglutinating antibodies. Until recently, practicing ophthalmologists have been compelled to rely upon the Sabin-Feldman dye test, which is performed in relatively few laboratories and which entails the additional risks of handling and maintaining living strains of the parasite. For this reason facilities have in the past been inadequate for the testing of patients' sera, and certain laboratories have had to restrict the acceptance of serum specimens to tests on pregnant women and newborn infants.

Lunde and Jacobs[28] have shown that their hemagglutination test generally parallels the Sabin-Feldman test in titer. The difference in titer between the two tests was usually not more than one fourfold dilution. Some doubt has been cast on this issue by Mitchell and Green,[30] who found the hemagglutination tests positive in some 20 patients in whom simultaneous dye tests were negative. In general, it is felt that the hemagglutination test is somewhat more sensitive than the dye test; and if there is a difference in the titers, it is usually the hemagglutination test that gives the higher value. Some of the patients in Mitchell and Green's series may represent borderline cases in which the hemagglutination test showed the presence of antibody when the dye test did not. On the other hand, Reuss[37] was able to establish complete agreement between the hemagglutination test and the dye test as far as negative sera were concerned; and 89.9% of his dye test positive sera showed correspondingly positive hemagglutination tests, with only minor differences in titer.

Precipitin test

O'Connor[32] in 1957 first demonstrated the presence of precipitating antibodies to *Toxoplasma* in the blood and aqueous humor of certain patients suspected of having toxoplasmosis. He demonstrated these antibodies by the use of Ouchterlony's[34] double-diffusion technique in agar. According to this method, antibodies placed in a hole or reservoir in a layer of clear agar are allowed to diffuse toward a source of *Toxoplasma* antigen, located in the same layer of agar at a given distance from the antibody reservoir. As diffusion proceeds and the antibody comes into contact with the antigen, an insoluble grayish white precipitate is laid down in the agar. This takes the form of a thin straight line, which is always laid down at right angles to an imaginary line constructed between the centers of the respective antigen and antibody reservoirs.

Using an antigen solution derived from the peritoneal exudate of infected mice, O'Connor[33] was able to demonstrate multiple lines of precipitation, each corresponding to a separate antigen-antibody system. This showed that the *Toxoplasma* parasite actually elaborated at least five antigens, each of which stimulated the formation of a separate precipitating antibody in the host. The author's work has subsequently been confirmed by Uminski and Wawrzkiewicz[44] and by Strannegård,[42] who was able to show a time-relation curve correlating the appearance of precipitating antibodies, dye test antibodies, and complement-fixing antibodies in sera of rabbit and human subjects. In general, it can be said that precipitating antibodies appear in the serum early in the course of the disease, being most plentiful between 6 weeks and 2 months after onset. It is rare to find circulating precipitins later than 2 years after onset of the disease, although dye test antibodies may still be present in high titer. Thus the appearance and duration of precipitating antibodies seem to run approximately parallel with complement-fixing antibodies. In any case, a given serum might show as many as five types of precipitating antibodies or none at all, depending on the phase of the disease and the individual capacity of the patient to produce precipitins. It is likely that precipitating antibodies represent entirely different types of molecules from dye test antibodies. On the other hand, some precipitating antibodies are likely to be complement fixing.

The functions of the different antigenic components of the organism, analogous perhaps to the multiple antigens of the hemolytic *Streptococcus*, have not yet been elucidated. It may be that some of them are enzymic in nature, corresponding to the antigenic streptolysin O derived from the beta-hemolytic *Streptococcus*. It is likely, in any case, that there is a serum antibody corresponding to each of the antigenic components of *Toxoplasma* and that the individual antibodies may one day be assayable in the same way that antistreptolysin activity is currently measurable in the sera of patients with streptococcal disease.

One of the chief advantages of the precipitin method is that relatively small quantities are required for testing. For example, as little as 0.05 ml of serum, spinal fluid, or aqueous humor can be placed in the central hole of a standard Ouchterlony agar plate and tested simultaneously against five or six different antigens. In addition, specific precipitates can be differentiated from one another by means of the so-called reaction of identity. In this reaction, lines of precipitate from adjacent antigen reservoirs containing a common antigen join each other to form a smooth, rounded angle; whereas two different antigens give rise to lines that cross over each other. This principle is illustrated in Fig. 11-8. Here an unknown serum suspected of containing precipitins to either *Toxoplasma* or *Streptococcus* was in fact found to contain antibodies to both organisms.

The application of the agar-diffusion method to the study of aqueous humor ap-

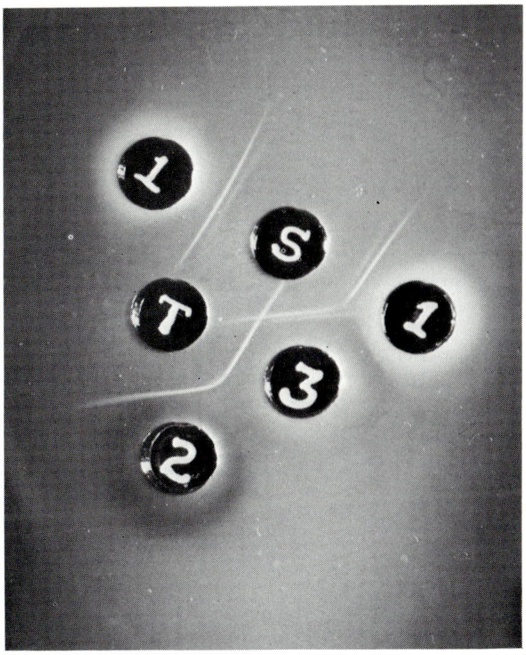

Fig. 11-8. Testing for precipitins by the agar-diffusion technique. S, Reservoir containing streptococcal antigens; *T*, *Toxoplasma* antigen; *1*, serum known to contain antibodies to *Strepotcoccus*, negative for *Toxoplasma; 2*, serum known to contain antibodies to *Toxoplasma*, negative for *Streptococcus; 3*, unknown serum, contains antibodies to both *Toxoplasma* and *Streptococcus*.

pears to be particularly promising. In 1957 O'Connor[33] demonstrated precipitating antibodies to *Toxoplasma* in 11 out of 63 human aqueous specimens tested. Of these 63 specimens, 32 came from patients seriously suspected of having ocular toxoplasmosis on the basis of high serum dye tests, positive skin tests, and "classical" or compatible lesions in the eye. Of particular interest was the fact that 7 out of 11 positive cases showed precipitating antibodies in their aqueous humor, where none could be detected in the serum. This suggested that the formation of antibody may very well take place in the eye itself; and if this is indeed the case, the testing of aqueous humor may be much more specific than the testing of blood. A positive test in the aqueous is of particularly great significance when simultaneous findings in the serum are negative. If, however, both are positive for precipitating antibodies, it should still be possible to differentiate the portion of the antibody molecules that was elaborated in the eye itself from the portion that might have seeped into the eye because of altered permeability of the blood-aqueous barrier. If analyses of the gamma globulin content of both blood and aqueous humor are performed simultaneously, it should be possible to calculate the amount of antibody present per mg of gamma globulin; and this, as Witmer[47] points out, is the really significant measurement. A quotient expressing the titer divided by the amount of gamma globulins per ml can be calculated separately for both the aqueous humor and the serum. If the value of the quotient found for the aqueous humor divided by the quotient for the serum exceeds 1.0, it may be assumed that there is a greater amount of antibody in the anterior chamber than could be accounted for on the basis of seepage through the blood-aqueous barrier alone. Witmer[47] has shown that this value often exceeds 1.0 in experimental leptospiral uveitis, and he has cited this as evidence for formation of antibody within the eye itself. These determinations have recently been performed by Desmonts[7] in cases of human toxoplasmic uveitis, where it is likely that a similar situation obtains.

The agar-diffusion method of Ouchterlony offers the possibility of testing a relatively small amount of fluid (20 to 100 μl) against multiple antigens simultaneously. Heretofore, extensive testing of the aqueous has always been hampered by the small volumes of test fluid that could be collected at any one time. However, one should not allow himself to become overly optimistic about this or other methods involving the direct examination of the aqueous humor in cases of toxoplasmic uveitis. The fact is that the majority of cases, at least in the subacute or chronic stages, involve the posterior portion of the eye exclusively. It is often true that no cells or flare can be seen in the anterior chamber despite rather fulminating disease in the retina or posterior vitreous. In the experience of the author, tests for antibody in the aqueous humor are of no avail unless there is at least some degree of flare in the anterior chamber, as seen on slit-lamp examination.

Flocculation test

Siim and Lind[41] have described a flocculation test for the detection of antibodies to *Toxoplasma.* The test involves the coating of polymethyl meta-acrylic particles with soluble antigen derived from the peritoneal exudates of infected mice. The patient's serum, suitably diluted in a solution consisting of 2% normal human serum in saline, is mixed with a 1:20 suspension of the coated particles on a glass slide and allowed to stand overnight at 4° C. The tests are read the next day, the final titer representing the reciprocal of that serum dilution which gives rise to a standard degree of flocculation.

According to Siim and Lind, 39 out of 40 sera with dye tests in the range of 1:250 to 1:6,250 showed flocculation titers in the range of 1:40 to 1:1,240. Five out of 18 sera negative for the dye test showed titers in the range of 1:10 to 1:40 for the flocculation test.

At present only preliminary reports are available on this technique, and the test is not as yet in general use.[28,41] It seems, however, that this method might be of particular use where (1) only small quantities of material are available (aqueous humor), (2) limitations of space or personnel preclude the constant maintenance of *Toxoplasma* strains, or (3) rapid screening of large segments of the population is desirable on a mass-production basis.

Fluorescein techniques

One of the most important landmarks in the field of applied immunology was passed when Coons and his co-workers[5] developed a method for labeling antibodies with fluorescein. These investigators found that they could couple fluorescein with antibodies of various types without the loss of specific immunologic activity.

The original method, involving the use of fluorescein-4-isocyanate, was both tedious and dangerous. In recent times, however, a more stable compound called fluorescein isothiocyanate has become commercially available. It is no longer difficult to prepare fluorescein-antibody conjugates by the use of this product.

Goldman[10] has labeled anti-*Toxoplasma* antibodies with fluorescein isothiocyanate and has demonstrated the fluorescence of the organisms on fixed smears after staining with the fluorescein-antibody conjugate. A layer of fluorescent antibody is actually laid down on the surface of the cell membrane, which then appears to glow as a greenish golden capsule when viewed microscopically under ultraviolet light (Fig. 11-9). Aside from its aesthetic aspects, which are considerable, the technique has great diagnostic possibilities.

Goldman[11] has also described a test for antibodies to *Toxoplasma* based on the inhibition of specific staining. If smears of the organism are first coated with the patient's serum and then treated with fluorescein-labeled antibody, the labeled antibody will not stick to the organism in those cases where the patient's serum is positive. The test is based on the assumption that there is a limited number of receptor sites on the surface of the organism. If these become occupied by specific antibodies from the patient's serum, they will no longer be able to bind the labeled antibodies that may be applied to them subsequently. Negative sera, on the other hand, will not adhere to the receptor sites; and after gentle washing with saline and application of fluorescein-labeled antibodies, the organisms will be rendered brilliantly fluorescent. In fact, Goldman has shown that the inhibition of staining is just as efficient if the patient's serum and the labeled serum are applied together in a mixture. The explanation for the efficiency of such a mixture must be that natural human antibodies are more successful in the competition for receptor sites on the organism than are the fluorescein-labeled antibodies.

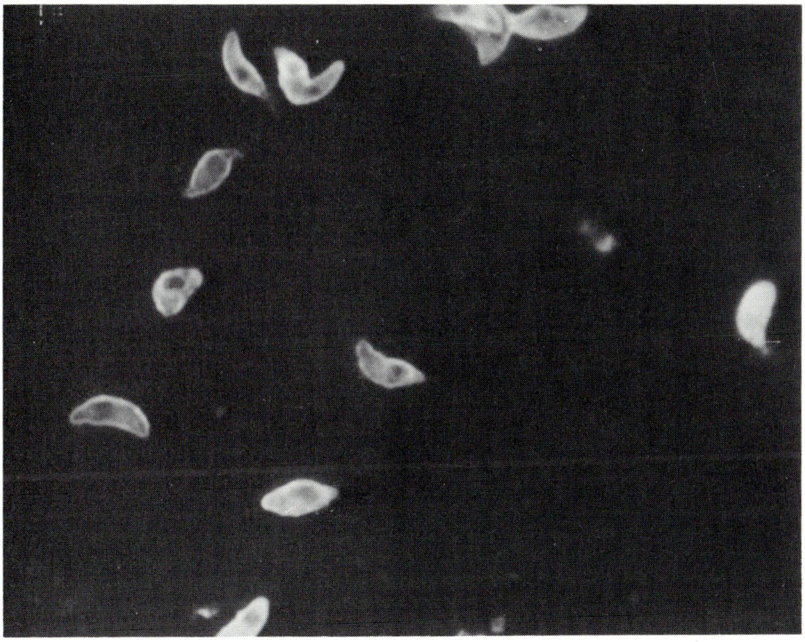

Fig. 11-9. Fixed smear of *Toxoplasma* organisms stained with fluorescein-tagged antibody. Ultraviolet light microscopy. (×1,000.)

Dallenbach and Piekarski[6] have used fluorescein-labeled antibodies to *Toxoplasma* to detect the organisms in tissue sections. The parasite has been detected in lymph node, spleen, and liver preparations from both infected mice and guinea pigs. These investigators noted, moreover, that the organisms stained much more brilliantly in acute infections and that the effectiveness of the labeled antibody preparation was directly proportional to its dye test. The method has not yet been applied to ocular tissues, but it is clear that its greatest usefulness will be in the sphere of necropsy or biopsy examinations.

Another ramification of this method has been employed in the laboratories of the Institute of Ophthalmology.* Here an indirect, or "sandwich," technique has been used to demonstrate antibodies in patients' sera. Smears of *Toxoplasma* organisms obtained from the peritoneal cavities of infected mice were first exposed to serial dilutions of sera, aqueous humor, or spinal fluid from patients thought to have toxoplasmosis. After about 30 minutes the tissues were washed and stained with fluorescein-labeled antibody to human gamma globulin. This antibody was obtained by serial intravenous injections of alum-precipitated human gamma globulin into rabbits. The smears of *Toxoplasma* that had been exposed to serum or eye fluid containing specific antibodies to *Toxoplasma* bound these antibodies and were then stained by the fluorescein-labeled antihuman gamma globulin. The organisms fluoresced in ultraviolet light, and they resembled in appearance the organisms illustrated in Fig. 11-9, which had been stained directly with fluorescent-labeled antibody to *Toxoplasma gondii.*

One hundred sera, in addition to 5 aqueous humor and 3 spinal fluid specimens,

*The author is indebted to Miss Mary-Alice Neville for most of the data presented in this study. Thanks are also due Dr. Elliot Osserman of the Francis Delafield Hospital for supplying the purified human gamma-globulin material and Drs. Beatrice Seegal and Konrad Hsu of the College of Physicians and Surgeons for their advice and help in preparing fluorescein conjugate.

Table 11-1. Results of tests for the presence of antibody to *Toxoplasma* in 100 sera, 5 aqueous humor specimens, and 3 spinal fluid specimens

Source of suspected *Toxoplasma* antibody	Precipitin test	Hemagglutination test	Indirect fluorescein test
Sera 1-7	Positive	Positive	Positive
Sera 8-56	Negative	Positive	Positive
Sera 57-65	Negative	Negative	Positive
Sera 66-100	Negative	Negative	Negative
Aqueous humor 1-3	Negative	Negative	Positive
Aqueous humor 4-5	Negative	Negative	Negative
Spinal fluid 1	Negative	Positive	Positive
Spinal fluid 2-3	Negative	Negative	Negative

have been tested simultaneously for the presence of *Toxoplasma* antibodies by the precipitin, hemagglutination, and fluorescein techniques (Table 11-1). Sera of 7 patients showed positive reactions in all 3 of these tests; sera of 48 patients were negative for precipitating antibody but positive for the other 2 tests (Table 11-1). Another 7 sera were negative for both the precipitin and hemagglutin test but positive for the fluorescein test. Finally, 35 specimens were negative for all the tests. Three of 5 aqueous humor specimens were positive for the fluorescein test, as was 1 of 3 spinal fluids. Thus it is seen that the fluorescent antibody test is sensitive and also provides a technique that can be particularly useful in testing aqueous humor. That volumes as small as 5 μl can be used to coat tiny fixed smears of *Toxoplasma* is a distinct advantage. Serial dilutions can also be carried out with relative ease. The resulting smears are clearly stained with the fluorescent material and are even easier to read than those prepared with human serum. In aqueous humor there may be less interference from viscous proteins, such as albumin, which are present in such large amounts in serum.

Radioactive methods

O'Connor[33] showed that antibodies to *Toxoplasma gondii* could be coupled with I^{131} and still retain their activity when tested subsequently on an Ouchterlony plate. It was hoped that this method might be useful in the localization of unbound antigen in tissues, such as those of the eye, where access of circulating antibody to the affected area is relatively limited. In experimental retinal lesions (in the rabbit) no significant uptake of intravenously injected radioactive antibody could be demonstrated either by scanning techniques or by radioautography of the sectioned eyes. The technique of using radioactive antibody is potentially useful, however, and a wide field is left in this area for further investigative work.

Conclusions on the diagnosis of Toxoplasma gondii infection

It is generally thought that toxoplasmosis accounts for 30% to 50% of all posterior uveitis. Under the best of circumstances the diagnosis of ocular toxoplasmosis is a difficult one to make, particularly where adult patients are concerned. There are many pitfalls, and of these the most common is that of placing too much confidence in a single blood test. It is sometimes difficult to remember that blood taken from an arm vein contains antibodies from the general circulation and that diseases such as toxoplasmosis and syphilis are *systemic* diseases. An acutely rising dye test titer, for example, is actually more likely to be associated with an active focus of toxoplasmic lymphadenitis at some remote point in the body than with an exacerbation of inflammatory changes in the retina. The ophthalmoscopic picture of the disease is often said

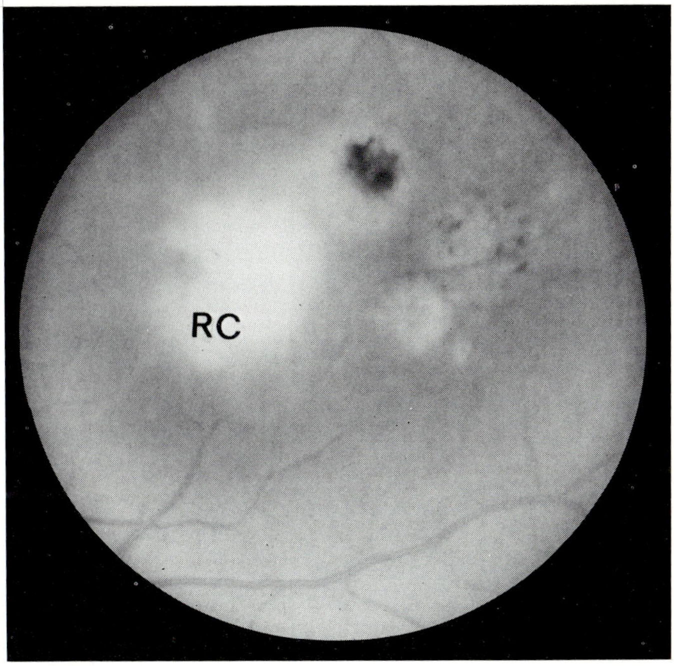

Fig. 11-10. Typical fundus picture of acute recurrent toxoplasmosis. Vitreous overlying the fresh retinochoroiditic lesion (*RC*) is slightly cloudy. Note adjacent healed, pigmented "satellite" lesions.

to be pathognomonic. It is well known, however, that certain of the granulomatous uveitises can mimic the clinical picture of other uveitises. Toxoplasmosis and tuberculosis, for example, have often been confused with each other in the past.

If we assume that the fundus and vitreous pictures (Fig. 11-10) are compatible with toxoplasmosis, what steps should then be taken to establish the diagnosis? In general, one should follow the clinical leads presented by the patient. A careful history should be taken. In many of the proved cases of acquired toxoplasmosis in adults, histories of chronic malaise, muscular aches, chronic low-grade fevers, and swollen lymph glands have been elicited. These symptoms closely resemble those of infectious mononucleosis, and indeed many cases of "infectious mononucleosis" with negative heterophile reactions have subsequently been proved to be toxoplasmosis.

The question of late, previously undetected congenital toxoplasmosis always arises. Inquiries into possible illness of the patient's mother during her pregnancy are singularly unrewarding in the author's experience. Rarely, the disease can be traced in this manner, particularly if the mother had lymphadenopathy or a skin rash during pregnancy; from this point of view, such questioning is worthwhile. If positive or suggestive information is obtained about the patient's mother, serologic tests should be performed on her as well as on the patient.

A baseline serologic test for toxoplasmosis should be performed, whether it be the dye test, the hemagglutination test, or the fluorescein-inhibition test. It should be repeated at least once for confirmation, especially if it is highly positive (over 1:1,024) or completely negative. If the test is positive, further attempts should be made to determine the stage or acuteness of the disease; the complement-fixation and precipitin tests are both helpful in this regard. In the opinion of most authors, a consistently negative dye test rules out the possibility of toxoplasmosis. A differential blood count should be performed. In proved cases of toxoplasmosis, leukopenia with a relative neutropenia has been seen, as well as large "abnormal" lymphocytes. Eosinophilia is variable.

The anterior chamber should be examined for the presence of cells and flare. If either or both is present, a diagnostic paracentesis is indicated. The specimen should be centrifuged and a smear made for routine Gram staining and Giemsa staining. Habegger[13] has found *Toxoplasma* organisms in the aqueous humor of a 2-month-old infant, but it should be emphasized that this is indeed a rare experience. In any case the small amount of effort expended in examining a Giemsa smear is certainly justified, if only to document the type of inflammatory cells present. Approximately 0.2 ml of aqueous humor usually suffices for both a dye test (initial dilution 1:4) and an agar-diffusion test for precipitating antibody. The indirect fluorescein test can be performed as an alternate procedure. In the deep-frozen state, aqueous humor can be stored in sealed glass capillary tubes almost indefinitely; serologic examination of the specimen therefore can be postponed if desired. In addition, precipitating antibodies and dye test antibodies are heat stable, and test samples can be sent through the mail.

If lymph nodes are palpable or inflamed, the patient should be urged to undergo a lymph node biopsy. Prior arrangements should be made with a well-equipped laboratory for isolation studies on the lymph node as well as routine histopathologic examination. Injection of minced lymph node tissue into the peritoneal cavity of a mouse seems, by all odds, to be the most reliable method for making an isolation. A great deal of information has been gained from lymph node studies, and parallel success in isolation has been achieved with muscle (gastrocnemius) biopsies.

Skull x-rays for intracerebral calcification may be of help, especially in suspected late congenital cases. In the few cases where this has been justified, there has usually been a long-standing history of visual impairment, strabismus, or mental deficiency.

The skin test (intradermal injection of toxoplasmin) may be employed as a confirmatory measure. Dermal hypersensitivity to *Toxoplasma* antigens usually cannot be detected until about 6 months after infection. For this reason the test is not useful in detecting early infections. It must be remembered, too, that a certain number of patients, particularly in the older age groups, will always be anergic to skin test antigens, or relatively so.

In the diagnosis of congenital toxoplasmosis among infants we stand on somewhat firmer ground. In addition to the ophthalmoscopic findings there are often other associated signs of disease, such as hydrocephalus, mental retardation, neurologic defects, and microphthalmia. Skull x-ray films sometimes show the presence of intracerebral calcifications. There may also be associated cardiovascular disease, skin rash, and lymphadenopathy. Cytomegalic inclusion disease in infants has often been observed to run a parallel course with toxoplasmosis. The reason for this association is not yet clear, although it may be linked with pathologic changes in the host's cellular defense mechanisms.

Serologic studies on both the mother and the patient are particularly important. If both react positively, attention should be directed to the type of antibody present. Remington and his associates[36] have shown that macromolecules at the 19S type will not cross the normal placenta. If an infant suspected of having toxoplasmosis shows antibody to *Toxoplasma* that is of the 19S type, it may be assumed that he himself has the disease. Smaller antibodies of the 7S type cross the placental barrier easily. If an infant's positive dye test is caused by 7S antibodies alone, it may be assumed that he has received a passive transfer of antibodies from his mother.

Finally, a word of caution should be inserted about the confirmation of the diagnosis by therapeutic trial. Although numerous studies now seem to suggest that pyrimethamine (Daraprim), particularly when given in combination with the sulfa drugs, is effective in the treatment of both the systemic and ocular forms of the disease, these effects have always been more easily demonstrable in animal experiments and tissue culture than in humans. But even if we grant that these drugs are effective, all forms of uveitis, toxoplasmosis included, undergo certain phases of spontaneous exacerbation and remission. To say that the improvement in a given patient was necessarily correlated with specific therapy is indeed spurious. Often the diagnosis itself is so uncertain that even if the retinopathy were improved by the drug therapy, it would still be difficult to ascribe the eye disease to toxoplasmosis. We must look to the future for more exact methods of diagnosis *upon the eye itself* before we can expect to make etiologic diagnosis a practical reality.

REFERENCES

1. Ansari, N., and Minou, A.: Présence de toxoplasmes dans des frottis de conjunctive palpébrale humaine, Bull. Soc. Path. Exot. **41**: 463, 1948.
2. Boyden, S. V.: The adsorption of proteins on erythrocytes treated with tannic acid and subsequent hemagglutination by antiprotein sera, J. Exp. Med. **93**:107, 1951.
3. Bringmann, G., and Holz, J.: Licht und elektronenmikroskopische Untersuchungen zum Sero-Farbtest auf Toxoplasmose nach Sabin und Feldman, Z. Ges. Hyg. **138**:151, 1953.
4. Bringmann, G., and Holz, J.: Die Bewegungsorganellen des Toxoplasma gondii, Z. Tropenmed. Parasit. **5**:54, 1954.
5. Coons, A. H., Creech, H. J., Jones, R. N., and Berliner, E.: The demonstration of pneumococcal antigen in tissues by the use of fluorescent antibody, J. Immun. **45**:159, 1942.
6. Dallenbach, F., and Piekarski, G.: Über den Nachweis von Toxoplasma gondii im Gewebe mit Hilfe markierter fluorescierender Antikörper (Methode nach Coons), Virchow Arch. Path. Anat. **333**:607, 1960.
7. Desmonts, G.: Definitive serological diagnosis of ocular toxoplasmosis, Arch. Ophthal. **76**: 839, 1966.
8. Feldman, H. A.: The clinical manifestations and laboratory diagnosis of toxoplasmosis, Amer. J. Trop. Med. **2**:420, 1953.
9. Frenkel, J. K., and Jacobs, L. J.: Ocular toxoplasmosis: pathogenesis, diagnosis and treatment, Arch. Ophthal. **59**:260, 1958.
10. Goldman, M.: Staining Toxoplasma gondii with fluorescein-labeled antibody: the reaction in smears of peritoneal exudate, J. Exp. Med. **105**:549, 1957.
11. Goldman, M.: Staining Toxoplasma gondii with fluorescein-labeled antibody: a new test for antibodies to Toxoplasma based upon inhibition of specific staining, J. Exp. Med. **105**: 557, 1957.
12. Goldman, M., Carver, R. K., and Sulzer, A. J.: Reproduction of Toxoplasma gondii by internal budding, J. Parasit. **44**:161, 1958.
13. Habegger, H.: Toxoplasmose humaine: mise en évidence des parasites dans les milieux intra-oculaires (humeur acqueuse, exsudat rétro-rétinian), Arch. Ophthal. **14**:470, 1954.
14. Hogan, M. J.: Ocular toxoplasmosis; clinical and laboratory diagnosis; evaluation of immunologic tests; treatment, Arch. Ophthal. **55**:333, 1956.
15. Hogan, M. J., Yoneda, C., Feeney, L., Zweigart, P., and Lewis, A.: Morphology and culture of Toxoplasma, Trans. Amer. Ophthal. Soc. **58**:167, 1961.
16. Hogan, M. J., Yoneda, C., and Zweigart, P.: Growth of Toxoplasma strains in tissue culture, Amer. J. Ophthal. **51**:920, 1961.
17. Hogan, M. J., Zweigart, P., and Lewis, A.: Recovery of Toxoplasma from a human eye, Arch. Ophthal. **60**:548, 1958.
18. Jacobs, L. J.: Biology of Toxoplasma, Amer. J. Trop. Med. **2**:365, 1953.
19. Jacobs, L., Cook, M. K., and Wilder, H. C.: Serologic data on adults with histologically diagnosed toxoplasmic chorioretinitis, Trans. Amer. Acad. Ophthal. Otolaryng. **58**:193, 1954.
20. Jacobs, L., Fair, J., and Bickerton, J.: Adult ocular toxoplasmosis: report of parasitologically proven case, Arch. Ophthal. **52**:63, 1954.
21. Jacobs, L., and Lunde, M. N.: A hemagglutination test for toxoplasmosis, Parasitology **43**:308, 1957.
22. Jacobs, L., Naquin, H., Hoover, R., and Woods, A. C.: A comparison of the toxoplasmin skin test, the Sabin-Feldman dye test, and the complement fixation test for toxoplasmosis in various forms of uveitis, Bull. Johns Hopkins Hosp. **99**:1, 1956.
23. Jacobs, L. J., Woke, P., and Jones, F. E.: Studies on the transmission of Toxoplasma gondii, J. Parasit. **36**:36, 1950.
24. Jankû, J.: Pathogenesis and pathologic anatomy of colomboma of macula lutea in eye of

normal dimensions and in microphthalmic eye, with parasites in retina, Cas. Lek. Cesk. **62**:1021, 1054, 1081, 1111, 1138, 1923.
25. Kaufman, H. E., Remington, J. S., and Jacobs, L.: Toxoplasmosis: the nature of virulence, Amer. J. Ophthal. **46**:255, 1958.
26. Ludvik, J.: Verschiedene elektronoptische Untersuchungen am Toxoplasma gondii und Sarcocystis nevilla, Zbl. Bakt. (Orig.) **166**:60, 1956.
27. Lunde, M. N., and Jacobs, L.: A comparison of results of hemagglutination and dye tests for toxoplasmosis in a survey of Trinidad natives, Amer. J. Trop. Med. **7**:523, 1958.
28. Lunde, M. N., and Jacobs, L.: Evaluation of a latex agglutination test for toxoplasmosis, J. Parasit. **53**:933, 1967.
29. Maloney, E. D., and Kaufman, H. E.: The rapid and convenient detection of Toxoplasma antibodies using formaldehyde-treated human erythrocytes, Amer. J. Ophthal. **50**:945, 1960.
30. Mitchell, R. G., and Green, C. A.: The hemagglutination test for Toxoplasma antibodies, J. Clin. Path. **13**:331, 1960.
31. Nicolle, C., and Manceaux, L.: Sur un protozoaire nouveau du gondi, C. R. Acad. Sci. [D] (Paris) **148**:369, 1909.
32. O'Connor, G. R.: Anti-Toxoplasma precipitins in aqueous humor: new application of the agar-diffusion technique, Arch. Ophthal. **57**: 52, 1957.
33. O'Connor, G. R.: Precipitating antibody to Toxoplasma: a follow-up study on findings in the blood and aqueous humor, Amer. J. Ophthal. **44**(4):75, 1957.
34. Ouchterlony, Ö.: Antigen-antibody reactions in gels, Acta Path. Microbiol. Scand. **26**:507, 1949.
35. Park, H. K.: Toxoplasma hemagglutination test using alcohol-formalin fixed sensitized lyophilized erythrocytes, Arch. Ophthal. **65**: 184, 1961.
36. Remington, J. S., Miller, M. J., and Brownlee, I.: IgM antibodies in acute toxoplasmosis: diagnostic significance in congenital cases and a method for their rapid demonstration, Pediatrics **41**:1082, 1968.
37. Reuss, K.: Untersuchungen zur Hemagglutinationsreaktion and Toxoplasmose nach Jacobs und Lunde, Immunitätsforschung **121**:75, 1961.
38. Sabin, A. B., Eichenwald, H., Feldman, H. A., and Jacobs, L.: Present status of clinical manifestations of toxoplasmosis in man, J.A.M.A. **150**:1063, 1952.
39. Sabin, A. B., and Feldman, H. A.: Dyes as micro-chemical indicators of a new immune phenomenon affecting a protozoan parasite (Toxoplasma), Science **108**:660, 1948.
40. Sabin, A. B., and Ruchman, I.: Characteristics of the Toxoplasma neutralizing antibody, Proc. Soc. Exp. Biol. Med. **51**:1, 1942.
41. Siim, J. C., and Lind, K.: A Toxoplasma flocculation test, Acta Path. Microbiol. Scand. **50**:445, 1960.
42. Strannegård, Ö., University of Göteborg, Sweden. Personal communication.
43. Strannegård, Ö.: An electronmicroscopic study on the immunoinactivation of Toxoplasma gondii, Acta Path. Microbiol. Scand. **71**:463, 1967.
44. Uminski, J., and Wawrzkiewicz, J.: Preliminary results of investigations concerning the application of the precipitation reaction in a gel medium for the diagnosis of toxoplasmosis, Wiadomosci Parazytologiczne Rok VII **2**:423, 1961.
45. Warren, J., and Sabin, A. B.: The complement fixation reaction in toxoplasmic infection, Proc. Soc. Exp. Biol. Med. **51**:11, 1942.
46. Wilder, H. C.: Toxoplasma chorioretinitis in adults, Arch. Ophthal. **48**:127, 1952.
47. Witmer, R. N.: Experimental leptospiral uveitis in rabbits, Arch. Ophthal. **53**:547, 1955.
48. Wolf, A., and Cowen, D.: Granulomatous encephalomyelitis due to encephalitozoan (encephalitozoic encephalomyelitis): new protozoan disease of man, Bull. Neurolog. Inst. N. Y. **6**:306, 1937.

12

Ocular toxocariasis

HAROLD W. BROWN AND DAVID H. BROWN

Ocular toxocariasis results primarily from invasion of the eye by the larval stage of *Toxocara canis,* the common roundworm of man's best friend, the dog. *Toxocara cati* of the domestic cat may also cause infection, though invasion of the eye has not been reported. The predominance of *T. canis* as opposed to that of *T. catis* in human infection may be because of the fastidious toilet habits of the cat. *T. canis* is widely distributed throughout the world, and unrecognized human infections with the larvae are probably more widespread than the few hundred reported ocular infections suggest. The adult worm lives in the small intestine of the dog, and its microscopic eggs are passed in its stools. After a short incubation period in the soil, the eggs contain infective larvae (Fig. 12-1). When eaten by a dog, they liberate their larvae in its small intestine; and after a bloodstream invasion and a pulmonary migration, they grow to maturity in the small intestine. In man, an aberrant host, the larvae hatching from the ingested embryonated *Toxocara* eggs penetrate the intestinal mucosa and by way of the bloodstream reach the liver, lungs, brain, eye, and other organs of the body. These larvae, strangers in a strange land, do not mature, but wander in the tissues for many months before dying.[4]

Ocular toxocariasis has been reported in 245 patients ranging from 2 to 31 years of age. Unfortunately, for the sake of ready diagnosis the leukocytosis and eosinophilia, which are pathognomonic of visceral larva migrans, are not usually present in uncomplicated ocular toxocariasis. The typical visceral larva migrans syndrome consists of hepatic enlargement and tenderness, cough, fever, central nervous system disturbances, marked leukocytosis, and eosinophilia. Larval overflow into the eyes may cause ocular toxocariasis. However, very few of the patients with ocular toxocariasis experienced recognizable generalized larval invasion of the body, or such involvement was not sufficient to produce symptoms of visceral larva migrans. Only 5 of the 245 patients with ocular toxocariasis had a typical visceral larva migrans syndrome before or during the ocular disease. Table 12-1 summarizes the clinical differences between ocular and visceral *T. canis* disease.[1]

PATHOLOGY

The *Toxocara* larvae probably enter the eye by way of the retinal artery. The most characteristic lesion of ocular toxocariasis is a white, elevated, circular tumor approximately one to two disk diameters, usually in the macular area or temporal to the optic disk (Plate 3, *C*). Dark areas in the lesion represent the site of the larva. The surrounding retina may be relatively normal in appearance, although tension folds may radiate from the lesion and retinal

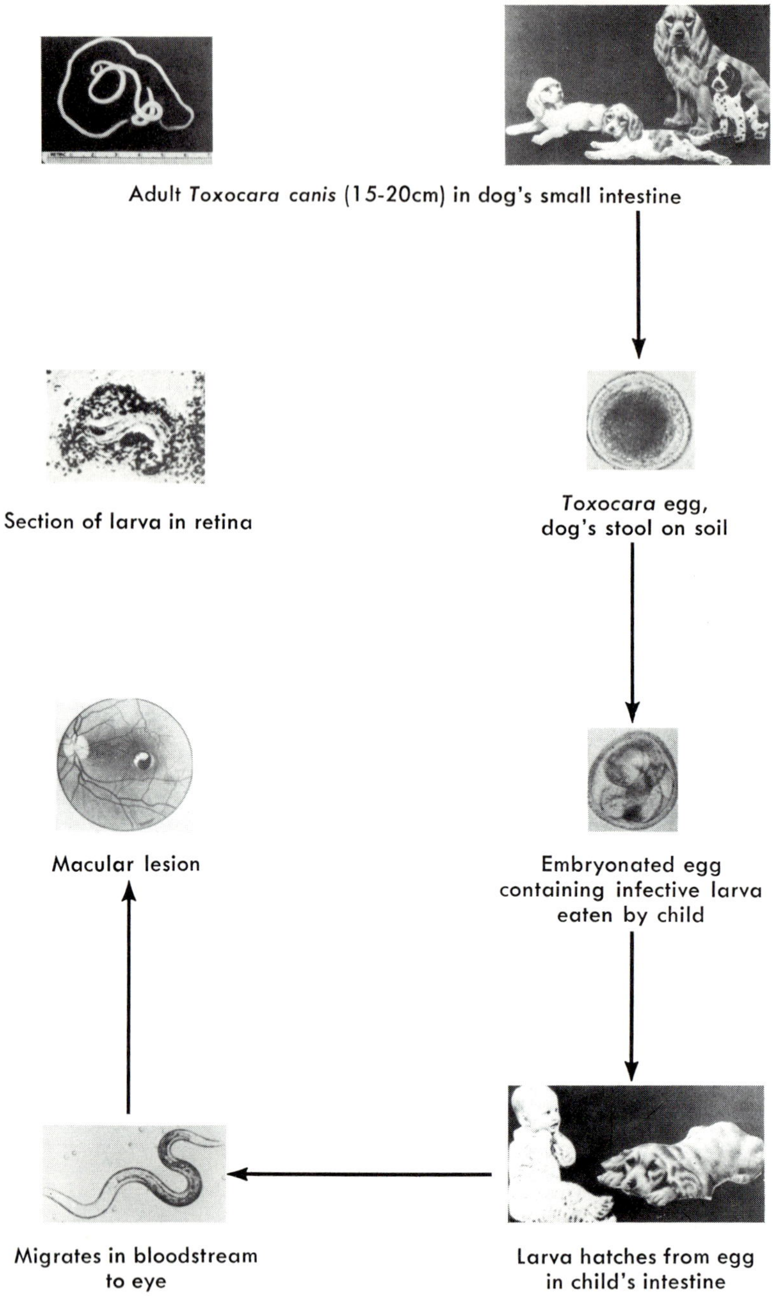

Fig. 12-1. Ocular *Toxocara canis* infection. (From Brown, D. H.: J. Pediat. Ophthal. 7:182, 1970.)

vessels may invade and disappear into it. Complete detachment of the retina may occur. Less commonly, the larva is situated anteriorly in the fundus and is accompanied by chronic endophthalmitis, iridocyclitis, and posterior synechiae. Although vision is grossly impaired, the eye appears normal outwardly. In 6 of the 245 ocular infections there was a possibility of bilateral infections. Optic neuritis has been reported in one pathologically proved infection. *T. canis* probably accounted for 10%

Table 12-1. Clinical differences between ocular *Toxocara canis* disease and visceral larva migrans

	Ocular *Toxocara canis* disease	**Visceral larva migrans**
Average age of patient	7.5 years	2 years
WBC	Normal	Elevated
Eosinophilia	Normal	Elevated (>30%)
Hepatomegaly	None	Usually present
Splenomegaly	None	Usually present
Ocular findings	Posterior pole lesion, endophthalmitis, uveitis	Very rare

From Brown, D. H.: Ocular Toxocara canis, J. Pediat. Ophthal. **7**:190, 1970.

of the 150 cases of childhood uveitis reported by Perkins,[8] all of which were unilateral.

The characteristic histologic lesion includes an eosinophilic granuloma with plasma cells and lymphocytes, as well as eosinophils and necrotic fibrinoid material. Epithelioid and giant cells containing fragments of the larva are diagnostic. Table 12-2 lists the data reported by various authors on the pathologic findings in 143 of the 245 cases of *T. canis* ocular infection that have been indicated in the literature.

DIAGNOSIS

The presenting signs and symptoms of the patient, in order of frequency, are strabismus, failing vision, blind eye, and leukokoria. The clinical observations, in order of frequency, are solid retinal tumor, endophthalmitis, uveitis, chorioretinitis, retinal detachment, corneal larva, cyclitic membrane, iritis, iris granuloma, nummular keratitis, cataract, massive retinal fibrosis, and optic neuritis.

Only one out of eight patients that have been reported gave a history of contact with a dog or cat. This to a large degree represents a failure to question the patient or his parents about such contact. The majority of patients who were questioned about contact with dogs or cats gave an affirmative answer.

Ocular toxocariasis is difficult to diagnose clinically because of its resemblance to retinoblastoma, endophthalmitis, and Coats's disease. A sensitive specific serologic test would be of great value. Such tests are of some value in the diagnosis of visceral larva migrans with its extensive organ involvement.[6] However, when only the eye is invaded by larvae, the serologic tests presently available are of little value. A recent summary of serologic data on repeated sera from a patient whose eye was removed and *Toxocara* larva demonstrated showed that all tests were negative. Serologic tests with purified *Ascaris* antigen also were negative, as were passive cutaneous anaphylaxis tests. No specimens revealed an increase of IgA or IgM levels. The patient had type O blood and no significant titer to A or B erythrocytes. Thus, neither specific nor nonspecific antibodies

Table 12-2. Pathologic findings in 143 cases of ocular *Toxocara canis* infection

Slide specimens of eye	*Toxocara canis* second-stage larva	53
	Toxocara species	3
	Nematode larva	20
	No larva found, eosinophilic granuloma	60
Slide specimens of liver biopsy	*Toxocara canis* second-stage larva	1
	No larva found, eosinophilic granuloma	1
Slide specimen of corneal trephine button	*Toxocara canis* second-stage larva	1
In vivo	Nematode larva	4

From Brown, D. H.: Ocular Toxocara canis, J. Pediat. Ophthal. **7**:188, 1970.

were detected in this proved case of ocular toxocariasis.[7]

Clinical data obtained from examination of patients seen in the children's tumor clinic at the Institute of Ophthalmology, Columbia-Presbyterian Medical Center (IOCPMC) are summarized in Table 12-3. Most of the patients were referred for the purpose of ruling out retinoblastoma; thus no laboratory data was gathered, and the diagnosis depended upon the findings in the eye and on the history of the case. As is seen from the table, 10 eyes were enucleated because of continued suspicion of retinoblastoma. Microscopic study of the eye sections was done at the IOCPMC, and the pathologic findings are listed. Typical eosinophilic granulomas were found in 5 of the 10 cases, but these are only suggestive of *T. canis* since no larvae were found. Finding larvae often requires serial sections, which have not yet been made on these patients. The series indicates the difficulty in making a definitive diagnosis of *T. canis* even in enucleated eyes. Since patients with *T. canis* infection should not have the eye enucleated, it is most important to establish a helpful laboratory test. Brown[2] has shown that *T. canis* contains human blood group A antigen. As *T. canis* stimulates some production of anti-A antibodies in man, the possibility of using a test for rising antibody to group A antigen as a diagnostic tool is being further explored.

Table 12-3. Summary of 43 cases of presumed ocular *Toxocara canis* infection in the children's tumor clinic of the IOCPMC

Age	Average	4.4 years	
	Range	3 months to 11 years	
	0.4 years	23	
	5-8 years	18	
	9-12 years	2	
Sex	Male	26	
	Female	17	
Dog or cat contact		27	
Pica (geophagia)		7	
Original complaint			
	Strabismus	19	
	Failing vision	5	
	Leukokoria	3	
	Routine exam	3	
	Blind eye	1	
	Fixed pupil	1	
	Red eye	1	
Clinical observations			
	Solid retinal tumor	23	
	Posterior pole	18	
	Periphery	5	
	Vitreous mass or vitreous haze (fundus not seen)	12	
	Retinal detachment	10	
	Cataract	2	
	Chorioretinitis	1	
	Iris heterochromia	1	
	Microphthalmos	1	
Visceral larval migrans syndrome			0
Possible bilateral lesions			1
Pathology: patients 43 enucleation 10			
	Toxocara canis second stage larva		0
	No larva found, eosinophilic granuloma		5
	Congenital anomalies		2
	Coats's disease		1
	Retinoblastoma		1
	Toxoplasmosis		1

From Brown, D. H.: Ocular Toxocara canis, J. Pediat. Ophthal. **7**:189, 1970.

THERAPY

Therapy of ocular toxocariasis is neither specific nor satisfactory. Steroid therapy consisting of prednisone, 40 mg daily for several weeks, is of value, especially when organs other than the eye are involved. A patient harboring an adult intraretinal nematode was treated with 40 mg of prednisone daily for 3 weeks and 2 gm of thiabendazole daily for 5 days with good results.[3] The larva disappeared from the fundus within 24 hours after the initiation of therapy, and a linear retinal hemorrhage remained where the larva was last seen. Although the chemotherapy of visceral larva migrans with thiabendazole has given equivocal results, its recent 15- to 30-day use in *Capillaria* infections suggests an extended course, if necessary, in *Toxocara* infections. Light coagulation and cryotherapy are alternative treatments that might be given a trial in ocular toxocariasis.

PREVENTION

Close contact with infected dogs and cats should be avoided. Since puppies and kittens are more commonly and more heavily infected and may carry *Toxocara* eggs on their fur, small children should be protected against them. Animals under 6 months old should be dewormed with piperazine every month and older ones every 2 months. Worms passed as a result of treatment should be destroyed. Dog and cat feces passed in children's play areas should be buried; and sandboxes, which offer attractive animal defecating areas, should be covered when not in use.

REFERENCES

1. Brown, D. H.: Ocular Toxocara canis, J. Pediat. Ophthal. **7**:182, 1970.
2. Brown, D. H.: Ocular Toxocara canis: experimental immunology, Ann. Ophthal. **3**:907, 1971.
3. Brown, H. D.: Antiparasitic drugs: IV 2(4'-thiazolyl)-benzimidazole, J. Amer. Chem. Soc. **83**:1764, 1961.
4. Brown, H. W.: Basic clinical parasitology, New York, 1969, Appleton-Century-Crofts, p. 343.
5. Duquid, I. M.: Chronic endophthalmitis due to Toxocara, Brit. J. Ophthal. **45**:75, 1961.
6. Duquid, I. M.: Features of ocular infestation by Toxocara, Brit. J. Ophthal. **45**:789, 1961.
7. Kagan, I. G.: Serologic diagnosis of visceral larva migrans, Clin. Pediat. **7**:508, 1968.
8. Perkins, E. S.: Pattern of uveitis in children, Brit. J. Ophthal. **50**:169, 1966.
9. Rubin, M. L., Kaufman, H. E., and Tierney, J. P.: An intraretinal nematode, Trans. Amer. Acad. Ophthal. Otolaryng. **72**:855, 1968.

13

Fungal infections of the eye

with **ARTHUR GERARD DeVOE AND MARGARITA SILVA-HUTNER**

Interest in the possible role of fungi as ocular pathogens was evident in a few areas as early as the middle of the eighteenth century, according to Professor Theodor Leber, who in 1879 published the first report of keratomycosis in man. Leber (Fig. 13-1), an ophthalmologist, made many contributions to the field, among the more notable of which were his studies on the physiology of the circulation of the eye and on inflammation. He distinguished inflammatory response caused by physical or chemical trauma from that caused by infection. His early training in botany may have given him the interest and skill to isolate and identify the etiologic agent in a case of mycotic ocular infection. The patient was a farmer who sustained an injury to the eye from oat chaff while working with a threshing machine. During the next few days the eye became painful; there was a loss of visual acuity; and on the fifth day a corneal ulcer measuring 4 to 5 mm in diameter, with a grayish, turbid base and slightly raised edge, was found. Pus in the anterior chamber reached the level of the lower edge of the ulcer and was associated with intense chemosis. During the next 5 days the ulcer enlarged, and a membrane lifted from the upper border was found to be thickly overgrown with mycelial elements. With the assistance of Professor Reincke, a botanist, Leber identified the organism as *Aspergillus glaucus.* Leber contaminated corneal wounds of rabbits with small bits of mycelium from pure cultures of the *Aspergillus* and injected rabbit corneas with suspensions of the *Aspergillus* spores. In both instances the fungus grew with surprising swiftness and in 2 days penetrated the thickness of the cornea.[31]

Despite Leber's classic paper. only scattered accounts of mycotic infections of the eye appeared during the next 70 years. Chick and Conant[11] in their review of the literature found 148 case reports of corneal mycotic infections following Leber's observation, but 84 of these occurred between 1951 and 1962. They point out that this was an era of intensive antibiotic and steroid therapy. The fungi most frequently isolated were members of the genus *Aspergillus.* However, inspection of Table 13-1, a list of the fungi known to have caused corneal ulcers, shows that at least 95 species in 44 genera have been reported. A few, indicated by an asterisk, are known to be potential pathogens of man; but the great majority of these fungi have their normal habitat in the soil and vegetable matter as saprophytes that produce disease only when some damaging circumstance promotes their infectivity. Such fungi are referred to as opportunists.

Various conditions listed in Table 13-2 give opportunity to potential pathogenic and saprophytic fungi alike to overcome man's natural resistance to mycotic infec-

Table 13-1. Genera and species of fungi isolated in cases of keratomycosis

Genera	Species
Absidia	*A. corymbifera, A. ramosa, Absidia* species
Acremonium	*Acremonium* species
Acrostalagmus	*A. cinnabarinus*
Acrothecium	*A. hominis*
Allescheria	*A. boydii**
Alternaria	*Alternaria* species
Aspergillus	*A. flavus,* A. fumigatus,* A. glaucus, A. nidulans,* A. niger, A. niveus, A. ochraceus, A. versicolor, Aspergillus* species
Beauveria	*B. brumptii*
Blastomyces	*B. dermatitidis*
Botrytis	*B. cinerea, Botrytis* species
Candida	*C. albicans,* C. guilliermondii, C. krusei,* C. mycoderma,* C. parapsilosis,* C. pseudotropicalis,* C. tropicalis,* Candida* species
Cephalosporium	*C. arcuatum, C. curtipes, C. serrae,* Cephalosporium* species
Cryptococcus	*C. laurentii,* C. neoformans**
Curvularia	*C. geniculata, C. lunata, Curvularia* species
Fusarium	*F. conglutinans, F. oxysporum, F. nivale, F. solani, Fusarium* species
Fusidium	*F. terricola*
Gibberella	*G. fujikuroi*
Glenospora	*G. graphii*
Helminthosporium	*Helminthosporium* species
Hormodendrum	*Hormodendrum* species
Lasiodiplodia	*Lasiodiplodia* species
Microsporum	*M. canis**
Monosporium	*M. apiospermum* (imperfect state of *Allescheria boydii*)
Mucor	*M. cornealis, M. mucedo, M. racemosus, Mucor* species
Oospora	*O. floccosa, Oospora* species
Paecilomyces	*Paecilomyces* species
Penicillium	*P. citrinum, P. columnaris, P. crustaceum, P. chrysogenum, P. glacum, P. lilacidum, P. notatum, P. spinulosum, Penicillium* species
Periconia	*P. keratitidis*
Phialophora	*P. verrucosa**
Phycomyces	*Phycomyces* species
Rhizomucor	*R. parasiticus*
Rhizopus	*R. equinus, R. nigricans, R. parasiticus, Rhizopus* species
Rhodotorula	*Rhodotorula* species
Scopulariopsis	*S. brevicaulis,* S. mastigocladium, Scopulariopsis* species
Sporothrix	*S. schenkii**
Sporotrichum	*S. fonsecia, Sporotrichum* species
Sterigmatocystis	*S. nigra*
Tetraploa	*Tetraploa* species
Trichoderma	*Trichoderma* species
Trichophyton	*T. schoenleinii,* T. tonsurans,* Trichophyton* species
Trichosporon	*T. rugosi*
Tritirachium	*T. brumpti, T. roseum*
Ustilago	*U. zeae*
Verticillium	*V. graphii, V. rubrum, Verticillium* species†

Compiled from many published reports and unpublished data from 1879 to 1970. In addition to these isolates, which were classified as to genus and species, three authors reported five cases of keratomycosis by fungi belonging in the order Mycelia sterila (no reproductive structures known).
*Known to be pathogenic for man.
†The term species throughout indicates an isolate that was identified as to genus only.

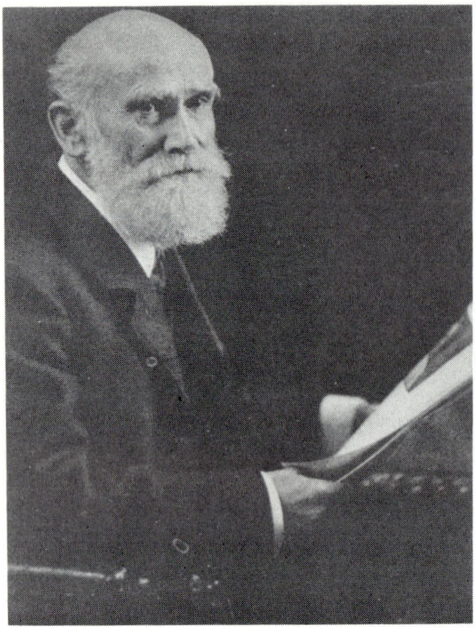

Fig. 13-1. Theodor Leber (1840-1917), biologist and physician. He was introduced to ophthalmology by Hermann Knapp, and his early training was guided by Helmholz, Professor of Physiology at Heidelberg, by Ludwig in Vienna, and by Virchow in Berlin. After years spent with Liebreich in Paris, he went to Berlin with Albrecht von Graefe and later became the Director of the University Eye Clinic in Gottingen and thereafter the director in his own university at Heidelberg. (From Festschrift zur Feier des Siebzigsten Geburtstages Herrn Geheimrat Professor Dr. Th. Leber in Heidelberg, Gewidmet von Dankbaren Schülern, Graefes Arch. Ophth. **74**:1910.)

Table 13-2. Factors that may promote mycotic ocular infections

Physical injuries	
	Abrasions
	Lacerations
	Penetrating wounds
Occupational hazards	
	Rural living
	Agricultural workers, gardeners, foresters, telephone linemen, and others have higher incidence of ocular trauma
Surgical procedures	
	Repair of retinal tear
	Keratoplasty
	Cataract extraction
	Removal of intraocular foreign body
Therapeutic regimens	
	Broad-spectrum antibiotics used over long periods of time singly or with local or systemic steroids
	Infected eye drops
Preceding nonfungal infections	
	Bacteria
	Viruses
	Trachoma
Miscellaneous causes	
	Incomplete removal of foreign bodies
	Inadequate care after surgery
	Extension to eye from infected contiguous area
	Trichiasis
	Exposure keratitis
	Bullous keratitis

tion. First among these predisposing factors are traumatic wounds to the eye. Chick and Conant[11] stated that trauma preceded keratomycosis in 77 of the 148 patients whose case histories they reviewed. Antibiotics and steroids probably have favored fungal eye infections recently. Clinical and experimental evidence, to be described later, supports this hypothesis.[32,36,66] It has been estimated that three quarters of fungal corneal ulcers have developed in eyes treated with steroids and broad-spectrum antibiotics.[13] These figures are probably similar today in many parts of the world because diagnosis of mycotic infection is so often made late, after these therapeutic measures have been tried.

Occupational hazards exert an important influence on the incidence of fungal infection. Fig. 13-2, taken from Blake's 1969 study of ocular hazards in agriculture, presents the cause and incidence of trauma in 416 cases of eye injuries seen at the Eye and Ear Hospital in Dublin over the period 1958 to 1967.[9] Agriculture engages but one third of Ireland's workers, yet 58.5% of the injuries were those that would be expected among workers in the field and forest. It will be seen later that because ocular injuries that become infected with a fungus occur more frequently in agricultural communities, they are not unexpected and therefore may be diagnosed more rapidly; thus the added hazard of nonspecific anti-

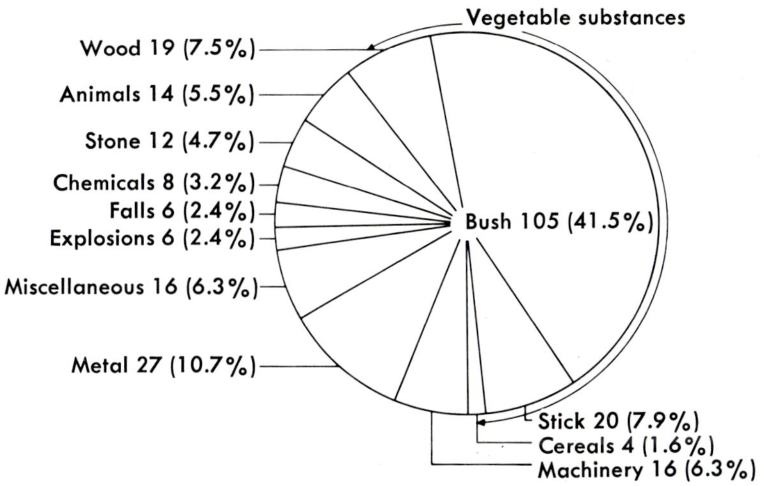

Fig. 13-2. Causes of serious injuries to the cornea. (From Blake, J.: Ophthalmologica **158**:126, 1969. S. Karger, Basel, New York.)

biotics and steroids may be reduced. Other factors that may promote fungal infections, such as preceding nonfungal infection, surgical procedures, and miscellaneous causes (Table 13-2) were encountered infrequently by Blake.

FUNGI CARRIED BY HEALTHY MAN

Information about the source of infections caused by any group of microorganisms is essential as a first step toward the control of such infections. What is the normal habitat of the organism? Does man carry it, and if so, how? Does it always cause disease when present in the tissues, or do accessory factors promote its pathogenicity?

Several studies of the distribution of fungi in the eye and body of man have been reported. A list of fungi isolated from the normal eye is presented in Table 13-3. Eighty-three species belonging to 49 genera have been grown from the normal eye by several investigators. The great majority of these fungi are considered to have their normal habitat in soil and vegetable matter. This is also true for the fungi, listed in Table 13-1, that have been recovered from patients with keratomycosis. A comparison of the findings given in Table 13-1 with those in Table 13-3 shows that 38 species from 25 genera, grown from fungal infections of the cornea, have also been grown from the normal eye. Such findings are compatible with the hypothesis that fungi found in some ocular infections may have been carried by the patient. This is, however, still speculation, since no cultures prior to mycotic ocular infection have been reported. Percebois and Raspiller[44] and Wilson and his associates[65] took repeated cultures of normal eyes at intervals of days and found either a varying mycotic flora or none on such serial examinations. They surmise that the fungal population of the normal eye is inconstant. Percebois and Raspiller report great fluctuations in the number of colonies isolated at each testing. The conclusion that might be drawn from these observations is that the condition of an eye at a moment of trauma may determine the likelihood of endogenous infection.

In association with the late Dr. Rhoda W. Benham we have studied the incidence of fungi in healthy eyes of 508 young people 10 to 18 years old and of 1,347 adults 19 to 80 years old. The results are presented in Table 13-4. This series of studies revealed the following information: (1) fungi were less frequently present in

Table 13-3. Genera and species of fungi isolated from adult normal eyes

Genera	Species
Acremonium	*Acremonium* species
Acrostalagmus	*A. cinnabarinus*
Acrothecium	*A. hominis*
Alternaria	*Alternaria* species
Aspergillus	*A. flaviceps, A. fumigatus, A. glaucus, A. niger, A. terreus, Aspergillus* species
Aureobasidium	*A. pullulans*
Botrytis	*B. cinerea, Botrytis* species
Candida	*C. albicans, C. guilliermondii, C. krusei, C. parapsilosis, C. pseudotropicalis, C. pulcherima, C. tropicalis, Candida* species
Cephalosporium	*Cephalosporium* species
Circinella	*C. minor*
Cladosporium	*C. herbarum, C. mansoni, Cladosporium* species (see also *Hormodendrum*)
Closterosporium	*Closterosporium* species
Cryptococcus	*C. albidus, C. laurentii, Cryptococcus* species
Curvularia	*C. geniculata, C. lunata, Curvularia* species
Debaryomyces	*D. hansenii*
Dematium	*Dematium* species
Eurotium	*Eurotium* species
Fusarium	*Fusarium* species
Geotrichum	*Geotrichum* species
Gliocladium	*Gliocladium* species
Haplographium	*Haplographium* species
Helminthosporium	*Helminthosporium* species
Heterobotrytis	*Heterobotrytis* species
Hormodendrum	*H. algeriensis, Hormodendrum* species (*Hormondendrum* now a synonym of *Cladosporium*)
Isaria	*Isaria* species
Madurella	*Madurella* species
Monilia	*M. sitophila*
Monosporium	*M. apiospermum, Monosporium* species
Mucor	*Mucor* species
Nigrospora	*Nigrospora* species
Oospora	*O. penicillioides, Oospora* species
Paecilomyces	*P. varioti, Paecilomyces* species
Papulaspora	*Papulaspora* species
Penicillium	*P. citrinum, P. commune, Penicillium* species
Pestalotia	*Pestalotia* species
Pullularia	*Pullularia* species
Rhizopus	*Rhizopus* species
Rhodotorula	*R. mucilaginosa, R. rubra, Rhodotorula* species
Saccharomyces	*S. cerevisiae, S. fragilis, Saccharomyces* species
Schizosaccharomyces	*S. hominis*
Scopulariopsis	*S. brevicaulis, S. mastigocladium, Scopulariopsis* species
Sporotrichum	*Sporotrichum* species
Stachybotrys	*S. atra*
Sterignatocystis	*S. nigra*
Torula	*T. chartarum, Torula* species
Torulopsis	*T. glabrata, Torulopsis* species
Trichoderma	*T. viride, Trichoderma* species
Trichophyton	*Trichophyton* species
Trichothecium	*T. roseum*

Compiled from many published reports and unpublished data. In addition to these isolates, which were classified as to genus and species, some authors reported fungi belonging in the order Mycelia sterila (no reproductive structures known).

Table 13-4. Incidence of fungi cultured from clinically healthy eyes of 508 young people 10 to 18 years of age and in 1,347 adults 19 to 80 years of age

Fungus isolated	Number of subjects positive age 10 to 18 years		Number of subjects positive age 19 to 80 years	
	Conjunctiva	Eyelid	Conjunctiva	Eyelid
Aspergillus species	—	—	10	12
Aspergillus niger	—	—	1	1
Candida species	2	4	3	8
Candida albicans	1	1	1	1
Cephalosporium species	1	2	4	7
Cryptococcus species	—	1	5	7
Fusarium species	1	1	7	10
Geotrichum species	1	1	—	3
Hormodendrum species	—	—	1	5
Penicillium species	—	1	2	2
Pullularia species	—	—	4	5
Rhizopus species	—	—	1	3
Rhodotorula species	—	—	9	11
Rhodotorula rubra	1	2	7	9
Saccharomyces species	1	2	4	7
Total number positive	8	15	59	91
Percent positive	1.5	2.9	4.4	6.7

Developed in collaboration with the late Dr. Rhoda W. Benham, Columbia-Presbyterian Medical Center.

the eyes of young people (1.5% as opposed to 4.4% in adults); (2) *Aspergillus,* the fungus most commonly cultured from adult eyes, was missing from the eyes of healthy young people; (3) the eyelids were more likely to contain fungi than were the conjunctivas; and (4) in the adult population the genera *Aspergillus* and *Rhodotorula* accounted for almost half the fungi isolated.

Some similar observations have been made in other parts of the world. Williamson and his associates[63] in Glasgow, reporting on 553 patients from newborns to those 70 years old and older, stated that children up to 9 years of age had an incidence of only 0.8% of fungi in the conjunctiva; and in those 10 to 20 years old the incidence was 1.4%, whereas the average for the older group was 9%. Wilson and his coworkers[65] in Florida found a higher incidence of fungi on the eyelids than in the conjunctiva. This latter observation indicates the need for care in culturing the conjunctiva to avoid contact with the eyelid, which might become a source of contamination for the conjunctiva. High figures (36%) for carriage rate of fungi are reported by Olson[40] in California, but examination included eyelid cultures.

The incidence of fungi in clinically normal eyes of adults reported from various areas of the world is presented in Table 13-5. The percent of cases showing positive cultures varies from 2.45% to 52%. When the figures were examined, it was found that the number of species of fungi identified by the various investigators ranged from 3 to 29. Furthermore, there was a disparity in the predominating fungus found in different geographical areas. The incidence of *Penicillium* species (27%) was twice that of any other fungus reported by Fazakas. The figures from the Columbia-Presbyterian Medical Center (CPMC) placed *Aspergillus* species at the head of the list, whereas the studies of Janke and Schwab[27] showed that 50% of the fungi were *Candida* species. Some of the differences in incidence and classification of fungi in normal eyes probably were caused by climate and occupation. On the whole, the lower carriage rates were in northern

Table 13-5. Incidence of fungi in conjunctivas of normal adult eyes in various areas of the world

Geographic area	Number people cultured	Percent positive	Reported by
Armenia, USSR: Erevan	250	2.45	Ovsepian and Osipian, 1965
Austria: Vienna	171	11.1	Janke and Schwab, 1961
England: Oxford	43	27.9	Ainley and Smith, 1965
Hungary: Debrecen	160*	24.3	Fazakas, 1935
	456*	25.65	Fazakas, 1938
	992*	25.5	Fazakas, 1953
India: Calcutta	112	13.4	Sinha and Das, 1968
Alligarh	100	22.2	Nema and associates, 1966
New Delhi	100	6.0	Agarwal and Khosla, 1963
Japan: Kumamoto	65	18.4	Mitsui and Hanabusa, 1955
Philippines: Manila	232	3.5	de Ocampo and associates, 1965
Scotland: Glasgow	553	2.9	Williamson and associates, 1968
Spain: Santiago de Compostela	42	52.0	Vasquez de Parga and Pereiro, 1965
USA: Little Rock, Arkansas	156	10.3	Hammeke and Ellis, 1960
Miami, Florida	158	22.1	Wilson and associates, 1969
New York, N.Y.	1,347	4.4	Locatcher-Khorazo and Benham, 1968

*Number of eyes cultured.

and urban areas. In the 180 individuals studied by Nema and his co-workers,[38] 92 were urban dwellers, of which 18.5% carried fungi in the eye, whereas 88 were living in the country, of which 25.4% carried fungi. Fazakas[17] found that 80% of harvest workers, when tested after returning from threshing, harbored fungi in the eye. The variety of fungi (Table 13-3) and the variability in their incidence in the eyes of healthy people around the world is not surprising when the ubiquitous nature of these organisms is considered. For example, 55 genera of airborne fungi have been identified in different parts of the world, 27 of which have been reported to dwell in the eyes and/or the body of healthy man.

All reports on ocular mycosis in relation to steroid and antibiotic therapy stress the likelihood that these agents, alone or in combination, promote fungal infection, as was first suggested in 1953 by Thygeson and his associates.[60] Mitsui and Hanabusa[36] were the first to obtain information on the effect of antibiotics and steroids on the flora of the healthy eye (Table 13-6). Hydrocortisone ointment applied for 3 weeks resulted in the emergence of fungi in the eyes of 9 out of 18 individuals who had shown no fungi before treatment. In experiments lasting for 1 week only Williamson and his co-workers found no change in the incidence of fungi in eyes treated with betamethasone; but when neomycin was added to the steroid, the carrier rate increased from 2% to 22%. Nema and his associates treated the eyes of one group of individuals previously free of fungi with hydrocortisone and another group with tetracycline for 4 weeks. The carrier rate of fungi in the first group rose to 41% and in the second group to 29%. Both Mitsui and Hanabusa and Nema and his associates present considerably more confirming data on series of individuals from whom no cultures were grown previous to the treatment but who carried substantially more organisms after treatment than those seen in healthy control groups. It may also be noted that among the fungi isolated in the experiments shown in Table 13-6, *Aspergillus*, *Penicillium*, and *Candida* predominated.

Summary

The data arising from the study of the normal mycotic flora in man have certain

Table 13-6. Effect of topical application of steroids alone or in combination with an antibiotic on mycotic flora of the healthy eye

Type of treatment	Number of subjects	Number positive before treatment	Number positive after treatment	Number fungi after treatment	Reported by
Hydrocortisone ointment 5-6 times daily for about 3 weeks	18	None	9	1 *Aspergillus* species 1 *Dematium* species 1 *Hyalopus* species 4 *Penicillium* species 2 *Rhodotorula* species	Mitsui and Hanabusa, 1955
Betamethasone disodium phosphate for 1 week	86	1 *Aspergillus* species 1 *Rhodotorula* species	3	1 *Aspergillus* species 1 *Penicillium* species 1 *Saccharomyces* species	Williamson and associates, 1968
Betamethasone disodium phosphate and neomycin sulfate for 1 week	52	1 *Candida albicans*	10	3 *Aspergillus* species 3 *Candida albicans* 3 *Penicillium* species 1 *Trichoderma* species	
Hydrocortisone 1% for 4 weeks	34	None	15	1 *Alternaria* species 4 *Aspergillus* species 1 *Candida* species 2 *Penicillium* species 1 *Helminthosporium* species 2 *Hormodendrum* species 1 *Monosporium* species 1 *Curvularia* species 1 *Mucor* species 1 *Trichothecium* species	Nema and associates, 1969
Tetracycline 1% for 4 weeks	37	None	18	1 *Alternaria* species 1 *Aspergillus* species 2 *Candida* species 1 *Fusarium* species 1 *Helminthosporium* species 1 *Penicillium* species 1 *Trichothecium* species	

relevance to mycotic infections of the eye, which may be summarized as follows:

1. Many species of fungi are found in the conjunctival sac of a portion of the healthy population, free of ocular disease. A larger number are carried in other parts of the body and in the air.
2. Many of the fungi found as transients or colonizers in normal man are among those known to be associated with ocular mycosis.
3. The carrier rate of fungi reported from various parts of the world varies from 2.45% to 52%. The reasons for this great spread in incidence of fungi are not certain; but a warm, moist climate, a rural agricultural environ-

ment, and advanced age may be associated with an increase in the number of people yielding positive fungal cultures.

4. It has been shown experimentally that both antibiotics and steroids increase the number of fungi isolated from the healthy eye.

INCIDENCE OF MYCOTIC OCULAR DISEASE

External eye

At the Institute of Ophthalmology, Columbia-Presbyterian Medical Center (IOC-PMC) from 1938 to 1968 there were 3,358 patients with disease of the external eye that appeared to be caused by infection but from which no bacterial pathogen was isolated. Smears and scrapings were stained, and exudates were cultured for fungi. The late Dr. Rhoda W. Benham gave early supervision and assistance in the isolation and identification of these organisms. The results of these studies are summarized in Table 13-7, where the area of infection and the fungi involved are recorded. Inspection of the table shows that a diagnosis of fungal infection was established in 114 instances. Only 10 of these infections occurred before 1950. The eyelids were involved in 37 infections, the lacrimal apparatus in 26, the conjunctiva in 13, and the cornea in 16. There also were 21 infections of the socket and one endogenous uveitis. In all infections except keratomycosis, *Candida* was the fungus most frequently recovered, with *Aspergillus* a poor second. Corneal ulcers were produced by *Candida* organisms in 8 instances, and the remainder were caused by 7 other fungi. In this group of 114 cases from which fungi were grown, smears and/or scrapings revealed the presence of fungi.

The sparsity of fungal infections of the eye is apparent in this New York series. During the same time (1938 to 1968) some 33,000 bacterial infections of the eye were seen (Chapter 5), 3,532 of which were corneal ulcers of proved bacterial origin. There are two other studies of fungal infection of the eye, covering a period of several years, which present somewhat the same picture. The first of these was made by Fazakas[17] in Hungary in the years 1934 to 1953. He found that in a total of 2,241 diseased eyes cultured for fungi there were 38 fungal infections.* Halde and Okumoto[23] report a series of fungal infections of the eye recognized during 1952 to 1966 at the Francis I. Proctor Foundation in San Franciso. In this period 13,500 cases of external eye disease were examined, in which 30 mycotic ulcers and 13 other various cases of ocular mycosis were identified.† Table 13-8 has been constructed so that the fungi found to cause external ocular disease in these three rather distantly spaced areas of the world might be compared. The fungi causing disease are listed at the left, and the number of infections caused by each fungus as found by Fazakas,[17] Locatcher-Khorazo and associates,[34] and Halde and Okumoto,[23] are indicated in the proper space. The findings for keratomycosis, mycosis of the conjunctiva, mycosis of the lacrimal apparatus, and mycosis of the eyelid are recorded. Study of the table reveals some interesting similarities and differences:

1. Keratomycosis was caused by a wider range of fungi than were found in other parts of the eye. This may be because of the almost constant association of some sort of preceding trauma. Fig. 13-3 illustrates the only case of corneal ulcer caused by *Verticillium* species (Fig. 13-20 shows a culture of the organism). The patient was diabetic.

2. *Aspergillus* accounted for 10 of the 29 cases of keratomycosis reported from

*Nine cases caused by *Actinomyces* organisms are omitted from the totals given by Fazakas, since these are now classified with the bacteria.

†Five cases of corneal ulcers are omitted from the totals given by Halde and Okumoto because they were caused by *Nocardia,* which is now classified with the bacteria. Thirty-four infections caused either by *Nocardia* or *Actinomyces* are deleted from the other ocular infections for the same reason (Chapter 5).

Table 13-7. Fungi causing ocular infection observed at the IOCPMC: 1938-1968

Clinical diagnosis	Number patients studied	Number fungal infections	Genera	Fungi isolated (species and number)
Infected eyelid	22	7	*Candida*	*C. albicans* (2)
				C. parapsilosis (4)
			Trichophyton	*T. mentagrophytes* (1)
Meibomitis	48	16	*Candida*	*C. albicans* (5)
				C. parapsilosis (6)
				C. tropicalis (2)
				C. pseudotropicalis (1)
			Cryptococcus	*C. neoformans* (2)
Chronic blepharitis	356	14	*Candida*	*C. albicans* (6)
				C. parapsilosis (4)
				C. mortifera (3)
			Aspergillus	*A. fumigatus* (1)
Lacrimal canaliculitis	124	15	*Candida*	*C. albicans* (6)
				C. parapsilosis (5)
				C. tropicalis (3)
				C. pseudotropicalis (1)
Lacrimal obstruction	356	11	*Candida*	*C. albicans* (3)
				C. parapsilosis (4)
				C. tropicalis (3)
			Aspergillus	*Aspergillus* species (1)
Chronic conjunctivitis	1,203	13	*Candida*	*C. albicans* (5)
				C. parapsilosis (4)
				C. tropicalis (4)
Corneal ulcer	922	16	*Candida*	*C. albicans* (6)
				C. pseudotropicalis (1)
				C. tropicalis (1)
			Cephalosporium	*Cephalosporium* species (2)
			Alternaria	*Alternaria* species (1)
			Monosporium	*M. apiospermum* (1)
			Fusarium	*Fusarium* species (1)
			Verticillium	*Verticillium* species (1)
			Cryptococcus	*C. laurentii* (1)
			Rhizopus	*Rhizopus* species (1)
Infected socket	326	21	*Candida*	*C. albicans* (5)
				C. parapsilosis (4)
				C. tropicalis (3)
				C. pseudotropicalis (1)
				C. pseudotropicalis (2)
			Aspergillus	*A. fumigatus* (4)
				A. niger (2)
Endogenous uveitis	1	1	*Aspergillus*	*A. fumigatus* (1)

Table 13-8. Summary of results from three long-term studies of mycotic infections of the eye

Species*	Keratomycosis			Mycosis of the conjunctiva			Mycosis of the lacrimal apparatus			Mycosis of the eyelids		
	(1)	(2)	(3)	(1)	(2)	(3)	(1)	(2)	(3)	(1)	(2)	(3)
Achorion schoenleinii (*Trichophyton schoenleinii*)										1		
Acrothecium hominis				1						1		
Acrostalagmus cinnabarinus	2									1		
Alternaria species		1	1									
Aspergillus flavus	2			1								
Aspergillus fumigatus	6		1								1	
Aspergillus species	2		1					1				
Candida albicans		6			5			9			13	
Candida mortifera		1									3	
Candida parapsilosis					4			9	1		14	
Candida pseudotropicalis								1			1	
Candida tropicalis		1			4			6			2	
Candida species			12						5			2
Cephalosporium species		2	1									
Coccidioides immitis						2						
Cryptococcus hominis (*C. neoformans*)	1											
Cryptococcus laurentii		1										
Cryptococcus neoformans											2	
Fusarium solani			4									
Fusarium species		1	4									
Hormodendrum algeriensis	1											
Microsporum fellineum (*M. canis*)										1		
Monosporium apiospermum		1										
Mucor cornealis	2											
Mucor species	1											
Oospora floccosa	1											
Penicillium crustaceum	3			1								
Penicillium lilacinum			1									
Penicillium species							1					
Periconia keratitidis	2											
Rhizomucor parasiticus	2											
Rhizopus species		1										
Scopulariopsis mastigocladium	1						2					
Scopulariopsis brevicaulis	2											
Sporotrichum councilmanni										1		
Sterigmatocystis niger	1											
Trichosporon rugosum							1					
Trichophyton species										2	1	
Verticillium species		1										

Sources of data are: (1) Fazakas, 1934-1953; (2) Locatcher-Khorazo, Benham, and Silva-Hutner, 1938-1968; (3) Halde and Okumoto, 1952-1966.

*Only fungi identified by culture are included. Figures to the side of names of fungi indicate number of cases.

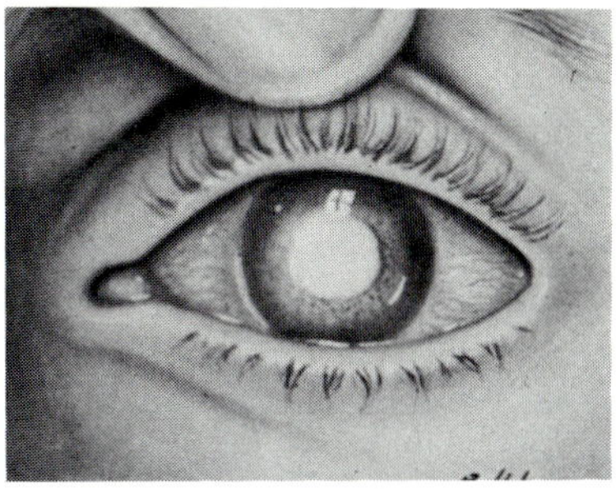

Fig. 13-3. Corneal ulcer caused by *Verticillium* species. (Courtesy Dr. C. Perera.)

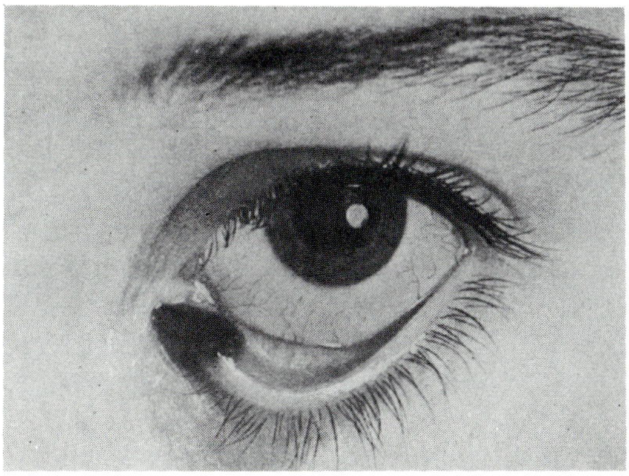

Fig. 13-4. Involvement of the lower punctum, inferior canaliculus, and palpebral conjunctiva by *Aspergillus niger*. (From Donahue, H. G.: Amer. J. Ophthal. **32**:207, 1949.)

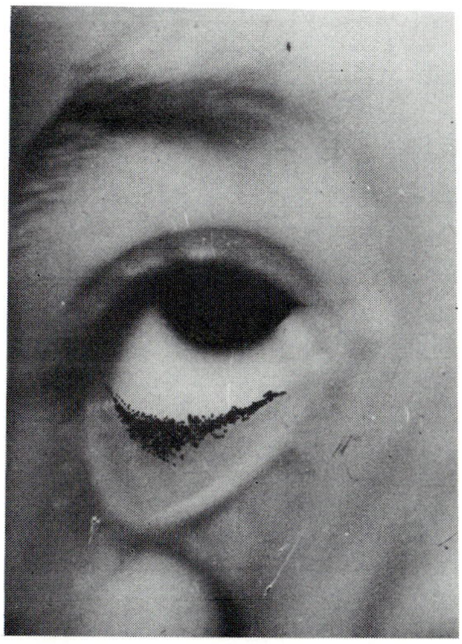

Fig. 13-5. Involvement of the conjunctiva by *Aspergillus niger*. (From Abboud, I. A., and Hanna, L. S.: Brit. J. Ophthal. **54**:480, 1970.)

Hungary but for only 2 of 40 cases from the East and West coasts of the United States. Other areas of the United States, however, have had a number of cases caused by *Aspergillus*. Figs. 13-4 and 13-5 show the eyes of two patients infected with *Aspergillus niger*, unique in that it may suggest the diagnosis on inspection.

3. *Candida* infection played the most important role in the production of keratomycosis in both the New York and San Francisco areas. Fig. 13-6 shows a hypopyon ulcer caused by *Candida albicans*. (Fig. 13-13 illustrates the primary culture from this case, and Fig. 13-15 the PAS-stained direct scraping.)

4. The number of ocular infections in the other parts of the eye as reported from Hungary and San Francisco were considerably fewer than those reported from New York, and *Candida* was the fungus most frequently found.

Other variations in the incidence of mycotic ocular disease have been sought by a survey of reported fungal corneal ulcers around the world. Table 13-9 presents data on the incidence of culturally identified keratomycosis involving 444 patients from 25 countries. The genera of fungi most frequently causing corneal ulcers proved to be *Aspergillus*, 33.3%; *Candida*, 16.4% *Fusarium*, 14.2%; *Cephalosporium*, 6.8%; and *Penicillium*, 6.7%. The remaining 105 patients (23.6% of the total) had infections

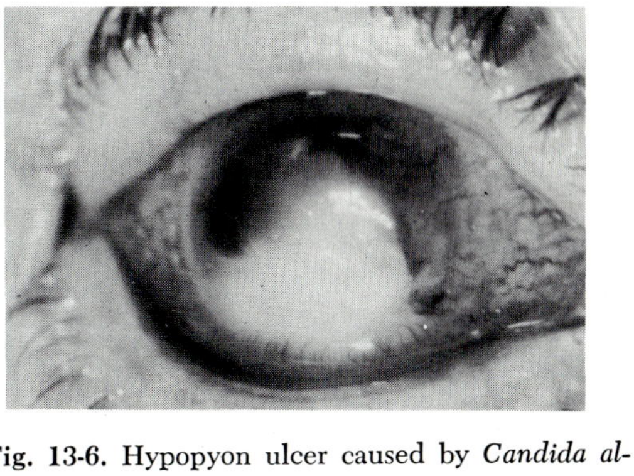

Fig. 13-6. Hypopyon ulcer caused by *Candida albicans*.

Table 13-9. Keratomycosis in various areas of the world, verified by cultures: 1879-1970

Geographic area	Number of fungi grown	Genera of fungi recovered (number)*						Total number
		Aspergillus	*Candida*	*Fusarium*	*Cephalosporium*	*Penicillium*	Others	
North America								
Canada	2							
United States	130	15	31	49	10	3	24	132
South America								
Argentina	2							
Brasil	4							
Peru	3	—	—	3	1	—	5	9
Europe								
Austria	3							
Bulgaria	8							
England	5							
Finland	1							
France	11							
Germany	21							
Greece	1							
Hungary	29							
Ireland	1							
Italy	15							
Poland	9							
Spain	9							
Switzerland	2							
USSR	26	76	17	1	3	8	36	141
Egypt	1	—	—	—	—	—	1	1
Ceylon	3							
India	91	37	7	7	4	12	27	94
China	5							
Japan	48							
Philippines	14	20	18	3	12	2	12	67
Total number of species		148 (33.3%)	73 (16.4%)	63 (14.2%)	30 (6.8%)	25 (5.7%)	105 (23.6%)	444 (100%)

Compiled from many published reports.
*Six more fungal cultures are recorded than there were patients. Nine patients had dual infections.

caused by one of the 37 other genera of fungi listed in Table 13-1. The United States, India, Japan, and Hungary had the largest series of cases. The reasons for the relatively large number of infections in these areas appeared to differ. In the United States the reports were made by 25 teams of investigators from 24 different cities spread over the country, including some in Hawaii. The largest series of cases were those from San Francisco and New York, described in Table 13-8, and a review of 39 cases reported from Miami in 1970 by Jones and his co-workers.[28] Otherwise there were 16 single cases reported, and the remaining 10 publications described 2 to 10 mycotic corneal ulcers. This variation in the apparent incidence of fungal infection in various parts of the United States may be because of concentration of interest and competence in the recognition of fungi in certain parts of the country.

Ninety-one proved cases of keratomycosis from India have been described, and it is apparent that the situation is different from that in the United States. Fungi cause a sizeable proportion of corneal ulcers in India. For example, Balakrishnan[7] of Madras states that in a 2-year period, October 1960 to November 1962, he saw 60 suspected mycotic ulcers among approximately 780 hypopyon ulcers, and in 30 of the 60 cases he identified the fungus by culture. Puttana[45] identified the fungus in 20 cases of keratomycosis seen in a 4-year period in Bangolore. Rao and Ramakrishnan,[46] from Manipal, in the period December 1965 to September 1966, saw 40 cases of corneal ulcers and 6 cases of conjunctivitis with lacrimal canaliculitis; all eyes were carefully investigated for fungi. In 13 of the ulcers (33%), fungi were isolated, and in another case a fungus was seen on the smear but not grown. Fungal infection was the cause of 4 of the 6 cases of canaliculitis. Only 8 teams of investigators made the reports on fungal infection in India. It seems, however, that fungal diseases of the eye are familiar to the physician, since diagnosis is made relatively soon and treatment is started early.[12a,13a,44a]

The 48 cases of keratomycosis from Japan were reports of single cases or small groups of not more than 5 patients. Thirty of the patients' histories were collected from the literature of 1910 to 1969 by Okuda, Matsuura, and Okabe.[39] Fazakas described 28 of the 29 cases from Hungary, which are reported in Table 13-8. They are a tribute to the energy and skill of one man.

Two other pieces of information entered in Table 13-9 are provocative. The small number of cases of mycotic infection of the cornea recorded in South America probably does not give an accurate estimate of the amount of infection caused by fungi in this area. De Almeida[4] from Brazil has given an account of 77 cases of infection following cataract extraction, of which 13 were caused by fungi. It is likely that where there are so many postoperative fungal infections there also must be keratomycosis. The single case of keratomycosis from Egypt was recognized by Lichaa in 1932.[33] He made the clinical diagnosis but sent the culture to the laboratory of Professor Brumpt in Paris where Dr. Langeron discovered that the fungus was a new species of the genus *Beauveria: Beauveria brumptii.* Other reports of keratomycosis from Egypt have not been found, although the climate and agricultural activities of the country seem to favor the disease.

The spotty distribution of the reported cases of keratomycosis in various parts of the world indicate that fungal infections of the eye probably are much more common than the published figures indicate. This point of view is supported by other data. For example, Ball,[8] Ophthalmic Surgeon of the St. Louis City Hospital, stated in 1926 that locality probably had much to do with the frequency of keratomycosis caused by *Aspergillus,* "Dr. C. F. Brieglеb of St. Clair, Mo., having met with fifty cases within twenty years." The only case of the disease that Ball had seen "came from the same vicinity." Ball's case is illustrated in Fig. 13-7. Since we were not able to locate Briegleb's report, these possible 50 examples of *Aspergillus* keratitis have been omitted from Table 13-9. Kinnas[29] of Greece reported in 1965 on a corneal ulcer caused by *Acremonium* species and stated that he had treated 33 clinically similar cases, which were not cultured.

There are, furthermore, some substantial data from which one may conclude that cultures of fungi can be negative even when subsequent histologic findings show that the disease was of fungal origin. Salceda and his associates[51] in the Philippines saw 17 patients, 12 of them manual workers, all with a history of corneal trauma, who presented a picture considered typical of fungal keratitis. In 13 cases a fungus was isolated and identified, but in 4 no fungus could be grown. In these latter cases, however, fungi were identified in keratectomy

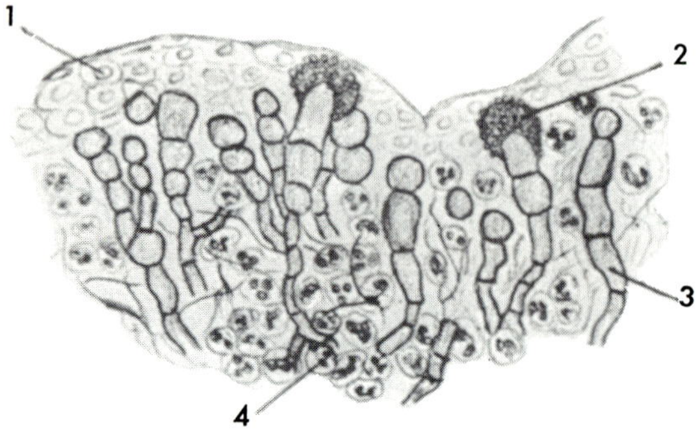

Fig. 13-7. Microscopic section of growth in keratitis caused by *Aspergillus*. *1*, Epithelium of the cornea; *2*, sporangia; *3*, mycelium; *4*, pus corpuscles. (Original drawing by Dr. Carl Fisch. From Ball, J. M.: Modern ophthalmology, vol. 1, Philadelphia, 1926, F. A. Davis Co., p. 479.)

Table 13-10. Incidence of keratomycosis in the material of the Armed Forces Institute of Pathology

Time interval	Kerato-mycosis cases	Number intact enucleated globes	Incidence
1933-1951	3	33,987	1:11,329
1952-1956	14	5,783	1:413
1957-1961	21	4,814	1:229
1962-1966	13	4,515	1:347

From Naumann, G., Green, W. R., and Zimmerman, L. E.: Mycotic keratitis: a histopathologic study of 73 cases, Amer. J. Ophthal. **64**:668, 1967.

sections. Presumably the reason for failing to grow the fungus was the difficulty of obtaining material from the active area of infection or prior death of the fungus.

There is other evidence that mycotic keratitis often is not diagnosed until histologic examination is made. Naumann and his co-workers[37] have published the results of a study of 73 cases of primary mycotic keratitis proved by means of histologic examination. Table 13-10 presents the data on 51 of these patients from whom surgically enucleated whole eyes were submitted directly to the Armed Forces Institute of Pathology. The table shows that histologic examination of 33,987 enucleated globes in the years 1933 to 1951 revealed only 3 cases of keratomycosis, or one in 11,329 cases. A combination of the figures for the remaining 15 years gives a total of 48 globes with keratomycosis among 15,112 eyes examined, or about 1 in 315 cases. This represents a 36-fold increase in incidence in recent years. The diagnosis of keratomycosis in the other 22 eyes was made from portions of eyes previously studied in other laboratories or from corneal buttons from cases treated by keratoplasty.

Naumann and his associates have supplied additional useful data from the series of 73 patients with mycotic keratitis. Ages ranged from 9 to 87 years, and one half of the patients were 51 years old or older. Men outnumbered women 51 to 16. Information was obtained in 51 instances as to the time of year in which the infection began. Particularly in the posttraumatic cases the majority occurred in the warmer months. Approximately two thirds of the specimens were contributed to the Armed Forces Institute of Ophthalmology from southern or southwestern states of the USA or from tropical countries of South America or Africa. The paper also lists the frequency of the various causes of trauma or eye diseases that preceded these cases of keratomycosis. Among the 33 cases with initial corneal trauma, 14 were caused by vegetable matter; in 6 the type of foreign body was unknown; while the remaining injuries were caused by a variety of other objects. Glaucoma with related complications preceded 10 of the infections, and 15 infections followed other miscellaneous corneal diseases. In 15 cases no preceding disease or trauma had been reported.

The histopathology of keratomycosis as described in this series of cases included ulceration of the epithelium and Bowman's membrane with migration of leukocytes into the corneal parenchyma around the organisms and into the anterior chamber. There was frequent formation of multiple abscesses separated from the main lesion. The fungi typically were found throughout the entire thickness of the cornea. Less fre-

Table 13-11. Incidence of *Pityrosporum orbiculare* in various ocular infections and in clinically healthy eyes

Clinical diagnosis	Total number of cases	Percent with seborrheic dermatitis	Percent with *Pityrosporum orbiculare* in eyelid margin scrapings
Seborrheic blepharitis	1,001	80.1	91.6
Seborrheic blepharoconjunctivitis	376	32.9	80.5
Blepharoconjunctivitis	1,201	40.4	80.1
Chronic blepharitis	1,626	25.5	74.3
Squamous blepharitis	326	0.1	27.8
Ulcerative blepharitis	216	0.6	25.4
Allergic conjunctivitis	258	—	34.8
Follicular conjunctivitis	220	—	27.2
Corneal ulcers	144	—	26.3
Chronic conjunctivitis	2,466	0.8	25.8
Keratitis	107	—	25.2
Patients awaiting ocular surgery	1,408	11.5	42.6
Normal controls	1,202	11.8	32.9

In the early days of this investigation the identification of the fungi was carried out in association with Dr. Rhoda W. Benham.

quently they were seen only in the middle or deeper layers. The corneal surface and the crater of the ulcer were usually free of fungi, although there was a profuse growth of hyphae on the surface in a few cases.

The incidence of mycotic infections in the other parts of the external eye—the eyelids, the lacrimal apparatus, and the conjunctiva—as seen at the Columbia-Presbyterian Medical Center, by Fazakas, and by Halde and Okumoto have been given in Tables 13-7 and 13-8. There are several additional reports of infection of the lacrimal canal, which add four more genera of fungi: *Rhinosporidium, Glenospora, Hyalopus,* and *Torulopsis.* According to François and his associates,[20] infection of the lacrimal sac by *Blastomyces, Sporotrichum, Cephalosporium,* and *Trichophyton* may occur as well. The series of cases of fungal conjunctivitis reported in Tables 13-7 and 13-8 are the most extensive ones that have been observed. This condition may precede or be concomitant with canaliculitis, blepharitis, meibomitis, or keratomycosis.

The series of cases of fungal infections in these parts of the eye, as reported in Table 13-7, showed equal distribution between sexes; only 6 of the patients were under 12 years of age. In 22 instances the infections were apparently acquired from neighboring areas, namely, the nose, nasopharynx, the sinuses, and adjacent skin.

Seborrheic blepharitis and blepharoconjunctivitis are associated in a high percentage of cases (Table 13-11) with the presence of a fungus, *Pityrosporum orbiculare,* which is found in 100% of cases of seborrheic dermatitis. This disease involves the eyebrows, hair, and external ears of most patients with seborrheic blepharitis and blepharoconjunctivitis (Fig. 13-8, *A*). Scrapings of the affected areas show yeast-like organisms ranging in size from 2 to 10 μ (Fig. 13-8, *B*). The organisms are most abundant when the eyelid scrapings are obtained from a site with marked inflammation. As may be seen from Table 13-11, normal eyes or eyes of people with other categories of disease had neither a high rate of seborrheic dermatitis nor as high an incidence of *Pityrosporum* on the eyelid margins. The numbers of organisms seen in the smears of scrapings was sharply decreased. Definite proof that the association of the *Pityrosporum* group of fungi with seborrheic conditions establishes an etiologic role has not been given. Gots, Thy-

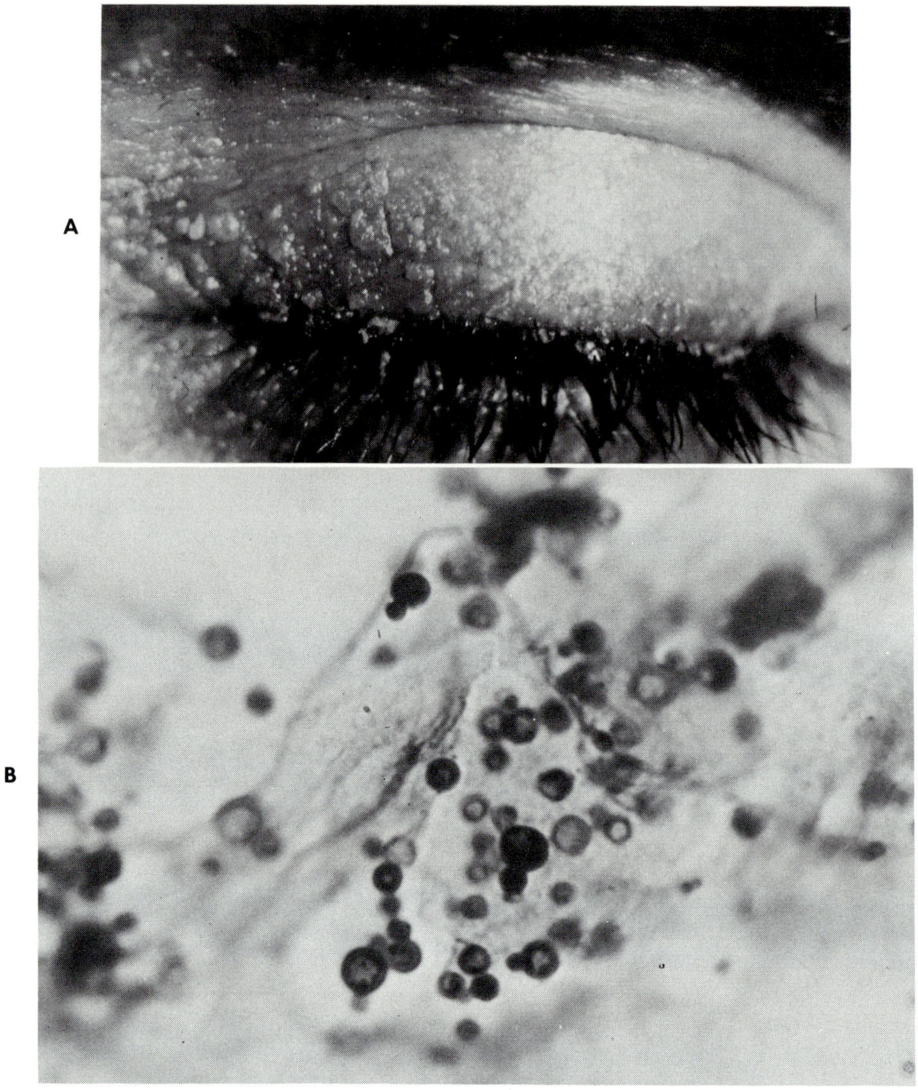

Fig. 13-8. A, Seborrheic blepharitis. (Courtesy U. S. Department of Health, Education, and Welfare.) **B,** Direct scraping from eyelid margins from patient shown in **A.** Note mostly spherical forms, some budding cells, singly or in pairs, of *Pityrosporum orbiculare.*

geson, and Waisman[21] in 1947 reported that their investigation did not result in conclusive evidence that *Pityrosporum* was pathogenic for the eye and its adnexa. However, the following results were suggestive of an etiologic relationship: (1) constant presence of yeastlike organisms in the lesions, (2) the apparent relationship between the number of the organisms found in the scrapings and the severity of the clinical disease, and (3) the absence of the organisms or their presence in only small numbers in clinically normal eyes. Thygeson and Vaughan[61] in 1955 found *Pityrosporum* in 98% of lesions in patients with seborrheic blepharitis, in 86% of lesions with mixed types of blepharitis, and in 46% of patients with staphylococcic blepharitis. In normal eyelids in patients in a hospital for the mentally ill, the organisms were present in 58% of the cases and in 20% of the cases in a series of private patients.

Table 13-12. Mycotic ocular infections following ocular surgery: summary of cases identified by cultures

Type of surgery	Day of onset first symptoms	Causative agent	Final outcome	Reported by
Cataract extraction				
OD	9 days	*Volutella cinerescens*	47th day, enucleation	Foster and associates, 1958
OS	31 days	*Volutella cinerescens*	Blind eye	
Cataract extraction		*Volutella cinerescens*	Enucleation	
Cataract extraction	15 days	*Cephalosporium* species	3½ months, enucleation	Fine and Zimmerman, 1959
Cataract extraction	2 months	*Hyalopus bogolepofii*	2½ months, enucleation	Paiva and associates, 1960
Cataract extraction	40 days	*Volutella* species	92 days, enucleation	Theodore and associates, 1961
Cataract extraction	15 days	*Cephalosporium* species	No useful vision	
Cataract extraction	14 days	*Neurospora sitophila*	Light perception	Theodore and associates, 1962
Cataract extraction	10 months	*Aspergillus fumigatus*	1 year, enucleation	Diamond and Kirk, 1962
Cataract extraction	24 days	*Sporothrix schenkii*	6 weeks, enucleation	Küper, 1962
Cataract extraction	2 weeks	*Cephalosporium* species	4 weeks, enucleation	
Cataract extraction	10 months	*Hormodendrum* species	10 months and 8 days, enucleation	François and associates, 1962
Cataract extraction	6 months	*Sporothrix schenkii*	Enucleation	
Cataract extraction	24 hours	*Cladosporium* species	Enucleation	de Azevedo, 1962
Cataract extraction	2 months	Mycelia sterila	Enucleation	
Cataract extraction	7 days	*Aspergillus niger*	5 months, enculeation	Queiroga, 1961 Cited by de Rezende, 1962
Cataract extraction	24 hours	*Cladosporium* species	8 days, enucleation	Lobo, 1961 Cited by de Rezende, 1962
Cataract extraction	5 months	*Candida lipolytica*	Enucleation	Graf, 1964
Lamellar keratoplasty (for a stromal herpes infection)	5 weeks	*Cephalosporium* species	Enucleation 5 weeks after 2nd graft	Hoffman and Naumann, 1963
Cataract extraction	2½ months	*Scopulariopsis brevicaulis*		Strampelli and Maggi, 1963
Cataract extraction	28 days	*Cephalosporium* species	Visual result poor	Green and associates, 1965
Cataract extraction		*Cephalosporium* species		Halde and Okumoto, 1966
Postoperative vitreous abscess		*Candida* species		
Keratoplasty (2 cases)		*Candida* species		
Lamellar graft for corneal dystrophy	7 days	*Aspergillus nidulans*	3 weeks, lamellar graft removed; second graft successful	White, 1969
Lamellar graft		*Pullularia pullulans*	Both cleared up with antifungal treatment	
Lamellar graft		*Trichophyton rubrum*		
Cataract extraction	35 days	*Cephalosporium* species	7 weeks, enucleation	Albesi, 1969
Cataract extraction	1 month	*Cephalosporium* species	Enucleation	

On the contrary, Parunovic and Halde[43] in 1967 reported that microscopic examination of eyelid margins demonstrated that *Pityrosporum orbiculare* was present in as many subjects with normal eyelid margins as in those with seborrheic lid margins.

Treatment that removes the *Pityrosporum* from the lid margins in cases of blepharitis and blepharoconjunctivitis results in considerable improvement in the condition of the eye. If this fungus is not acting as an etiologic agent in the disease, it is at least a very irritating factor in the eye.

Internal eye

The largest number of fungal infections that penetrate to the internal structures of the eye must undoubtedly arise from keratomycosis. In the absence of early diagnosis and treatment, hypopyon is almost inevitable, and endophthalmitis is the result in the majority of cases. This aspect of keratomycosis is considered later.

Among the remaining internal mycotic infections, those of greatest concern to the ophthalmologist follow ocular surgery. Surgical skill, careful observation of asepsis, and presurgical preparation of the eye are such that relatively few postsurgical infections occur, and of these only a small portion are caused by fungi. In their book on ocular mycosis, François and his associates[20] have included 64 examples of postoperative infection, seen from 1914 to 1965, which were proved by culture and/or histologic examination. From the literature 9 more cases, also proved by culture, have been added. Table 13-12 gives data on 29 cases in which the fungi were identified by culture. An outstanding characteristic of postoperative infection is the irregular and usually long latent period between surgery and the onset of symptoms of the infection. In the cases presented in Table 13-12 the latent period varied from 7 days to 10 months. The indolent way in which postoperative infections begin is an important diagnostic aid. The data given in column four of Table 13-12 established the fact that significant sight was the end result in only 3 cases of lamellar graft surgery. Eighteen eyes were enucleated.

The fungi involved in these postsurgical infections differed from those found in keratomycosis in the following respects: 5 cases involved *Volutella, Hyalopus, Neurospora* (Fig. 13-9), *Cladosporium,* and *Pullularia,* genera of fungi that had not been recovered from cases of keratomycosis; *Cladosporium* had been reported in the normal eye. The incidence of *Cephalosporium* was higher in postoperative infections than in keratomycosis, whereas that of *Aspergillus* and *Candida* was lower. Both *Fusarium* and *Penicillium* were absent. In such a small number of widely distributed infections these differences may not be significant, but they alert the mycologist to include a wider range of fungi among possible pathogens or opportunists.

A very few intraocular mycotic infections have followed penetration of the eye by trauma. François and his associates[20]

A

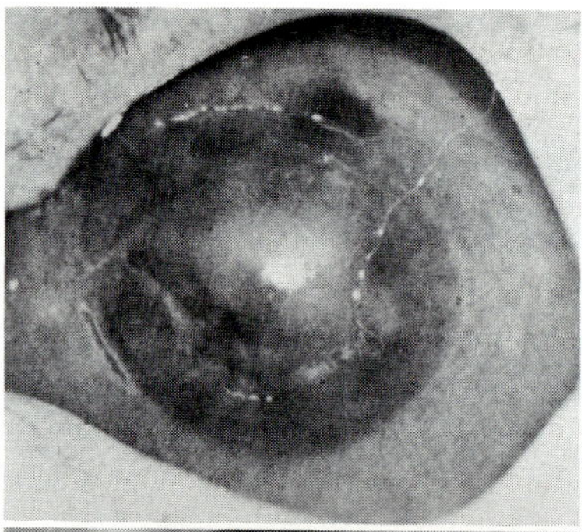

B

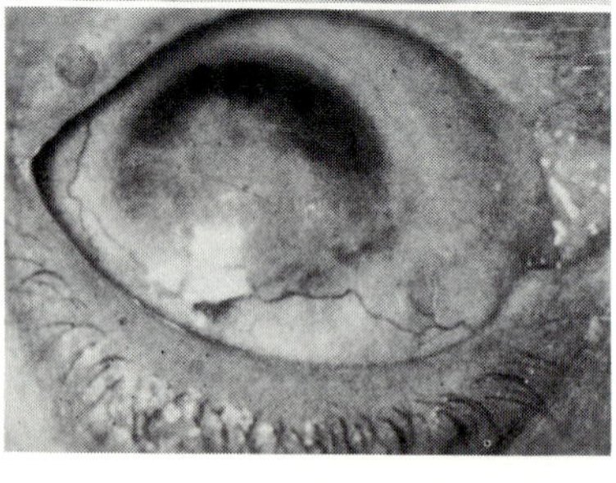

Fig. 13-9. A, Endophthalmitis, following cataract extraction, caused by *Neurospora sitophila;* 48 days after operation. **B,** Photograph of eye seen in **A,** 6 months after operation. (From Theodore, F. H., Littman, M. L., and Almeda, E.: Amer. J. Ophthal. **53**:35, 1962.)

have collected 21 examples from the years 1898 to 1968. Only 2 of these, both caused by *Aspergillus fumigatus,* were diagnosed by culture, the remainder being examined histologically. In the 3 instances in which the data were given, there was a long latent period between the trauma and the signs of infection: 11 days, 2 weeks, and 1 month.

A larger group of intraocular infections arise from a variety of endogenous sources: direct extension from the brain or opposite eye, debilitating infections, or other disease leading to generalized mycosis or focal mycosis elsewhere in the body. François has also tabulated 98 cases from the literature covering the period 1910 to 1968. Diagnosis was made by culture in 44 cases and by histologic examination in the remainder. The fungi involved were predominantly *Aspergillus, Candida,* and *Crytococcus,* the last as a sequela of cerebral or pulmonary infection. *Coccidioides immitis* was recorded 10 times; and in the 6 infections where the original site of infection was recorded, it was either generalized or in the lungs. François gives one reference to a case of retinal spots caused by *Histoplasma capsulatum* and states that more than 100 others have been described. However, the cultural identification of *Histoplasma* in the eye is recorded only by Hoefnagels and Pijpers.[26a] The mycotic infections included in this group of intraocular infections are usually seen first by the internist.

CLINICAL ASPECTS OF MYCOTIC INFECTIONS OF THE EYE

Because the distribution of fungi is so widespread and preventing contamination by them is nearly impossible, it is remarkable that serious infection of the eye or its appendages is relatively rare. Fortunately, the fungi, whose role in nature is apparently to break down dead and devitalized tissue of all kinds, have relatively little virulence when placed on normal, healthy human tissue. Numerous studies have been made concerning the incidence of fungi in normal conjunctival sacs. Variations from 2% to 80% have been noted, the higher figure being obtained from agricultural workers in the field at harvest time. Under normal circumstances the fungi do not invade, but injury with resulting devitalization of tissue can be followed rather rapidly by invasion of ocular structures. Fungal infections are much less common in an urban population with similar injuries, presumably because the size of the inoculum is so much smaller.

Mycotic infections of the conjunctiva are uncommon but may be of either superficial or granulomatous appearance. A thrushlike conjunctivitis may be caused by *Candida albicans* and by the ringworm group, such as *Microsporum* and *Trichophyton.* The role of *Pityrosporum orbiculare* in seborrheic conjunctivitis is somewhat questionable. Probably the commonest external mycotic problem seen by the opthalmologist is *Actinomyces israelii* infection of the lacrimal drainage system. This organism is classified at the present time among the higher bacteria rather than among the fungi. As such, it is more amenable to chemotherapeutic attack. The firm yellowish granules that plug the lacrimal canaliculus and sac require surgical removal. This is ordinarily done by slitting the lower punctum and removing material with a chalazion curette.

Atypical papillomatous lesions in the conjunctiva should always arouse suspicion of mycotic invasion as well as neoplasia, syphilis, tuberculosis, and leprosy. *Aspergillus, Blastomyces, Coccidioides,* and *Rhinosporidium* have been implicated in such lesions. All are rare in the northern part of North America but become increasingly common the further south one goes.

The two most common types of mycotic infection seen by the clinical ophthalmologist are those involving the cornea and those seen after intraocular surgery. Both have characteristics that tend to differentiate them from bacterial and viral infections. Keratomycosis is rarely if ever found in a healthy individual who has suffered no injury to the cornea.

The typical history of keratomycosis may be one of several types. Probably the most common is one of prolonged corneal infection, usually herpes simplex, which has been treated for months with steroids, antibiotics, and every medication available without effecting a cure. There may be a rather precipitous turn for the worse with a localized gray infiltration of the anterior stroma, totally refractory to all ordinary therapy, and slowly but relentlessly extending in depth and width. Characteristically, the inflammatory reaction of the entire globe is much less than one would anticipate with a similar bacterial infection. There may be small satellite lesions extending out from the main area of invasion. These are almost diagnostic of mycotic superinfection. If the individual has a serious systemic and debilitating disease, such as generalized carcinomatosis, diabetes, tuberculosis, or chronic alcoholism, one's suspicions should be increased.

Diagnosis is not always simple. At the first suspicion of mycotic invasion, one should immediately attempt to obtain material for histologic inspection. Superficial scraping or use of applicators will not be sufficient. We prefer to use the operating microscope and to remove first superficial necrotic tissue. This is then followed by deep and aggressive removal of tissue at the base and under the overhanging margins of the ulcer. The material is examined immediately in a saline or 10% sodium hydroxide drop so that it is frequently possible to establish the diagnosis at once. The presence of a negative result in a clinically suspicious case requires repeated and more vigorous tissue removal. On occasion this may mean the use of a trephine with lamellar keratectomy in order to obtain an adequate specimen. The material is then utilized not only for culture but for histologic section. It has been our experience that this technique is not only valuable in diagnosis but is also an effective adjuvant to therapy. Although all of the currently available antibiotics and chemotherapeutics known to have some effect upon the various fungi are of relatively little help in curing advanced disease, they may be effective when the major mass of diseased tissue is removed so that the drug can reach the deep tissues. It is our feeling, however, that antibiotics are relatively futile when used alone in advanced keratomycosis. Total excision is rarely possible, but we have repeatedly seen recovery following subtotal resection of the involved cornea. We have even salvaged the one remaining eye in a patient with a large, perforated, *Cephalosporium*-caused ulcer with extruded lens, hypopyon, and severe diabetes. The entire cornea was removed with a 10 mm trephine and replaced with a full-thickness graft. Even though it was possible to culture organisms from the vitreous face, the graft was retained and the globe salvaged without further evidence of intraocular invasion. If a major part of the involved tissue is removed, there is a reasonable chance that infection can be controlled.

Recently a technique has been devised by which specific antibody to a fungus has been conjugated with fluorescein and instilled into the eyes of animals that have been infected with *Candida albicans*. The stained antigen-antibody complex is then treated with the argon laser, destroying the fungal element. So far, this has been accomplished only in animals, but the principle offers some promise. It seems highly doubtful to us that any of the systemic antibiotics effective against fungi have much practical use, since these antibiotics are highly toxic. None has been effective enough in our experience to justify the hazard. In addition to the commonly used antibiotics (such as amphotericin B, nystatin, and pimaricin), grenz rays, ultraviolet light, cryocautery, and thermocautery have been used without dramatic improvement. The use of the thermophore unfortunately requires a temperature that destroys not only the fungus but also the corneal stroma.

Acute endophthalmitis following cataract surgery is rare, the incidence being somewhere in the order of one per thousand. Viral infections other than the presumed release of virus in needling and aspiration of rubella cataract must be extremely uncommon. The possibility exists, however, that they may be the cause of certain apparently sterile inflammatory reactions after cataract operation. Bacterial intraocular infections are characterized by acute inflammatory onset within 24 to 48 hours after surgery. If, after uneventful surgery, the eye is apparently well on the road to healing and at about the fourth or fifth week begins to develop a progressively severe low-grade inflammatory reaction, one's suspicion should turn to fungus invasion. Diagnosis here is perhaps even more difficult than in corneal infections. As soon as infection is suspected, an anterior chamber tap should be performed and suitable culture media inoculated. Direct examination of the fluid may be positive. There is no really satisfactory therapy available for mycotic endophthalmitis. If the virulence of the organism is low or the inoculum small, it is possible that with the usual supporting methods of therapy common to any ocular inflammation, the body may be able to withstand the invasion and overcome it. In general, however, the prognosis is extremely poor.

Endogenous endophthalmitis of mycotic origin is being reported with increasing frequency. Blastomycosis, actinomycosis, aspergillosis, mucormycosis, and cryptococcosis, among others, have all been described. Although cures have been reported, not only is the eye usually lost but not infrequently the disease is lethal.

Orbital cellulitis, not obviously explained by direct injury or sinusitis of bacterial origin, should alert the clinician to the possibility of fungal invasion of the orbit. The most commonly reported offender has been *Mucor*. In by far the majority of cases, approaching 90%, the patients have been either severely diabetic or overwhelmed by wasting disease. Invasion of the orbit can

A

B

C

D

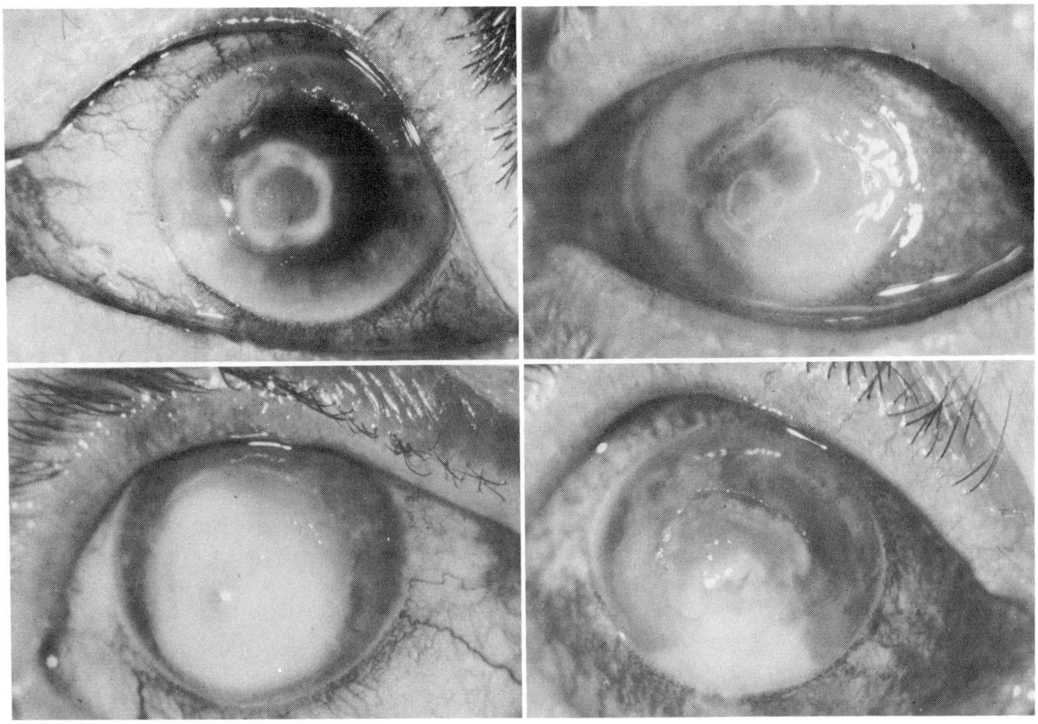

Fig. 13-10. A, Keratitis caused by *Candida tropicalis;* **B,** keratitis caused by *Alternaria;* **C,** keratitis caused by *Fusarium;* **D,** keratitis caused by *Monosporium apiospermum.*

be either by the bloodstream or more commonly by direct extension from the nose through the sinuses and then the orbit. Such orbital disease usually implies a widespread involvement, and many of these situations end fatally. Systemic antibiotics are essential in their management of the disease.

The clinical ophthalmologist should be aware that any structure of the eye can be invaded by fungi, that such infections are apt to be obscure and puzzling, and that not infrequently the diagnosis may be missed for a considerable period. Therefore, one should be on the alert to suspect such invaders in unusual clinical problems and particularly in individuals who have a systemic disorder that has resulted in severe debilitation. One must be prepared for the fact that treatment is frequently unsatisfactory.

Fig. 13-10, *A-D* illustrates keratitis produced by four genera of fungi: *Candida tropicalis*, *Alternaria* species, *Fusarium* species, and *Monosporium apiospermum*. Fig. 13-21 illustrates a fresh preparation from a culture of the *Alternaria* keratitis, and Fig. 13-19 shows a similar culture of *Monosporium apiospermum* from the patient shown in Fig. 13-10, *D*.

TREATMENT OF MYCOTIC KERATITIS

Various chemical or physical agents have been reported effective in the management of both clinical and experimental mycotic keratitis. They include nystatin, amphotericin B, pimaricin, potassium iodide, heat, cryotherapy, laser beam, and surgical curettage. These agents were used alone or in combination with one of the others listed.[11a]

THE LABORATORY DIAGNOSIS OF MYCOTIC KERATITIS

Collection of specimens

The fungus producing ophthalmic keratitis is confined to the base of the ulcer where it is firmly embedded in a layer rarely exceeding 0.5 mm. For this reason a cutting instrument such as an ophthalmic curette should be employed, rather than a cotton swab, in collecting a sample. The sample does not have to be larger than the head of a pin, but it should be collected aseptically and kept moist or rehydrated with sterile water at the time of examination and culture.

To avoid introducing contaminants, one should collect the sample in a draft-free room and take strict aseptic precautions, which should be maintained from the time of collection throughout the entire process of transport to and subsequent handling in the mycology laboratory.

For this purpose, sterile glass Petri dishes of standard size (10 cm in diameter and 1 cm deep) are employed at the Columbia-Presbyterian Medical Center. The dishes are wrapped individually in paper before sterilization and kept in this sterile envelope to protect the dish from air currents and the ever present aerosol of spores of contaminating bacteria and fungi. Care is taken in opening and closing the dish, which is always handled within the confines of its own loosened sterile paper wrapper.

These extra aseptic precautions are necessary because of the slow growth of pathogenic fungi. Since cultures will have to be incubated at times for several weeks, any accidental airborne contaminant will have an opportunity to develop and outgrow the pathogen.

The wet sample is deposited directly from the curette into the center of the bottom dish either by rubbing the instrument against the glass bottom of the dish or by detaching the sample with the aid of a sterile needle or another sterile curette. The lid of the dish is replaced gently, the paper wrapper pressed firmly but slowly against the surface of the closed dish, and the sample is taken to the laboratory without delay to avoid drying.

Direct microscopic examination

Immediately upon arrival at the laboratory the sample is rehydrated with a drop

Table 13-13. Guide to the recognition in tissue and isolation in cultures of fungi most frequently implicated as causes of mycotic keratitis

Genus or species	Parasitic morphology	Conditions for isolation: Culture media	Conditions for isolation: Temperature
Aspergillus fumigatus	Septate branching hyphae, 2-6 μ wide, often in clusters; occasional conidial heads (Fig. 13-1)	Sabouraud's glucose agar	45° and 37° C
Candida albicans	Oval-to-elongate budding cells, 2-3 × 3-7μ, plus hyphae and pseudohyphae	Sabouraud's glucose agar, Mycosel agar*	Room temperature and 37° C
Fusarium *Cephalosporium* *Penicillium* *Monosporium* *Verticillium* *Alternaria*	Sparse septate branching hyphae, 2-4 μ, with occasional intercalary chlamydospores	Sabouraud's glucose agar	Room temperature or 23-25° C

*Sabouraud's glucose agar plus chloromycetin and cycloheximide.

of sterile distilled water. A small portion of the sample—no larger than one-fourth its total volume—is separated by means of the cutting edge of a specially flattened, stiff nichrome wire (mycologic needle) and transferred to a sterile slide. A sterile coverslip is then gently lowered over this portion of the specimen; and after the preparation is flattened with firm but gentle pressure, the slide is examined *without further additives* directly under a compound light microscope. Scanning with the low power permits locating filamentous or unicellular structures of presumably fungal nature. These can appear as hyphae or conidia or as clusters of budding cells, depending on the genus or species. Higher magnification will permit confirming the suspicion and at the same time enable preliminary identification of the fungus. Table 13-13 describes the morphology of the fungal genera and species most frequently implicated as agents of mycotic keratitis.

The successful demonstration of the invading fungus in a wet sterile preparation of a portion of the specimen will accomplish two objectives: it confirms the tentative clinical diagnosis that the lesion was indeed a mycotic infection, and it permits a preliminary identification of the particular fungus causing the problem. This information will be useful to the physician in choosing the most specific therapy available and to the mycologist in choosing the best media, temperature, and atmosphere for the cultural isolation of the disease-causing fungus.

Should microscopic examination of the first slide be negative, one or two additional fractions of the sample should be similarly mounted and examined. In the event that only one of the small fragments examined has been positive, the coverslip can be lifted and the specimen returned to the Petri dish for further subdivision before culturing. The reason for using a sterile slide and coverslip now becomes apparent, for they permit culturing the area of the specimen, which contains fungal elements.

Special stains

To help reveal the fungus in those cases where microscopic examination of wet preparations has been negative, and also to keep a permanent record of positive cases, certain microbiologic and histologic stains are useful. These are enumerated below.

GRAM STAIN. For smears or exudates, the Kopeloff and Beerman modification of the Gram stain should be employed. This is a buffered stain, recommended by the Stain Committee of the American Society of Microbiology, to reveal gram-positive microorganisms in exudates. For actinomycetes in histologic sections, the Brown and Brenn modification of the Gram stain is essential. The more widely employed Gram-Weigert stain is unsuitable. Although all fungi are gram positive, this stain should be employed only for yeast cells and actinomycetes. Filamentous fungi do not stain well with Gram stain, and other stains should be employed (see below).

PERIODIC ACID, SCHIFF REAGENT STAIN. The PAS stain and its many modifications (Gridley's, for example) are useful in helping reveal those fungi that do not stain well with H & E in histologic sections. The Gridley modification is useful for staining smears as well.

GOMORI SILVER METHENAMINE STAIN. Although a prolonged procedure, the Groccot modification of the silver methenamine stain has great sensitivity as a detector of fungi and actinomycetes in histologic sections and is the preferred procedure in screening for their presence on any suspected lesion.

FITE-FARACO STAIN. As a stain to demonstrate acid-fast organisms the Fite stain, as modified by Faraco, is unexcelled in sensitivity. Hansen's bacillus and other mycobacteria are often revealed by this stain where Ziehl-Neelsen's has failed. The Coates modification has been particularly devised for *Nocardia asteroides*.

Primary cultures

Besides the culture media listed in Table 13-13, others useful in culturing systemic fungal pathogens from the eye include Littman's oxgall agar and brain-heart infusion agar to which may be added 10% whole blood and chloromycetin or gentamicin.

As already discussed, small pieces of the sample can be deposited individually on various spots on the surface of the agar media, avoiding the edges. Streaking is seldom necessary.

Purification of cultures

As soon as a fungal colony has reached a diameter of 2 to 5 mm, it should be subcultured to fresh media to avoid overgrowth by contaminants that may be present in the primary culture. The pathogen can usually be recognized by its slower growth and by the fact that several similar colonies will appear simultaneously at various inoculated sites. If subcultures are carried out early enough, one can usually obtain a pure culture for further study. At this time, a teased mount can be made for preliminary identification of the fungus.

Identification of cultures

The criteria employed in identifying genera and species of fungi include (1) gross colony morphology; (2) microscopic morphology, with particular emphasis on the type of sporulation; (3) biochemical reactions; (4) serologic reactions; and (5) animal pathogenicity. In order for one to be able to observe all these, special media and methods are required, which are described below.

Cultural characteristics of fungi most frequently invading the eye

GENUS ASPERGILLUS. This genus has been found to be the cause of 33% of fungal eye lesions, as seen in a survey of the world literature (summarized in Table 13-9). The generic name *Aspergillus* is descriptive of its conidiophores (Fig. 13-11), whose vesicle resembles an aspergillum, a perforated globe used to sprinkle holy water in church. The most frequent pathogen in this genus is the species *fumigatus* (Figs. 13-11 and 13-12). The specific name *fumigatus* describes the smoky color of the colony, which is a grayish yellow-green when its conidia have reached maturity. This generally occurs in less than 48 hours if cultures are incubated at 45° C, the op-

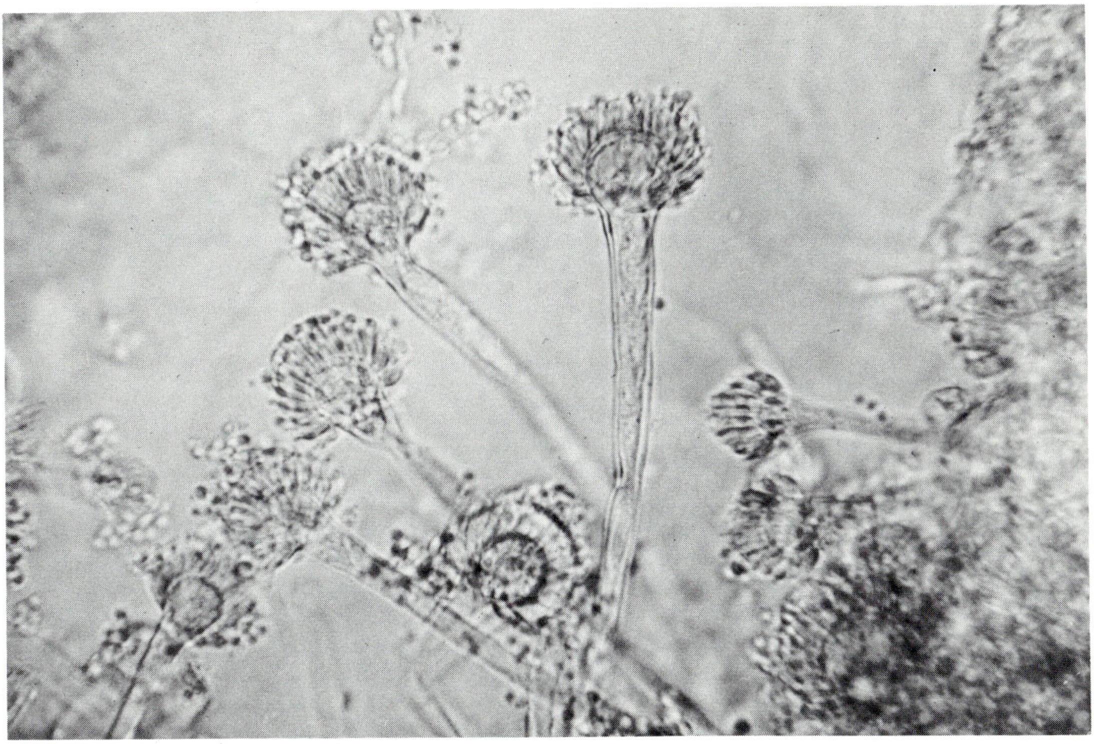

Fig. 13-11. *Aspergillus fumigatus* (sputum isolate) showing conidiophores with typical clavate vesicles and uniserate sterigmata (phialids) after 48 hours' growth on Sabouraud's glucose agar at 45° C. (approx. ×600.)

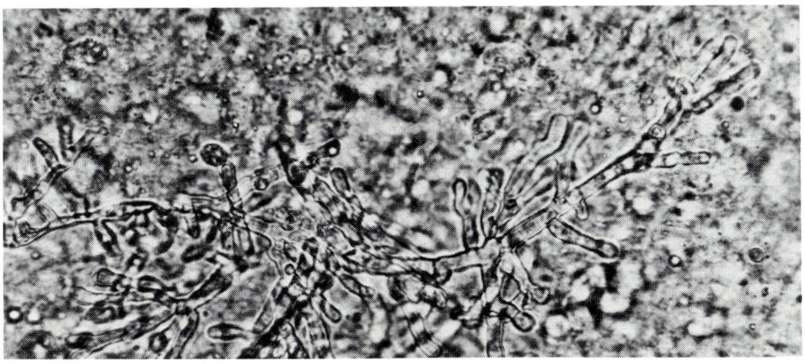

Fig. 13-12. Typical cluster of branching septate hyphae of *Aspergillus fumigatus* in a fresh preparation of sputum mounted in distilled water. (×430.)

timal temperature for growth of this thermophilic species. On Sabouraud's glucose agar, the entire surface of the slant will be covered by the fungus in a day or two. The border of a growing colony and its undersurface remain white because of the absence or immaturity of the conidia.

The species is identified by the following criteria.

The morphologic characteristics of infected tissues consist of compact aggregates of septate hyphae of uniform thickness (4 to 6 μ in diameter), exhibiting a characteristic coralloid pattern with dichotomous branching and rounded, sometimes swollen, hyphal tips (Fig. 13-12).

Microscopic examination reveals clavate vesicles with single layers of phialids on

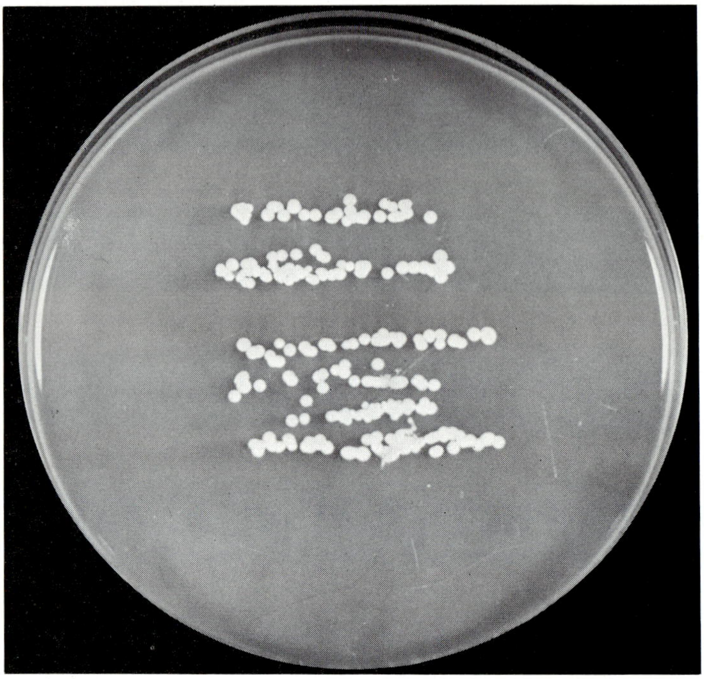

Fig. 13-13. *Candida albicans* colonies in primary culture of corneal scraping on Sabouraud's glucose agar. (×½.)

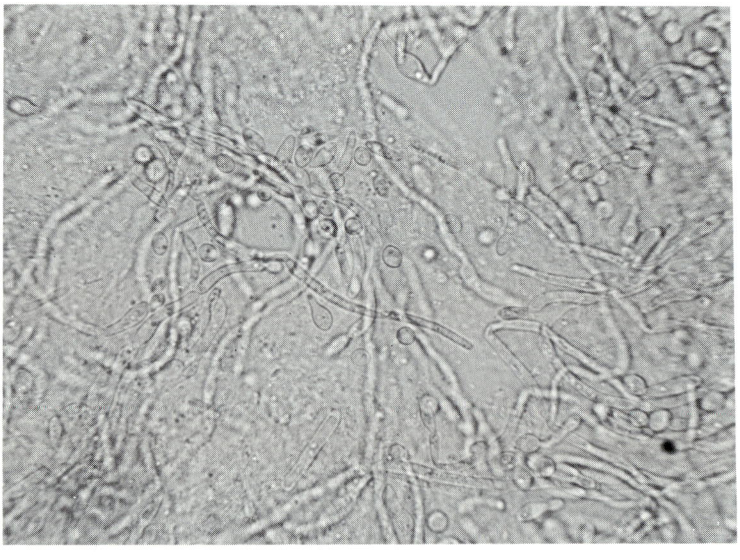

Fig. 13-14. *Candida albicans* from corneal ulcer. Budding cells, hyphae, and pseudohyphae in unstained wet preparation of direct scraping. (×400.)

their upper hemispheres from which conidia are abstricted repeatedly, forming parallel chains that adhere to each other and give the sporulating head a characteristic columnar appearance.

Aspergillus has the ability to grow at a temperature as high as 50 to 55° C; the optimal temperature is 45° C.

Besides *A. fumigatus,* the species *flavus, glaucus,* and *niger* have been reported from corneal ulcers. For a key to their specific identification, the reader is referred to Raper and Fennell's monograph *The Genus Aspergillus.*[47]

These additional specific names are descriptive of the species' conidial pigments (flavus, yellow; glaucus, white, and niger, black). All three have spherical, rather than clavate, vesicles at the sporulating end of their conidiophores; and one or two layers of phialids (uniseriate or biseriate) may extend all over the surface of the vesicle from which conidial chains radiate to give the sporulating head a spherical, rather than columnar, shape.

Genus Candida. The genus *Candida* includes a group of fermentative yeasts, which, besides reproducing vegetatively by budding, are also capable of producing pseudohyphae and true hyphae but no ascospores. The most frequent pathogen in this genus is the species *albicans,* whose description follows.

Colonies are pasty to creamy, buff colored, hemispherical in outline, and rarely exceed 2 to 3 mm in diameter during the first week of growth (Fig. 13-13). Microscopically, surface growth on Sabouraud's agar consists of oval budding cells (blastospores) of medium size (2 × 3 μ). Subsurface growth on cornmeal and Wolin-Bevis agar shows pseudohyphae and true hyphae along whose length spherical clusters of blastospores are strung at regular intervals (Fig. 13-14). Toward the ends or tips of these filaments chlamydospores are produced. These are diagnostic for the species and are spherical in shape, 8 to 10 μ in diameter, with heavy, double-contoured walls and large droplets of lipid and glycogen in their cytoplasm (Fig. 13-15).

C. albicans can also be identified by the ability of its blastospores (budding cells) to round up and germinate or extrude filamentous outgrowths when suspended in human or other mammalian blood serum and incubated at 37° C for 1 to 4 hours. Other characteristics used in its identification are: (1) resistance to cycloheximide; (2) ability to grow on various media at 37° C as well as at room temperature; (3) ability to ferment, with gas production, the sugars glucose, maltose, and sucrose, but not lactose; (4) inability to split urea or to utilize KNO_3; and (5) pathogenicity for the mouse and rabbit, causing death with miliary renal abscesses in less than 1 week.

Fig. 13-16 illustrates a smear from a culture of *C. parapsilosis.*

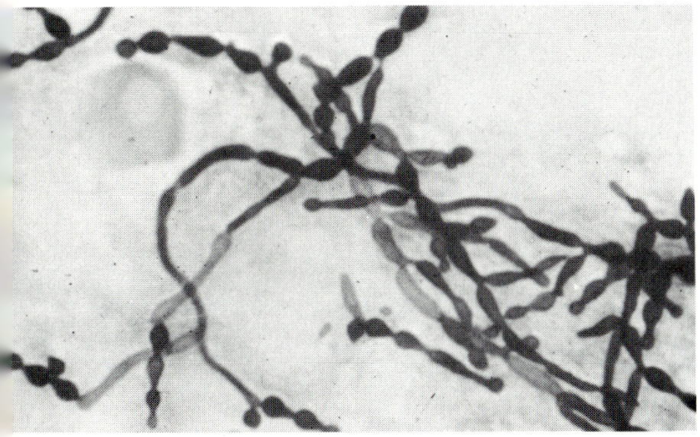

Fig. 13-15. *Candida albicans* from direct corneal scraping. Budding cells and young pseudohyphae. PAS stain. (×400.)

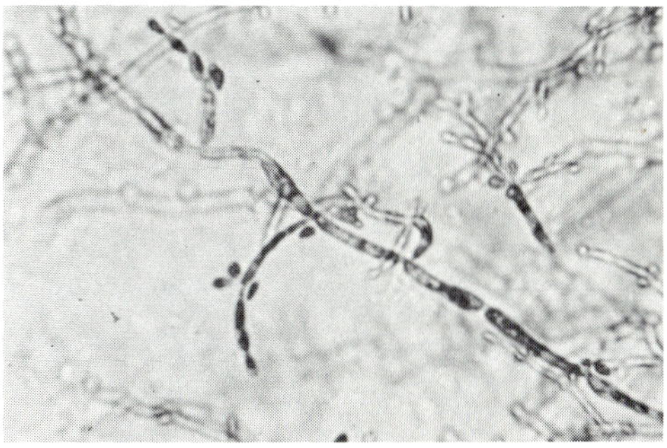

Fig. 13-16. *Candida parapsilosis.* Giant pseudohyphae in culture on cornmeal agar. From a patient with meibomitis. (×400.)

GENUS FUSARIUM. This genus produces colonies that are cottony in texture, and lavender, pink, or yellow. Their conidia are produced in clusters from phialids in palisade arrangement along the aerial (fertile) hyphae and are of two types: unicellular and multicellular. The unicellular ones, called microconidia, are oval to crescent-shaped; the multicellular ones, called macroconidia, are longer, curved into long crescents, and septate. Since all the septa are at right angles to the long axis of the spores, these macroconidia are said to resemble canoes. Clusters of conidia are often compared to bunches of bananas; they are frequently held together in a gelatinous substance by the conidiophores.

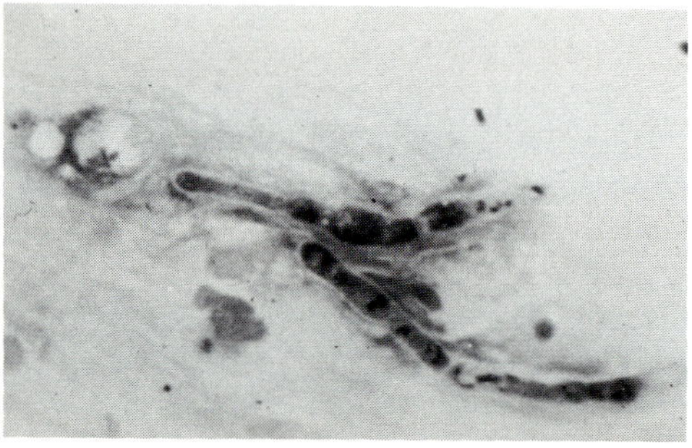

Fig. 13-17. *Cephalosporium* species. Hyphae in direct scraping from corneal ulcer, showing septa and intercalary chlamydospore. Giemsa stain. (×400.)

Fusarium is a very large genus containing numerous species, most of which are parasitic on fruit trees and other crops. Because of its importance to agriculture, the genus has been extensively studied and monographed. A good reference is Snyder and Hansen's article, published in 1940.[54]

Perhaps because of its wide distribution in nature, *Fusarium* is a frequent air contaminant. This fact plus its association with erosive vegetable particles may account for its frequent incidence in eye lesions.

GENUS CEPHALOSPORIUM. The name of this genus describes its conidiophores, borne singly as erect tapering stalks on whose apex conidia are clustered as heads. When grown slightly below room temperature and in short periods of daylight, *Cephalosporium* (Figs. 31-17 and 13-18) can also produce conidia in enclosed cushionlike structures called sporodochia. Taxonomically, this event requires transferring the species to the genus *Volutella* in the family Tuberculariaceae (other filamentous fungi mentioned thus far are in the family Moniliaceae [Saccardo's classification]). This taxonomic information is given here because several cases of *Cephalospor-*

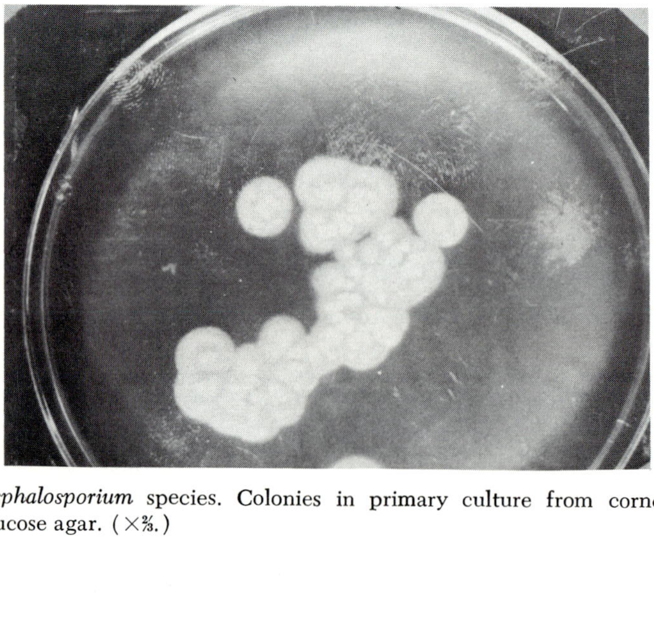

Fig. 13-18. *Cephalosporium* species. Colonies in primary culture from corneal scraping on Sabouraud's glucose agar. (×⅔.)

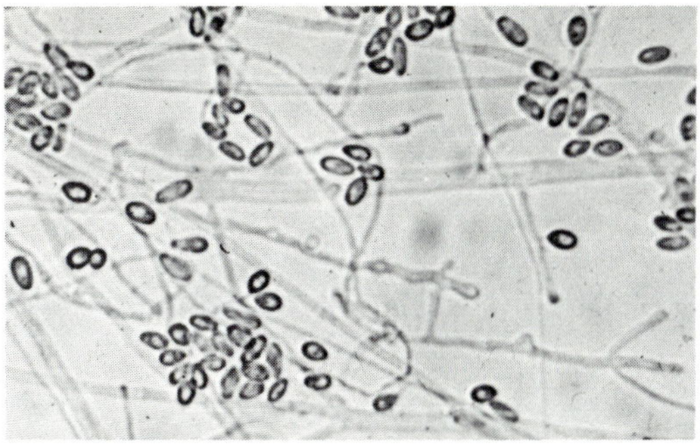

Fig. 13-19. *Monosporium apiospermum.* Conidia in culture, lactophenol mount. From a corneal ulcer. (×400.)

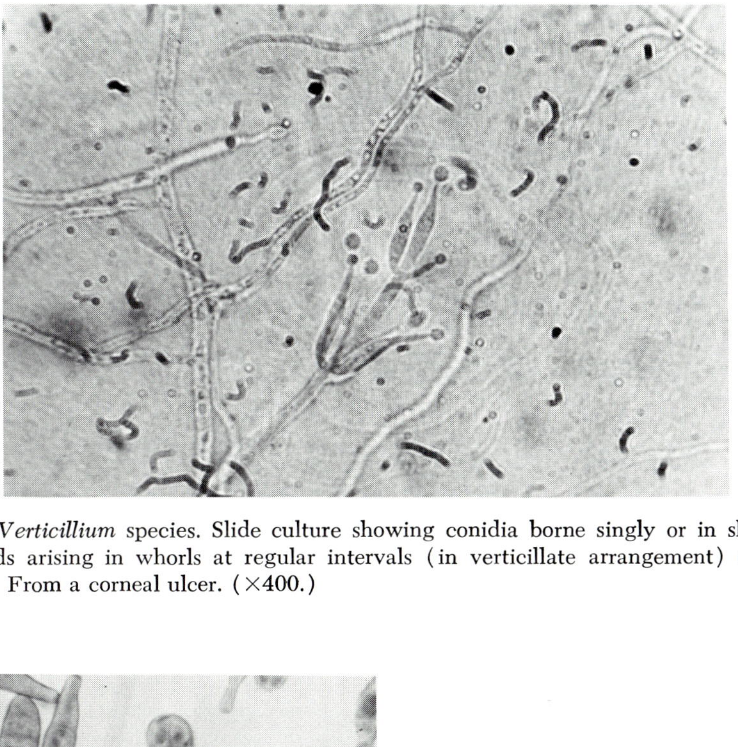

Fig. 13-20. *Verticillium* species. Slide culture showing conidia borne singly or in short chains from phialids arising in whorls at regular intervals (in verticillate arrangement) on the conidiophores. From a corneal ulcer. (×400.)

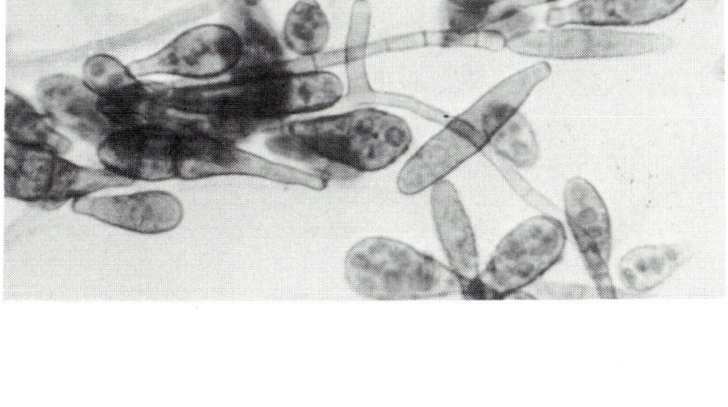

Fig. 13-21. *Alternaria* species. Typical dematiaceous (brownish) multiseptate conidia with septa in two planes (dyctiospores). From a corneal ulcer. (×1,000.)

ium and *Volutella* corneal ulcers have been described, and it is important to know that we are dealing with the same isolates grown under different environmental conditions. *Cephalosporium* (or *Volutella*) organisms have also been isolated from the cortisone eye drops used by patients.

Colonies of these two genera are velvety to fluffy, but may be membranous in species producing sparse aerial mycelium with moist conidiophores.

GENUS PENICILLIUM. This genus is closely related botanically to *Aspergillus*, but differs from it in morphologic characteristics. Its colonies are more finely powdery than those of *Aspergillus*, with shades of dark blue-green or blue-gray predominating. Colony color here, too, is the color of the mature conidia, which are also produced from phialids. These, however, are not on a vesicle but in branched conidiophores whose terminal cells (metulae) are not inflated. The conidial head therefore resembles a fine painter's brush (penicillus) rather than a dust mop or aspergillum (Plate 3, *D*). Species on this genus, of which *P. notatum* (producer of penicillin) is a well-known example, are widely distributed in nature as fruit and leather spoilers. Citrus fruits, peaches, and plums, as well as shoes, belts, and suitcases, are often seen covered with the bluish mold dust of *Penicillium* conidia.

• • •

Figs. 13-19, 13-20, and 13-21 illustrate the appearance of other fungi that have been cultured from patients with corneal ulcers.*

---

*For further information on identification of fungi involved in keratitis, see references 10, 25, 35, 48, 49, and 54.

REFERENCES

1. Agarwal, L. P., and Khosla, P. K.: Organismal conjunctival flora in Indians, Orient. Arch. Ophthal. **1**:145, 1963.
2. Ainley, R., and Smith, B.: Fungal flora of the conjunctival sac in healthy and diseased eyes, Brit. J. Ophthal. **49**:505, 1965.
3. Albesi, E. J.: Infeccion micotica ocular, Arch. Oftal. B. Air. **44**:101, 1969.
4. de Almeida, A. A.: Infecção pós-operatória—Bacteriana e micótica, Rev. Brasil. Oftal. **22**:53, 1963.
5. Arnold, R., and Whildin, J.: Rhinosporidiosis of the conjunctiva, Amer. J. Ophthal. **25**:1227, 1942.
6. de Azevedo, M. L.: Investigações preliminares sôbre a microflora ocular, Arq. Brasil. Oftal. **25**:41, 1962.
7. Balakrishnan, E.: Mycotic keratitis. In XIX International Ophthalmological Congress Acta 11, 1242, New Delhi, 1962.
8. Ball, J. M.: Modern ophthalmology, vol. 1, Philadelphia, 1926, F. A. Davis Co., p. 479.
9. Blake, J.: Ocular hazards in agriculture, Ophthalmologica (Basel) **158**:125, 1969.
10. Barron, G. L.: The genera of Hyphomycetes from soil, Baltimore, 1968, The Williams and Wilkins Co.
11. Chick, E. W., and Conant, N. F.: Mycotic ulcerative keratitis: a review of 148 cases from the literature, Invest. Ophthal. **1**:419, 1962.
11a. DeVoe, A. G.: Keratomycosis, Amer. J. Ophthal. **71**:406, 1971.
12. Diamond, M. A., and Kirk, H. Q.: Postoperative intraocular aspergillosis, Amer. J. Ophthal. **54**:1124, 1962.
12a. Dieckhues, B.: Die Behandlung der Keratomykose mit Nystatin und Pimaricin, Klin. Mbl. Augenheilk. **148**:895, 1966.
13. Editorial: Fungal corneal ulcers, J.A.M.A. **179**:649, 1962.
13a. Ellison, A. C., Newmark, E., and Kaufman, H. E.: Chemotherapy of experimental keratomycosis, Amer. J. Ophthal. **68**:812, 1969.
14. Fazakas, A.: Über die von Bindehaut, Hornhaut, Lidrand und Tränenwegen gezüchteten Pilze, Graefes Arch. Ophth. **133**:461, 1935.
15. Fazakas, A.: Über die Schimmelpilze des gesunden und kranken Auges, Graefes Arch. Ophth. **138**:416, 1938.
16. Fazakas, A.: Zusammenfassender Bericht über meine ophthalmologischen Pilzuntersuchungen, Ophthalmologica (Basel) **126**:91, 1953.
17. Fazakas, A.: Zusammenfassender Bericht über meine im Rahmen der Akademischen Arbeitsgemeinschaft durchgeführten ophthalmologischen Pilzuntersuchungen, Ophthalmologica (Basel) **128**:163, 1954.
18. Fine, B. S., and Zimmerman, L. E.: Exogenous intraocular fungus infections with particular reference to complications of intraocular surgery, Amer. J. Ophthal. **48**:151, 1959.
19. Foster, J. B. T., Almeda, E., Littman, M. L., and Wilson, M. E.: Some intraocular and conjunctival effects of amphotericin B in man and in the rabbit, Arch. Ophthal. **60**:555, 1958.
19a. François, J., DeVos, E., Hanssens, M., and

Elewaut-Rysselaere, M.: Mycoses intra-oculaires, Ann. Oculist. **195**:97, 1962.

20. François, J., Elewaut-Rysselaere, M., and De Vos, E.: Les mycoses oculaires, Paris, 1968, Masson et Cie.
21. Gots, J. S., Thygeson, P., and Waisman, M.: Observations on Pityrosporum ovale in seborrheic blepharitis and conjunctivitis, Amer. J. Ophthal. **30**:1485, 1947.
22. Graf, K.: Postoperative intraokulare Mykosen nach Kataraktoperation, Klin. Mbl. Augenheilk. **144**:309, 1964. (Abstract.)

22a. Green, W. R., Bennett, J. E., and Goos, R. D.: Ocular penetration of amphotericin B.: a report of laboratory studies and a case report of postsurgical Cephalosporium endophthalmitis, Arch. Ophthal. **73**:769, 1965.

23. Halde, C., and Okumoto, M.: Ocular mycosis: a study of 82 cases. In Proc. XX International Congress of Ophthalmology, part 2, 705, 1966. International Congress series no. 146. Excerpta Medica Foundation.
24. Hammeke, J. C., and Ellis, P. P.: Mycotic flora of the conjunctiva, Amer. J. Ophthal. **49**:1174, 1960.
25. Hazen, E., Gordon, M. A., and Reed, C.: Laboratory identification of pathogenic fungi simplified, ed. 3, Springfield, Ill., 1970, Charles C Thomas, Publisher.
26. Hoffmann, D. H., and Naumann, G.: Ein Beitrag zur Pilzinfektion der Hornhaut, Klin. Mbl. Augenheilk. **142**:286, 1963.

26a. Hoefnagels, K. L. J., and Pijpers, P. M.: Histoplasma capsulatum in a human eye, Amer. J. Ophthal. **63**:715, 1967.

27. Janke, R. G., and Schwab, F.: Zur Frage der Pilzflora der normalen Bindehaut des Menschen, Wien. Med. Wschr. **111**:859, 1961.

27a. Jones, B. R., Richards, A. B., and Morgan, G.: Direct fungal infection of the eye in Britain, Trans. Ophthal. Soc. U. K. **89**:727, 757, 1969.

28. Jones, D. B., Sexton, R., and Rebell, G.: Mycotic keratitis in South Florida: a review of 39 cases, Trans. Ophthal. Soc. U. K. **89**:781, 1969.
29. Kinnas, J. S.: Ophthalmic disease caused by a mycete of the giant cane, Brit. J. Ophthal. **49**:327, 1965.
30. Küper, J.: Zur Klinik postoperativer intraokularer Mykosen, Klin. Mbl. Augenheilk. **140**: 827, 1962.
31. Leber, T.: Keratomycosis aspergillina als Ursache von Hypopyonkeratitis, Graefes Arch. Ophth. **25**:285, 1879.
32. Ley, A. P., and Sanders, T. E.: Fungus keratitis: a report of three cases, Arch. Ophthal. **56**:257, 1956.
33. Lichaa, E.: Mycose oculaire primitive due au "Beauveria Brumpti–Langeron et Lichaa," Bull. Ophthal. Soc. Egypt **26**:91, 1933.
34. Locatcher-Khorazo, D., Benham, R. W., and Silva-Hutner, M.: Incidence of fungi from clinically healthy eyes of 508 young people 10-18 years of age and in 1,347 adults 19-80 years of age. Unpublished data.
35. Lodder, J., editor: The yeasts, a toxonomic study, Amsterdam, 1970, North Holland Publishing Co.
36. Mitsui, Y., and Hanabusa, J.: Corneal infections after cortisone therapy, Brit. J. Ophthal. **39**:244, 1955.
37. Naumann, G., Green, W. R., and Zimmerman, L. E.: Mycotic keratitis: a histopathologic study of 73 cases, Amer. J. Ophthal. **64**:668, 1967.
38. Nema, H. V., Ahuja, O. P., Bal, A., and Mohapatra, L. N.: Mycotic flora of the conjunctiva, Amer. J. Ophthal. **62**:968, 1966.
39. Okuda, K., Matsuura, K., and Okabe, S.: A case of keratomycosis caused by Cephalosporium sp. (light and electron microscopic observations), Folia Ophthal. Jap. **21**:285, 1970.
40. Olson, C. L.: Ocular mycosis, Gen. Practice **40**:78, August, 1969.
41. Ovsepian, T. L., and Osipian, L. L., Mycologic flora of the conjunctival sac, Zh. Eksp. Klin. Med. **5**:78, 1965.
42. Paiva, C., Chaves Batista, A., and Gomes, A.: Endoftalmite micótica pós-operatoria por Hyalopus bogolepofii, Rev. Brasil. Oftal. **19**: 193, 1960.

42a. Parfenov, L. K.: Fungal infections of the eyes in the Astrakhan region, Vestnik Oftal. **76**:17, 1963.

43. Parunovic, A., and Halde, C.: Pityrosporum orbiculare: its possible role in seborrheic blepharitis, Amer. J. Ophthal. **63**:815, 1967.
44. Percebois, G., and Raspiller, A.: Flore fongique de la conjonctive humaine, Bull. Soc. Ophtal. Franc. **48**:626, 1968.

44a. Polack, F. M., Kaufman, H. E., and Newmark, E.: Keratomycosis: medical and surgical treatment, Arch. Ophthal. **85**:410, 1971.

45. Puttanna, S. T.: Mycotic infections of the cornea, J. All India Ophthal. Soc. **15**:11, 1967.
46. Rao, P. N. S., and Ramakrishnan, T. S.: Studies on the fungus diseases affecting man in and around Manipal, Indian J. Path. Bact. **11**:53, 1968.
47. Raper, K. B., and Fennell, D. I.: The genus Aspergillus, Baltimore, 1965, The Williams and Wilkins Co.
48. Raper, K. B., and Thom, C.: Manual of the Penicillia, Baltimore, 1949, The Williams and Wilkins Co.
49. de Rezende, C.: Ocular mycosis. In XIX Concilium Ophthalmoligicum, New Delhi, 1962. Acta **1**:299, 1962.

50. Sachsenweger, R.: Klinische Befunde und experimentelle Untersuchungen üeber Augenerkrankungen durch saprophytär wachsende Pilze, Klin. Mbl. Augenheilk. **127**:721, 1955.
51. Salceda, S. R., Nievera, L.-F., and Abendaño, R.: Keratomycosis: a clinical, laboratory and therapeutic evaluation of 17 cases, Philippine J. Ophthal. **1**:31, 1969.
52. Sanders, N.: Penetrating keratoplasty in treatment of fungus keratitis, Amer. J. Ophthal **70**:24, 1970.
52a. Scholer, H. J., and Saubermann, G.: Aspergillose der Hornhaut, vol. 2, Diskussion von 90 Fällen der Literatur, Basel, 1959, S. Karger, p. 23.
53. Sinha, B. N., and Das, M. S.: Bacterial and fungal flora of the conjunctival sacs in healthy and diseased eyes, J. Indian Med. Ass. **51**:217, 1968.
54. Snyder, W. C., and Hansen, H. N.: The species concept of Fusarium, Amer. J. Bot. **27**:64, 1940.
55. Strampelli, B., and Maggi, C.: Endoftalmite micotica post-operatoria, Riv. Ital. Trachome Patol. Ocul. Esot. **15**:168, 1963.
56. Theodore, F. H., Littman, M. L., and Almeda, E.: The diagnosis and management of fungus endophthalmitis following cataract extraction, Arch. Ophthal. **66**:163, 1961.
57. Theodore, F. H., Littman, M. L., and Almeda, E.: Endophthalmitis following cataract extraction due to Neurospora sitophila, a so-called non-pathogenic fungus, Amer. J. Ophthal. **53**:35, 1962.
58. Thomas, C. I.: The cornea, Springfield, Ill., 1955, Charles C Thomas, Publisher.
59. Thygeson, P.: Etiology and treatment of blepharitis: a study in military personnel, Arch. Ophthal. **36**:445, 1946.
60. Thygeson, P., Hogan, M. J., and Kimura, S. J.: Cortisone and hydrocortisone in ocular infections, Trans. Amer. Acad. Ophthal. Otolaryng. **57**:64, 1953.
61. Thygeson, P., and Vaughan, D. G., Jr.: Seborrheic blepharitis, Trans. Amer. Ophthal. Soc. **52**:173, 1955.
62. Vasquez de Parga, A. S., and Pereiro, M.: Flora micotica de la conjunctiva, Arch. Soc. Oftal. Hisp. Amer. **25**:168, 1965.
63. White, J. H.: Fungal contamination of donor eyes, Brit. J. Ophthal. **53**:30, 1969.
64. Williamson, J., Gordon, A. M., Wood, R. Dyer, A., and Yahya, O. A.: Fungal flora of the conjunctival sac in health and disease, Brit. J. Ophthal. **52**:127, 1968.
65. Wilson, L. A., Ahern, D. G., Jones, D. B., and Sexton, R. R.: Fungi from the normal outer eye, Amer. J. Ophthal. **67**:52, 1969.
66. Zimmerman, L. E.: Keratomycosis, Survey Ophthal. **8**:1, 1963.

14

The Chlamydia: trachoma and inclusion conjunctivitis

Trachoma, a disease of the conjunctiva and cornea, is clinically defined by four stages. These start with granular conjunctivitis and epithelial keratitis. Follicular hypertrophy, particularly in the conjunctiva of the upper eyelid, is followed by pannus formation, which is most constant in the upper segment of the cornea; but when the disease is severe, the whole cornea becomes involved. Healing takes place with varying degrees of cicatrization, which determine the extent of visual impairment. Trachoma is considered a disease limited to the eye, spontaneously transmitted only from one eye of man to another. It is to be differentiated from inclusion conjunctivitis, which in the newborn is acquired from an infection of the mother's birth canal and in the adult from contact with infected material from the genitourinary tract as in swimming pools before chlorination or, rarely, from infected eyes. Initially somewhat similar in appearance to the *early* stages of stages II or IIb,[17] inclusion conjunctivitis is mild, does not produce gross pannus formation, and heals without cicatrization. But certain common features between trachoma and inclusion conjunctivitis, which are currently being investigated, make it more relevant at present to treat the two diseases in parallel in order to help clarify their relationship to each other.

EPIDEMIOLOGY

Trachoma

Trachoma is apparently as old as recorded history. According to Kugelmass,[15] the disease was known in China in the twenty-seventh century BC and was endemic in Mesopotamia in the twentieth century BC. The Ebers Papyrus, written about 1550 BC, mentions a disease whose description is consistent with that of trachoma. In the fifth century BC trachoma was common in Greece. As noted in Chapter 1, Celsus in 14 AD recorded the roughness of the eyelids, and Aetus of Amida in 550 AD described the four stages of the disease.[7] Trachoma is now endemic around the world, as may be seen in Table 14-1, which shows the distribution and prevalence of the disease in 1962.[4,5] The areas of highest concentration of trachoma lie around the Mediterranean, especially Africa, and in parts of Iran, India, and Indochina. In the United States trachoma is found in some Indian reservations in the West and among some rural groups in the Appalachian mountains. It is estimated that about 400 million people are infected with the trachoma agent and that about 20 million are blind.[6]

Trachoma is spread from eye to eye by contact with contaminated hands, towels, and other intermediate carriers. Being con-

Table 14-1. Geographic distribution of trachoma*

Majority of population affected with trachoma	Trachoma highly widespread (20%-50%)	Trachoma quite common (1%-20%)	Trachoma prevalent sporadically	Trachoma practically extinct
Egypt	Aden	Argentina	Baltic states	Austria
Eritrean highlands	Africa (equatorial East, and South—(among the native populations	Australia (among the aboriginal tribes)	Chile	Belgium
Israel (Arab population)	Borneo	Africa (West)	Finland	Canada
Kuwait	Burma	Balkan states	France (imported cases only)	Denmark
Lybia	Cambodia	Brazil	Guatamala	England
Some districts of	China (mainland)	Bulgaria	Honduras	Germany
Algeria	India (areas)	Ceylon	Ireland	Holland
China	Indonesia	Greece	Italy (central and northern)	Iceland
India (northern)	Iran	Hungary	Panama	Norway
Iran	Iraq	India (areas)	Paraguay	Scotland
Iraq	Jordan	Israel	Peru	Switzerland
Lebanon	Laos	Italy (southern)	Philippines (areas)	
Morocco	Lebanon	Japan	Salvador	
Saudi Arabia	Morocco	Korea	Sweden	
Syria	Pakistan (West)	Lebanon	Uruguay	
Tunisia	Sudan	Mediterranean Islands	United States (non-Indian populations)	
Vietnam	Syria	Mexico	Venzuela	
	Thailand	New Zealand (among the Maoris)		
	Tunisia	Pacific Islands		
	Turkey (southern)	Pakistan		
	Vietnam (South)	Poland		
		Portugal		
		Rumania		
		Spain (Mediterranean coast)		
		Turkey (central and northern)		
		USSR (southern and central)		
		United States (among the American Indians)		

*From surveys published in 1962 and 1967.[4,5]

cerned with the spread of the disease in the army, Vetch in 1807 prevented the use of common towels by a group of soldiers, some of whom had the disease, while permitting common use of towels by another similar group.[14] He observed that fresh cases of the disease were much more frequent in the latter group. Transmission of trachoma with follicular material to two human volunteers was accomplished in 1823 by Werneck, who established an incubation period of 9 days in one volunteer and 14 days in the other.[14]

Thus, more than 150 years ago information was available, which if used could reduce the spread of the disease. But this information preceded the discovery of bacteria and antisepsis, and attempt at control of trachoma was hardly exercised. The disease spread under conditions of poverty, overcrowding, and cultural patterns that opposed hygienic measures. It was not until 1907, when Halberstaedter and von Prowazek[11] (Fig. 14-1, *A* and *B*) saw viruslike inclusion bodies in the eptihelial cells from

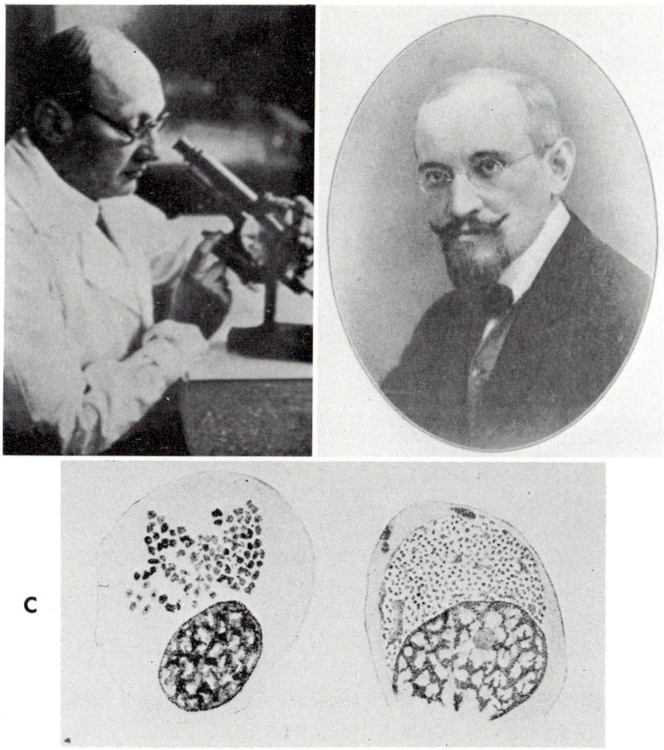

Fig. 14-1. A classic observation in trachoma was made jointly by a German, Halberstaedter (1877-1949), **A**, and an Austrian, von Prowazek (1875-1910), **B**. Both of these physicians were famous for other reasons. Halberstaedter was a pioneer radiologist who developed much of the important groundwork in this field. Von Prowazek worked in the field of rickettsial infections, and the causative organism of typhus fever is named *Rickettsia prowazekii* in his honor. Like Ricketts, he died from typhus fever. When on a joint expedition to Java to study syphilis, Halberstaedter and von Prowazek noted that severe conjunctivitis of trachoma was common. Scrapings of these conjunctivas, **C**, revealed small granular intracellular bodies that stained red with Giemsa stain and lay in a blue matrix. They believed these to be the cause of trachoma, and when the bodies were present in heavy masses, they called them inclusion bodies. They were successful in producing infection in the eyes of the orangutan with their scrapings. (**A** from Finzi, N. S.: Brit. J. Radiol. **22**:347, 1949; **B** from Olpp, G.: Charakterkopfe der Tropenmedizin, Berlin, 1936, Verlag Die Brücke Zur Heimat, p. 60; **C** from Halberstaedter, L., and von Prowazek, S.: Deutsch. Med. Wschr. **33**:1285, 1907.)

trachomatous eyes (Fig. 14-1, *C*), that the modern history of the cause and control of trachoma began.

Inclusion conjunctivitis

Awareness of the disease inclusion conjunctivitis arose in this century. In 1903 Morax[18] described a disease of the eyes of the newborn that occurred in the absence of pathogenic bacteria. Stargardt[22] and Schmeichler[21] in 1909 saw, in epithelial cells of nongonorrheal conjunctivitis of the newborn, inclusion bodies that appeared identical to those found in trachoma. Halberstaedter and von Prowazek looked for evidence of inclusion body disease in the birth canals of those mothers who had infants with inclusion conjunctivitis and found typical inclusions in the epithelial cells.[7] Lindner[16] confirmed these observations and showed that material from both the venereal disease and the conjunctivitis of the newborn proved to be infectious for the eye of the baboon. Lindner named the disease of the infants inclusion blennorrhea.

As in the case of trachoma, under natural conditions the agent of inclusion conjunctivitis is spontaneously pathogenic only for man but has been transmitted to a few primates. This disease of the newborn resembles gonococcal ophthalmitis epidemiologically in that it is acquired from the mother's birth canal. Venereal transmission probably maintains the organism as a human pathogen. The genital infection in the female is seldom recognized, since the cervix is the area of infection and there are no symptoms. However, about 40% of nongonorrheal urethritis in men is found to be of chlamydial origin.[8] The exudate is largely made up of the polymorphonuclear leukocytes that do not have inclusion bodies and of a few epithelial cells with inclusion bodies. Thygeson has commented that infection of the adult eye with the agent of inclusion conjunctivitis has become more frequent with the advent of the sexual revolution. Transmission from infants' eyes is unusual, although obstetricians and nurses may become infected.[12,30] Cases of adult eye infection that used to occur from contaminated swimming pools is now relatively rare because of chlorination.

ETIOLOGY

The organisms that cause trachoma and inclusion conjunctivitis have offered one of the most interesting problems in identification and classification. Halberstaedter and von Prowazek, who saw and first pictured the inclusion bodies of trachoma (Fig. 14-1), gave the name *Chlamydozoen* (mantle body) to these organisms. The similarity of the inclusion bodies of trachoma to those found in psittacosis was noted by Thygeson[24] in 1934. Nicolle and his associates,[19] Thygeson and Proctor,[31] and Julianelle[14] demonstrated the filterability of the infectious agents and transmission of the diseases to monkeys, apes, and man. Despite all this information and the use of the ever increasingly successful methods for cultivation of similar types of obligate intracellular parasites, the agent of trachoma was not successfully cultured until 1957. T'ang and his co-workers[23] substituted streptomycin for penicillin in the preparation of the infectious material for injection in the chick embryonic yolk sac and were successful in the cultivation of the infectious agent. They found that a mixture of streptomycin and penicillin might also be used but yielded fewer positive cultures. Now both the trachoma and inclusion conjunctivitis agents (TRIC agents) have been grown in many laboratories in various areas around the world. Their cultivation characteristics and classification are documented by Jawetz[12] in an article on the history of this milestone in microbiology.

The generic term *Chlamydia* includes the psittacosis group primarily infecting birds; the human pathogens causing lymphogranuloma venereum, trachoma, and inclusion conjunctivitis; and finally a wide variety of other mammalian agents producing such diseases as feline pneumonitis and bovine encephalitis. The various chlamydia are morphologically similar. The infectious particle, or elementary body, is 0.2 to 0.3 $m\mu$ in diameter.[32] When these particles enter a cell they change, after a lag period, to the larger (0.7 μ), much less infectious initial bodies. These in turn give rise to elementary bodies that increase in numbers and finally burst from the cell to infect fresh cells. Both DNA and RNA have been demonstrated in these bodies, and they further resemble rickettsiae and bacteria in having a cell wall, similar to that of gram-negative bacteria, which derives its rigidity from mucopeptide containing the amino sugar muramic acid.

A question still unsettled is the relation of the trachoma (TR) agent to the inclusion conjunctivitis (IC) agent. Since they are culturally identical, the effort to distinguish them has been directed toward a classification based on antigenic difference. This has been a difficult problem because of a major antigen or antigens that are common to many of the chlamydia. The most successful test has proved to be the mouse toxicity prevention test. Mice are immunized against a variety of TRIC strains, and their immunity to lethal doses of unknown strains are tested.[3] By this technique six types are currently recognized. Most of the strains (62 of 64) from eyes diagnosed ocular trachoma have been placed in types A, B, or C. Two strains from clinical trachoma and 16 strains from sources other than ocular trachoma belong to types D, E, or F.[1] This type of classification will undoubtedly be extended since, besides the theoretical importance, the whole problem of prophylactic vaccination depends on the choice of suitable antigens.

In an effort to understand the relationship of trachoma to inclusion conjunctivitis, many investigators have conducted studies of the lesions produced in man and animals by experimental infection with these agents. Thygeson and his associates[27,29] have shown that *Chlamydia* organisms isolated from trachoma produce a less severe disease in monkeys than do *Chlamydia* organisms isolated from inclusion conjunctivitis. Wang and Grayston,[33] in experimental infection carried out on 451 *Macaca cyclopis* monkeys, presented data indicating that TRIC agents derived from both trachoma and inclusion conjunctivitis may cause the clinical picture of trachoma in the eyes of these animals. The disease appeared to be more severe, and pannus formation more prominent, when the animals had a relatively high antibody titer against the organism, and it was concluded that "hypersensitivity to homologous or heterologous TRIC agents is an important part of the host response in the pathogenesis of pannus formation." Tarizzo and his co-workers,[23a] using 13 human volunteers, found that cultured inclusion conjunctivitis agents could elicit corneal as well as conjunctival changes normally considered peculiar to trachoma. The role of partial immunity in this clinical picture is also discussed by Tarizzo and his co-workers. In the natural infection in man the clinical distinction between trachoma and inclusion conjunctivitis is usually quite clear. But whether further investigations will show that the agents of these diseases are independent of one another or that one represents a mutation or that the condition of the host determines the type of infection still remains open. Immunologic data favor two distinct agents.

CLINICAL DIAGNOSIS

Trachoma

According to the classification presented by MacCallan,[17] there are four stages in the evolution of trachoma. In children the onset may be insidious with minimal symptoms.[26,28] For these reasons it is often overlooked. In the adult stage I begins 5 to 12 days after infection and is characterized by the presence of immature follicles on the upper tarsal plate. There is only slight papillary hypertrophy, little if any conjunctival exudate, and the disease is often relatively asymptomatic. The bulbar conjunctiva may not be inflamed. Epithelial keratitis is always present but usually can be seen only with the aid of some magnification and best with the biomicroscope. Fig. 14-2, *A* and *B* illustrates the developing follicles in the upper tarsal conjunctivas in the early and advanced stage I, respectively. Plate 3, *E* illustrates the eye of another patient with early lesions of the tarsal conjunctiva. This phase of the disease may last 3 months to 3 years. In Stage IIa (Fig. 14-2, *C*) the tarsal conjunctiva is swollen with sago-grainlike follicles that are mature, soft, and easily expressed, which is diagnostic of trachoma, since the follicles found in some other ocular diseases are firm and not expressible. Discharge continues to be minimal and symptoms are mild, but the keratitis has advanced and may be visible without magnification. Pannus formation (Fig. 14-3) proceeds, and limbal follicles may be present. In both stages I and II, scrapings of the affected areas will yield epithelial cells containing the characteristic inclusion bodies, which are illustrated in Fig. 14-4 and Plate 1, *E*. The discharges present in stages I and IIa are rich in neutrophils in contrast to lymphocytes found in viral eye infections. The material ex-

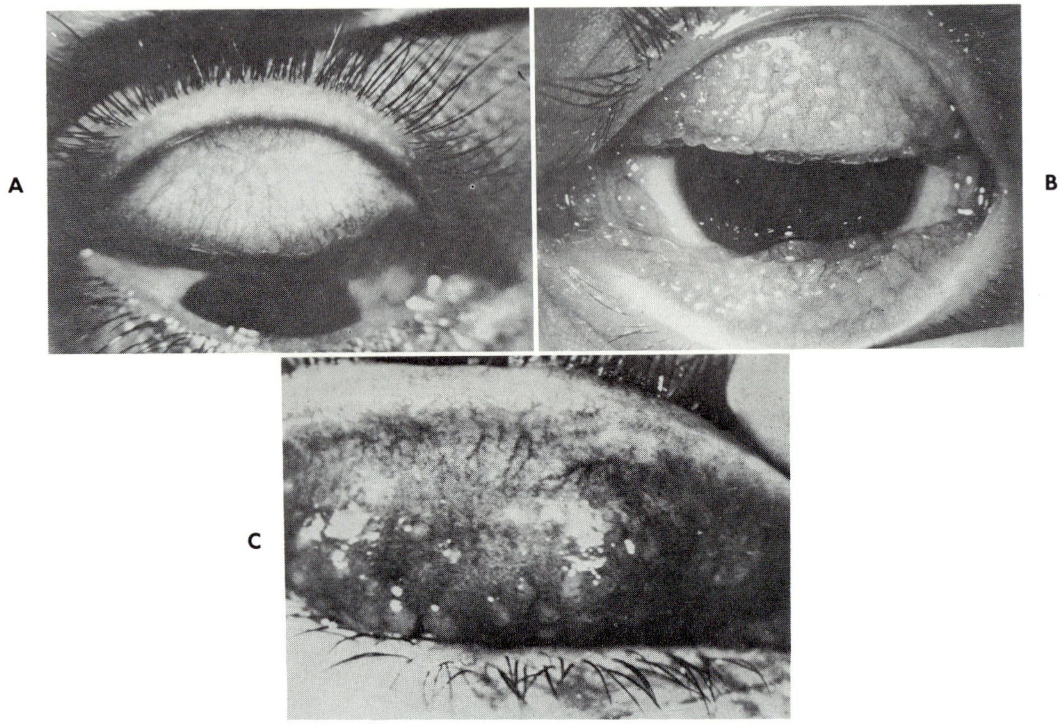

Fig. 14-2. A, Stage I trachoma, showing immature follicles in the upper tarsal conjunctiva. B, Stage I trachoma in transition to stage IIa, showing immature follicles in the upper tarsal conjunctiva and mature follicles in the fornices and lower tarsal conjunctiva. C, Stage IIa trachoma, showing sago-grainlike mature follicles in the upper tarsal conjunctiva. (From Thygeson, P.: Trachoma manual and atlas, Public Health Service Publication No. 541, Washington, D. C., 1960, U. S. Department of Health, Education, and Welfare.)

pressed from the follicles shows poorly staining lymphoid elements, bare nuclei, scattered cytoplasmic fragments, and numerous large mononuclear phagocytes filled with cell debris (Fig. 4-14). Stage IIa may last from 3 months to 2 to 3 years.

In some instances of highly virulent trachoma or of trachoma complicated by a bacterial infection, a stage IIb is produced in which the follicles may be masked by intense cellular infiltration and papillary hypertrophy. This condition may subside into stage IIa or pass directly into stage III.[7,25]

The time of arrival at stage III with its scar formation varies considerably. Usually progression in children is slower than in adults. Beginning scar formation is recognized with the aid of the biomicroscope. Signs of activity of the infection decrease as cicatrization progresses. With severe disease and rapid cicatrization, the scars become visible (Fig. 14-5). As the follicles undergo necrosis, they are replaced by connective tissue. Interference with blood supply may produce further necrosis and shrinking of the conjunctiva, leading to the development of trichiasis and entropion.

Pannus formation progresses through stages I and II, for the cornea is always involved early. The upper half of the cornea is involved first. The severity of the pannus usually is a measure of the severity of the disease. Corneal ulcers caused by the breakdown of trachoma pustules are often seen. Their healing may result in thick scar formation. Herbert's peripheral pits result from cicatrization of limbal follicles; and in the process, a dimple is formed, filled with transparent epithelium giving the ap-

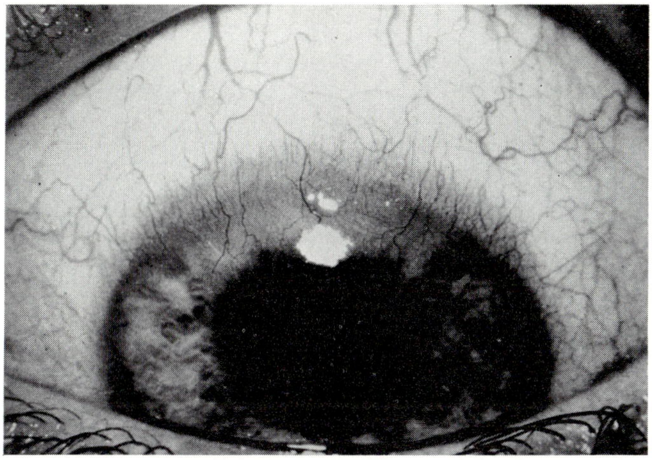

Fig. 14-3. Early pannus formation. (Courtesy Dr. P. Thygeson.)

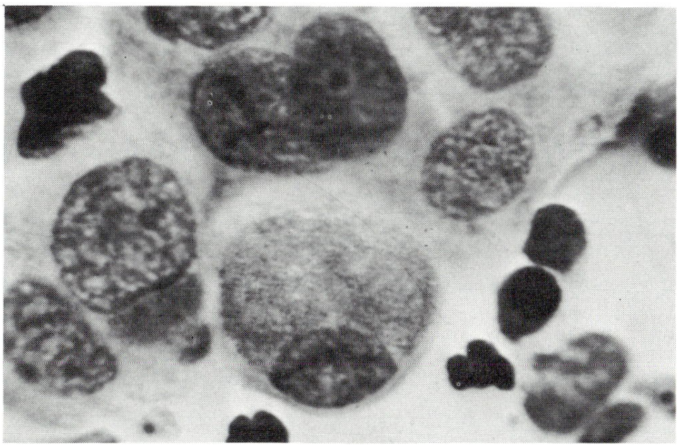

Fig. 14-4. Epithelial conjunctival scraping from a patient with acute trachoma (Plate 3, *E*), showing inclusion bodies in the cytoplasm of two epithelial cells.

pearance of a pit. These are characteristic of trachoma as seen in half the cases among American Indians.[25,30] Stage III may last for several years; but especially in children, if healing occurs spontaneously or following the use of drugs, the scars may be visible only with magnification.

Stage IV may exist indefinitely without symptoms if there are no complications such as tear deficiency and secondary bacterial infection. The biomicroscope can be used to detect the healing. If the cornea is free of subepithelial infiltrates and fluorescein will not stain the cornea, it is presumed that healing has taken place. This can be further established if treatment with topical steroids fails to exacerbate the disease. When extensive pannus formation and ulceration and cicatrization have occurred, the end result is severe impairment of the eye, which sometimes may be helped by restorative surgery.

Inclusion conjunctivitis

Inclusion conjunctivitis is a relatively mild disease that may be considered in two forms, inclusion blennorrhea (inclusion conjunctivitis) in the newborn and inclusion conjunctivitis in other age groups. The untreated disease in the newborn is char-

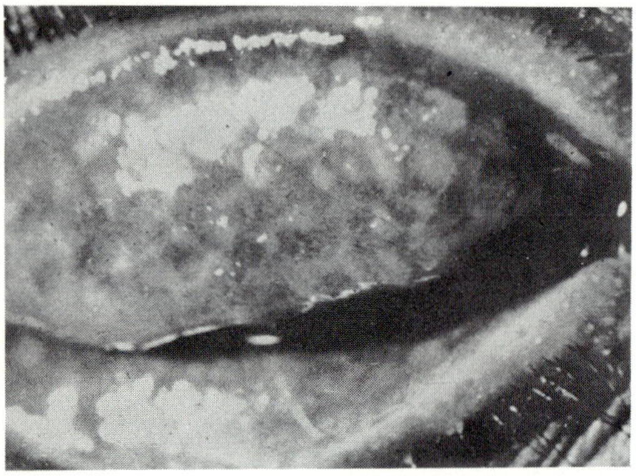

Fig. 14-5. Stage III, cicatrizing trachoma. Follicles in process of cicatrization can be seen clearly. (From Thygeson, P.: Trachoma manual and atlas, Public Health Service Publication No. 541, Washington, D. C., 1960, U. S. Department of Health, Education, and Welfare.)

acterized by a incubation period of 5 to 12 days, followed by the onset of intense inflammation of the conjunctiva and profuse discharge (Plate 3, *F*). The exudate contains many neutrophils and epithelial cells showing cytoplasmic inclusion bodies similar to those found in conjunctival epithelial cells in trachoma. In the untreated disease follicular conjunctivitis develops, but the cornea is not involved except for minor epithelial keratitis. In a matter of months the lesions heal spontaneously without residual damage. Prompt treatment with sulfonamides or antibiotics or both results in cure within a week or so, before the folliculitis occurs.

Inclusion conjunctivitis of older children and adults appears as an acute follicular conjunctivitis without major keratitis and with only moderate involvement of the conjunctiva of the upper tarsus. Untreated, it may run a course of 3 to 12 months. It too is readily treated with sulfonamides and antibiotics. The primary source for both examples of this infection is the genitourinary tract. In the female there is a subclinical cervicitis and in the male a nonspecific urethritis. The newborn becomes infected as he passes through the mother's birth canal. At one time children and those of older age groups acquired the disease most often from using swimming pools that presumably had been contaminated from the genitourinary tracts of the swimmers. This gave the name of swimming pool conjunctivitis to the disease. Today adequate chlorination of the water has almost eliminated this source of infection. Nurses or nurses aides or members of the family sometimes acquire the disease from the infant or the mother, but the source of infection is still primarily the genitourinary system.

DIFFERENTIAL DIAGNOSIS

Trachoma

Other types of follicular conjunctivitis may be mistaken for trachoma. These include pharyngoconjunctival fever, usually caused by adenovirus type 3; epidemic keratoconjunctivitis, caused by adenovirus type 8; acute primary herpetic keratoconjunctivitis; and conjunctivitis resulting from Newcastle disease caused by a paramyxovirus disease of chickens. None of these present a difficult diagnostic problem (Chapters 17, 18, and 19). The exudates from these infections lack cells containing inclusion bodies and show a predominance of lymphocytes over neutrophils. Chronic follicular conjunctivitis (Axenfeld type), a disease of unknown etiology, is the one most likely to be confused with trachoma, since this type of conjunctivitis occasionally has follicles in the upper tarsal conjunctiva. It is distinguished because of the lack of inclusion bodies; the character of the scanty exudate, which has mostly mononuclear cells; its benign course, without cicatrization or pannus, progressing to spontaneous healing in a year or two; and its failure to respond to chemotherapeutic agents.

There are three types of toxic follicular conjunctivitis to be distinguished from trachoma. The presence of molluscum nodules in the lid margins identifies the first of these: molluscum contagiosum conjunctivitis. The second is a conjunctivitis arising from the prolonged use of idoxuridine (IDU) in patients with herpetic disease and of eserine and other miotics in glaucoma patients. They may develop a follicular conjunctivitis that, if neglected, can simulate trachoma even to pannus formation and scarring. A third follicular conjunctivitis may arise in susceptible children in response to various irritants, such as ordinary bacterial conjunctivitis or Parinaud's oculoglandular conjunctivitis caused by *Leptothrix buccalis*. Finally, there is a folliculosis of unknown etiology associated with noninflammatory follicular hyperplasia of the nasopharynx, a chronic but self-limited disease distinguished from trachoma because of slight or no involvement of the upper tarsal conjunctiva. These categories of disease to be differentiated from trachoma are reviewed in the World Health Organization Technical Report Series.[9]

Inclusion conjunctivitis

The differential diagnosis of inclusion blennorrhea presents few difficulties. The incubation period of several days, the failure to detect a bacterial agent in the profuse exudate, and the presence of epithelial inclusion bodies in scrapings make the diagnosis in the newborn; and the relatively benign course and response to sulfonamides and tetracycline confirm it. In the child or adult the diagnosis may present some difficulties. A history of the possible source of infection, together with the characteristic involvement of the lower tarsal conjunctiva and the failure to compromise the cornea seriously, differentates the infection from trachoma.

EXPERIENCE WITH THE TRIC AGENTS AT THE IOCPMC

Since trachoma is not indigenous to New York City, the patients seen at the IOCPMC were for the most part people who were in transit. Diagnosis of this disease depended on the results obtained from the examination of scrapings. Table 14-2 summarizes the findings. The table shows that of 1,367 patients examined because of possible trachoma, 223 had cells containing inclusions, which were considered characteristic of the active stages of trachoma, and in 32 the findings were compatible with chronic trachoma. Inclusion blennorrhea was suspected in 1,585 newborns, 362 of which had scrapings confirming this diagnosis. In a few instances scrapings of the mother's cervix were taken, and all were positive for inclusions. Ocular scrapings were examined in 1,077 patients with a questionable diagnosis of inclusion conjunctivitis, and 201 cases showed cytoplasmic inclusions.

The predominating bacteria found in eyes of patients with acute trachoma were (1) *Staphylococcus aureus* with diphtheroids, (2) *Diplococcus pneumoniae*, and (3) *Klebsiella pneumoniae*. Fewer organisms were found in the 32 patients with chronic trachoma; but in 14 of these, *Mor-*

Table 14-2. Incidence of trachoma and inclusion conjunctivitis at the IOCPMC: 1938-1968

Number of patients examined	Diagnosis in question	Laboratory diagnosis as determined by conjunctival epithelial scrapings	Number of patients positive
1,367	Acute trachoma	Inclusions characteristic of *Chlamydia* infection; polymorphonuclear neutrophils present	223
	Chronic trachoma	Cytoplasmic inclusions very rare; presence of lymphocytes and macrophages	32
1,585	Inclusion blennorrhea	Cytoplasmic inclusions identical with those in trachoma; polymorphonuclear cells and a few lymphocytes	362
1,077	Inclusion conjunctivitis (adult)	Cytoplasmic inclusions as in trachoma; polymorphonuclear cells and lymphocytes	201

axella species were isolated in a flora that also contained S. *aureus.*

LABORATORY DIAGNOSIS

The growth of TRIC agents in the chick embryo and on cultured cells[2,8,10] is technically too complicated to be useful as a routine diagnostic tool. Two laboratory procedures, however, are of practical value. The first is the time-honored examination of conjunctival scrapings. Details for the technique of preparing and staining these smears are given in Chapter 4. The scrapings for acute trachoma and inclusion conjunctivitis are similar (Table 14-3). The differential diagnosis of these diseases, as already stated, depends upon the character of the follicular conjunctivitis and upon the involvement of the cornea.

The immunofluorescein technique for the recognition of inclusion bodies in scrapings containing epithelial cells from trachomatous eyes is accurate, fast, and yields a higher percentage of positive tests than can be obtained by other techniques. The principal of the test is to label antibody to TRIC agents or cross-reacting lymphogranuloma antibody with fluorescein, to "stain" smears of the exudate, scrapings, or cultured cells under question with the labeled antibody, and to examine the preparation under ultraviolet light. The antibody is bound to those areas in the cell harboring the TRIC agent, and the attached fluorescein gives a bright yellow-green fluorescence that stands out brilliantly against a darker background (Plate 3, *G*).[20] In this way a rare infected cell is readily seen. The test requires the use of a source of ultraviolet light, a trained technician, and a room with greatly reduced light for the examination. Since the test is useful for the identification of viruses and often of bacteria as well, it can become a valuable part of the equipment of a microbiology laboratory in a department of ophthalmology.

The fluorescein test is only as specific as the antibody employed. As yet it has proved difficult to obtain sera that can readily be used to classify the subdivisions of the TRIC agents, and even the subdivisions of the *Chlamydia;* so as yet much remains to be done in sharpening immunologic diagnostic procedures for this group of organisms.

PROPHYLAXIS AND THERAPY

Attempts at prophylaxis for trachoma are centered about the development of a vaccine useful in preventing or ameliorating

Table 14-3. Diagnosis of stained scrapings from patients with TRIC infection

Selective affinity of TRIC agents	Sites for obtaining scrapings	Results of staining smears from scrapings	Cytoplasmic structures that may be mistaken for inclusions
		Trachoma	
Confined to epithelium	Upper tarsal conjunctiva, fornix, cornea	Intracytoplasmic inclusions present in high percentage in early phase and in acute exacerbations of late disease; polymorphonuclear cells; difficult to find inclusions in later chronic stages; in trachomatous follicular expression, macrophages contain broken-down debris, which is abundant; pale-staining large mononuclear cells; some plasma cells	Pseudoinclusion bodies Pigment granules Aggregates of nonspecific granular cytoplasm Aggregates of bacteria
		Inclusion conjunctivitis	
	Lower tarsal conjunctiva	Intracytoplasmic inclusions, polymorphonuclear cells	

the disease. The investigators at best have claimed only some reduction in the attack rate for short periods and at worst some accentuation of the disease apparently caused by acquired hypersensitivity.[13] It seems necessary to find a key antigen associated with infectivity that can stimulate a protective antibody. On theoretical grounds it is a difficult problem, since trachoma, even after years of activity, produces no lasting immunity.

The transmission of trachoma is favored by poor hygiene. According to Jawetz,[12] transmission of the disease is highest in the homes of the poor, where there is overcrowding, sharing of common towels and other possessions, and little knowledge of hygiene. In the Middle East, North Africa, and the Orient, seasonal epidemics of bacterial conjunctivitis caused by such organisms as *Hemophlius aegypticus, Neisseria gonorrhoeae, Moraxella lacunata,* and staphylococci often occur. These infections exacerbate trachoma and increase its spread by the profuse conjunctival exudate. The history of the lessening or disappearance of trachoma from most of Europe before the introduction of specific therapy must reflect the importance of such factors.

Therapy of trachoma and inclusion conjunctivitis are the same. For trachoma, sulfonamides are given orally for about 3 weeks or less. Local application of a 1% concentration of a broad-spectrum antibiotic, usually tetracycline, is given twice daily or more for 1 to 3 months. Tetracyclines taken orally make good substitutes for sulfonamides when a patient is sulfa sensitive. The period of treatment necessary for inclusion conjunctivitis is considerably less than that needed for trachoma. Though the treatment of trachoma may seem simple on paper, in practice, unless conditions of living can be improved, reinfection often occurs.

REFERENCES

1. Alexander, E. R., Wang, S. P., and Grayston, J. T.: Further classification of TRIC agents from ocular trachoma and other sources by the mouse toxicity prevention test, Amer. J. Ophthal. **63**(Suppl.):1469, 1967.
2. Al-Hussaini, M. K., Jones, B. R., and Dunlop, E. M. C.: Genital infection in association with TRIC virus infection of the eye: cytology (preliminary report), Brit. J. Vener. Dis. **40**:25, 1964.
3. Bell, S. D., Jr., and Theobald, B.: Differentiation of trachoma strains on the basis of immunization against toxic death of mice, Ann. N. Y. Acad. Sci. **98**:337, 1962.
4. Bietti, G. B., Freyche, M. J., and Vozza, R.: La diffusion actuelle du trachome dans le monde, Rev. Int. Trachome **39**:113, 1962.
5. Bietti, G., and Werner, G. H.: In Kugelmass, I. N., editor: Trachoma: prevention and treatment, Springfield, Ill., 1967, Charles C Thomas, Publisher.
6. Davis, B. D., Dulbecco, R., Eisen, H. N., Ginsberg, H. S., and Wood, W. B.: Microbiology, New York, 1967, Harper and Row, Publishers.
7. Duke-Elder, S.: System of ophthalmology, Diseases of the outer eye, vol. 8, part 1, St. Louis, 1965, The C. V. Mosby Co., pp. 260, 300.
8. Dunlop, E. M. C., Hare, M. J., Darougar, S., Jones, B. R., and Rice, N. S. C.: Detection of Chlamydia (Bedsonia) in certain infections of man: clinical study of genital tract, eye, rectum and other sites of recovery of Chlamydia, J. Infect. Dis. **120**:463, 1969.
9. Expert Committee on Trachoma: World Health Organization technical report series no. 234, third report, 1962.
10. Gordon, F. B., Harper, I. A., Quan, A. L., Treharne, J. D., Dwyer, R. St. C., and Garland, J. A.: Detection of Chlamydia (Bedsonia) in certain infections of man: laboratory procedures: comparison of yolk sac and cell culture for detection and isolation, J. Infect. Dis. **120**:451, 1969.
11. Halberstaedter, L., and von Prowazek, S.: Zur aetiologie des Trachoms, Deutsch. Med. Wschr. **33**:1285, 1907.
12. Jawetz, E.: Agents of trachoma and inclusion conjunctivitis, Ann. Rev. Microbiol. **18**:301, 1964.
13. Jawetz, E.: Summary of discussion of papers 67-73, Amer. J. Ophthal. **63**:1654, 1967.
14. Julianelle, L. A.: Etiology of trachoma, New York, 1938, The Commonwealth Fund, pp. 42, 148.
15. Kugelmass, I. N., editor: Trachoma: prevention and treatment, Springfield, Ill., 1967, Charles C Thomas, Publisher.
16. Lindner, K.: Gonoblennorrhöe, Einschlussblennorrhöe und Trachom, Graefes Arch. Ophth. **78**:345, 1911.

17. MacCallan, A. F.: Trachoma, London, 1936, Butterworth and Co.
18. Morax, V.: Sur l'etiologie des ophthalmies du nouveau-né et la déclaration obligatoire, Ann. Oculist. **129**:346, 1903.
19. Nicolle, C., Blaisot, L., and Cuénod, A.: Le magot animal réactif du trachome: filtrabilité du virus; pouvoir infectant des larmes, C. R. Acad. Sci. **155**:241, 1912.
19a. Nichols, R. L., editor: Trachoma and related disorders caused by chlamydial agents: proceeings of a symposium held in Boston, Massachusetts, 17-20 August 1970, Amsterdam, 1971, Excerpta Medica Foundation.
20. Nichols, R. L., Bobb, A. A., Haddad, N. A., and McComb, D. E.: Immunofluorescent studies of the microbiologic epidemiology of trachoma in Saudi Arabia, Amer. J. Ophthal. **63**: 1372, 1967.
21. Schmeichler, L.: Üeber Chlamydozoenbefunde bei nichtgonorrhoischer Blennorrhöe der Neugeborenen, Berl. Klin. Wschr. **46**: 2057, 1909.
22. Stargardt, K.: Über Epithelzellveränderungen beim Trachom und andern Conjunctivalerkrankungen, Graefes Arch. Ophth. **69**:525, 1909.
23. T'ang, F., Chang, H., Huang, Y., and Wang, K.: Studies of the etiology of trachoma with special reference to isolation of the virus in chick embryo, Chin. Med. J. **75**:429, 1957.
23a. Tarizzo, M. L., Nataf, R., and Nabli, B.: Experimental inoculation of thirteen volunteers with agent isolated from inclusion conjunctivitis, Amer. J. Ophthal. **63**:1120, 1967.
24. Thygeson, P.: The nature of the elementary and initial bodies of trachoma, Arch. Ophthal. **12**:307, 1934.
25. Thygeson, P.: Trachoma manual and atlas, U. S. Department of Health, Education, and Welfare, Public Health Service Publication No. 541, 1960.
26. Thygeson, P.: Corneal changes in TRIC agent infections, Amer. J. Ophthal. **63**:1278, 1967.
27. Thygeson, P., and Crocker, T. T.: Observations on experimental trachoma and inclusion conjunctivitis, Amer. J. Ophthal. **42**:76, 1956.
28. Thygeson, P., and Dawson, C. R.: Trachoma and follicular conjunctivitis in children, Arch. Ophthal. **75**:3, 1966.
29. Thygeson, P., Dawson, C., Hanna, L., Jawetz, E., and Okumoto, M.: Observations on experimental trachoma in monkeys produced by strains of virus propagated in the yolk sac, Amer. J. Ophthal. **50**:907, 1960.
30. Thygeson, P., and Hanna, L.: TRIC agents. In Lennette, E. H.,. and Schmidt, N. J., editors: Diagnostic procedures for viral and rickettsial infections, ed. 4, New York, 1969, American Public Health Association, p. 904.
31. Thygeson, P., and Proctor, F. I.: The filtrability of trachoma virus, Arch. Ophthal. **13**: 1018, 1935.
32. Thygeson, P., Proctor, F. I., and Richards, P.: Etiologic significance of the elementary body in trachoma, Amer. J. Ophthal. **18**:811, 1935.
33. Wang, S., and Grayston, J. T.: Pannus with experimental trachoma and inclusion conjunctivitis agent: infection of Taiwan monkeys, Amer. J. Ophthal. **63**:1133, 1967.

15

Rickettsiae in relation to infection of the eye

THE RICKETTSIAE

The generic term *Rickettsia* belongs to a group of agents of disease, first discovered by Dr. H. T. Ricketts[23] (Fig. 15-1) in 1906. They appear under the light microscope as coccobacillary or bacillary forms usually about $0.3 \times 0.5\ \mu$ in size; they divide by binary fission. Fig. 15-2 shows massive multiplication of these organisms in a macrophage infected with rickettsiae causing Q fever. Typhus *Rickettsia* organisms growing in the yolk sac of a chick embryo are seen by electron microscopy in Fig. 15-3, where variations in form are apparent. Although these organisms seem structurally similar to bacteria, and like bacteria contain both DNA and RNA, most of them are unable to survive except in living cells. They are further remarkable because they have a wide host range and are transmitted from host to host by insect or arachnoid vectors—namely, lice and fleas or ticks and mites. Table 15-1 presents some of the characteristic features of the seven *Rickettsia* species that are important human pathogens and that also produce noteworthy infection of the eye. Many mammals are susceptible to strains pathogenic for man and act as reservoirs of the organisms. A number of possible vectors are available for most strains, and some vectors are also hosts to the organisms, passing them on to their offspring. Rickettsiae, because of their mode of division, possession of DNA and RNA, and their chemical composition and metabolic activities, are considered obligately parasitic, true bacteria.[13] In most instances, they require living cells for growth.

Rickettsial diseases of man are undoubtedly of long standing. Typhus is thought to have existed at the time of Hippocrates, and tsutsugamushi disease was described in a Chinese medical book of the sixth century A.D.[30] Nevertheless, Ricketts was the first to transmit one of this group of diseases, Rocky Mountain spotted fever, to laboratory animals and to describe the organism. He injected the blood of patients, drawn during the first few days of their illness, into monkeys and guinea pigs, which proved susceptible to infection. Ricketts then demonstrated that a tick transmitted the disease to man, and in 1907[24] he reported that the "virus" was hereditary in the tick. Descriptions of the organisms of Rocky Mountain spotted fever were given by Ricketts in 1909,[24] and descriptions of the organisms of Mexican typhus were given by Ricketts and Wilder in 1910.[25] By cross-immunity experiments these investigators showed that the two diseases were distinguishable immunologically. At the age of 39, Ricketts died of typhus fever in Mexico.

The rickettsial diseases of man usually are characterized by a lesion at the site of the insect bite, which produces an eschar. The onset of symptoms occurs after 1 to 2 weeks' incubation, and the diseases are characterized by high fever, severe headache, and general malaise. In a few days a macular rash or maculopapular rash appears on the trunk and extends over much of the body. In the case of Rocky Mountain spotted fever there is a petechial rash, and in Q fever the lesion is in the lungs and only rarely is there a cutaneous rash. In this latter disease, transmission is principally by inhalation of infected droplets from expired air or contaminated dust, and here there is no eschar. The organisms in man are found chiefly in endothelial cells of capillaries, arterioles, and venules. The distribution of the lesions is widespread, but the skin and central nervous system are more severely affected. Thrombi form, followed by hemorrhage and perivascular infiltration. The organisms also may be present in smooth muscle cells of the media of some arterioles. On this basic pattern the various rickettsiae exhibit certain individual characteristics, which will be mentioned later, since they are relevant to the eye.

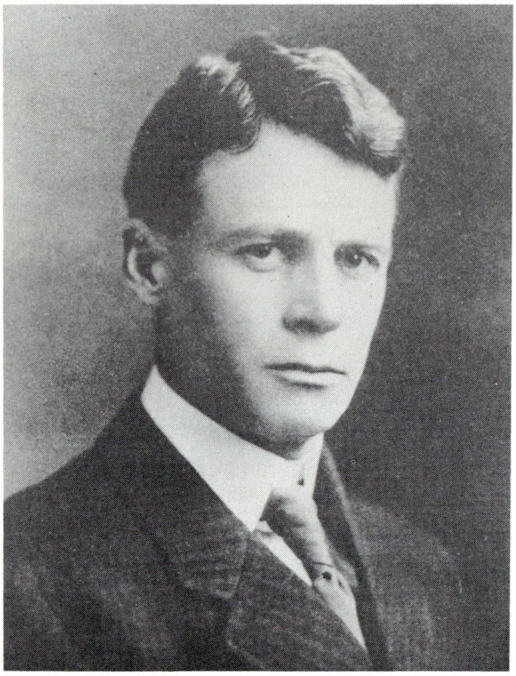

Fig. 15-1. Dr. Howard Taylor Ricketts (1871-1910). (From Olpp, G.: Charakterkopfe der Tropenmedizin, Berlin, 1936, Verlag Die Brücke Zur Heimat, p. 60.)

The rickettsiae, which are demonstrable in the cytoplasm and sometimes in the nuclei of cells, may be seen by staining with Giemsa stain, in which they appear bluish purple, or with Macchiavello's stain, after which they are bright red. The organism can be found in the saliva and gut of vectors and in the bloodstream and vascular endothelium of the host. Monkeys, rabbits, guinea pigs, mice, and rats are among the

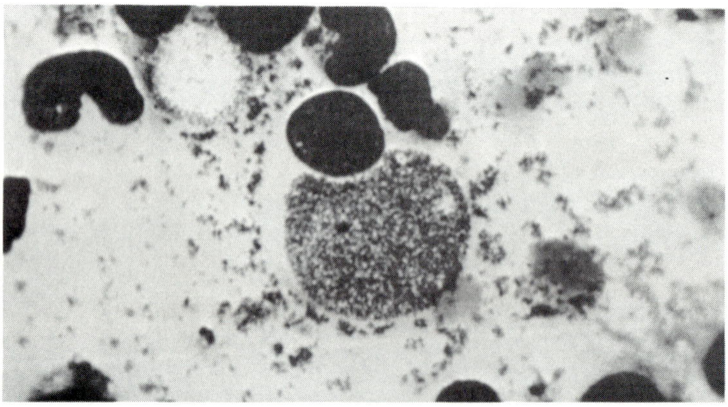

Fig. 15-2. Rickettsiae of Q fever in a smear of skin exudate. Note the macrophage packed with enormous numbers of rickettsiae. (× 1,125.) (From Burrows, W., and others: Textbook of microbiology, ed. 19, Philadelphia, 1968, W. B. Saunders Co., p. 829.)

Table 15-1. Rickettsiae producing ocular disease

Disease produced	Etiologic agent	Natural cycle: Arthropod	Natural cycle: Mammal host range	Susceptable laboratory animals	Positive Weil-Felix test	Complement-fixation test	Immunity	Geographical distribution
Typhus								
Epidemic	*Rickettsia prowazekii*	Human body louse—*Pediculus corporis*	Man only	Guinea pig—fever only	OX-19	Positive, group and type specific	For many years	Worldwide
Endemic murine	*Rickettsia mooseri*	Rat louse—*Polyplax spinulosa*; Rat flea—*Xenopsylla*	Wild rats, rodents, field mice	Guinea pig—fever, scrotal swelling	OX-19	Positive, group and type specific	For many years	Worldwide
Spotted fever								
Rocky Mountain spotted fever	*Rickettsia rickettsii*	Ticks: wood tick—*Dermacentor andersoni;* dog tick—*Dermacentor variabilis* and other species	Dogs, wild rodents	Guinea pig—fever, scrotal necrosis	OX-19 OX-2	Positive, group and type specific	High degree of immunity	Western hemisphere, Brazil, Colombia
Boutonneuse fever South African tick bite fever	*Rickettsia conori*	Ticks: *Rhipicephalus sanguineus* and a number of others	Dogs, wild rodents	Guinea pig—fever, scrotal swelling	OX-19 OX-2	Positive, group and type specific	Present	Mediterranean countries of Europe, Asia, Africa
Scrub typhus	*Rickettsia tsutsugamushi*	Several species of trombiculid mites	Wild rodents, many species	Mouse—rough fur, inactive, ascites	OX-K	Positive in about 50% of patients	Second attack may occur within a few years after initial disease	Australia, Pacific Islands, Asia
Epidemic Q fever	*Coxiella burnetti*	Ticks: number of species	Very broad; wild and domesticated animals, birds	Guinea pig—fever only	Negative	Positive, group and type specific	Second attacks have been reported	Worldwide
Trench fever	*Rickettsia quintana*	Human body louse—*Pediculus humanus*	Man	—	Negative	None available	Partial immunity	Europe, Africa, North America

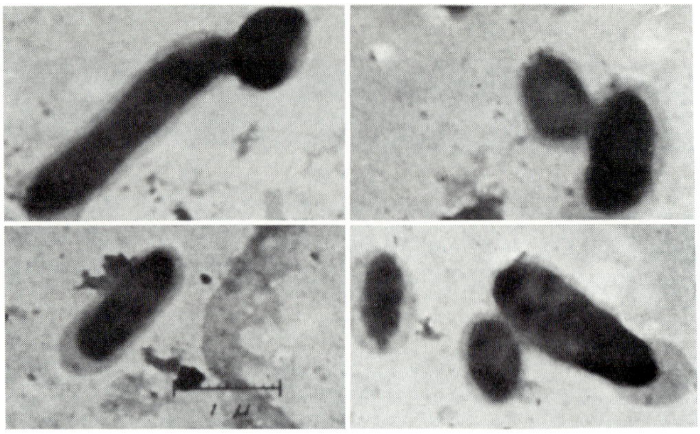

Fig. 15-3. Electron micrographs of typhus rickettsiae from egg yolk culture. Note the variability in size, ranging from cocco-bacillary to bacillary forms, and the capsular material surrounding the individual cells. (Courtesy Lilly Research Laboratories.)

mammals that can be infected experimentally with various strains of rickettsiae that are pathogenic for man. The rickettsiae may be cultivated in tissue-cultured cells or in the yolk sac of 5- to 7-day-old chick embryos. Isolation is quite difficult, however, and of only limited use in diagnosis.[9]

Immunologic classification of rickettsiae may be made by complement-fixation (Table 15-1), agglutination, and neutralization tests. Though sharing some common antigens, the rickettsiae are immunologically distinguishable, and immunity to infection is strain specific. The rickettsiae also carry antigens shared in common with certain strains of the *Proteus* group of bacilli—namely OX-19, OX-2, and OX-K. Patients suffering from one of the various diseases produced by the rickettsiae develop agglutinins to one or two of the three strains of *Proteus* involved, or to none at all. After performing an agglutination test, the Weil-Felix test, and using the patient's serum and suspensions of the *Proteus* bacilli, one should look for rising titers of antibodies during the course of the disease. This series of tests is most useful and avoids the necessity of using the rickettsiae as antigens.

Recovery from an attack of most rickettsial diseases results in lasting immunity, perhaps because of the persistence of the organisms in the human host. Brill's disease, however, is a relapse seen in some who have had epidemic typhus fever. This is a relatively mild disease, when compared with the original attack, and is thought to result from the prolonged survival of *R. prowazekii* in some tissue of the body in a latent form. It occurs many years after the initial attack.

The fact that infection with rickettsiae produces lasting immunity suggests that vaccines should be successful prophylactic agents, and this has proved to be correct in some of the diseases. In practice, however, the more practical public health measure against epidemic attacks of typhus fever is to eradicate the vector. DDT has been used with excellent results in areas where typhus is prevalent. The hairy areas of the body, which harbor lice, are sprayed with DDT, thus killing the vector and breaking the cycle.

When untreated, rickettsial infections may cause a high mortality rate; in epidemic periods the mortality for typhus has run as high as 70%. Both chloramphenicol and tetracyclines have been effective in the treatment of rickettsial disease in man.

Epidemic typhus, murine typhus, Rocky Mountain spotted fever, boutonneuse fever, African tick typhus, scrub typhus, Q fever, and trench fever may be associated with lesions of the eye. Table 15-2 presents features of the ocular lesions produced by each

Table 15-2. Ocular diseases caused by rickettsial infections

Etiologic agent	Primary disease	Incidence of ocular involvement in various parts of the eye, clinical features, and complications that may occur	References
Rickettsia prowazekii	Epidemic typhus fever	Systemic infection can be acquired through conjunctival route; conjunctivitis and conjunctival hyperemia; subconjunctival hemorrhages; photophobia; corneal ulcers; chorioretinitis and retinal hemorrhages; optic neuritis; uveitis; vitreous opacities	Brooks and Fineberg[3]* Duke-Elder[8] Lebas and Bernaerts-Lebas[15] Rouher and others[26]
Rickettsia mooseri	Endemic murine typhus	Mild conjunctivitis; systemic infection may result through conjunctiva as portal of entry; uveitis; perivascular chorioretinitis	Lebas and Bernaerts-Lebas[15] Rouher and others[26]
Rickettsia rickettsii	Rocky Mountain spotted fever	Conjunctivitis and conjunctival hyperemia; photophobia; iridocyclitis	Lebas and Bernaerts-Lebas[15] Venable and Pollack[29]
Rickettsia conori	Boutonneuse fever South African tick bite fever	Primary lesion and infection of conjunctiva results from direct contamination after squashing tick or spurting blood from crushing tick between fingers; initially, lesion is ulcerative or granulomatous; extensive involvement of preauricular and submaxillary nodes; chorioretinitis and iridocyclitis; in systemic infection, a mild preeruptive conjunctivitis	Audoueineix[2] Clavel and Hamart[5] Duke-Elder[8] Lebas and Bernaerts-Lebas[15] Rhodes and van Rooyen[22]
Rickettsia tsutsugamushi	Scrub typhus	Conjunctival hyperemia; subconjunctival hemorrhages sometimes associated with ecchymosis of eyelids; eschar on eyelid; corneal ulcers; retinal edema and hemorrhages; uveitis; vitreous opacities; engorgement of veins; nystagmus; if primary lesion appears on eyelids, a black escharotic ulcer develops with a violent conjunctival reaction and lymphadenopathy	Ahlm and Lipshutz[1] Lebas and Bernaerts-Lebas[15] Scheie[27]
Coxiella burnetti	Endemic Q fever	Infection may be transmitted through human conjunctiva; violent conjunctival hyperemia, gangrene of eyelids, uveitis, chorioretinitis, episcleritis, optic neuritis result; ocular involvement in the course of the usual disease may be associated with retroorbital pain, photophobia, and injection of conjunctiva	Audoueineix[2] Calmettes and others[4] Lebas and Bernaerts-Lebas[15]
Rickettsia quintana	Trench fever	Conjunctivitis; hyperemia of conjunctiva; retinitis	Lebas and others[15]

*Superscript numbers indicate references at end of chapter.

A

B

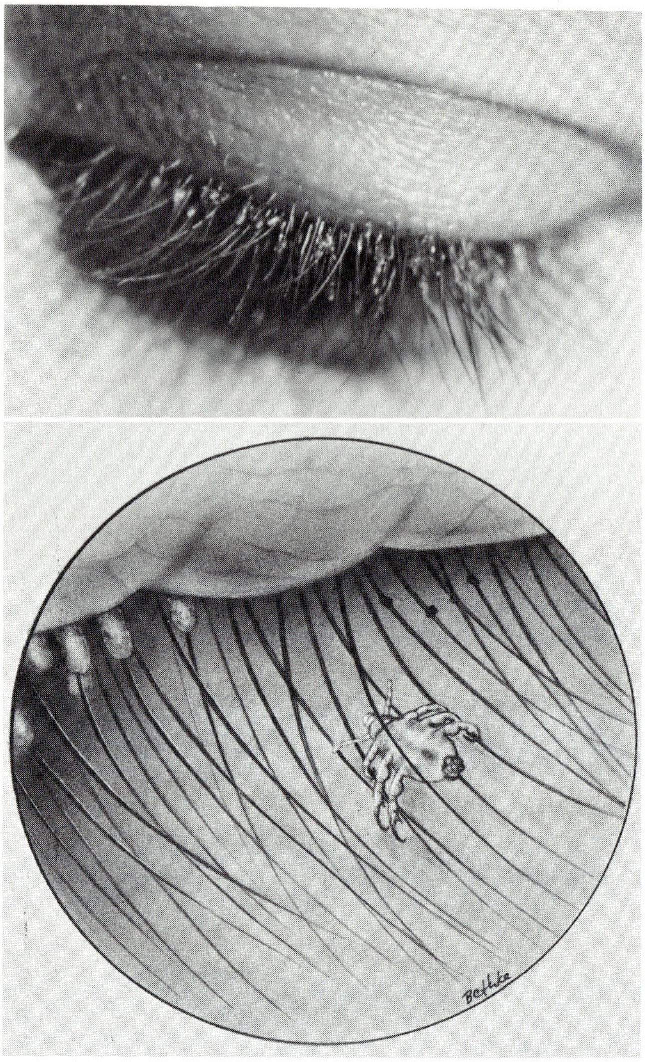

Fig. 15-4. A, Pediculosis of the eyelid. **B,** *Phthirus pubis* on eyelashes seen in **A.** (Courtesy Dr. R. Castroviejo.)

organism. Since rickettsial organisms are spread throughout the body via the bloodstream, ocular manifestations of rickettsial diseases are, in a majority of cases, an expression of the widespread distribution of the organisms in the end arterioles, capillaries, and venules. As previously stated, the inflammation produced in these vessels causes thrombus formation with leukocytic infiltration, hemorrhage, and focal necrosis. Any part of the eye may be involved, a fact that accounts for the great variety of ocular lesions reported in Table 15-2.

Infections of the eye, in rare instances, may be acquired by the primary introduction of the rickettsial organism into the eye tissue. This can come from a bite on the eyelid by the arthopod vector. Fig. 15-4, *A* illustrates the presence of lice on the lid margin and eyelashes of a patient seen at the IOCPMC. Fig. 15-4, *B*, is a drawing of an individual louse. In such circumstances the bite of an infected louse produces an initial lesion, which develops as an eschar on the lid. Infection of the eye may also occur if an individual rubs his eye after he contaminates his fingers with infected blood or feces by crushing a tick or louse or by scratching a bite on the skin. The disease spreads from the initial site to produce the generalized infection characteristic of rickettsial disease. Further involvement of the eye may then develop later in the course of the disease.

TYPHUS FEVER

Epidemic typhus fever, caused by *R. prowazekii* (named to honor von Prowazek who, like Ricketts, died of typhus fever while studying the disease), is associated with poverty, overcrowding, war, famine, and all other conditions that favor the human body louse. Between 1918 and 1922 Eastern Europe and Russia were ravaged, and some 30 million people were infected; mortality was 10%.[30] In World War II, typhus fever complicated military operations in Europe; and in the Far East, Japan, and Korea, outbreaks of typhus also developed. Deaths from typhus fever have been greater among medical personnel than among other groups, and laboratory infestions have occurred frequently.

Epidemic typhus fever is a severe febrile disease that arises spontaneously only in man. Man is both the host and the reservoir of this infection. The human body louse, *Pediculus humanus* var. *corporis*, is the most important vector, although *Pediculus capitis* may also transmit the infection. The rickettsiae fill the intestinal tract of the louse and are deposited on the person's skin when the louse draws blood. The bite causes itching, and man scratches the feces into the bite. After an incubation period of 10 to 14 days there is an abrupt onset of chills and fever with prostration. A maculopapular rash appears in 5 to 7 days first on the trunk and later on the extremities. Only in severely ill patients is the face involved. *R. prowazekii* is found in the blood of the patient during the febrile period and is infective for lice feeding on the patient during the first 10 days of the illness.

A review of ocular manifestations in typhus fever was made by Brooks and Fineberg[3] in 1951. While reviewing the literature from 1867 to 1943, they collected reports of 2,031 cases of eye involvement caused by typhus. Their paper opens with a quotation from Larionow: ". . . man solle die Augen typhöser Kranker öfter untersuchen."[14*] The great variety of lesions reported indicates that this advice should be carefully followed. Their report covers every area of the eye, and their table carries 38 types of pathologic conditions. The commonest disease reported was optic neuritis (395 examples, or 19.75%). This is followed by 274 cases of constructed visual fields (13.95%), 144 cases of retinal hyperemia (7.20%), 136 cases of retinal edema (6.80%), 110 cases of papillary hyperemia (5.10%), and 85 cases of conjunctivitis (4.20%). The cornea was involved in the disease in 31 instances; the pupils in 44; the uveal tract in 33; the media in 29; the optic nerve in addition to neuritis and papillary hyperemia in an additional 19 instances. Besides retinal hemorrhage and edema, there were 32 instances of other retinal pathologic conditions. Blood vessels of the eye were visibly implicated 26 times; and in addition to constriction of visual fields, the function of the eye was impaired in various other ways 33 times. The authors point out that, with the possible exception of constricted visual fields, most of the eye complications are those reflecting change in the circulation; and the authors conclude that in typhus one should search for changes in the eye that can result from involvement of the circulation of the eye.

In Duke-Elder's discussion of ocular manifestations in typhus fever, the role of conjunctivitis, with or without hemorrhages, is stressed.[8] He states that conjunctival hyperemia is invariable and that in some 10% of the cases, catarrhal conjunctivitis with slight secretion occurs.

The above manifestations of ocular involvement in typhus are those that take place during the acute disease and that

---

*"One should frequently examine the eyes of the patient with typhus fever."

fade with convalescence. P. V. Morax and his associates[18] have reported on 15 patients, 9 with uveitis and the remainder with uveitis and additional complications. The only sign pointing to the possible cause was the presence of antibodies in the patients' sera, which agglutinated one of the preparations of rickettsial antigens used for the microagglutination test (a test that is credited with a high degree of specificity).[13] Appropriate antibiotic treatment improved or cured the ocular condition and also eliminated the positive agglutination tests. Four of the patients had antibodies to *R. prowazekii.* The idea that latent rickettsial infections might produce uveitis many months later is reasonable, since it has a counterpart in Brill's disease, an exacerbation of a latent infection with *R. prowazekii,* which may occur many years after the acute manifestations have subsided.

MURINE TYPHUS

Murine typhus is an endemic disease that has been reported in many parts of the world and that clinically is similar to mild typhus fever. *R. mooseri,* the etiologic agent, resembles *R. prowazekii* in shape and staining properties. The two share a common soluble antigen, but each has immunologically distinct toxins; infection with one does not protect against the other disease. *R. mooseri* finds a reservoir in rats, and both the rat louse and the rat flea carry the infection from rat to rat. The disease is transmitted from rat to man by the rat flea and from man to man by the body louse. It is possible that food soiled with rat urine may also be a source of infection.

The incubation period of murine typhus, like that of typhus fever, is 1 to 2 weeks. An eschar is found at the site of the infecting bite, and the patient develops fever, generalized pains, and headache. The macular rash comes about 5 days after the onset of fever and spreads from the trunk to the limbs. Usually all symptoms are milder than those seen in typhus fever, and there are a smaller number of complications and a lower death rate. However, a severe case of murine typhus will simulate typhus fever. As in other rickettsial diseases, chloramphenicol or tetracycline or both are effective in treatment. Infection establishes long-term immunity.

The involvement of the eye in this disease is slight when compared with that seen in typhus fever (Table 15-2). Usually it is limited to a mild conjunctivitis. It is possible, however, for one to infect the conjunctiva directly by rubbing the eye with fingers contaminated by feces of the carrier flea. This produces a severe conjunctivitis, and the generalized infection develops from this local site. As in typhus fever the organisms are present in the blood for several days, and such blood will transmit infection to laboratory animals or chick embryos.

In this disease, as well as in typhus fever, late ocular lesions may occur—namely, uveitis with perivascular chorioretinitis. The evidence that these conditions are late sequelae of the rickettsial disease has been based on the presence of significant titers of agglutinating antibodies in the patient's serum.

ROCKY MOUNTAIN SPOTTED FEVER

Rocky Mountain spotted fever was first reported in 1873 from the Rocky Mountain areas. As has been described earlier, Ricketts found that the infection was transmitted to man by the wood tick, and he infected guinea pigs and monkeys with the blood of patients with Rocky Mountain spotted fever. He found the agent in blood smears from man, guinea pigs, and monkeys, and in the tissues of the ticks. The ticks transmit the agent to their progeny. Rocky Mountain spotted fever often is an occupational disease, seen among hunters, foresters, highway engineers, maintenance crews, and other individuals exposed to wood ticks. It is prevalent in all parts of the world. In the USA it extends to the Atlantic Coast and is found in the southeastern states. Thirteen cases from the Cape Cod area, with two deaths, were reported in 1969.[11]

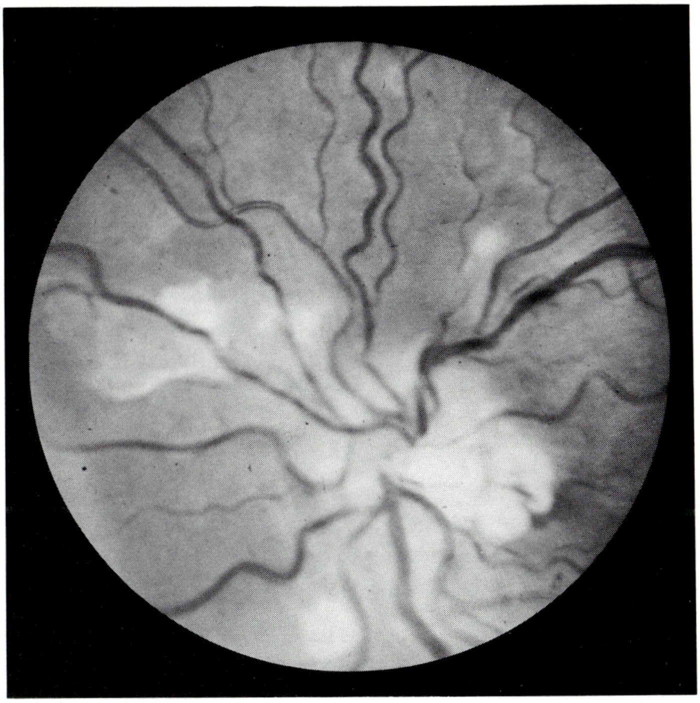

Fig. 15-5. Fundus changes in Rocky Mountain spotted fever. Eye showing papilledema, cotton-wool exudates, small, flame-shaped hemorrhages, tortuosity of the vessels, and venous engorgement. (From Presley, G. D.: Amer. J. Ophthal. **67**:263, 1969.)

The etiologic agent of Rocky Mountain spotted fever is similar in morphologic and cultural characteristics to *R. prowazekii.* It has the characteristic predilection for endothelial cells of small vessels. The incubation period of the disease is rather short, usually 4 to 8 days; the onset is abrupt, characterized by fever, chills, headache, and muscle and bone pains. In 2 to 14 days a generalized rash develops, which may be petechial or hemorrhagic. Unlike the rash of typhus fever, it usually starts on the extremities and moves centripetally; the palms of the hands and the soles of the feet are also involved. The disease seen in the western United States is carried by the wood tick, *Dermacentor andersoni,* that in the Atlantic area by the dog tick, *D. variabilis.* Immunity develops in man and in laboratory animals after recovery from infection. Effective vaccines were first employed in the prophylaxis of this disease.

The ocular manifestations of infection with *R. rickettsii* include a conjunctivitis characterized by hyperemia with photophobia and mild catarrh.[29] Iridocyclitis, occurring as a late sequela, has been described by Lebas and Bernaerts-Lebas.[15] Presley[20] in 1969 examined 6 children, 5 to 14 years old, in the acute stage of the disease at the Division of Ophthalmology, University of North Carolina. All but one showed lesions of the fundus (Fig. 15-5), which included engorgement of retinal veins, papilledema, retinal edema, cytoid bodies, flare-shaped hemorrhages, Roth spots, and an arterial occlusion. A similar case has been reported by Raab and his associates.[21]

BOUTONNEUSE FEVER AND SOUTH AFRICAN TICK BITE FEVER

Rickettsia conori was recognized and first described by Conor and Bruch in 1910 in Tunisia.[6] The disease caused by this agent is known as boutonneuse fever. The name boutonneuse refers to a local nodule, the black buttonlike necrotic primary lesion, tache noir, usually observed on the leg. *R. conori* is also the cause of South African tick bite fever. *R. conori* belongs to the Rocky Mountain spotted fever group and is morphologically and immunologically similar to but separable from *R. rickettsii*, by toxin neutralization tests and other serologic methods.

Infected tissue cells may exhibit intranuclear as well as intracytoplasmic rickettsiae, but the latter predominate. *R. conori* has been cultivated in yolk sacs of the developing chick embryo; the organisms multiply intranuclearly when growing in the chorioallantoic membrane of the fertile egg. The animal reservoirs of infection are the dog, rodents, and mice; the disease is transmitted by ticks.

Following the incubation period, which lasts 5 to 7 days, the infection is characterized by fever, chills, headache, and malaise. The lesions are similar to those seen in typhus. The generalized maculopapular rash, involving most of the body, including face, palms, and soles, appears on the fourth day. The Weil-Felix test becomes positive during the second week, and complement-fixing antibodies appear shortly thereafter. The diagnosis is established by the clinical picture, including the tache noir, positive serologic tests, and geographic location.

Ocular disease seen in boutonneuse fever (as outlined in Table 15-2) is, according to Duke-Elder,[8] probably the most interesting of the rickettsioses, from the ophthalmologic point of view, for the conjunctival infection is characteristically acquired by direct contamination. The dog tick is the vector, and infection of the eye comes about by contamination after squashing the tick.

In the case of the patient with South African tick bite fever, shown in Fig. 15-6, infected blood had squirted into the eye. Pronounced edema of the lid and soft tissues below the eye are seen.[22] Rubbing an eye with contaminated fingers will also in-

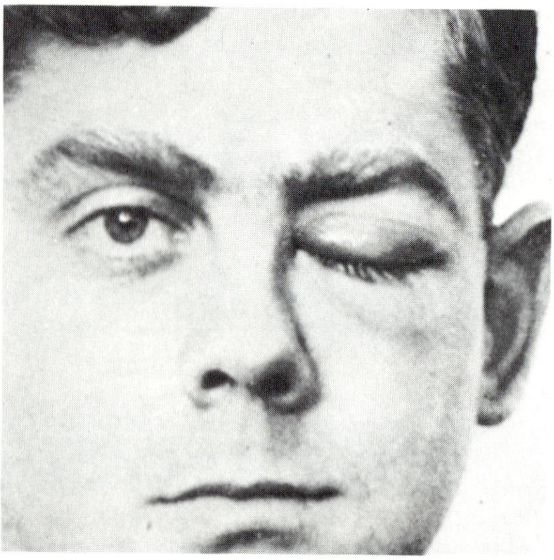

Fig. 15-6. South African tick typhus. Primary lesion on conjunctiva following spurting of blood from crushing an infected dog tick between the fingers. (Courtesy Dr. J. H. S. Gear. From Rhodes, A. J., and van Rooyen, C. E.: Textbook of virology for students and practitioners of medicine, ed. 4, Baltimore, 1962, The Williams & Wilkins Co.)

fect the conjunctiva. The initial lesion is ulcerative or granulomatous, and the preauricular and submaxillary nodes are rapidly involved. Chorioretinitis and paramacular hemorrhages, as well as iridocyclitis, may develop. The systemic disease manifests itself in about 5 days. A mild conjunctivitis is present during the systemic infection.

SCRUB TYPHUS

Scrub typhus, or tsutsugamushi disease, was originally described in Japan and is also found in many of the islands of Southwest and Eastern Asia and in India and Australia. The disease occurred in military units in the Asiatic-Pacific area during World War II. The animal reservoirs of the disease are the field mouse and other rodents, and the vectors are the trombiculid mites. These, like the tick vectors of the spotted fever group, transmit the rickettsiae transovarially to succeeding generations of mites.

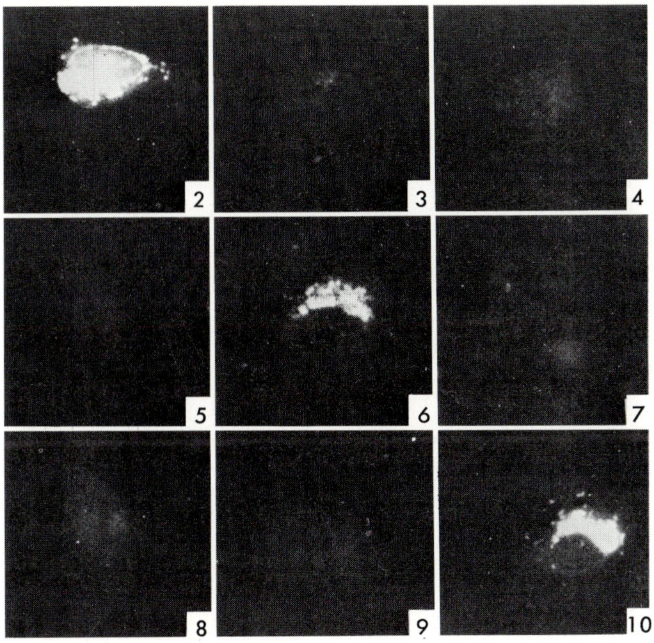

Fig. 15-7. Illustration of the use of fluorescein-labeled antibody to identify strain differences in the *R. tsutsugamushi* organism. Gilliam, Karp, and Kato strains were used to immunize guinea pigs. Immune sera obtained against all three strains were labeled with fluorescein and used to stain peritoneal exudates from infected mice. Slides 2 to 4 were prepared from mice infected with the Gilliam strain, 5 to 7 with the Karp strain, and 8 to 10 with the Kato strain. All were treated with a 1:4 dilution of the labeled antisera to Gilliam, Karp, and Kato strains, respectively. Organisms were stained only with specific antibody. (From Iida, T., Kawashima, H., and Kawamura, A.: J. Immun. **95**:1129, 1965. © 1965 The Williams & Wilkins Co., Baltimore.)

R. tsutsugamushi is characterized by variation in antigenic composition. Shishido[28] has differentiated three antigenically distinct groups: the Gilliam, Karp, and Kato strains. Fig. 15-7 illustrates the use of specific fluorescein-labeled antisera to differentiate the three groups. Slides prepared from peritoneal exudate of infected mice were stained with antibodies specific to each of the three strains; each fluorescent antibody bound only to its specific strain.[12]

The incubation period of this rickettsial disease is 6 to 21 days. A generalized maculopapular rash appears at the end of the first week. The rise of agglutinins in the patient's serum to *Proteus* OX-K strain, as determined by the Weil-Felix test, is considered the most useful diagnostic measure in scrub typhus. Immunity to this disease lasts only a few years.

Various ocular changes may occur in infection caused by *R. tsutsugamushi.* Congestion of the conjunctiva has been observed in the acute phase of the infection so constantly that it is considered a clinical feature. Sheie[27] in 1947 recorded ocular changes in the routine examination of 451 patients suffering from scrub typhus and noted the incidence of ocular pathologic characteristics as follows:

Conjunctival injection	38 %
Subconjunctival hemorrhages	6.4%
Ecchymosis of eyelids	1 %
Eschar of eyelid	0.5%
Engorgement of veins	67 %
Fixation nystagmus	0.5%
Retinal edema	36 %
Retinal hemorrhages	6.6%
Exudates	4.9%
Uveitis	1.3%
Vitreous opacities	4.6%

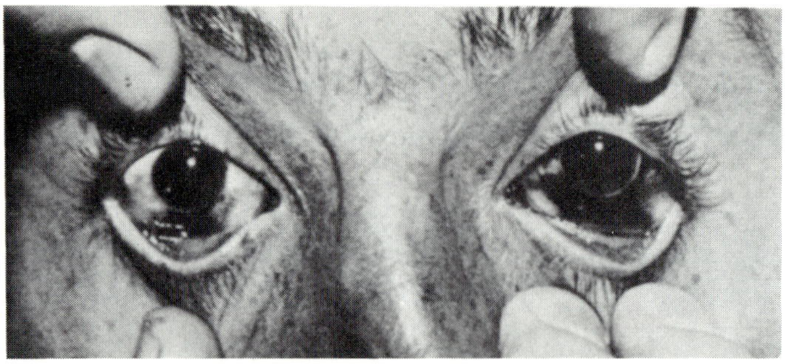

Fig. 15-8. Bilateral subconjunctival hemorrhages in patient with scrub typhus. (From Scheie, H. G.: Trans. Amer. Ophthal. Soc. **45**:637, 1947.)

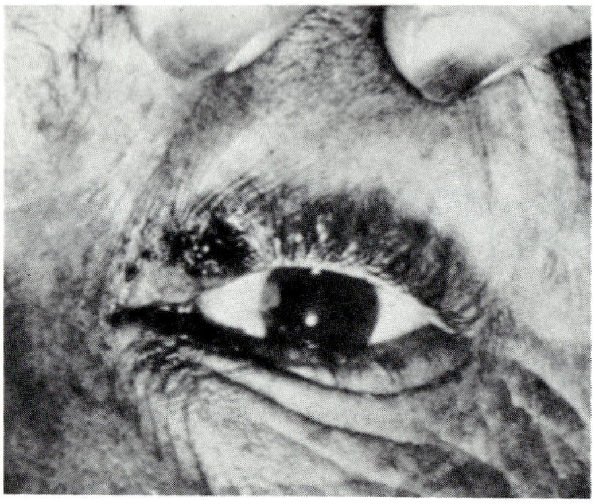

Fig. 15-9. Primary lesion of eyelid in patient with scrub typhus. (Courtesy H. G. Scheie.)

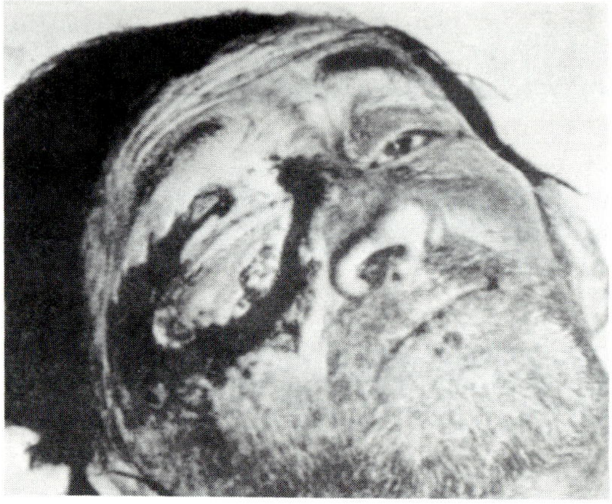

Fig. 15-10. Q fever. Shows widespread ulceration in the region of eyelids with preauricular adenopathy in a 64-year-old patient. (From Calmettes, L., Deodati, F., and Bec, P.: Bull. Mem. S. F. O. **73**:509, 1960, Masson et Cie, Paris.)

Figs. 15-8 and 15-9, from Scheie's report, illustrate bilateral subconjunctival hemorrhage and a primary lesion of the eyelid in the area where mites might like to rest. Pathologic studies of the eyes obtained at autopsy showed subacute diffuse choroiditis to be the basic lesion. As may be seen in Table 15-2, retinal hemorrhage and corneal ulcer have been added to this list by other investigators. In addition, Macaskill[17] has reported bilateral optic atrophy in one patient 6 months after the acute illness.

Q FEVER

Q fever is a self-limited infection caused by *Coxiella burnetti.* The symptoms of this disease are more characteristic of influenza or atypical pneumonia than of typhus. This is caused in part by the mode of transmission, which typically is inhalation or ingestion. Ticks transmit the agent to cattle, sheep, and goats. Cows develop a chronic infection of the udder, and rickettsiae are excreted in the milk. The placenta of cows and sheep also contain the organisms, and parturition creates infectious aerosols. Dust becomes contaminated. Thus, Q fever patients rarely give a history of tick bite. Patients and animals develop agglutinins and complement-fixing antibodies, but man does not produce agglutinins to *Proteus* antigens. The unique resistance of *C. bur-*

netti to prolonged exposure in nature contributes to the spread of the agent.

After an incubation period of 9 to 20 days following respiratory exposure, there is abrupt onset of fever, headache, muscle pain, and malaise. The temperature remains elevated with fluctuations for a period of about 3 weeks. In contrast to the other rickettsial infections, there is no rash.

General infection with *C. burnetti* may be acquired through the conjunctiva. It is characterized by violent conjunctival hyperemia and occasionally gangrene of the eyelids.[19] Uveitis, chorioretinitis, episcleritis, and optical neuritis may occur. Fig. 15-10 illustrates ulceration in the region of the eyelids with preauricular adenopathy. Harvey and his co-workers[10] in 1951 described a small outbreak of Q fever in East Kent. The ocular features in these patients consisted of retroorbital pain with photophobia and some injection of the conjunctiva.

TRENCH FEVER

Trench fever is a self-limited louse-borne rickettsial disease characterized by intermittent fever and generalized aches and pains. The agent, *R. quintana,* grows extracellularly in the louse intestine and is excreted in louse feces. The organisms can be cultivated on agar enriched with 10% fresh blood. Transmission occurs by rubbing louse feces into skin abrasions produced by the bite of the louse. The incubation period varies from 5 to 38 days, but usually is 2 to 4 weeks. History of contact with lice within this period is a useful diagnostic aid. Trench fever is associated with headache, exhaustion, fever, a roseolar rash, and relapses. This disease may show exacerbation over a period of a year.

Ocular features of infection caused by *R. quintana* include conjunctivitis, hyperemia of the conjunctiva, photophobia, and retinitis. Deduit[7] in 1963 described a case of iridocyclitis in a patient suffering from paresis. The patient was inoculated with a strain of *R. quintana* for therapeutic purposes and developed iridocyclitis and later a small focus of retinitis.

REFERENCES

1. Ahlm, C. E., and Lipshutz, J.: Tsutsugamushi fever in the Southwest Pacific Theater, J.A.M.A. **124**:1095, 1944.
2. Audoueineix, M. E.: Les complications oculaires des rickettsioses dans la Sarthe, Bull. Soc. Franc. Ophthal. **73**:477, 1960.
3. Brooks, F., and Fineberg, R.: Ocular manifestations of typhus fever: a review of the literature from 1867 to 1943, Amer. J. Ophthal. **34**:605, 1951.
4. Calmettes, L., Deodati, F., and Bec. P. Gangrène des paupières d'origine rickettsienne, Bull. Soc. Franc. Ophtal. **73**:509, 1960.
5. Clavel, A., and Hamart: Manifestations oculaires au cours d'une fièvre boutonneuse méditerranéenne autochtone, Ann. Oculit **182**:232, 1949.
6. Conor, A., and Bruch, A.: Une fièvre éruptive observée en Tunisie, Bull. Soc. Path. Exot. **3**:492, 1910.
7. Deduit, Y.: Iridocyclite et bouton de rétinite au cours d'une rickettsiose thérapeutique a Rickettsia quintana, Ann. Oculist. **196**:934, 1963.
8. Duke-Elder, S.: System of ophthalmology. Diseases of the outer eye, vol. 8, part 1, St. Louis, 1955, The C. V. Mosby Co., p. 244.
9. Elisberg, B. L., and Bozeman, F. M.: Rickettsiae. In Lennette, E. H., and Schmidt, N. J., editors: Diagnostic procedures for viral and rickettsial infections, ed. 4, New York, 1969, American Public Health Association, p. 826.
10. Harvey, M. S., Forbes, G. B., and Marmon, B. P.: An outbreak of "Q" fever in East Kent, Lancet **2**:1152, 1951.
11. Hazard, G. W., Ganz, R. N., Nevin, R. W., Nauss, A. H., Curtis, E., Bell, D. W. J., and Murray E. S.: Rocky Mountain spotted fever in the eastern United States, New Eng. J. Med. **280**:57, 1969.
12. Iida, T., Kawashima, H., and Kawamura, A.: Direct immunofluorescence for typing of tsutsugamushi disease Rickettsia, J. Immunol. **95**:1129, 1965.
13. Jawetz, E., Melnick, J. L., and Adelberg, E. A.: Review of medical microbiology, ed. 9, Los Altos, Calif., 1970, Lange Medical Publications, p. 263.
14. Larionow, N.: Erkrankungen des Sehorgans beim Typhus, Klin. Mbl. Augenheilk. **16**:487, 1878.
15. Lebas, M. P., and Bernaerts-Lebas, M. A.: Rickettsioses et affections oculaires, Bull. Soc. Belg. Ophtal. **135**:437, 1963.
16. Lennette, E. H., and Schmidt, N. J.: Diagnostic procedures for viral and rickettsial infections, ed. 4, New York, 1969, American Public Health Association.

17. Macaskill, J.: Some ocular complications of scrub typhus, Brit. J. Ophthal. **29**:537, 1945.
18. Morax, P. V., Saraut, H., Moday, S., and Coscas, G.: Les manifestastions oculaires des rickettsioses et des neorickettsioses, Ann. Oculist. **194**:929, 1961.
19. Perdriel, G., Michel, A., Guyard, M., and Hoel, J.: Les manifestations oculaires de la fièvre "Q," Ann. Oculist. **194**:957, 1961.
20. Presley, G. D.: Fundus changes in Rocky Mountain spotted fever, Amer. J. Ophthal. **67**:263, 1969.
21. Raab, E. L., Leopold, I. H., and Hodes, H. L.: Retinopathy in Rocky Mountain spotted fever, Amer. J. Ophthal. **68**:42, 1969.
22. Rhodes, A. J., and van Rooyen, C. E.: Textbook of virology, Baltimore, 1962, The Williams and Wilkins Co., p. 534.
23. Ricketts, H. T.: Further observations on Rocky Mountain spotted fever and Dermacentor occidentalis, J.A.M.A. **47**:1067, 1906.
24. Ricketts, H. T.: Further experiments with the wood-tick in relation to Rocky Mountain spotted fever, J.A.M.A. **49**:1278, 1907; and **52**:379, 1909.
25. Ricketts, H. T., and Wilder, R. M.: The etiology of the typhus fever (tabardillo) of Mexico City: a further preliminary report, J.A.M.A. **54**:1373, 1910; and **55**:309, 1910.
26. Rouher, F., Cluzel, P., Cantat, and Vaurs, M. R.: Kératite recidivante et rickettsies, Bull. Soc. Franc. Ophtal. **63**:86, 1963.
27. Scheie, H. G.: Ocular changes in scrub typhus: a study of 451 patients, Trans. Amer. Ophthal. Soc. **45**:637, 1947.
28. Shishido, A.: Identification and serological classification of the causative agent of scrub typhus in Japan, J. Med. Sci. Biol. **15**:308, 1962.
29. Venable, M. P., and Pollock, F. J.: Rickettsias in ophthalmolgoy, Arch. Ophthal. **30**:362, 1943.
30. Wolbach, S. B.: The rickettsial diseases, a general survey. In Virus and Rickettsial diseases, Cambridge, 1940, Harvard University Press.

16

Introduction to viral ocular infections

VIRAL AGENTS OF DISEASE

In 1948 Rivers' definitive textbook on viral and rickettsial infections of man brought together under one cover the current knowledge concerning these agents of human disease.[18] At that time 31 viruses and rickettsiae had been propagated in the chick embryo. Tissue-culture methods were only in the developmental stage.

An early criterion for the identification of a virus was its inability to grow in the absence of living cells. It was apparent that viruses depended heavily on the apparatus of cells for their propagation. Just how this was controlled to favor the virus was unknown. Viruses were characterized in part by their particle size, determined by filtration through materials of known pore diameter. Iwanowski[11] was the first to recognize the filterability of these agents under conditions that kept back bacteria. A tentative classification of the viruses on the basis of size was made possible through the development of methods of filtration through graded collodion membranes.[7] Passage of viruses through filters was determined by the infectivity of the filtrates.

Microscopic examination of stained preparations of lesions found in known or suspected viral diseases had shown the presence of inclusion bodies, small intracellular structures in nuclei, cytoplasm, or both. Woodruff and Goodpasture[22] demonstrated that inclusion bodies seen in fowlpox produced typical fowlpox disease when inoculated into the skin of hens.

Small bits of information were pieced together from cultural requirements, size, and inclusion body formation, but were not sufficient to establish any sort of classification comparable to that by which bacteria were recognized. Many viruses went only by the name of the disease they caused; and in many cases the virus etiology, though suspected, was not proved by culture. For example, epidemic keratoconjunctivitis (Chapter 17) was thought to be produced by a virus, since mice or rabbits injected intracerebrally with material from the early lesions developed fatal encephalitis in about a week, though no bacteria were found. Rabbits inoculated in the cornea developed keratitis. A relationship to the herpes simplex virus (Chapter 18) was suspected, as herpes simplex was known at times to produce meningoencephalitis as well as keratoconjunctivitis in man. Several years were to pass before the etiologic agent of keratoconjunctivitis was identified as a member of the adenovirus group. Trachoma and inclusion conjunctivitis were accepted as diseases of viral origin because of the presence of inclusion bodies in the cells involved in the pathogenic process and the transmissibility of the diseases by filtered material gathered from the lesions. Another 10 years went by before the infectious agents were isolated and classified in a group apart from the viruses (Chapter 14).

Today the viruses are in some respects as well known as the bacteria. Fourteen

Table 16-1. Classification of viruses into groups based on chemical and physical properties

Nucleic acid core	Capsid symmetry	Virion enveloped or naked	Ether sensitivity	Number of capsomers	Virus particle size (nm)*	Molecular weight nucleic acid virion ($\times 10^6$)	Number of genes	Virus group
DNA	Icosahedral	Naked	Resistant	12 or 32	18–24	1.5	7	Parvovirus
				42 or 72	40–55	2–4	10	Papovavirus
				252	70–80	23	50	Adenovirus
		Enveloped	Sensitive	162	180–250 (110)†	40–84	150	Herpesvirus
	Unknown	(Complex)	Resistant		230×300	160–240	400	Poxvirus
RNA	Icosahedral	Naked	Resistant	32	18–30	2	10	Picornavirus
				92	70–75	10	50	Reovirus‡
	Unknown§	Enveloped	Sensitive	32§	50–60 (35)§	2	10	Togavirus§
					110			Tacaribe-LCM‖
					80–120			Coronavirus¶
	Helical	Enveloped	Sensitive		80–200	2–5	10	Myxovirus
					100–300	7–10	40	Paramyxovirus
					60×225	3–4	10	Rhabdovirus
	Unknown	Enveloped	Sensitive		100	10–12	50	Leukovirus#

Table prepared by J. L. Melnick. From Jawetz, E., Melnick, J. L., Adelberg, E. A.: Review of medical microbiology, ed. 9, Los Altos, Calif., 1970, Lange Medical Publications, p. 278.

*Diameter, or diameter × length.

†The naked virus, that is, the nucleocapsid, is 110 nm in diameter; however, the enveloped virion varies from 180 to 250 nm.

‡Recent evidence indicates that reovirus is one of a large group of viruses possessing double-stranded RNA (diplornaviruses).

§Included in the togavirus group are arboviruses of subgroups A and B. Rubella virus and lactic dehydrogenase (LDH) virus of mice have similar properties. One togavirus that has been studied in detail (Sindbis) has been shown to have a nucleocapsid 35 nm in diameter, containing 32 capsomers in an icosahedral surface lattice with a triangulation number of T = 3. The enveloped virion is about 50 to 60 nm in diameter.

‖Lymphocytic choriomeningitis virus recently has been shown to be identical morphologically, and to cross-react serologically, with arboviruses of the Tacaribe complex, which includes the Junin and Machupo viruses of South American hemorrhagic fevers. A new taxonomic group of these RNA-containing, enveloped viruses has been proposed: the Tacaribe-LCM group.

¶Included in this group of viruses with petal-shaped surface projections are a number of new human respiratory viruses, avian infectious bronchitis virus (IBV), and mouse hepatitis virus.

#The leukovirus group refers to leukemia viruses of avian, feline, and murine species, since a human leukemia virus has not yet been described.

major groups, which contain hundreds of immunologically distinct types (or species) pathogenic for man or animals or both, have been established (Table 16-1).[9,12,20] Other viruses are awaiting classification. In addition to these groups there is a large and important number of viruses infecting plants. It is probable that viruses are responsible for at least 50% of all infectious diseases of man and animals, as well as for some forms of cancer. The rapid growth of knowledge concerning these agents was made possible in great measure by the introduction of the monolayer growth of cultured cells on glass by Enders and his associates.[7] This provided a relatively simple method for the cultivation of large quantities of virus. Antibiotics also contributed much to viral cultivation by cutting down on bacterial contamination of both embryonated eggs and cell cultures. Initial isolation of viruses taken from contaminated areas became possible.

Structure of viruses

The physical features of animal viruses are schematically illustrated in Fig. 16-1. The core of a virus, the nucleic acid genome, is made up of either ribonucleic acid (RNA) or deoxyribonucleic acid (DNA). The capsid is a symmetric protein coat enclosing the nucleic acid genome. The capsomers are clusters of the structural units, the basic building blocks of the capsid. Some more complicated virions (complete, infective viral particles) may have one or more additional membranes. Fig. 16-2, *1* is an electron micrograph of a varicella virus particle in its enveloping membrane with a centrally placed capsid. On the right such a virus particle with ruptured membrane shows the hollow capsomers on the surface of the capsid.

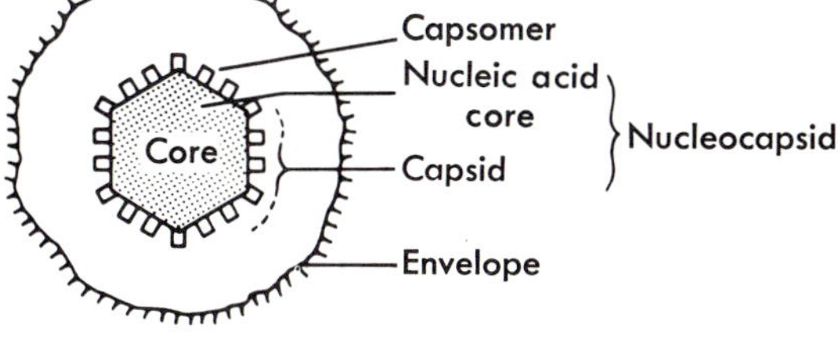

Fig. 16-1. Components of a complete virus particle, or virion. (From Horne, R. W.: Sci. Amer. **208:** 50, 1963.)

The size of viruses, still a basic criterion for classification, is now measured by electron microscopy, ultracentrifugation, or ionizing radiation, as well as by filtration. Fig. 16-3 illustrates the relative size, determined by electron microscopy, of 4 viruses that contain DNA and 4 that contain RNA in their core. These are representatives of the 14 major groups of viruses so far classified (Table 16-1). The variation in size is even more striking if it is expressed in terms of volume. The poxvirus has a mass 1,000 times greater than that of the picornavirus. By contrast, the mass of a small bacterium is 50,000 times greater than the picornavirus.

Table 16-1 presents the physical characteristics of the 14 groups of viruses listed. This table shows that specific information is available in most instances about the size, shape, and structure of the elements of the virion, including the molecular weight of the nucleic acid core and the number of genes. Ether sensitivity, included in this table, is believed to depend on the presence of lipids in the membrane.

Some of the most exciting work in micro-

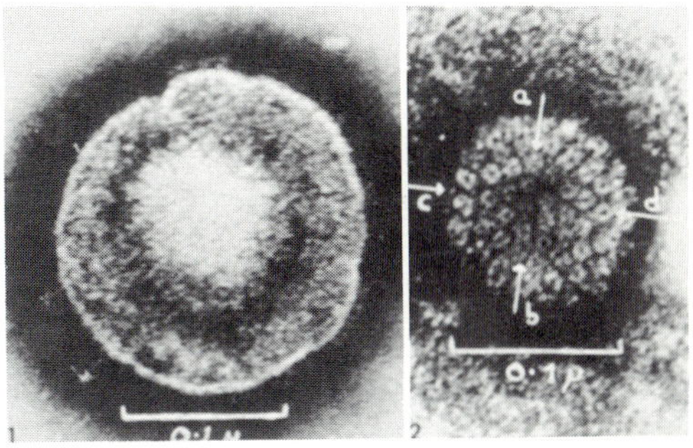

Fig. 16-2. *1*, Intact varicella virus particle showing enveloping membrane with projections and centrally placed capsid. *2*, Particle in which the envelop had ruptured, showing structure of capsid more clearly. (From Almeida, J. D., Howatson, A. F., and Williams, M. G.: Virology **16**(3): 353, 1962. Copyright © Academic Press, Inc.)

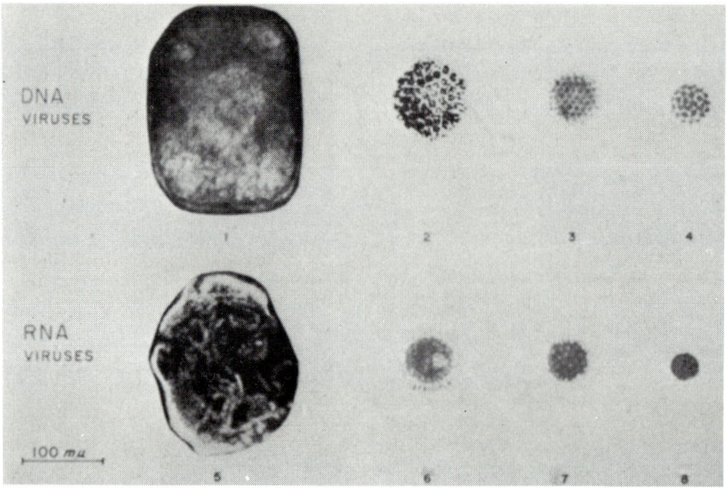

Fig. 16-3. Relative sizes of animal viruses (negative-stained virus particles). *1,* Poxvirus group (vaccinia virus); *2,* herpesvirus group (herpes simplex); *3,* adenovirus group; *4,* papovavirus group (papilloma virus); *5,* paramyxovirus group (Sendai virus); *6,* myxovirus group (influenza A virus); *7,* reovirus group; *8,* picornavirus group (polio virus). (From Hsiung, G. D.: Bact. Rev. **29**:470, 1965.)

biology deals with the studies on the manner in which viruses replicate their structure. For reviews of the subject, Erikson[7a] and Jawetz and his coauthors[12] may be consulted.

Viral antigens and antibodies

The structural proteins of the viral capsids are important for a number of reasons. They form a compact and stable, structured symmetry that protects the genome, and they play a part in the attachment of some viruses to susceptible cells. To the immunologist and physician, however, the most important characteristic of viral protein is its antigenic specificity, which permits identification of viral groups and types, thus enabling precise diagnosis of the infectious agent of a viral disease. A corollary to this is the ability to utilize preparations of living or dead viruses as vaccines to stimulate active immunity in man or to provide from animals antibodies that are useful both in therapy and in viral identification. Antibody response also may influence the type of immunopathologic reaction. The absence of immunologic response may result in enhanced susceptibility to infection on the one hand or to inapparent infection or the carrier state on the other.[12]

Antibodies are used to recognize viruses by one or more of the following procedures:

1. Myxovirus, paramyxovirus, and poxvirus groups of viruses agglutinate red blood cells of man and some animals. The source and method of operation of the hemagglutinin varies with the group, but in each case the agglutinating agent is antigenic. The antibodies produced will specifically prevent the hemagglutinating activity. Hemagglutination neutralization is a useful diagnostic test.
2. Antiviral sera fix complement in the presence of viral antigens. Some viruses produce a group-specific soluble antigen that stimulates early antibody production. The detection of the antibody by the complement-fixation test may have considerable diagnostic value.
3. Infectious virus particles induce the production of a virus-neutralizing antibody, which may protect against the transmission of the disease or prevent its develment in man. Virus-neutralizing anti-

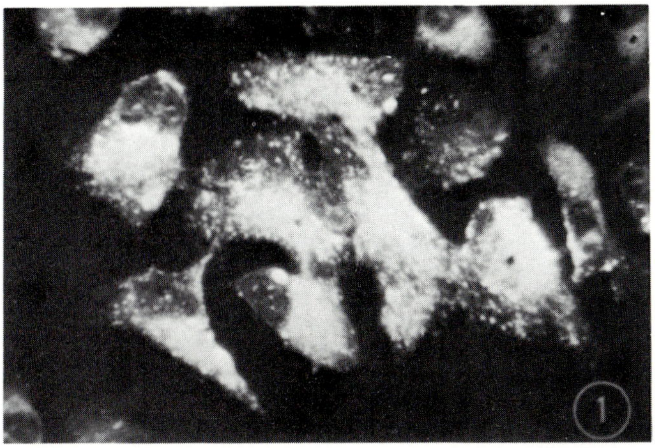

Fig. 16-4. Infection of human conjunctiva cells with cytopathogenic line of Dunai strain mumps virus. Stained with fluorescent antibody 30 hours after inoculation. Mumps virus antigen is distributed throughout the cytoplasm in small and large granules. (× 500.) (From Walker, L., and Hinze, H. C.: J. Exp. Med. **116**:750, 1962.)

body can also be used to protect tissue-cultured cells. Viruses growing in tissue culture usually produce cellular destruction, proliferation, or some other gross abnormality called cytopathogenic effect (CPE). This cellular damage will be prevented by specific neutralizing antibody. Individuals who have had viral infection develop this antibody. If it has not been possible to isolate the cause of a given infection but a virus is suspected, serum from the patient, drawn 2 or more weeks after symptoms have developed, may be used to establish a diagnosis. Such a serum is added to a series of cultured cells together with one of the several viruses that might have been the cause of the patient's disease. If the CPE of any one of the viruses tested is prevented, it is assumed that this virus was the cause of the disease.

One very important control is necessary. A sample of blood taken when the patient is first ill, the acute phase sample, must be tested simultaneously with the convalescent serum to rule out the possibility that the patient is carrying an antibody to a virus acquired during a previous exposure but unrelated to the illness under question.

4. It is possible to couple fluorescein isothiocyanate with immune globulins without impairing the immunologic activity of the globulin.[13] Such coupled virus-specific antibodies may be added to infected cultured cells, exudates, or pieces of tissue taken by biopsy from a site of infection. After a short period to permit reaction between the immunoglobulin and the specific virus in the specimen, the excess of labeled globulin is washed away. The preparation is examined with a microscope using ultraviolet light. The area where the immune globulin is bound fluoresces, emitting a yellow-green light, thus showing the presence of the virus in cells. Fig. 16-4 illustrates the appearance of mumps virus growing in cultured human conjunctival cells, examined by the fluorescein technique. The infected cells had been grown on coverslips, dried, fixed in acetone, and stained with fluorescein-labeled rabbit antibody to measles virus. The illustration shows that this virus is irregularly distributed in the cytoplasm of the cells.

A similar use of labeled antibody has been introduced into electron microscopy.[21] The antibodies are labeled with electron-

A 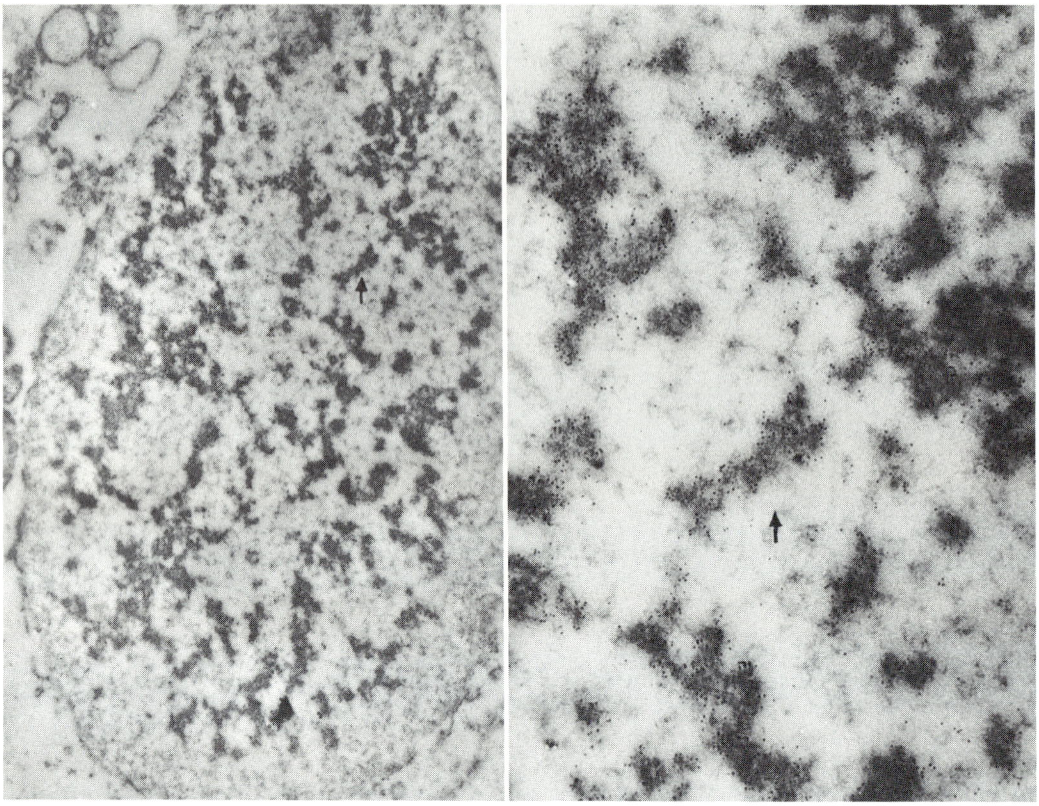 B

Fig. 16-5. A, Nucleus of a cell infected with influenza virus, containing aggregates of dense material (arrow). The chromatin is sparse, and the nuclear membranes have disrupted. (× 26,000.) **B,** Part of the nucleus seen in **A** (arrow), viewed at higher magnification. Ferritin-conjugated antibody to the influenza virus is present within the aggregates of dense material (arrow). The intervening nuclear matrix is nearly devoid of ferritin. (× 97,000.) (From Morgan, C., Hsu, K. C., Rifkind, R. A., Knox, A. W., and Rose, H. M.: J. Exp. Med. **114**:833, 1961.)

opaque ferritin. The tissue containing the virus is treated in a manner analogous to that used for fluorescein examination, and ultrathin sections are prepared for electron microscopic examination. The potentialities of the technique can be illustrated by influenza virus. In Fig. 16-5, *A*, the nucleus of a cell infected with this virus shows collections of amorphous electron-opaque material. Ferritin-labeled antibody to the nucleocapsid antigen of the virus was applied to the tissue prior to fixation for electron microscopic study. Fig. 16-5, *B*, a higher magnification of a portion of this nucleus, illustrates the presence of ferritin particles in the amorphous aggregates. Their presence indicates that the ferritin-labeled antibody to nucleocapsid antigen has been bound to the aggregates, which therefore must contain nucleocapsid antigen made in this area. Complete viral particles, however, are found only on or near the surface of the cell, as can be seen in Fig. 16-6. Thus the ferritin-labeled antibody identifies specific antigens of the virus. These studies and other related investigations are helping to distinguish the areas of the cell where parts of the viruses may be made or put together.

Pathogenesis of viral disease

The modes of entry of viruses into the human body are as numerous as those used by bacteria. They are: (1) inhalation

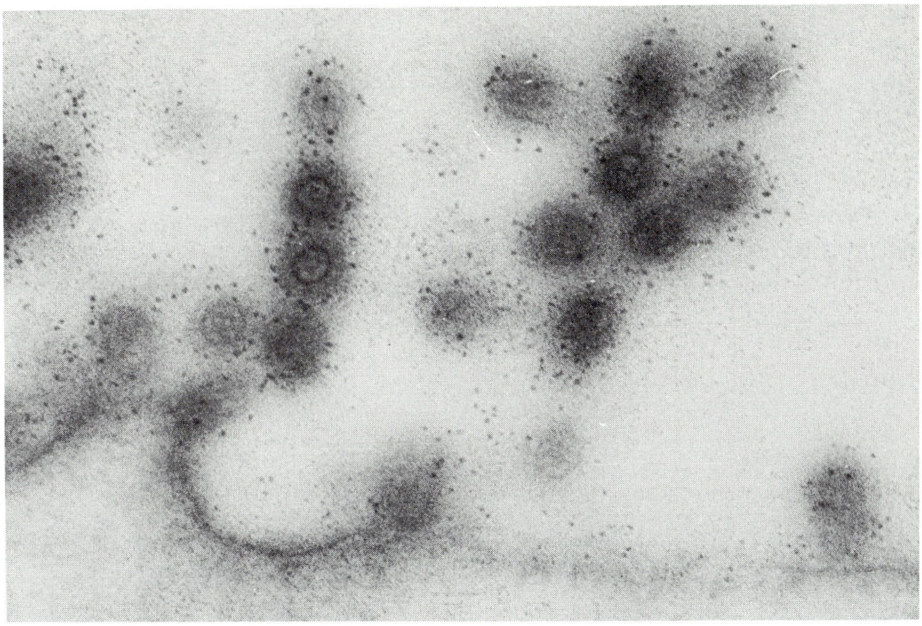

Fig. 16-6. Influenza virus at the surface of a chick chorioallantoic membrane. The surface of the cell has been cut obliquely, and cytplasm occupies the lower border of the field. It is of interest that, in addition to fully formed virus, ferritin has tagged particles in the process of budding from the cell. (× 135,000.) (Courtesy Dr. C. Morgan.)

of airborne droplets or dust, (2) ingestion, (3) direct contact, (4) bite of an infected animal, and (5) bite of an insect or arthropod. Some of the viruses inhaled and some ingested appear to remain localized either in the upper respiratory tract or the intestinal canal. The majority seem to travel rather freely via the circulation, though a predilection for a specific tissue is common.

Virus usually can be cultured from infected areas or the bloodstream only during the first few days of acute infection. Nevertheless, it has long been conjectured that a virus may persist in the host after recovery has taken place, since many viral infections are followed by lasting immunity. Evidence for the carriage of a virus in healthy cultured cells and in the tissues of some animals has been reported.[12,19] Such evidence is not as readily obtained in man. However, there is a chronic degenerative brain disorder—Dawson's inclusion body encephalitis—seen in some who have had measles a number of years previously. Measles virus has been isolated from such a case.[17] More data are needed, however, before the role of a carrier state in the maintenance of protection from infection is established.

An apparent exception to prolonged immunity afforded by viral infection is the common cold. Colds are caused by various members of the picornavirus group, including a number of enteroviruses and rhinoviruses. Since many types within the groups have been involved and immunity to some affords no protection to others, man is always potentially vulnerable to new strains.

The immune response of the body to the presence of a virus over a period of months or years may be of great importance in the pathogenesis of some viral diseases. The most familiar examples are found in the herpesvirus group. Latent infection (the carrier state) with herpes simplex can last for many years even when circulating antibodies are demonstrable. Varicella virus, a member of this group, produces chicken-

Table 16-2. Viruses causing ocular infection

Virus group and subgroups or types	Primary diseases	Ocular diseases
Papovavirus group		
Papilloma virus	Warts; tumorlike papilliform proliferations	Warts of lid margins; bulbar conjunctiva and opposite lid; verrucose conjunctivitis and keratitis
Adenovirus group		
Type 8	Epidemic keratoconjunctivitis	Epidemic keratoconjunctivitis
Type 3 (predominately)	Pharyngoconjunctival fever and other upper respiratory tract diseases	Pharyngoconjunctival fever
Types 1-11, 14-17, 20, 22, 26, 27	Fever; pharyngitis with involvement of neighboring areas	Follicular conjunctivitis; keratoconjunctivitis
Herpesvirus group		
Herpes simplex	Systemic infection at birth or herpetic stomatitis; chronic recurrent infections	Herpetic keratitis and keratouveitis
Varicella-zoster	Chickenpox in childhood; shingles in adulthood	Rare involvement of conjunctiva and cornea; conjunctivitis; keratitis; scleritis; iridocyclitis; and optic neuritis
Cytomegalo virus	Cytomegalic inclusion disease of newborn and young children; in adults 80% positive serology	Ocular involvement rare, usually includes lacrimal gland, uveal tract, and sometimes retinal changes
Poxvirus group		
Variola	Smallpox	Exanthematous, catarrhal conjunctivitis; superficial infiltration of cornea
Vaccinia	Spread of infection from vaccinated area	Ranges from uncomplicated blepharoconjunctivitis in immune person to purulent conjunctivitis and disciform keratitis
Molluscum contagiosum	Molluscum contagiosum disease characterized by small epithelial tumors	Molluscum tumors may occur on lids and palpebral conjunctiva, leading to conjunctivitis and sometimes keratitis
Picornavirus group		
Rhinovirus of cattle	Foot-and-mouth disease of cattle transmitted to man	A rare disease, in association with ulcerative condition of mouth; severe keratoconjunctivitis arises
Togavirus group		
Rubella virus	German measles	Catarrhal or follicular conjunctivitis; mild keratitis
Arbovirus B, yellow fever virus	Yellow fever, transmitted by mosquito	Intense conjunctival injection; subconjunctival hemorrhages; edema and swelling of face
Arboviruses B, dengue fever virus	Dengue fever, transmitted by mosquito	Conjunctival injection (bulbar); edema of lids; lacrimation; retrobulbar pain
Arbovirus (ungrouped), sandfly fever virus	Sandfly fever, transmitted by *Phlebotomus papatasi*	Injection of bulbar conjunctiva limited to exposed part; burning pain; lacrimation
Myxovirus group		
Influenza viruses	Influenza	Catarrhal, occasionally acute follicular conjunctivitis

Table 16-2. Viruses causing ocular infection—cont'd

Virus group and subgroups or types	Primary diseases	Ocular diseases
Paramyxovirus group		
Measles virus	Measles	Eye lesions precede exanthem; mucopurulent conjunctivitis; papules and pale spots (Koplik's spots) on mucous membrane; caruncle; punctate keratitis in severe disease
Mumps virus	Mumps	Simple conjunctivitis common; edema of bulbar conjunctiva; may develop episcleritis, keratitis
Newcastle disease virus	Primarily pathogenic for fowl; an occupational disease of man primary to the eye	Mild conjunctivitis with itching, burning, or mild gelatinous swelling with follicles, palpebral edema

pox in children; and herpes zoster, indistinguishable from varicella, produces shingles in adults. Herpes zoster can also be a source of chickenpox in children. Adults exposed to chickenpox may develop herpes zoster. The question to be answered is whether long residence in the body changes tissue response to infection by the same virus.

"Slow virus diseases," where the incubation period is a matter of several years and there is no preliminary acute phase, are under intensive investigation and offer one of the most important areas for the study of the relation of immune response to pathology. In these diseases virus-antibody complexes may circulate for long periods of time. Trapping of these complexes in affected organs may serve to initiate the pathologic sequences. Among the human diseases under investigation for such an etiologic agent are spongiform encephalopathies, kuru, amyotropic lateral sclerosis, polymyositis, and progressive leukoencephalopathy.[12]

VIRUSES INFECTING THE EYE

Eight of the 14 major groups of animal viruses described in Table 16-1 are known to contain strains that produce ocular disease. Table 16-2 lists these viruses, the primary illnesses they cause, and the nature of the lesions found in the eyes. The table shows that viruses infecting the eye come from the upper respiratory tract and the skin in most instances, though three of the viruses are first introduced into the circulation by the bite of an insect. Each of the eye infections is considered in one of the three succeeding chapters.

Diagnosis of viral infections of the eye

Although each virus requires some special handling (choice of cultured cells, length of incubation, and so on, which will be discussed in the next few chapters), there are four basic methods for diagnosis, one of which may be handled in a routine laboratory if the necessary equipment is available (see also pp. 270-272). These methods are: (1) the immunofluorescein technique, in which specific viral antibodies labeled with fluorescein isothiocyanate are used to stain smears of scrapings from the suspected lesion; (2) the hemagglutination inhibition test, in which a series of known antiviral antibodies are used in an attempt to inhibit hemagglutination produced by the unknown virus; (3) the cytopathogenic neutralization test, in which known antiviral sera are tested for their ability to neutralize or prevent the cytopathogenic effect produced by the unknown virus in tissue-cultured cells; and (4) the retrospective diagnostic test, used when the attempt to grow the unknown virus has been unsuccessful. In this test a sample of the patient's serum drawn during his convalescence is compared with an early acute phase sample for the presence of antiviral antibodies, usually determined by the hemagglutination inhibition test, cytopathogenic neutralization test, or by the complement-fixation test.[12a]

The test that can be used without having a laboratory equipped for the cultivation of viruses utilizes the immunofluorescein technique to stain smears of scrapings. Since this technique requires several control slides, it is almost impossible to apply it to the small samples available from scrapings of the eye. This technique is much more successfully used when the virus is grown in tissue-cultured cells (Fig. 16-4). However, in some instances early cases of epidemic keratoconjunctivitis, probably caused by adenovirus type 8, or corneal ulcers, probably caused by herpesvirus infection, may be confirmed by staining scrapings from the lesions with fluorescein-labeled antibodies to the suspected viral antigen. The scrapings must be obtained as early as possible in the infection.

If there are no facilities available in association with the microbiology laboratory for growing viruses, the ophthalmologist may send the material to a virology laboratory. Since viruses can be isolated from the affected tissues only in the first few days of the disease, early cases alone are suitable for culturing. If there is abundant exudate, it may be taken on a cotton swab moistened with tissue-culture fluid or broth. A scraping from the lesion or vesicle fluid is more likely to contain the virus, since it grows in living cells. The scrapings are kept moist in a tube containing a drop of tissue-culture fluid or broth. Both specimens are sent to the laboratory immediately. If they are to be forwarded to a diagnostic center, they should be packed in dry ice to preserve the virus and prevent proliferation of contaminating bacteria. They should be accompanied by the following data:

Date of onset of disease
Date of obtaining specimen
Capsule history and clinical diagnosis
Recent travel

All specimens must be accompanied by a tube of clotted blood. This blood specimen (acute phase) should be obtained within 3 to 4 days of the onset of illness. The blood is needed to attempt a retrospective diagnosis in case no viral growth is obtained. This technique requires that the blood must be drawn again 2 to 4 weeks later in order to test for a rising titer of antibodies to one of the group of stock viruses. The history and clinical diagnosis that accompany the swab and serum sample assist the laboratory in choosing which group of antisera or viruses to use in identifying the unknown virus or in looking for serum antibodies.

SUMMARY

A few points may be stressed again.

1. Viral structure, content, physiology, and antigenicity are being documented, and it is now possible to speak of viruses with some of the same familiarity formerly reserved only for bacteria.
2. There are hundreds of viruses that can be identified because of their unique antigens. Most of them have been classified in 1 of 14 groups.
3. If it has not been possible to isolate a virus, retrospective diagnosis of viral infections can be made, using the patient's newly formed antibodies.
4. The immunologic response of the host to invading viruses may establish the pathologic manifestations of the disease.
5. Viruses known to cause ocular disease are listed. They come from 8 viral groups. In only 2 instances is the ocular disease primary to the eye.

REFERENCES

1. Almeida, J. D., Howatson, A. F., and Williams, M. G.: Morphology of varicella (chickenpox) virus, Virology **16**:353, 1962.
2. Andres, G. A., Hsu, K. C., and Seegal, B. C.: Immunoferritin technique for the identification of antigens by electron microscopy. In Weir, D. M., editor: Handbook of experimental immunology, Oxford, 1967, Blackwell Scientific Publications.
3. Beale, A. J., Doane, F., and Ormsby, H. L.: Studies on adenovirus infections of the eye in Toronto, Amer. J. Ophthal. **43**:26, 1957. (Symposium on Viral Keratoconjunctivitis)
4. Davis, B. D., Dulbecco, R., Eisen, H. N., Ginsberg, H. S., and Wood, W. B.: Microbiology, New York, 1967, Harper and Row, Publishers.
5. Duke-Elder, St.: System of ophthalmology. Diseases of the outer eye, vol. 8, part I, St. Louis, 1965, The C. V. Mosby Co.
6. Elford, W. J.: A new series of graded collodion membranes suitable for general bacteriological use, especially in filterable virus studies, J. Path. Bact. **34**:505, 1931.
7. Enders, J. F., Weller, T. H., and Robbins, F. C.: Cultivation of the Lansing strain of poliomyelitis virus in cultures of various human embryonic tissues, Science **109**:85, 1949.

7a. Erikson, R. L.: Replication of RNA viruses, Ann. Rev. Microbiol. **22**:305, 1968.

8. Horne, R. W.: The structure of viruses, Sci. Amer. **208**:48, 1963.
9. Horsfall, F. L., and Tamm, I.: Viral and rickettsial infections of man, ed. 4, Philadelphia, 1965, J. B. Lippincott Co.
10. Hsiung, G. D.: Use of ultrafiltration for animal virus grouping, Bact. Rev. **29**:477, 1965.
11. Iwanowski, D.: Uber die Mosaik-Krankheit der Tabaksplanze, Bull. Acad. Imp. Sci. (St. Petersburg) **35**(N.S. 3):67, 1892.
12. Jawetz, E., Melnick, J. L., and Adelberg, E. A.: Review of medical microbiology, ed. 9, Los Altos, Calif., 1970, Lange Medical Publications.

12a. Lennette, E. H.: General principles underlying laboratory diagnosis of viral and rickettsial infections. In Lennette, E. H., and Schmidt, N. J., editors: Diagnostic procedures for viral and rickettsial infections, ed. 4, New York, 1969, American Public Health Association, p. 1.

13. Liu, C.: Fluorescent antibody technics. In Lennette, E. H., and Schmidt, N. J., editors: Diagnostic procedures for viral and rickettsial infections, ed. 4, New York, 1969, American Public Health Association, p. 179.
14. Morgan, C., Howe, C., Rose, H. M., and Moore, D. H.: Structure and development of viruses observed in the electron microscope: viruses in the RI-APC group, J. Biophys. Biochem. Cytol. **2**:351, 1956.
15. Morgan, C., Hsu, K. C., Rifkind, R. A., Knox, A. W., and Rose, H. M.: The application of ferritin-conjugated antibody to electron microscopic studies of influenza virus in infected cells: the cellular surface, J. Exp. Med. **114**:825, 1961.
16. Morgan, C., Hsu, K. C., Rifkind, R. A., Knox, A. W., and Rose, H. M.: The application of ferritin-conjugated antibody to electron microscopic studies of influenza virus in infected cells: the interior of the cell, J. Exp. Med. **114**:833, 1961.
17. Payne, F. E., Baublis, J. V., and Itabashi, H. H.: Isolation of measles virus from cell cultures of brain from a patient with subacute sclerosing panencephalitis, New Eng. J. Med. **281**:585, 1969.
18. Rivers, T. M.: Viral and rickettsial infections of man, Philadelphia, 1948, J. P. Lippincott Co.
19. Walker, D. L., and Hinze, H. C.: A carrier state of mumps virus in human conjunctiva cells: observations on intracellular transfer of virus and virus release, J. Exp. Med. **116**: 751, 1962.
20. Wilner, B. I.: A classification of the major groups of human and other animal viruses, ed. 4, Minneapolis, 1969, Burgess Publishing Co.
21. Woodruff, C. E., and Goodpasture, E. W.: The infectivity of isolated inclusion bodies of fowl-pox, Amer. J. Path. **5**:1, 1929.

17

Ocular infections caused by adenovirus and papovavirus groups

ADENOVIRUS INFECTION OF THE EYE

Adenoviruses are common and widespread parasites of man. Many may be found in the absence of disease, but most if not all of the 33 types so far isolated from man can act as pathogens. The commonest disease produced by members of the adenovirus group is acute febrile pharyngitis. In civilian life young children are more susceptible than adults. Among military groups, however, the incidence of adenovirus infection of the upper respiratory tract may be high; the infection goes by the name of acute respiratory disease. The eye is often involved, in which case the disease is called pharyngoconjunctival fever. Ocular disease—either acute follicular conjunctivitis or epidemic keratoconjunctivitis—may be the primary finding.

Discovery

Rowe and his associates[82] were the first to isolate and describe a member of this group of viruses. The new agent was obtained from explanted adenoid tissues, which had been removed from children during the winter and spring of 1952 to 1953, and was cultured by the chicken plasma clot technique. Thirty-three of the 53 cultured tissues demonstrated a characteristic rounding of the peripheral epithelium after 1 to 4 weeks. When inoculated into fresh preparations of adenoids, human embryonic tissue, or HeLa cells, the culture fluids produced characteristic changes in the epithelium of the recipient cultures. When a concentrated inoculum of the culture fluid was transmitted to HeLa cells, clumping and rounding of these cells appeared in 2 or 3 days. The authors report that Dr. Henry Pinkerton examined preparations of infected embryonic tracheal epithelium and described both nuclear and cytoplasmic inclusions.

Almost simultaneously with Rowe's experiments, Hilleman and Werner[35] recovered a similar, viruslike agent from nasopharyngeal secretions of military recruits with acute respiratory disease. Huebner and his co-workers[40] reported the isolation of 6 immunologically distinct types of virus from adenoid and tonsilar tissues removed surgically from nasopharyngeal or conjunctival secretions or from feces of persons with respiratory infections. Thus, confirmation of earlier findings followed rapidly, and it was soon apparent that the isolates constituted a group of infectious agents. Following the recommendation of these early workers,[23] further investigators proposed the name adenovirus to designate this rapidly growing family or viruses, which at that time numbered 12 serologically distinct types. In the past 15 years numerous papers have appeared in many areas of the world describing isolation from man of old and new members of this group of viruses. Table 17-1 presents the original source of the 33 immunologically distinct types of adenoviruses that have been obtained from human sources. The first 14 isolates were made in the United States, while 11 of the remaining types were found in the Netherlands, Saudi Arabia, and England. The viruses have been recovered predominantly

Table 17-1. Discovery of the types of adenoviruses of human origin

Types	Geographic origins	Sources	Clinical conditions	References
1	United States	Adenoid	Hypertrophied tonsils, adenoids	Rowe and others, 1953[82]* Huebner and others, 1954[40]
2	United States	Adenoid	Hypertrophied tonsils, adenoids	Huebner and others, 1954[40] Rowe and others, 1955[83]
3	United States	Nasal washing	Common cold (volunteer)	Huebner and others, 1954[40] Rowe and others, 1955[83]
4	United States	Throat washing	Primary atypical pneumonia	Hilleman and Werner, 1954[35]
5	United States	Adenoid	Hypertrophied tonsils, adenoids	Huebner and others, 1954[40] Rowe and others, 1955[83]
6	United States	Tonsil	Hypertrophied tonsils, adenoids	Huebner and others, 1954[40] Rowe and others, 1955[83]
7	United States	Throat washing	Pharyngitis	Berge and others, 1955[7]
7a	United States	Throat washing	Undifferentiated respiratory infection	Rowe and others, 1958[80]
8	United States	Corneal, conjunctival scraping	Epidemic keratoconjunctivitis	Jawetz and others, 1955[47]
9	United States	Stool	Rheumatoid arthritis	Kibrick and others, 1957[52]
10	United States	Eye swabbing	Conjunctivitis	Rowe and others, 1956[79]
11	United States	Stool	Paralytic poliomyelitis (type 1 polio virus recovered)	Kibrick and others, 1957[52]
12	United States	Stool	Nonparalytic poliomyelitis	Kibrick and others, 1957[52]
13	United States	Stool	Healthy child	Rowe and others, 1958[80]
14	Netherlands	Throat washing	Acute respiratory disease	van der Veen and Kok, 1957[88]
15-17	Saudi Arabia	Conjunctival scraping	Conjunctivitis (early trachoma in children under 15 years of age)	Murray and others, 1957[64]
18	United States	Anal swabbing	Niemann-Pick disease	Rowe and others, 1956[79]
19-24	Saudi Arabia	Conjunctival scraping	Trachoma in children from 7 months to 3 years of age	Bell and others, 1960[6]
25-28	United States	Anal swabbing	No specific illness	Rosen and others, 1961[76]
29, 30	United States	Anal swabbing	No specific illness	Rosen and others, 1962[77]
31	England	Anal swabbing	No specific illness	Pereira and others, 1965[70]
32, 33	United States	Anal swabbing	No specific illness	Blacklow and others, 1969[10]

*Superscript numbers indicate references at end of chapter.

Table 17-2. Adenovirus associated with epidemic and sporadic ocular infections

Clinical diagnosis	Adenovirus types	References
Follicular conjunctivitis	1, 2, 3, 4, 5, 6, 7, 8, 9, 10, 11, 14, 15, 16, 17, 20, 22	Murray and others, 1957[64]* Boniuk and others, 1966[13]
Follicular conjunctivitis with or without respiratory symptoms; may be associated with corneal opacities	2, 3, 4, 6, 7, 8, 9	Jawetz and others, 1956[46] Ormsby and others, 1957[68] Huebner and Rowe, 1957[41]
Pharyngoconjunctival fever with or without corneal opacities	1, 3, 4, 5, 6, 7, 7a, 9, 14	Bell and others, 1955[4] Beale and others, 1957[2] Evans, 1957[24] Huebner and Rowe, 1957[41] Kendall and others, 1957[51] Kimura and others, 1957[54] Oker-Blom and others, 1957[66] van der Veen and van der Ploeg, 1958[89]
Chronic superficial keratitis	2, 11	Koseki, 1960[56] Boniuk and others, 1965[12]
Keratoconjunctivitis	3	Fowle and others, 1955[27]
Punctate keratitis	3, 7, 8, 11	Koseki, 1960[56]
Epidemic keratoconjunctivitis, "infantile" form, with membranous conjunctivitis or pseudomembranous conjunctivitis	8	Mitsui and others, 1959[61] Mordhorst and Kjer, 1961[63]
Epidemic keratoconjunctivitis in adult	8, 11, 9	Jawetz and others, 1955[47] Koseki, 1960[56] Profeta and others, 1963[72]

*Superscript numbers indicate references at end of chapter.

from adenoids and tonsils, nasal and throat washings, corneal or conjunctival scrapings, and anal swabbings. Many apparently were not producing disease when isolated.

Additional types of adenovirus have been cultured from apes, monkeys, dogs, cows, pigs, mice, and chickens.[75]

Associated ocular diseases

Among the viruses first studied by Huebner and his co-workers[40] (Table 17-1), type 3 was isolated from several cases of acute nasopharyngitis and conjunctivitis during a winter outbreak of respiratory infection in a hospital ward and during a summer outbreak in a country day school. Jawetz and his associates[46] recovered type 8 in a conjunctival and corneal scraping from a merchant seaman who had just arrived from the Orient with epidemic keratoconjunctivitis. The table shows that types 10, 15, 16, 17, and 19 through 24 also were first isolated from the eye. All but type 10 of these latter viruses were found in Saudi Arabia. Table 17-2 lists the 18 types of adenoviruses that have been found in patients with ocular disease. Although there is no record as yet of spontaneous ocular disease produced by the other 15 types, there is some experimental evidence to indicate that at least a few are able to infect the eye under experimental conditions.

Induced ocular infections

Table 17-3 summarizes a number of studies on the production of ocular infections in human volunteers. Bell and his associates[5] showed that swabbing the lower

Table 17-3. Production of ocular infections with various adenoviruses in human volunteers

Adenovirus types	Methods of transmission	Clinical manifestations	References
1, 3, 4, 5	Swabbing conjunctiva only Swabbing lower palpebral conjunctiva and throat	Pharyngoconjunctival fever Follicular nonpurulent conjunctivitis	Bell and others, 1956[5]*
3, 4	Swabbing lower tarsal conjunctiva and posterior pharynx	Pharyngoconjunctival fever	Ward and others, 1955[91]
3	Inoculation into lower fornix of conjunctiva	Keratoconjunctivitis with diffuse centrally placed subepithelial opacities	Fowle and others, 1955[27]
8	Scraping lightly upper fornix of conjunctiva with sharp knife	Epidemic keratoconjunctivitis	Mitsui and others, 1957[60]
	Instillation of virus into conjunctival sac 5 times at 5 minute intervals; bandage then placed over eyes, removed following day	Acute follicular conjunctivitis with preauricular adenopathy and subepithelial opacities	Bietti and Bruna, 1957[9]
16	Stroking lower conjunctival sac 10 times with cotton swab previously immersed in 10^{-3} dilution of inoculum virus	An afebrile nonpurulent conjunctivitis associated in one case with slight corneal involvement	Kasel and others, 1963[49]
16, 17, 20	Dropping 0.05 ml of culture fluid into conjunctival sac, followed by gentle rubbing of inoculum into palpebral conjunctiva with a sterile cotton swab	Follicular conjunctivitis	Feng and others, 1959[26]
26, 27	Swabbing lower conjunctiva with a cotton swab soaked in tissue culture	Acute nonpurulent conjunctivitis	Kasel and others, 1963[49]

*Superscript numbers indicate references at end of chapter.

palpebral conjunctiva of human volunteers with cultures of adenoviruses types 1, 3, 4, or 5 resulted in infection (rarely associated with fever), which occurred after a latent period of 2 to 7 days and which generally persisted from 4 to 8 days. A rise in complement-fixing antibodies was demonstrable. The incidence of infection was influenced by the immunologic state of the volunteers, because those without detectable neutralizing antibodies developed conjunctivitis, whereas only 45 of 113 volunteers with detectable antibodies became infected. A nonpurulent, follicular conjunctivitis was produced; it frequently involved both the palpebral and bulbar conjunctiva and often was accompanied by blepharospasm. The cytologic examination of conjunctival scrapings revealed no cytoplasmic inclusions and only a lymphocytic response. Histopathologic examination of a conjunctival biopsy showed a conjunctivitis characterized predominantly by migration of lymphocytes into the submucosal tissue.

Other studies of the viruses listed in Table 17-3 confirm the above observations and give additional information. Fowle and her associates[27] inoculated a culture of type 3 virus from a case of keratoconjunctivitis into the lower fornix of the conjunctiva of the left eye of a volunteer. Five days after inoculation there was a sudden onset of a foreign-body sensation with profuse tearing. The preauricular node became enlarged and tender, and a pseudomembrane was observed on the lower conjunctiva. Conjunctival scraping revealed a lymphocytic response without inclusion bodies. The right eye became involved 5 days after onset of the disease in the left eye. At that time slit-lamp examination revealed 3 diffuse paracentral subepithelial opacities in the left eye and 1 in the right eye. Blurring of vision in the left eye persisted for 10 days.

Mitsui and his associates[60] used the following technique to transmit infection with type 8 adenovirus to 5 volunteers. The upper fornix of the conjunctiva was scraped lightly with a sharp knife after a local anesthetic was administered to the eye. The virus inoculum was then instilled into the conjunctival sac 5 times at 5-minute intervals. After the last instillation a bandage was placed over the eye for 24 hours. In 3 of the volunteers an acute follicular conjunctivitis and preauricular adenopathy developed. The secretion was fibrinous and contained mononuclear cells. Subepithelial punctate keratitis typical of epidemic keratoconjunctivitis appeared about 1 week after the onset of the conjunctivitis. The results corresponded to those of epidemic keratoconjunctivitis acquired by natural infection. There was a rise in neutralizing antibodies against adenovirus type 8 in the convalescent sera of these volunteers similar to that found in spontaneous epidemic keratoconjunctivitis. An acute follicular conjunctivitis resulted in the fourth volunteer, and the symptoms were those of mild epidemic keratoconjunctivitis without keratitis. In the fifth volunteer repeated inoculations with adenovirus type 8 were negative, and serologic findings suggested a partial immunity in this person.

Bietti and Bruna[9] also tested the infectivity of type 8 virus. They found that 6 volunteers inoculated with tissue-cultured material after scarification of the cornea developed follicular conjunctivitis similar to epidemic keratoconjunctivitis. Another 8 volunteers in whom the tissue-cultured material was merely dropped into the eye did not develop lesions.

Kasel and his co-workers[49] used adenovirus type 16 to infect 3 volunteers. The viral strain used to prepare the inoculum was isolated from an anal specimen of a young child. The inoculation of volunteers was performed by stroking the lower conjunctival sac of the eye 10 times with a cotton swab previously immersed in 1.5 ml of fluid containing a 10^{-3} dilution of culture inoculum. All 3 volunteers developed conjunctivitis with adenovirus type 16; in one a tender preauricular node was noted on the third day after inoculation. The acute phase of illness was associated with excessive lacrimation, photophobia, and foreign-body sensation. All 3 volunteers shed virus from the inoculated eyes and from the throat and rectum.

Adenovirus types 16, 17, and 20 grown from conjunctival scrapings from 2 patients with trachoma[6,64] produced acute follicular conjunctivitis in 3 blind children when 0.05 ml of culture fluid was dropped into the conjunctival sac and the inoculum gently rubbed into the palpebral conjunctiva with a sterile cotton swab. Viruses were reisolated in 2 of the 3 cases, whereas immunologic response was detected in all 3.

Kasel and his co-workers[48] cultured adenovirus types 26 and 27 from rectal specimens of children and infected the eyes of volunteers by swabbing the lower conjunctival sac with 0.1 ml of culture or instilling 0.5 ml in each nostril. An acute self-limited conjunctivitis developed. Virus was isolated from the inoculated eyes during the first week of infection, and sporadically from the throat and rectum during 2 to 3 weeks of convalescence, but never from urine or serum specimens. Nasal inoculation resulted in greater throat infection than that which followed eye inoculation, but both routes produced about the same degree of enteric infection. It is noteworthy that strains 26 and 27, so far as we know, have not produced spontaneous diseases of the eyes.

Thus, the findings described present experimental data to show: (1) the protective influence of natural immunity upon induction of adenovirus ocular infection, (2) the effect on the induction of disease exerted by the method of inoculation and the quantity of virus used, (3) the capability of experimental disease to extend to contiguous areas, such as the contralateral eye, the throat, and the preauricular lymph nodes, (4) the incubation period and progression of the disease, and (5) the resulting serologic responses. In addition, the data show that viruses not known to produce spontaneous disease nevertheless can produce experimental infection in man.

Characterization of adenovirus groups

Adenoviruses cultured from man and animals are categorized structurally in Table 16-1. Those arising from animals have come from simian, bovine, canine, murine, and avian sources. Three distinct hemagglutinins separate the human viruses into subgroups. Group 1 (types 3, 7, 11, 14, 16, 20, 21, 25, and 28) agglutinates rhesus but not rat erythrocytes; group 2 (types 8, 9, 10, 13, 15, 17, 19, 22, 23, 24, 26, 27, 29, and 30) agglutinates rat but not rhesus erythrocytes; group 3 (types 1, 2, 4, 5, 6, and 12) fails to agglutinate rhesus cells and only partially agglutinates rat cells. Types 18 and 31 have no hemagglutinating activity.

The diagnostic identification of these viruses depends largely on immunologic tests. The hexon antigen is found in the major subunits of the virus capsid, the capsomers. This antigen represents the group-reactive antigen common to all adenoviruses. Antibody to it will give a positive complement-fixation test with adenoviruses irrespective of type. Another viral antigen, penton antigen, is a complex antigen consisting of capsomers from the 12 vertices of the icosahedral virion together with their attached fibers. Penton antigen has a biologic activity that causes clumping and detachment of tissue-cultured cells. The fiber part of this penton antigen repre-

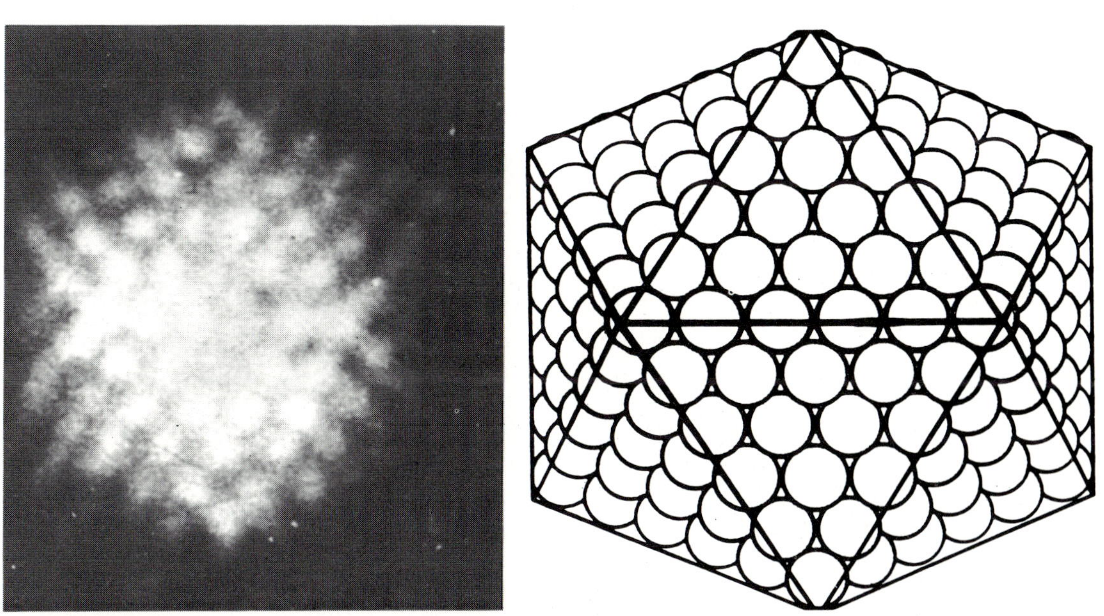

Fig. 17-1. Adenovirus is shown embedded in phosphotungstate, magnified about one million diameters (left). The drawing shows how the 252 surface subunits, or capsomers, are arranged with icosahedral symmetry. There are 12 on corners and 240 on faces or edges. (From Horne, R. W.: Sci. Amer. **208**:51, 1963.)

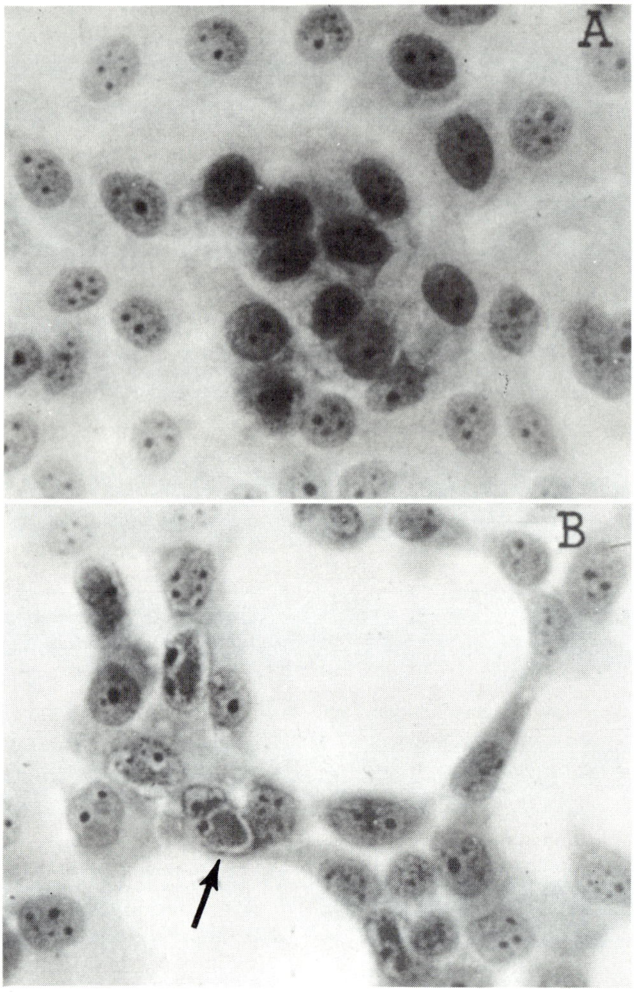

Fig. 17-2. A, Normal HeLa cells. Hematoxylin-eosin stain. (× 500.) **B,** HeLa cells 17 hours after infection with adenovirus type 3. Note aggregation of cells and nuclear inclusions (arrow). (From Beale, A. J., Doane, F., and Ormsby, H. L.: Amer. J. Ophthal. **43**:26, 1957.)

sents the *type*-specific component of the virion.[47a,75] Fig. 17-1 illustrates by electron microscopy and by schematic drawing the capsomers that compose these identifying antigens. The application of immunologic reactions to the identification and typing of adenoviruses is discussed on pp. 294-296.

The adenoviruses share certain cultural peculiarities. They have a predilection for epithelial cells, and primary isolation from human sources is readily carried out on HeLa cells derived from cervical carcinomas. Adenoviruses isolated from animals are best cultivated on epithelial cells from the specific susceptible host.[75] Characteristic cytopathogenic changes are produced in the nuclei of the infected HeLa cells by most types of these viruses. In local areas infected cells become rounded, enlarged, and show increased opacity. The cells tend to roll up and fall off the glass. Fig. 17-2 illustrates normal HeLa cells (*A*) and those infected 17 hours previously with adenovirus type 3 (*B*). The loss of some cells and the presence of inclusion bodies in surviving cells are seen in Fig. 17-2, *B*. Electron microscopic studies show that adenovirus types 3, 4, and 7 commonly

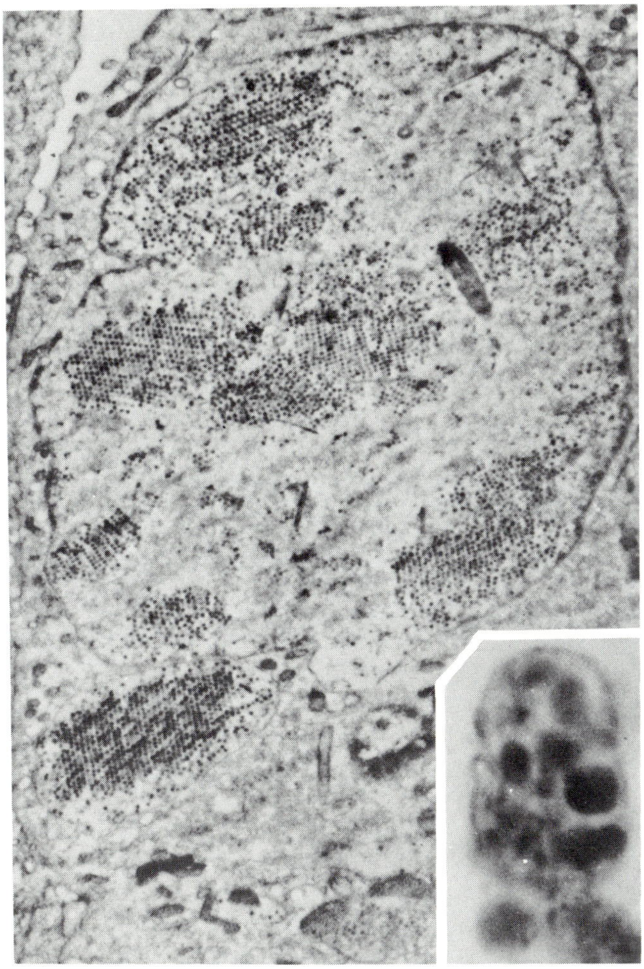

Fig. 17-3. Electron micrograph of a nucleus of a HeLa cell showing intranuclear aggregates and crystals composed of viral particles (adenovirus type 7). Each of the particles measures about 60 mμ in diameter. (× 14,000.) **Inset,** Adjacent thick section of the same nucleus after Feulgen staining, showing the aggregates seen in micrograph. Additional aggregates, which lie outside the plane of the thin section, appear in the thick section. Photomicrographs may show a slight loss of detail and quality because they have been reprinted from the original letterpress journal. (× 4,500.) (From Bloch, D. P., Morgan, C., Godman, G. C., Howe, C., and Rose, H. M.: J. Biophys. Biochem. Cytology 3:1, 1957.)

form viral crystals as they develop in cell nuclei. Fig. 17-3 is an electron micrograph showing aggregates and crystals of viral particles of type 7 in the nucleus of a cultured HeLa cell.

Epidemiology

Laboratory diagnosis of infection by viruses can be made by testing for a rising titer of specific antibodies in the serum of the patient. The application of this technique has led to surveys on the normal distribution of antibodies to adenoviruses. The results show the presence of adenoviral antibodies in most of the population at large. In adult life antibodies to one or more of these viruses are present in most normal individuals. These antibodies pass through the placenta and are demonstrable in the serum of infants for a few weeks.

Children then develop antibodies from exposure to the viruses, and before reaching their first year of life they often have been infected by at least one of the following types: 1, 2, 3, or 5. Although widely distributed, these viruses are of low pathogenicity; and primary infection occurring at an early age, as determined by a rising antibody titer, does not necessarily manifest clinical disease. About 10% of upper respiratory tract infections of children, however, are caused by adenoviruses. Less than 10% of adolescents are susceptible to these types.

The incidence of infections with adenoviruses in various age groups has been summarized by Ginsberg[30,31] in an attempt to present the natural history of man's relation to the virus. In the population as a whole about 2% to 5% of acute upper respiratory disease is caused by adenoviruses. Following primary infection, the virus may persist in the tonsils or adenoids and perhaps in other lymphoid tissues. The chronic viral infection appears as a result of parasitism of only a rare cell but is probably responsible for the presence of the base line of antibodies found in most adults.

Adenoviruses can be important pathogens for military personnel. As early as 1954 Hilleman and Werner[35] reported type 4 in military recruits, and Berge and his associates[7] isolated types 3, 4, and 7 from soldiers suffering from respiratory illness at Fort Ord in California. Tyrrell and his co-workers[87a] at this time recorded outbreaks of adenovirus infection in England in the Army and Royal Air Force. Recent studies show that adenovirus respiratory infections in induction centers may account for 70% to 80% of acute respiratory diseases among recruits. Following primary infection, lasting immunity often results.

Since antibodies to various types of adenoviruses are so readily demonstrated in sera of young adults and the disease is transmitted to relatively few contacts, vaccination appears possible and has been tried among military personnel. Both heat- and formaldehyde-inactivated type 3 virus tested by human volunteers stimulated neutralizing antibodies in 78% of those vaccinated. These immunized individuals were subsequently challenged with live virus and proved to be immune.[5]

Epidemic keratoconjunctivitis

For many decades epidemic keratoconjunctivitis (EKC) has occurred extensively in various areas throughout the world (Table 17-4). There are two phases in the history of this disease: in the first, the clinical entity was defined but the cause of the infection was obscure; in the second period, an adenovirus was identified as the causative agent.

Clinical diagnosis. Ernest Fuchs[29] (Fig. 17-4) gave the earliest description of this disease (Table 17-4). Fuchs was an ophthalmologist in Vienna who reported a form of "superficial punctate keratitis" in a group of 36 patients. In the same article he also described similar cases seen in December of 1885, in January of 1886, in March of 1887, and in the winter of 1888. The disease described by Fuchs was characterized by an acute onset, which involved only one eye in two thirds or more of the patients. At onset there was catarrhal conjunctivitis with marked ciliary injection; but within 3 to 14 days, pain, photophobia, lacrimation, and blepharospasm were predominant. The conjunctival secretion was characteristically thin and watery. Keratitis developed as conjunctivitis subsided, and corneal lesions appeared in a few days to a few weeks. These consisted of a number of gray, sharply defined punctate dots usually situated centrally rather than peripherally. These dots, about 0.5 mm in diameter, in many cases were arranged in rows or in irregularly scattered groups (Fig. 17-5). There often were as many as 100 of these lesions, although in some patients as few as 10 were seen. Some increased in size by coalescence of several adjacent foci. Each dot consisted of a number of fine points of opacity more closely aggregated at the center. The points were located just beneath Bowman's membrane; hence, they could

Table 17-4. Early records of epidemic keratoconjunctivitis in various countries (etiologic agent not yet known)

Geographic areas	Clinical observations and remarks	References
Austria	First classical description of superficial punctate keratitis	Fuchs, 1889[29]*
England	First report of superficial punctate keratitis	Gunn, 1890[32]
	Nonrecurrent superficial punctate keratitis of the Fuchs type, more common in winter than in summer	Doggart, 1933[22]
India	Superficial punctate keratitis thought to be associated with an encapsulated bacillus	Herbert, 1901[34]
	An epidemic of macular keratitis somewhat resembling superficial punctate keratitis; evidence of the contagious nature of disease	Kilpatrick, 1920[53]
	An epidemic form of superficial punctate keratitis; attempt made to transmit the disease by direct transfer of epithelial corneal scraping to healthy cornea of man and animals; histopathologic observations showed inclusion bodies	Wright, 1930[94]
	Epidemic superficial keratitis observed in families, among students in the same hostels	Sanyal, 1933[84]
	Epidemic superficial punctate keratitis; diagnosis confirmed by the minute spots on the cornea but could be missed unless examined with the corneal microscope	Kirwan, 1933[55]
Uruguay	Epidemic superficial punctate keratitis, generally bilateral; young adults affected	Iturburu, 1931[44]
Australia Tasmania	Superficial punctate keratitis with a record of a mild epidemic; frequency of bilateral involvement; complete examination of cornea with slit-lamp or corneal microscope recommended	Hamilton, 1941[33]
Malaya	"Acute kerato-conjunctivitis of unidentified origin, occasionally becoming epidemic"; susceptibility to infection greater following trauma or surgery	Viswalingam, 1941[90]
France	Superficial punctate keratitis; respiratory infection preceded onset of ocular disease	Fradkine, 1932[28]
Germany	Superficial punctate keratitis; epidemic nature of the disease thought to be caused by an unknown virus	Schneider, 1938[85] Zur Nedden, 1938[95]
Italy	Appearance of epidemic keratoconjunctivitis in 1942 coincided with arrival of German troups; disease was prevalent in Germany at that time	Bietti and Bruna, 1957[9]
China	Superficial punctate keratitis; half of the patients were exposed to swimming pool conjunctivitis	Ling, 1936[57]
Middle East Palestine	First report of epidemic superficial punctate keratitis in patients ages 26 to 67	Feigenbaum, 1939[25]
Japan	First record of superficial punctate keratitis in Orient	Inoue, 1894[43]
Java	Reported keratitis punctata tropica	Westhoff, 1912[92]

*Superscript numbers indicate references at end of chapter.

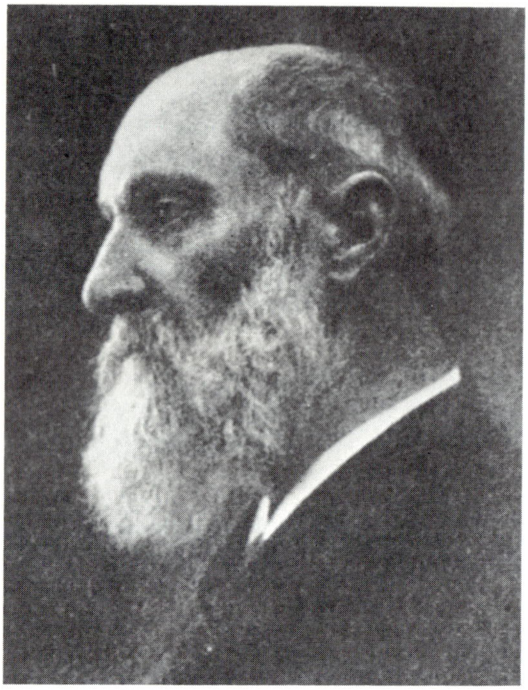

Fig. 17-4. Ernest Fuchs (1851-1930), an Austrian ophthalmologist, is credited with the original, classical description of superficial punctate keratitis, now known as epidemic keratoconjunctivitis (EKC). Though the cause was unknown then, the clinical picture was so clearly presented that the disease acquired a defined clinical identity. (From Amer. J. Ophthal. 14:1, 1939.)

not be removed by scraping the corneal epithelium. In 14 instances the corneal lesions remained for 6 to 10 months, and Fuchs stated that one could not be certain that the corneal lesions would disappear completely until after 1 to 2 years. Corneal sensitivity was diminished, and this also returned to normal only slowly. Fuchs observed that this punctate keratitis occurred in several members of one family, that the incidence increased in the winter time, that the onset might be associated with acute pharyngitis, and that young adults were commonly affected. Independently of Fuchs a number of Austrian ophthalmologists described the same clinical entity under different names. Apparently at that period of time epidemics existed in Austria, and the epidemic nature of this ocular disease was recognized by these early clinicians.

Since the original report by Fuchs, data have accumulated recording small, dispersed epidemics of a similar eye affection in the Orient and in the Western world. It appears that no nationality is immune from this infection and that there is no preference for sex or age. Table 17-4 lists early reports of this clinical syndrome in various countries other than the USA.

Wiener[93] in 1909 (Table 17-5) described the first case in the United States of the disease that was to be known as epidemic

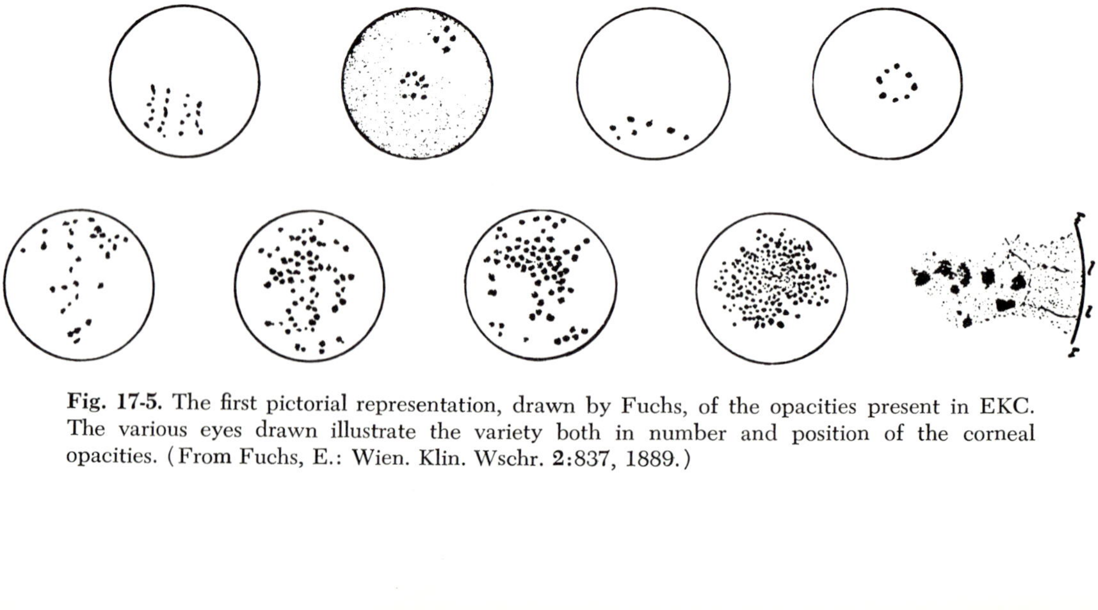

Fig. 17-5. The first pictorial representation, drawn by Fuchs, of the opacities present in EKC. The various eyes drawn illustrate the variety both in number and position of the corneal opacities. (From Fuchs, E.: Wien. Klin. Wschr. 2:837, 1889.)

keratoconjunctivitis. His patient, a young woman aged 21, developed irritation, lacrimation, and injection of the conjunctiva in November of 1907. This was followed by about 30 corneal opacities consisting of small round grayish dots 1 mm or less in diameter, which lasted about 6 weeks.

Hobson[36] reported an acute epidemic of superficial punctate keratitis in 16 patients at the Veterans Administration Hospital, San Fernando, California. Those affected included 2 members of the kitchen help and a number of ward attendants. All were living on the hospital grounds. The disease began with a violent conjunctivitis, unilateral in only one case and associated with pronounced photophobia and lacrimation. The ocular and palpebral conjunctiva became markedly red and edematous, but pain was not severe. Twenty to 100 minute, opaque, grayish dots were seen, involving, for the most part, the second layer of the cornea. In 4 of the cases there was a persisting reduction of visual acuity in one or both eyes, because absorption of deposits in these cases was incomplete and slight haziness of the cornea remained. There were no children in this series, which was equally divided between males and females.

EKC received considerable attention during World War II, when the disease was considered a major problem in some large industrial plants. Holmes[38] in 1941 in Oahu, Hawaii, reported a rapidly spreading type of conjunctivitis referred to by the patients and doctors as "pink eye." Repeated cultures and smears made from conjunctival scrapings and secretions failed to determine a causative agent. The ex-

Table 17-5. Some early records of epidemic keratoconjunctivitis in the United States

Prominent areas	Clinical observations and remarks	References
St. Louis	First record of superficial punctate keratitis; observed numerous small round grayish dots in the cornea	Wiener, 1909[93]*
California San Fernando	The first epidemic recorded under title "acute epidemic punctate keratitis"	Hobson, 1938[36]
Hawaii	Epidemic infectious conjunctivitis in a form of "pink eye"; extremely contagious	Holmes, 1941[38]
Spokane	Called the infection keratoconjunctivitis; swelling of the preauricular gland a frequent occurrence; etiology was believed to be a specific virus; trauma to the eye a predisposing factor	deRoetth, 1942[74]
Oregon	Acute conjunctivitis with corneal involvement in shipyard workers; unilateral, contagious; startling rapid spread	Rieke, 1942[73]
California San Francisco	Abbreviated as "EKC," the name epidemic keratoconjunctivitis was suggested and quickly adopted; infection occurred in shipyard workers; popular name "shipyard, or California, conjunctivitis" was attached to this disease	Hogan and Crawford, 1942[37]
Schenectady	Outbreak of epidemic keratoconjunctivitis in an industrial plant; report based on observations in several thousand cases	Perkins and others, 1943[71]
New York	Epidemic keratoconjunctivitis observed in over 2,000 cases from the New York area; convalescent plasma or sera seemed to be the treatment of choice	Braley, 1943[15] Braley, 1945[16]

*Superscript numbers indicate references at end of chapter.

treme contagiousness of this outbreak suggested that it might assume epidemic proportions, as had occurred in large outbreaks at the Pearl Harbor Navy Yard. At the end of June, the infection was fairly widespread; and people of all walks of life, irrespective of age, sex, and race, were affected. An estimated 10,000 to 25,000 cases occurred. The clinical picture was quite uniform. The most common complication was the development of the characteristic corneal infiltrates involving the second layer of the cornea. The number of dots varied from 1 to 100, and they were arranged in groups or rows, scattered irregularly, and commonly located on the central portion of the cornea. Other features occurring after a period of 2 to 5 days were profuse tearing, photophobia, and blepharospasm. The discharge was characteristically scant or absent. Multiple subconjunctival hemorrhages appeared on the tarsal portions of the conjunctiva and were so characteristic that they were considered almost pathognomonic of the disease. The eye remained irritable for 4 to 6 weeks or longer when corneal infiltrates developed. Preauricular adenopathy was noted in about 50% of the cases. A factor thought to contribute to the spread of the infection was rubbing of the eyes with unclean fingers. This hand-to-eye type of transmission was suggested by the involvement of the second eye in three fourths of the cases and by the presence in many instances of multiple cases in one family. Holmes stated that those who were infected in Hawaii were inclined to attribute the infection to foreign material lodging in or touching the eye: those working in canneries blamed it on drops of pineapple juice reaching the affected eye; the worker at the emery wheel was certain that his attack began when a piece of dust landed in the eye; those doing much swimming were convinced that the disease was caused by the contaminated water, and so on.

In 1942 deRoetth[74] reported 12 cases of a similar disease in Spokane, Washington, and used the term epidemic keratoconjunctivitis. The main clinical features were acute conjunctivitis followed by superficial punctate keratitis. Swelling of the preauricular gland was a frequent occurrence. Trauma of the eye was a predisposing factor. The etiology was unknown but was believed to be a specific virus.

Rieke[73] described an epidemic of ocular inflammation of unknown origin in the Oregon Shipbuilding Corporation yards at Portland, Oregon; the epidemic involved 600 cases in one shipyard. The clinical descriptions of Rieke's series closely resembled those already presented. The infection involved a small percentage of exposed men and usually attacked only one eye. It appeared that factors that influenced the epidemics were heavy concentration of men from all stations of life, poor ocular hygiene, and probably the virulence of the responsible agent. The author felt that the infection came from Hawaii.

Other examples of EKC were reported during the early years of the war by Hogan and Crawford[37] in San Francisco, Perkins and his co-workers[71] in Schenectady, New York, and Braley[16] in the New York City area. Bedell[3] described the distribution of epidemic keratoconjunctivitis in the United States. He noted the failure of the infection to appear in any of the great army mobilization centers and attributed this to the health of the men in service as well as to the high standard of sanitation in the camps. There were no epidemics in the shipyards on the Gulf of Mexico or along the Atlantic Coast, a fact proving that the infection was not a shipyard disease. Thygeson[87] in his review on the epidemiology of epidemic keratoconjunctivitis stated that during the later war years (1943 to 1946) only sporadic cases were observed. Contrary to expectations, the infection did not become a military problem.

In Canada, McGavin and his associates[59] reported that no evidence of the disease was observed until the winter of 1947 to 1948 when an epidemic of keratoconjunctivitis affected four plants of the Ford

Motor Company. The economic loss caused by this epidemic was severe.

Isolation of causative agent. The discovery of the etiologic agent of EKC came only about a year after the first isolations of types of the adenoviruses. Jawetz, Kimura, Hanna, Coleman, Thygeson, and Nichols[47] in a classic paper presented studies on a virus isolated from a merchant seaman traveling between the Orient and San Francisco. The patient was seen 12 days after the onset of the disease in his right eye. He showed "an intense conjunctivitis with pseudo-membrane formation and enlarged preauricular nodes. . . . The left eye became involved 4 days later." A virus, isolated on HeLa cells from each eye, proved to possess a complement-fixing antigen common to other human adenoviruses. But it was not typable with any antiserum then available and was classified by Dr. Huebner as type 8. Samples of sera were collected from patients with typical EKC in Canada, Philadelphia, Chicago, and California. All of the 25 patients with typical clinical manifestations of the disease showed neutralizing antibodies for the new type 8 after 19 days. These antibodies were demonstrable in only 1 of 5 patients with atypical keratoconjunctivitis or uveitis. Further studies by these and other workers demonstrated type 8 neutralizing antibodies, following EKC, in sera of patients from many parts of the world. An excellent correlation between clinical and laboratory diagnosis was demonstrable.

It may be seen from Table 17-2 that there are also two reports of EKC following infection with adenovirus types 9 and 11. Hence, the possibility that adenoviruses other than type 8 may sometimes produce EKC should be kept in mind.

The communicability of EKC is related to the ability of the virus to survive. Mordhorst and Kjer[63] studied an epidemic that occurred in Copenhagen in 1958. Type 8 virus was isolated from conjunctival swabbings of 5 patients taken within the first 6 days of symptoms. These swabbings were stored for 1 year before they were grown in cultured cells. Transmission of the infection has also been known to occur from contaminated tonometers, eye medicaments, and direct finger-to-eye contact. Offices, dispensaries, and hospitals may spread the infection.[8,18,18a,85a]

At the Institute of Ophthalmology, Columbia-Presbyterian Medical Center, over a thousand cases clinically diagnosed as epidemic keratoconjunctivitis have been seen in the past 30 years. Although the cases seen at the IOCPMC did not appear to be part of an epidemic, epidemics continue to occur in various areas of the country. One such epidemic, lasting from April through September of 1967, is of interest because of the hospital personnel and patients who were involved.[56a] It was the fourth largest epidemic in 18 years in the Philadelphia area. Virus isolation was accomplished in 38 of the 62 cases in which it was attempted. In an outbreak of EKC in and around Glasgow in the autumn of 1967 type 8 adenovirus was recovered from 57 of 186 patients, and the serologic reactions were positive in 21 additional infections.[3a]

Plate 3, *H* illustrates a severe follicular and membranous conjunctivitis in a 40-year-old Negro male with EKC. The patient was seen 13 days after onset of illness. In Plate 3, *I* an artist's drawing shows the appearance and position of subepithelial corneal infiltrates 3 weeks after onset of the disease in another patient.

Specific treatment for epidemic keratoconjunctivitis has not yet been discovered. The disease may impair vision for months or years, and in rare instances the corneal opacities never clear.

Pharyngoconjunctival fever

Pharyngoconjunctival fever is a highly infectious disease responsible for epidemic outbreaks in schools and military establishments. It also occurs in families as well as in sporadic form. Small epidemic outbreaks in civilian populations, private offices, dispensaries, hospitals, and among medical personnel have been recorded.

Probably the earliest report of a form of

acute follicular conjunctivitis, now called pharyngoconjunctival fever, was that made by Béal[1] in 1907. The characteristic feature of the disease was the presence of follicles, particularly on the palpebral conjunctiva and in the cul-de-sacs. The upper tarsal conjunctiva was not affected; the bulbar conjunctiva was edematous and hyperemic. Corneal changes were not seen. The conjunctival secretions were scanty, and mononuclear cells predominated. One third of Béal's patients had an associated acute upper respiratory tract infection. Enlargement of the preauricular and submaxillary nodes was noted. The infection was observed in several members of the same family; therefore, Béal believed that the disease was contagious. However, an etiologic agent was not determined. Morax[62] in 1933 described the disease under the name "acute follicular conjunctivitis, Béal's type." In this country, Thygeson[86] in 1935 reported a minor epidemic, occurring among students at the University of Iowa, of an acute follicular conjunctivitis that in all respects closely resembled the type described by Béal. Because of the absence of bacteria, Thygeson suggested that a virus was probably the etiologic agent. Derrick[20] in 1943 reported 3 cases of "swimming bath conjunctivitis" from Australia. Duke-Elder[22a] states that although the disease is characterized by the triad of fever, pharyngitis, and a nonpurulent follicular conjunctivitis often associated with regional lymphadenitis, these may occur singly or together and in all stages of severity.

In 1951 Cockburn[17] observed in Greeley, Colorado, an epidemic of a disease known as "Greeley disease," which occurred during the months of August and September. The clinical entity consisted of an unusual combination of features; acute, nonpurulent conjunctivitis with photophobia, follicular inflammation, and edema, sometimes followed by nonmembranous keratitis. Scrapings revealed mononuclear cells; no inclusions were observed. Usually one eye was involved initially, followed by infection of the other eye. Conjunctival scrapings revealed no viral inclusions, and no bacterial pathogens were isolated. Three weeks after onset, in 13 out of 54 cases slit-lamp examination revealed that the cornea had small whitish plaques, 1 mm or less in size. Other associated findings were vesicular pharyngitis, pyrexia, and severe muscle pain. The preauricular lymph nodes were not significantly enlarged, but the lymph nodes in the neck were involved. Conjunctivitis persisted from 3 days to 3 weeks. Many of the patients had all clinical features. All but 3 of the patients were under 21 years of age. One was a mother who became infected from her child. The sources of infection in the Greeley outbreak were either direct contact or association with swimming pools, since 25% to 50% of the children using the pools developed the disease. In some instances a diagnosis of poliomyelitis was made; but spinal puncture did not show any cells in the cerebrospinal fluid, and all the patients suspected of having the disease made an uneventful recovery.

Cockburn, Rowe, and Huebner[17] related the disease to adenovirus infection when they studied the sera that had been drawn from 11 patients during the Greeley epidemic in 1951. Ten of the 11 sera showed a rise in the complement-fixing antibody titer to the group antigen of adenovirus, and 8

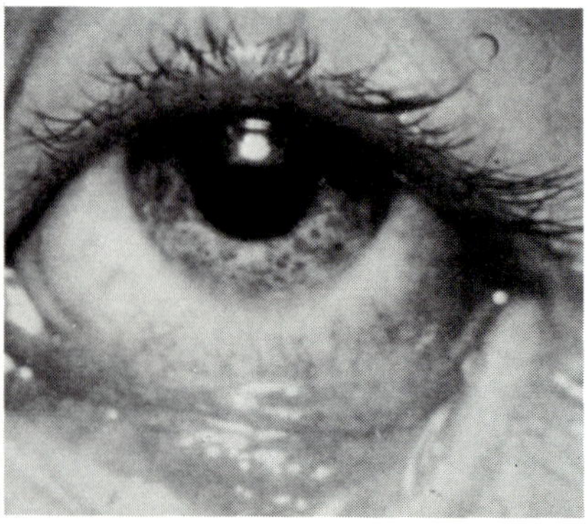

Fig. 17-6. Acute follicular conjunctivitis in pharyngoconjunctival fever caused by type 3 adenovirus. (From Thygeson, P.: Med. Clin. N. Amer. 43:1423, 1959.)

exhibited a rise in neutralizing antibody to adenovirus type 3. In 1955 blood samples were taken from several of the patients from the 1951 series to determine the persistence of neutralizing antibodies. These antibodies were again detected 41 months after the infection.

Fig. 17-6 illustrates pharyngoconjunctival conjunctivitis caused by type 3 adenovirus. Table 17-2 lists other types of adenoviruses (1, 4, 5, 6, 7, 7a, 9, and 14) that have been reported to cause the same clinical syndrome. Type 3 adenovirus has also been cultured from other ocular lesions (see Table 17-2), EKC excepted. In Table 17-6 some of the similarities and differences in EKC and pharyngoconjunctival fever are presented. Today infections of the eye with adenoviruses usually are classified in either of these two categories.

The clinical features of pharyngoconjunctival fever are varied but typically consist of acute nonmembranous follicular conjunctivitis associated with preauricular adenopathy, pharyngitis, fever, malaise, and sometimes diarrhea and muscle pains. Acute catarrhal inflammation, as seen in Fig. 17-6, occurs on the lower palpebral conjunctiva and may extend into the bulbar and upper palpebral conjunctiva. Hyperplasia of lymph follicles is most marked in the lower palpebral conjunctiva. Visual blurring may occasionally occur together with excessive lacrimation. Conjunctivitis may persist for only 3 to 4 days or last as long as 3 weeks and is followed by

Table 17-6. Epidemic keratoconjunctivitis and pharyngoconjunctival fever: similarities and differences

Epidemic keratoconjunctivitis	Pharyngoconjunctival fever
Described by Fuchs in 1889 in Vienna	Described by Béal in 1907 in France
Etiologic agent, adenovirus type 8, isolated in 1955	Etiologic agent, largely adenovirus type 3, isolated in 1955; also associated with other adenovirus infections, notably type 7
Frequently epidemic, worldwide	Frequently epidemic, worldwide
Incubation period 5 to 12 days	Incubation period 5 or 6 days
High incidence of epidemics in industrial plants, private offices, hospitals, and dispensaries; marked tendency to spread among medical personnel	Epidemics related to swimming pools and population density
Predilection for adults	Predilection for young children
Highly infectious	Highly infectious
Rarely associated with febrile systemic manifestations	Usually marked febrile and systemic manifestations
Preauricular lymphadenopathy usual	Lymphadenopathy variable
Acute follicular or membranous conjunctivitis	Acute severe follicular conjunctivitis
Corneal involvement constant; primary subepithelial infiltrates grossly visible	Corneal involvement rare and slight
Resolution 8 weeks to 2 years; permanent visual damage very rare	Resolution rapid: 1 to 3 weeks
Low incidence of antibodies to adenovirus type 8 in general population	High incidence of antibodies to various types of adenoviruses causing pharyngoconjunctival fever

complete recovery. Usually there is no corneal involvement associated with the conjunctivitis, and when keratitis is present it does not interfere with vision or last long.

Pharyngoconjunctival fever has a predilection for young children; older people appear to be less susceptible, presumably because of previous exposure to adenoviruses. Infected individuals are the common sources of spread, via the respiratory tract, from person to person. Swimming pools have been implicated as an important source of infection.[17,65,67] The incubation period is usually from 5 to 6 days; the virus, most frequently type 3, can be isolated in the first few days of the disease but is rarely found after the ninth day. Specific antibodies persist in the circulation for 3 or more years.[17] Immunity is type specific, and recovery from infection with one type does not result in resistance against infection with another type.

Acute follicular conjunctivitis

A number of adenoviruses have been isolated in acute follicular conjunctivitis (Table 17-2). The major clinical manifestations are as follows. Follicles are seen mainly in the palpebral conjunctiva and fornix of the lower lid. The bulbar conjunctiva is edematous and hyperemic; itching and burning are of moderate severity; lacrimation may be present in the absence of photophobia. As with the other adenovirus infections, conjunctival scrapings reveal a predominance of lymphocytes and no inclusions.

Laboratory identification of adenovirus in ocular infection

Two approaches are available for establishing the etiologic agent in ocular disease caused by one of the adenoviruses. The first is to isolate the virus and identify it by serologic means. The second method, a retrospective measure, is to obtain 2 or more samples of serum from the patient; the first taken during the early acute phase of the disease, and further serum to be taken during the convalescent months. A rising titer of specific antibody to one of the types of adenoviruses indicates the particular virus that caused the infection[21] (see also Chapter 16).

Isolation of the virus. Conjunctival washings or conjunctival and corneal scrapings (Chapter 4) are obtained within the first few days of infection. The material recovered is placed in Earle's balanced salt solution with 500 mg per ml of penicillin and 250 mg per ml of streptomycin added. If the material is not to be on culture medium within 6 hours, it may be stored at −20° C after it has been quick-frozen in a mixture of dry ice and butanol. For prolonged storage (more than a month), a temperature of −60° C should be maintained. The HeLa cell is commonly used today for the cultivation of adenoviruses, although some laboratories use other cell lines.[75] The sample is inoculated into two or more tubes of cultured cells and incubated at 37° C. If an adenovirus is present, a typical cytopathogenic effect usually will be seen in a few days; this effect characteristically consists of enlargement and increased opacity of the cells. These round up, clump together, and eventually fall off the glass. Such changes may be observed in a few days, depending on the amount of virus present in the test specimen. Subcultures will produce cytopathogenic changes more rapidly. The adenoviruses multiply within the nuclei of the susceptible cells (Figs. 17-2 and 17-3). If these cells are stained with Giemsa stain, nuclear inclusions can be seen by the light microscope. Fluorescein-labeled specific antibody will bind to the nuclear inclusions, which contain virus antigen; and under ultraviolet light, fluorescence can be seen (Fig. 17-7). Final identification of the virus depends upon establishing the ability of a known type-specific antiserum either to interfere with hemagglutination, to neutralize cytopathogenic change in cultured cells, or to prevent infection of cultured cells. Detailed instructions for carrying out these procedures are to be found in the chapter by Rose[75] in the text edited by Lennette and Schmidt.

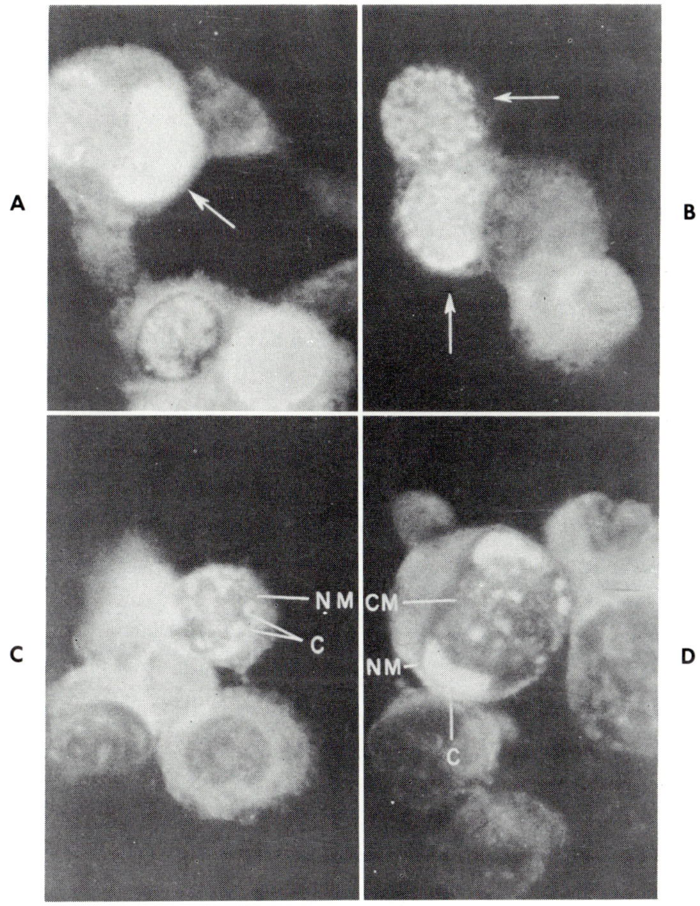

Fig. 17-7. A, HeLa cells 24 hours after infection with type 7 adenovirus stained by indirect fluorescent antibody technique demonstate intracellular virus antigen. Note intense fluorescence in infected nuclei. Cell indicated by arrow reveals diffuse nuclear staining of evenly spaced granules. **B,** HeLa cells in slightly later stage in sequence of infection. Note bright intranuclear staining (arrows) now appears in coarse aggregates. **C,** HeLa cell in still later stage, showing sharp-edged, brightly stained, crystallike masses (*C*) in nucleus. Denser central zone of nucleus can barely be distinguished. *NM* indicates site of nuclear membrane. **D,** HeLa cells late in course of infection (48 hours). Note large, sharply outlined crystalline masses (*C*) in peripheral nuclear zone and small fluorescent aggregates in central mass (*CM*). *NM* indicates site of nuclear membrane. Photomicrographs may show a slight loss of detail and quality because they have been reprinted from the original letterpress journal. (× 1,000.) (From Boyer, G. S., Denny, F. W., Jr., and Ginsberg, H. S.: J. Exp. Med. **110**:827, 1959.)

Test of rising antibody titer in serum from convalescent patients. Significant increases in complement-fixing and specific virus-neutralizing antibodies usually are found during convalescene. Initial acute phase sera must be examined to check the normal amount of antibodies present in each patient. Maximum serum levels of antibodies following infection are observed 2 or more weeks after onset of the disease. Titers then may decline, but in many individuals antibodies may be detected for more than a year. Identification of specific types is possible only in a virology laboratory that maintains many types and that is prepared to carry out extensive cultural and serologic work.[50,75]

Fluorescein-labeled antibody for identification of adenoviruses. Fluorescein-labeled antibodies to some of the commoner specific types of adenoviruses are now available commercially. They are useful in staining slides containing infected cells. The fluorescein technique for examining smears of ocular discharge or scrapings is complicated by the large number of types of adenoviruses. It is possible to make only a very limited number of smears from such material; therefore, even if the offending virus is highly suspected, as in the case of keratoconjunctivitis, it may be difficult to obtain a sufficient number of slides to set up the necessary controls. Another factor that may decrease the usefulness of direct smears or scrapings of the conjunctiva and cornea in studies with fluorescein-labeled antibody is the usual lack of demonstrable inclusion bodies in the cells of scrapings from patients with EKC and pharyngoconjunctival fever. It is these inclusions that bind the specific antibody in high concentration.[42] As is seen in Figs. 17-3 and 17-4, inclusion bodies are plentiful in tissue-cultured cells infected with adenoviruses. The usefulness of the fluorescein antibody technique in the study of infected cultured cells is well established. The fluorescein technique is presented by Liu[58] in the text edited by Lennette and Schmidt.

• • •

The story of the association of adenoviruses, especially type 8, with ocular disease has been described in more detail than is alloted to other viruses. There are several reasons for this. The first is the unique position that type 8 adenovirus occupies, because of its specific predilection for the eye. In contrast, the majority of the other types may often be associated with eye infections occurring spontaneously or produced experimentally. Perhaps the most compelling reason is that the story of the discovery of this group of viruses, their isolation from the normal and inflamed eye, and their identification has taken place through a brilliant series of studies by many investigators around the world. The first 30 of the known 33 types producing infection in man were isolated in a 10-year period, 1952 to 1962. A clear picture of the ocular disease produced and the epidemiology of the infections were largely established during this period, and much was learned of the physical structure and antigenic makeup of these agents. The immunologic responses of the host have been determined. The ophthalmologist has contributed a clinical description of the disease that, although it goes back almost a hundred years, has proved valid today. All of these facts, many of them established by our peers, provides a sense of participation in an exciting aspect of ocular disease.

PAPOVAVIRUS INFECTION OF THE EYE

The papovavirus group consists of small animal viruses that have only one representative typically infectious for man; the papilloma (wart) virus. Others of this group include the Shope rabbit papilloma, the polyoma virus of mice, and the vacuolating (SV 40) virus of monkeys. The name papovavirus is derived from the first two letters of these three viruses. They characteristically produce chronic infections in their hosts, and all are tumorigenic. Their structural characteristics are given in Table 16-1, which shows that they share several common traits with adenoviruses.

Papilloma, or wart, virus of man has been reported to produce proliferative changes in tissue-cultured cells of human embryonic skin and mucle. These are similar to tissue-culture changes produced by the rabbit papilloma virus.[5] In man the warts consist of irregular upgrowths of epidermis containing elongated papillae carrying blood vessels, and of thickened corneum. Most of the cells of the papilloma above the basal cells contain intranuclear inclusion bodies and characteristic cytoplasmic masses. Crystalline virus particles may be obtained from these warts. The extraction of elementary bodies and bits of crystals is carried out by a relatively simple procedure, which has been described by Melnick.[59a] Fig. 17-8 shows both individual elementary bodies and a three-dimensional array of

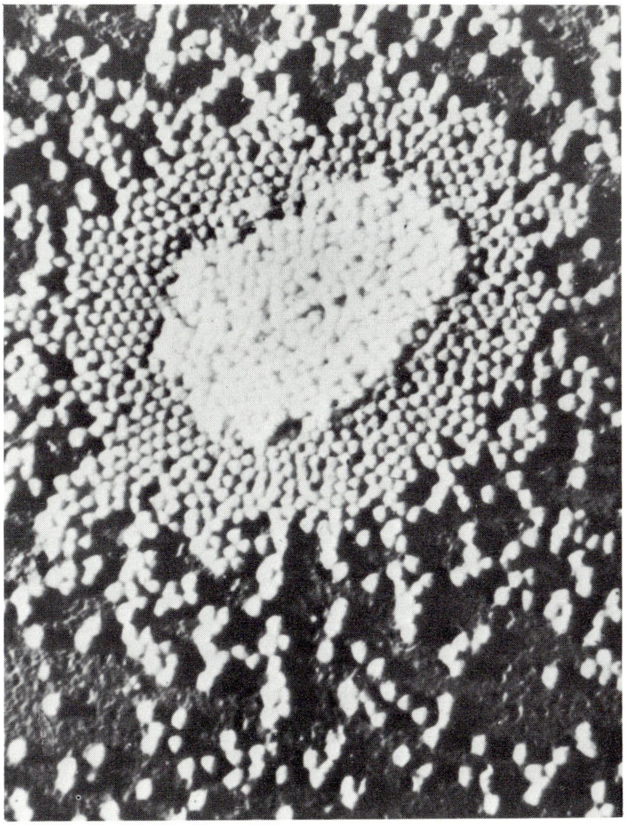

Fig. 17-8. Human wart virus, with particles showing the beginning of orderly arrangement into crystalline formation. Particles 50 mμ in diameter. (From Annals of The New York Academy of Sciences, volume 54, article 6, figure 6, p. 1216, J. L. Melnick et al. © The New York Academy of Sciences; 1952; reprinted by permission.)

these particles. This illustrates the first crystalline substance of this type obtained from any animal viral growth.

Warts, or verrucae, are spread through autoinoculation by scratching and by direct or indirect contact. Patients who are carrying warts have circulating antibody specific for the human papovavirus. This antibody is carried in the IgM fraction of the immunoglobulins.

When warts are situated on the margins of the lids between the eyelashes, a catarrhal conjunctivitis usually results, as was first described by deRoetth.[73a] It is subacute without much discharge. The scrapings fail to show inclusion bodies in the cells. The cornea also may be involved with multiple punctate erosions. Duke-Elder[22a]

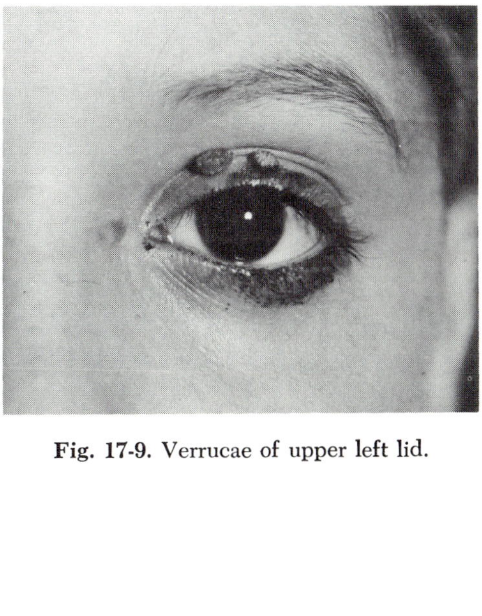

Fig. 17-9. Verrucae of upper left lid.

believes that the conjunctival and corneal lesions are probably either toxic or allergic in origin, since inclusion bodies so characteristic of the infection are not found and since removal of the warts by excision or fulguration results in prompt healing of the lesions of both the conjunctiva and cornea. Small warts may be difficult to see between the eyelashes and should be carefully searched for. Fig. 17-9 illustrates verrucae of the upper lid of a patient seen at the IOCPMC. These were associated with edema and tenderness. The verrucae were excised, and relief of the eye condition followed.

REFERENCES

1. Béal, R.: Sur une forme particulière de conjonctivite aigue avec follicules, Ann. Oculist. **87**:1, 1907.
2. Beale, A. J., Doane, F., and Ormsby, H. L.: Studies on adenovirus infections of the eye in Toronto, Amer. J. Ophthal. **43**:26, 1957.
3. Bedell, A. J.: Distribution of epidemic keratoconjunctivitis in the United States, J.A.M.A. **123**:1101, 1943.
3a. Bell, E. J., Martin, K. W., and Ross, C.A.C.: Laboratory diagnosis of epidemic keratoconjunctivitis, J. Med. Microbiol. **2**:125, 1969.
4. Bell, J. A., Rowe, W. P., Engler, J. I., Parrott, R. H., and Huebner, R. J.: Pharyngoconjunctival fever, epidemiological studies of a recently recognized disease entity, J.A.M.A. **157**:1083, 1955.
5. Bell, J. A., Ward, T. G., Huebner, R. J., Rowe, W. P., Suskind, R. G., and Paffenbarger, R. S.: Studies of adenoviruses (APC) in volunteers, Amer. J. Public Health: **46**:1130, 1956.
6. Bell, S. D., Jr., Rota, T. R., and McComb, D. E.: Adenoviruses isolated from Saudi Arabia: six new serotypes, Amer. J. Trop. Med. **9**:523, 1960.
7. Berge, T. O., England, B., Mauris, C., Shuey, H. E., and Lennette, E. H.: Etiology of acute respiratory disease among service personnel at Fort Ord, California, Amer. J. Hyg. **62**: 283, 1955.
8. Berg, R., and Ringstrom, C.-B.: Adenovirus type 8 associated follicular conjunctivitis and keratoconjunctivitis in patients subjected to tonometry, Scand. J. Infect. Dis. **1**:153, 1969.
9. Bietti, G. B., and Bruna, F.: Epidemic keratoconjunctivitis in Italy: some contributions to its clinical aspects, epidemiology and etiology (part II), Amer. J. Ophthal. **43**:50, 1957.
10. Blacklow, N. R., Hoggan, M. D., Austin, J. B., and Rowe, W. P.: Observations on two new adenovirus serotypes with unusual antigenic characteristics, Amer. J. Epidem. **90**: 501, 1969.
11. Bloch, D. P., Morgan, C., Godman, G. C., Howe, C., and Rose, H. M.: A correlated histochemical and electron microscopic study of the intranuclear crystalline aggregates of adenovirus (RI-APC virus) in HeLa cells, J. Biophys. Biochem. Cytol. **3**:1, 1957.
12. Boniuk, M., Phillips, C. A., and Friedman, J. B.: Chronic adenovirus type 2 keratitis in man, New Eng. J. Med. **273**:924, 1965.
13. Boniuk, M., Phillips, C. A., Hines, M. J., and Friedman, J. B.: Adenovirus infections of the conjunctiva and cornea, Trans. Amer. Acad. Ophthal. Otolaryng. **70**:1016, 1966.
14. Boyer, G. S., Denny, F. W., Jr., and Ginsberg, H. S.: Sequential cellular changes produced by types 5 and 7 adenoviruses in HeLa cells and in human amniotic cells: cytological studies aided by fluorescein-labelled antibody, J. Exp. Med. **110**:827, 1959.
15. Braley, A.: Epidemic keratoconjunctivitis, Med. Clin. N. Amer. **27**:1641, 1943.
16. Braley, A.: Epidemic keratoconjunctivitis, Arch. Ophthal. **33**:47, 1945.
17. Cockburn, T. A., Rowe, W. P., and Huebner, R. J.: Relationship of the 1951 Greeley, Colorado outbreak of conjunctivitis and pharyngitis to type 3 APC virus infection, Amer. J. Hyg. **63**:250, 1956.
18. Dawson, C., and Darrell, R.: Infections due to adenovirus type 8 in the United States (parts I and II), New Eng. J. Med. **268**: 1031, 1963.
18a. Dawson, C. R., Hanna, L., Wood, T. R., and Despain, R.: Adenovirus type 8 keratoconjunctivitis in the United States: epidemiologic, clinical, and microbiologic features, Amer. J. Ophthal. **69**:473, 1970.
19. Dean, A.: Superficial and punctate keratitis, Mich. State Med. Soc. **33**:295, 1934.
20. Derrick, E. H.: Swimming bath conjunctivitis, with a report of three probable cases and a note on its epidemiology, Med. J. Aust. **2**: 334, 1943.
21. Doane, F., Rhodes, A. J., and Ormsby, H. L.: Virological investigations in adenovirus infections of the conjunctiva, Toronto, 1955-56, Canad. Med. Ass. J. **77**:675, 1957.
22. Doggart, J. H.: Superficial punctate keratitis, Brit. J. Ophthal. **17**:65, 1933.
22a. Duke-Elder, S.: System of ophthalmology. Diseases of the outer eye, vol. 8, part 1, St. Louis, 1965, The C. V. Mosby Co., p. 348.
22b. Ellison, E. D., Kaufman, H. E., and Little,

J. M.: Comparison of methods for the laboratory diagnosis of ocular adenovirus type 3 infection, Invest. Ophthal. **8**:484, 1969.

23. Enders, J. F., Bell, J. A., Dingle, J. H., Francis, T., Jr., Hilleman, M. R., Huebner, R. J., and Payne, A. M. M.: "Adenoviruses," group name proposed for new respiratory-tract viruses, Science **124**:119, 1956.
24. Evans, A. S.: Acute respiratory disease in University of Wisconsin students, New Eng. J. Med. **256**:377, 1957.
25. Feigenbaum, A.: Note sur la kératite ponctuée superficielle épidémique en Palestine, Rev. Int. Trachome **16**:18, 1939.
26. Feng, M., Chang, R. S., Smith, T. R., and Snyder, J. C.: Adenoviruses isolated from Saudi Arabia: pathogenicity of certain strains for man, Amer. J. Trop. Med. **8**:501, 1959.
27. Fowle, A. M. C., Cockeram, A., and Ormsby, H. L.: Virus isolations from patients with keratoconjunctivitis, Amer. J. Ophthal. **40**:180, 1955.
28. Fradkine, J.: Trois cas de kératite ponctuée superficielle: étiologie-thérapeutique, Bull. Mem. Soc. Franc. Ophtal. **45**:135, 1932.
29. Fuchs, E.: Keratitis punctata superficialis, Wien. Klin. Wschr. **2**:837, 1889.
30. Ginsberg, H. S.: Newer aspects of adenovirus infections, Amer. J. Public Health **49**:1480, 1959.
31. Ginsberg, H. S., and Dingle, J. H.: The adenovirus group. In Horsfall, F. L., Jr., and Tamm, I., editors: Viral and rickettsial infections of man, ed. 4, Philadelphia, 1965, J. P. Lippincott Co., pp. 860-891.
32. Gunn, R. M.: Two cases of superficial punctate keratitis (Fuchs), Trans. Ophthal. Soc. U. K. **10**:79, 1890.
33. Hamilton, J. B.: A survey of superficial punctate keratitis in Tasmania with the record of a mild epidemic, Brit. J. Ophthal. **25**:1, 1941.
34. Herbert, H.: Superficial keratitis associated with an encapsulated bacillus, Ophthal. Rev. **20**:339, 1901.
35. Hilleman, M. R., and Werner, J. H.: Recovery of new agent from patients with acute respiratory illness, Proc. Soc. Exp. Biol. Med. **85**:183, 1954.
36. Hobson, L. C.: Acute epidemic superficial punctate keratitis, Amer. J. Ophthal. **21**:1153, 1938.
37. Hogan, M. J., and Crawford, J. W.: Epidemic kerato-conjunctivitis, Amer. J. Ophthal. **25**: 1059, 1942.
38. Holmes, W. J.: Epidemic infectious conjunctivitis, Hawaii Med. J. **1**:11, 1941.

38a. Horne, R. W.: The structure of viruses, Sci. Amer. **208**:48, 1963.

39. Horsfall, F. L., Jr., and Tamm, I., editors: Viral and rickettsial infections of man, ed. 4, Philadelphia, 1965, J. B. Lippincott Co., p. 872.
40. Huebner, R. J., Rowe, W. P., Ward, T. G., Parrott, R. H., and Bell, J. A.: Adenoidal pharyngeal-conjunctival agents: a newly recognized group of common viruses of the respiratory system, New Eng. J. Med. **251**: 1077, 1954.
41. Huebner, R. J., and Rowe, W. P.: Adenoviruses as etiologic agents in conjunctivitis and keratoconjunctivitis, Amer. J. Ophthal. **43**:20, 1957.
42. Imre, G., Korchmáros, I., Geck, P., Nasz, I. and Dán, P.: Antigenic specificity of inclusion bodies in epidemic keratoconjunctivitis, Ophthalmologica **148**:7, 1964.
43. Inouse, M.: Superficial punctate keratitis, Ganka Zasshi **1**:273, 1894.
44. Iturburu, J. C.: Queratitis punctata superficial de carácter epidémico, Rev. Otoneuro-oftal. (S. Amer.) **6**:500, 1931.
45. Jawetz, E., Hanna, L., Kimura, S. J., and Thygeson, P.: Clinical diseases of adults associated with sporadic infections of APC viruses, Arch. Intern. Med. **98**:71, 1956.
46. Jawetz, E., Hanna, L., Kimura, S. J., and Thygeson, P.: A new type of APC virus from follicular conjunctivitis, Amer. J. Ophthal. **41**: 231, 1956.
47. Jawetz, E., Kimura, S. J., Hanna, L., Coleman, V. R., Thygeson, P., and Nicholas, A.: Studies on the etiology of epidemic keratoconjunctivitis, Amer. J. Ophthal. **40** (5, part 2):200, 1955.

47a. Jawetz, E., Melnick, J. L., and Adelberg, E. A.: Review of medical microbiology, ed. 9, Los Altos, Calif., 1970, Lange Medical Publications.

48. Kasel, J. A., Evans, H. E., Spickard, A., and Knight, V.: Conjunctivitis and enteric infection with adenovirus types 26 and 27: responses to primary, secondary and reciprocal cross-challenges, Amer. J. Hyg. **77**:265, 1963.
49. Kasel, J. A., Loda, F., and Knight, V.: Infection of volunteers with adenovirus type 16, Proc. Soc. Exp. Biol. Med. **114**:621, 1963.
50. Katz, S., Jordan, W. S., Jr., Badger, G. F., and Dingle, J. H.: Studies of complement-fixing and neutralizing antibodies against certain adenoviruses, J. Immun. **73**:118, 1957.
51. Kendall, E. J. C., Riddle, R. W., Tuck, H. A., Rodan, K. S., Andrews, B. E., and McDonald, J. C.: Pharyngo-conjunctival fever school outbreak in England during the summer of 1955 associated with adenovirus types 3, 7, 14, Brit. Med. J. **2**:131, 1957.
52. Kibrick, S., Melendez, L., and Enders, J. F.: Clinical associations of enteric viruses with particular reference to agents exhibiting prop-

erties of the echo group, Ann. N. Y. Acad. Sci. **67**:311, 1957.

53. Kilpatrick, H.: An epidemic of macular keratitis, Brit. J. Ophthal. **4**:16, 1920.
54. Kimura, S. J., Hanna, L., Nicholas, A., Thygeson, P., and Jawetz, E.: Sporadic cases of pharyngoconjunctival fever, Amer. J. Ophthal. **43**:14, 1957.
55. Kirwan, E. O'G.: Epidemic superficial punctate keratitis in Bengal, Proc. All-India Ophthal. Soc. **3**:1, 1933.
56. Koseki, S.: Studies on adenovirus type 11, infection of the eye, Jap. J. Ophthal. **4**:92, 1960.
56a. Laibson, P. R., Ortolan, G., and Dupre-Strachan, S.: Community and hospital outbreak of epidemic keratoconjunctivitis, Arch. Ophthal. **80**:467, 1968.
57. Ling, W. P.: Keratitis punctata superficialis and swimming pool conjunctivitis, Chin. Med. J. **50**:1381, 1936.
58. Liu, C.: Fluorescent antibody techniques. In Lennette, E. H., and Schmidt, N. J., editors: Diagnostic procedures for viral and rickettsial infections, ed. 4, New York, 1969, American Public Health Association.
59. McGavin, M. F., Boley, J. P., and Ormsby, H. L.: Epidemic keratoconjunctivitis, Canad. Med. Ass. J. **69**:137, 1953.
59a. Melnick, J. L., Bunting, H., Banfield, W. G., Strauss, M. J., and Gaylord, W. H.: Electron microscopy of viruses of human papilloma, molluscum contagiosum, and vaccinia, including observations on the formation of virus within the cell, Ann. N. Y. Acad. Sci. **54**: 1214, 1952.
60. Mitsui, Y., Hanabusa, J., Minoda, R., and Ogata, S.: Effect of inoculating adenovirus (APC virus) type 8 into human volunteers, Amer. J. Ophthal. **43**:84, 1957. (Symposium on viral keratoconjunctivitis)
61. Mitsui, Y., Hanna, L., Hanabusa, J., Minoda, R., Ogata, S., Kurihara, H., Okamura, R., and Miura, M.: Association of adenovirus type 8 with epidemic keratoconjunctivitis, Arch. Ophthal. **61**:891, 1959.
62. Morax, V.: Les conjonctivites folliculaires, Paris, 1933, Maison et Cie, p. 108.
63. Mordhorst, C. H., and Kjer, P.: Studies on an epidemic of keratoconjunctivitis caused by adenovirus type 8: virus isolation in human amniotic cells and serological observations, Acta Ophthal. (Copenhagen) **39**:974, 1961.
64. Murray, E. S., Chang, R. S., Bell, S. D., Tarizzo, M. L., and Snyder, J. C.: Agents recovered from acute conjunctivitis cases in Saudi Arabia, Amer. J. Ophthal. **43**:32, 1957.
65. Okamura, R.: A Study of pharyngoconjunctival fever, Acta Soc. Ophthal. Jap. **64**:96, 1960.
66. Oker-Blom, N., Wager, O., Strandström, H., Makela, P., and Jansson, E.: Adenoviruses associated with pharyngoconjunctival fever, Ann. Med. Exp. Biol. Fenn. **35**:342, 1957.
67. Ormsby, H. L., and Aitchison, W. S.: The role of the swimming pool in the transmission of pharyngoconjunctival fever, Canad. Med. Ass. J. **73**:864, 1955.
68. Ormsby, H. L., Fowle, M. C., and Doane, F.: Canadian cases of adenovirus infections, 1951-1956, Amer. J. Ophthal. **43**:17, 1957.
69. Pereira, H. G., Allison, A. C., Niven, J. S. F.: Fatal infection of new-born hamsters by an adenovirus of human origin, Nature **196**:244, 1962.
70. Pereira, M. S., Pereira, H. G., Clarke, S. K. R.: Human adenovirus type 31, a new serotype with oncogenic properties, Lancet **1**:21, 1965.
71. Perkins, J. E., Korns, R. F., and Westphal, R. S.: Epidemiology of epidemic keratoconjunctivitis, Amer. J. Public Health **33**:1187, 1943.
72. Profeta, M. L., Verdi, G. P., and Orzalesi, N.: Epidemia di cheratocongiuntivite epidemica (CCE) da adenovirus tipo 9, Ann. Sclavo **5**:454, 1963.
73. Rieke, F. E.: Epidemic conjunctivitis of presumed virus causation, report of an estimated six hundred cases in one shipyard, J.A.M.A. **119**:942, 1942.
73a. de Roetth, A. F.: Common wart as an etiological factor in certain cases of conjunctvtis and keratitis Arch. Ophthal. **21**:409, 1939.
74. de Roetth, A. F.: Epidemic keratoconjunctivitis, superficial punctate keratitis, Northwest Med. **41**:246, 1942.
75. Rose, H. M.: The adenoviruses. In Lennette, E. H., and Schmidt, N. J., editors: Diagnostic procedures for viral and rickettsial Infections, ed. 4, New York, 1969, American Public Health Association.
76. Rosen, L., Baron, S., and Bell, J. A.: Four newly recognized adenoviruses, Proc. Soc. Exp. Biol. Med. **107**:434, 1961.
77. Rosen, L., Hovis, J. F., and Bell, J. A.: Further observation on typing adenoviruses and a description of two possible additional serotypes, Proc. Soc. Exp. Biol. Med. **110**:710, 1962.
78. Rowe, W. P., and Hartley, J. W.: A general review of the adenoviruses, comparative virology (Ar. 2), Ann. N. Y. Acad. Sci. **110**: 466, 1962.
79. Rowe, W. P., Hartley, J. W., and Huebner, R. J.: Additional serotypes of the APC virus group, Proc. Soc. Exp. Biol. Med. **91**:260, 1956.
80. Rowe, W. P., Hartley, J. W., and Huebner, R. J.: Serotype composition of the adenovirus

group, Proc. Soc. Exp. Biol. Med. **97**:465, 1958.

81. Rowe, W. P., Huebner, R. J., and Bell, J. A.: Definition and outline of contemporary information on the adenovirus group, Ann. N. Y. Acad. Sci. **67**:255, 1956-1957.
82. Rowe, W. P., Huebner, R. J., Gilmore, L. K., Parrott, R. H., and Ward, T. G.: Isolation of cytopathogenic agent from human adenoids undergoing spontaneous degeneration in tissue culture, Proc. Soc. Exp. Biol. Med. **84**: 570, 1953.
83. Rowe, W. P., Huebner, R. J., Hartley, J. W., Ward, T. G., and Parrott, R. H.: Studies of the adenoidal-pharyngeal conjunctival (APC) group of viruses, Amer. J. Hyg. **61**:197, 1955.
84. Sanyal, S.: Epidemic superficial keratitis, Amer. J. Ophthal. **16**:390, 1933.
85. Schneider, R.: Ueber eine epidemische keratokonjunktivitis in Munchen and Umgebung, Munchen. Med. Wschr. **85**:1981, 1938.

85a. Svartz-Malmberg, G., and Germanis, M.: Adenovirus type 8 associated keratoconjunctivitis: hospital infections and secondary spread in Stockholm, 1967, Scand. J. Infect. Dis. **1**:161, 1969.

86. Thygeson, P.: Acute follicular conjunctivitis, Beal's type, Arch. Ophthal. **13**:853, 1935.
87. Thygeson, P.: The epidemiology of epidemic keratoconjunctivitis, Amer. J. Ophthal. **32**: 951, 1949.

87a. Tyrrell, D. A. S., Balducci, D., and Zaiman, T. E.: Acute infections of the respiratory tract and the adenoviruses, Lancet **2**:1326, 1956.

88. van der Veen, J., and Kok, G.: Isolation and typing of adenoviruses recovered from recruits with acute respiratory disease in the Netherlands, Amer. J. Hyg. **65**:119, 1957.
89. van der Veen, J., and van der Ploeg, G.: An outbreak of pharyngoconjunctival fever caused by types 3 and 4 adenovirus at Waalwijk, the Netherlands, Amer. J. Hyg. **68**:95, 1958.
90. Viswalingam, A.: Epidemic superficial punctate keratitis in Malaya, Brit. J. Ophthtal. **25**:313, 1941.
91. Ward, T. G., Huebner, R. J., Rowe, W. P., Ryan, R. W., and Bell, J. A.: Production of pharyngoconjunctival fever in human volunteers inoculated with APC viruses, Science **122**:1086, 1955.
92. Westhoff, C. H. A.: Keratitis punctata tropica, Zbl. Pract. Augenhed. **36**:289, 1912.
93. Wiener, M.: Keratitis punctata superficialis with report of a case, Arch. Ophthal. **38**:120, 1909.
94. Wright, R. E.: Superficial punctate keratitis, Brit. J. Ophthal. **14**:257, 1930.
95. Zur Nedden: Üeber eine Epidemie von Keratitis superficialis punktata, Klin. Mbl. Augenheilk. **101**:567, 1938.

18

Ocular infections caused by the herpesvirus group

RICHARD W. DARRELL

Four of the more than twenty viruses within the herpesvirus group are known to affect man. Their major common denominator is their similar structure revealed by electron microscopy. They all have a central core of DNA enveloped in a protein coat. This coat exhibits an icosahedral symmetry and is covered in turn by an envelope containing lipids. The infectivity of herpesvirus can be destroyed by lipid solvents, such as ether, because of this lipid envelope. In addition, human herpesviruses have in common the ability to cause different types of infection in the nonimmune and immune host. Although the primary infection in a nonimmune host is usually subclinical, it may have acute manifestations. Thereafter the virus remains in the body in a latent state, from which occasional acute infections reappear years later.

The four human herpesviruses are:

1. Herpes simplex virus types 1 and 2
2. Varicella-zoster virus
3. Cytomegalovirus
4. EB virus

HERPES SIMPLEX VIRUS INFECTIONS

Herpes simplex virus is responsible for the majority of severe eye infections, at least in temporate climates, and demands our first consideration. Although acute herpes simplex keratitis can be suppressed by chemotherapy, the chronic forms of keratitis still present great problems in management.

Primary

Herpes simplex virus is widespread.[36] Adults periodically shed virus into saliva and tears, usually in the absence of clinical illness.[38,39,48] The spread of infection to susceptible children usually occurs within the family. Within closed populations, as in an orphanage, the spread of virus is relatively rapid. For example, in one group of 51 children under 3 years of age, 20 developed a primary stomatitis within a year's observation, at an average age of 14 months.[1] The period in which primary infection occurs outside institutions is usually early childhood or late adolescence. Jones[35] has suggested that kissing is important in spreading the infection because of this peak frequency of primary infections in early childhood, presumably caused by parental kisses, followed by a peak in late adolescence, coinciding with burgeoning interest in the opposite sex. The primary attack is subclinical in about 85% of the patients and is recognized only in the 15% who developed a variety of illnesses, ranging from mild stomatitis to severe gingivostomatitis and keratoconjunctivitis.

In newborn infants, herpes simplex virus can present a spectrum of disease. Microcephaly, seizures, and death can follow neonatal infection; type 2 herpes simplex virus (genital strain) is usually isolated.[70] Bleeding disorders, often with a fatal outcome, have been reported.[51] However, herpes simplex infection in the neonate can be confined to the cornea, as in a 24-day-old infant who developed a large epithelial dendrite without other signs.[7] The mother's cervix was negative for virus on culture, so the infection was probably acquired after birth. On the other hand, another neonate with vesicles on the lids developed keratitis and subsequently died of an overwhelming infection.[5] In addition to the cornea, the lens, retina, and choroid can be involved with subsequent congenital cataract and pigmentary changes in the peripheral retina.[15,16,29]

Infants are protected by antibodies received from their mothers during the first 6 months of life. The peak incidence of primary infection occurs after 6 months up to 5 years of age. Primary infection takes the form of gingivostomatitis, regional lymphadenitis, and follicular conjunctivitis, but fatalities are rare. Dendritic and disciform keratitis is occasionally seen. Diagnosis is made primarily by slit-lamp examination of the cornea, with help from frequent presence of fever blisters on the lip or eyelid, and by a history of recent blisters in a parent or sibling. Laboratory diagnosis is made by isolation of herpes simplex virus in tissue culture, by fluorescent antibody identification, or by demonstration of a rise in antibody titer compared with the serum taken in the acute stage of disease. Although primary herpes simplex infection usually occurs in childhood, in one series an adult of 48 developed a primary infection.[55]

Treatment of primary ocular herpetic infection in children depends in part on the age of the patient. Dendritic keratitis can be treated either by topical 5-iodo-2′-deoxyuridine (IDU), or by curettage of the entire corneal epithelium followed by ether scrub. With very young children slit-lamp examination is difficult, and administration of eye drops is uncertain. The medicine may not go into the eye or may be washed out by crying. A general anesthesia may be preferable to permit careful examination of the cornea under the operating microscope, followed by definitive treatment by epithelial curettage and ether scrub, should treatment be indicated. Appropriate material for laboratory diagnosis can also be taken.

In older children, who present no obstacles to careful examination and treatment, a trial of IDU is indicated. The relative advantages of curettage and of IDU depend in part on the location and character of the ulcer and are discussed later in this chapter.

Recurrent

Herpes simplex virus remains in some form within cells of the body following primary infection, in spite of the presence of circulating antibodies. Recurrent herpetic infection occurs when the balance between latent virus and host protective mechanisms is disturbed. Among the protective mechanisms, the level of serum antibody seems to be unrelated to timing of recurrences.[14] The amount of antibody in saliva shows no correlation with serum antibody level or recurrence of infection in the oral mucous membranes.[20] Similarly, there is little correlation between secretory antibodies in tears and recurrence of corneal herpetic infection. Virus proliferation periodically occurs within mucous membranes and secretory glands leading to the appearance of infectious virus in saliva and tears without any evidence of clinical illness.[38,39,45,48] Recurrences become manifest when acute fever blisters appear on the lids or lips or when the cornea becomes involved. An attack can be precipitated by a febrile illness, by menses, or by exposure to sunlight. An unusual trigger is surgical section of the fifth nerve ganglion for tic douloureux, which may be followed by crops of fever blisters on the skin supplied by that nerve.[24] Reactivation of virus shedding into tears has also been reported to follow injections of epinephrine in the rabbit.[44a] A clue to the mechanism by which epinephrine acts to stimulate virus shedding is provided by recent experiments in epinephrine-induced skin lesions.[69a] A characteristic purple-colored hemorrhage was produced in rabbits at the site of intradermal injection of 100 μg of epinephrine when herpes simplex virus had been injected on the same site 3 to 4 hours previously. Histologic examination showed that the purple-colored hemorrhagic spots were caused by marked capillary dilation with extravasation of erythrocytes. Systemic administration of epinephrine in rabbits may have a similar vascular effect at sites of chronic virus multiplication.

Although the dendritic figure is the one classical sign of ocular herpes simplex infection (Plate 4, *A*), corneal lesions may be atypical or even absent. A chronic follicular conjunctivitis alone may be the only sign of herpetic disease. Serial viral culture in a series of such cases established the diagnosis in spite of a normal cornea.[9] An acute florid conjunctivitis, often follicular, may precede the onset of herpetic keratitis by several days. Such a conjunctivitis should not be immediately treated with corticosteroids until it becomes clear from the clinical course that herpes simplex virus is not the cause.

If a dendritic lesion enlarges and develops rounded, rather than serpiginous edges, it is termed a geographic ulcer. In one study there was a relationship between prior use of corticosteroids and subsequent development of geographic ulcer.[55]

At a later stage an epithelial ulcer may persist for weeks or months in the absence of demonstrable virus proliferation in the epithelium; these ulcers have been called metaherpetic keratitis (Plate 4, *B*). The failure of the epithelium to re-cover the corneal stroma is thought to lie in a damaged basement membrane. The desmosomes of the basement membrane can be destroyed by infection, trauma, or caustic chemicals. Destruction of the desmosomes has been shown to occur in herpes simplex virus infection of the rabbit cornea.[18b,72] An analogous situation has been shown in a case of recurrent erosion, in which the corneal epithelium and superficial stroma were removed at therapeutic lamellar keratoplasty and studied by electron microscopy.[27] To protect the basement membrane, we prefer to use ether following epithelial curettage because it probably causes less damage to the desmosomes as compared with the use of iodine and because ether directly destroys the infectivity of the lipid-containing herpes simplex virus.

The stroma underlying the epithelial ulcer rapidly develops pathologic changes, which often spread in spite of healing of the epithelial lesion. The entire thickness of the corneal stroma is invaded by inflammatory cells, with development of corneal edema, decompensation of the endothelium, and stromal scarring.[32] This chronic form of ocular herpetic infection is often termed disciform keratitis because of the frequent disc-shaped area of stromal edema (Plate 4, *C*). At the present time the most important mechanism involved in disciform keratitis thought to be delayed hypersensitivity, which can be suppressed in part by corticosteroids.[2,9,42,68]

Although herpes simplex virus particles have been identified within corneal epithelium and stroma in disciform keratitis,[19,22,66,67] they rarely cause stromal disease by active multiplication, as is the case in epithelial disease. Rather, the presence of virus within the keratocytes of the diseased stroma causes a new antigen to appear on the infected cell's surface membrane. It is thought that these neoantigens provoke the delayed hypersensitivity mechanism.[2] In addition, the endothelium is probably directly damaged by herpes simplex virus infection, and infectious virus has been cultured from it.[33]

Recurrences of dendritic ulcers often occur immediately above or adjacent to an underlying stromal herpetic scar. Does the

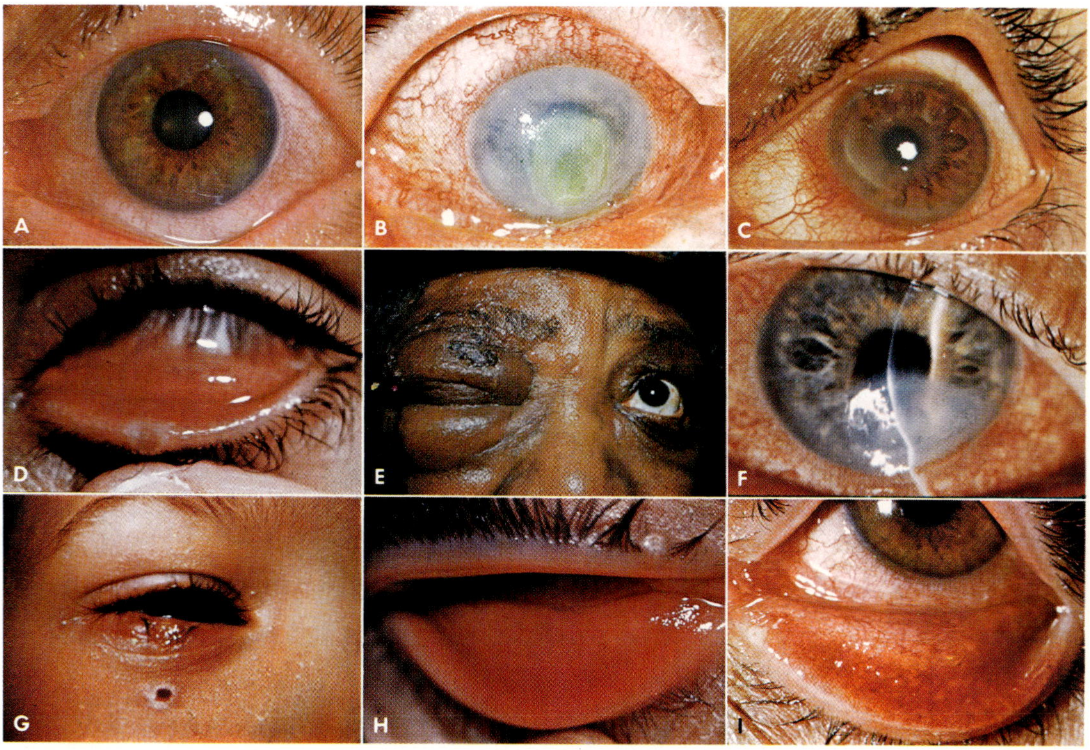

Plate 4. A, Acute herpetic keratitis with seven dendritic figures. **B,** Metaherpetic keratitis with persistent failure of epithelization. **C,** Disciform keratitis with semicircular Wessely ring. **D,** Varicella ulcer of lid margin. **E,** Herpes zoster ophthalmicus. **F,** Herpes zoster with corneal ulceration. **G,** Vaccinia of the eyelid. **H,** Molluscum contagiosum on lid, with secondary follicular conjunctivitis. **I,** Newcastle disease conjunctivitis in a laboratory worker.

virus responsible for a recurrence come from chronically infected superficial keratocytes, from inside out, or is the virus brought to the epithelium by the tear film? On clinical grounds the closeness of the old stromal and new epithelial disease often makes it logical to assume that virus from superficial keratocytes is responsible. There is ample evidence from electron microscopic studies of human stroma removed at keratoplasty at the convalescent stage of herpetic infection, that virus is present within keratocytes of chronically infected stroma.[19] To test the hypothesis that virus within keratocytes is responsible for recurrent epithelial disease, herpes-convalescent rabbit stroma was placed by penetrating keratoplasty into normal rabbit eyes and observed in vivo for up to 15 months. These grafts did not shed virus into tears and did not cause seroconversion in recipient rabbits.[18a] Thus, although virus can be found within keratocytes by electron microscopy, attempts at isolation of virus from chronically infected keratocytes have been unsuccessful both in vitro and in vivo.

Outside the cornea, other sites of latent virus infection have been found adjacent to the eye. Within the lacrimal and adnexal glands, virus has been identified by fluorescent antibody techniques; these glands must be the source of infectious virus shed into tears when the cornea has no ulceration[39,52] or is absent because of enucleation.[8]

Recent experiments have pointed out a third site of latent virus infection, within the sensory ganglia. Fifteen years ago recurrence of facial herpes was reported to follow surgical section of the trigeminal nerve for tic douloureux; 18 out of 26 patients treated in this way developed facial herpes over the denervated area.[24] The introduction of fluorescent antibody techniques and refinements in tissue culture have provided the tools to show latent herpes simplex virus infection in spinal ganglia. Following footpad injection of virus in mice, infection can be traced up the sciatic nerve to the sciatic ganglia, where a chronic virus infection is instituted.[64a] Similarly, even after herpetic keratitis resolves in rabbits, virus can still be isolated for up to 8 months by organ culture of the trigeminal ganglion, but not from the tear film.[64b] Chronic infection of the trigeminal ganglion is probably the dominant factor in recurrent ocular herpes.

Treatment of ocular disease

Dendritic keratitis. If there is only minmal stromal involvement accompanying acute dendritic keratitis, and particularly if corticosteroids have not been used, therapy either with IDU or by epithelial curettage and ether scrub yields equally good results. Following the initial report of the success of IDU in acute dendritic keratitis,[37] several double-blind trials confirmed its value.[12,46,54] There were some dissenting voices pointing out that up to 75% of the placebo group had spontaneous remissions.[34,49] Nevertheless, IDU has been established as an excellent treatment for acute dendritic keratitis. When IDU treatment is compared with curettage of the infected epithelium rather than with placebo drops, however, both IDU and curettage yield equally good results. In a recent double-blind study of 77 such cases, there was no statistical difference in results of treatment with IDU or by curettage.[55]

One major advantage of IDU over curettage is that treatment with IDU is painless. However, should the virus be resistant and treatment fail, the stromal disease may well become more extensive. The advantage of curettage is that the infected epithelium is immediately removed before irreversible stromal disease can be established. Unfortunately, after curettage there may be some pain, and a patch must be worn for a week. Visual acuity may not return to normal for a week or more, until the epithelium reestablishes a normal anterior smooth surface. Nevertheless, if the dendritic ulcer is located in the pupillary axis, immediate curettage is the treatment of choice, because it eliminates the risk of further stromal disease. In the pupillary axis, stromal disease cannot be risked. However, if the epithelial ulcer is not in the pupillary axis, a trial of IDU is certainly worthwhile. If the ulcer becomes smaller in 3 to 5 days, treatment should be continued; if not, curettage is indicated. Young children with recurrent herpetic infection may have to be examined under general anesthesia for accurate slit-lamp diagnosis, and at that time curettage of the corneal epithelium should be carried out.

Progression of a dendritic ulcer to a geographic ulcer can be caused by injudicious use of steroids. IDU is superior to curettage in treatment of these steroid-related geographic ulcers.[55] Dendritic ulcers that are unrelated to use of steroids, however, respond equally well either to IDU or to curettage.

METAHERPETIC KERATITIS. The corneal epithelium may fail to cover the cornea not because of active virus proliferation but because of severe damage to the basement membrane. The essential problem in such a case is lack of an epithelial barrier on the cornea against bacterial and fungal infection. Patching of the eye sometimes enhances epithelization, but more definitive steps are usually required. The epithelium can be replaced by a conjunctival flap, by lamellar keratoplasty, or by penetrating keratoplasty. We have had good results with lamellar keratoplasty to reestablish an anterior epithelium and basement membrane. Twelve months later, if the eye is quiet, penetrating keratoplasty through the previous lamellar graft often restores vision.

HERPETIC IRITIS. Herpes simplex virus has been identified in the iris stroma and cultured from the anterior chamber; clinically it can produce a very severe iritis.[56] The iritis may be the predominant problem, leading to endothelial decompensation, stromal edema, epithelial disease, and glaucoma. Although it is said that steroids should never be used in the presence of epithelial ulceration, exception must be made when the iritis is thought to be the major factor. Nonspecific epithelial ulceration with rounded edges may be secondary to an edematous stroma. When the iritis is controlled by mydriatics and steroids, the epithelial ulceration often heals. A cover of IDU is, of course, also used.

STROMAL KERATITIS. The most challenging problem for therapy is stromal herpesvirus infection, which presents in a variety of forms from limited anterior stromal disease, to larger, but delineated disciform opacity, and finally to total corneal edema, inflammatory reaction, and scarring. Shortly after the introduction of the corticosteroids 20 years ago, the initial clinical enthusiasm was sharply tempered by a growing feeling that steroids make herpetic keratitis worse.[40,43,68,69] They were then contraindicated in herpetic infection until IDU was introduced and the various stages of herpetic keratitis were more carefully delineated. Steroids are still inadvisable in simple dendritic keratitis associated at the most with minimal stromal disease. Beyond that, steroids are often essential in treatment, particularly if combined with IDU.[2,41,42] The risk of recurrent epithelial disease that has been associated with use of steroids is clearly reduced by concomitant use of IDU, as shown definitely by a recent double-blind trial. Patients receiving both IDU and steroids had 66% fewer recurrences of epithelial keratitis as compared with patients treated with steroids alone.[55] One way IDU works is by reducing the amount of infectious virus in the tear film. Although infectious virus can be isolated by a conjunctival swab from 75% of untreated patients who have dendritic keratitis, positive isolations number less than 4% in patients previously treated with IDU.[17] Steroids are indicated whenever the primary problem is inflammatory stromal disease and iritis in the absence of dendritic ulceration; small nonspecific epithelial ulcers are not a contraindication if steroid treatment is judged essential. Unfortunately, curettage and ether scrub are often unsuccessful in the presence of stromal keratitis.

Stromal herpetic infection may be difficult to diagnose in the absence of prior history or documentation of dendritic ulceration. For example, one patient presented with vessels on Descemet's membrane and deep stromal keratitis in association with a moderate iritis. Epithelial disease was completely absent. For 7 years she was maintained in moderate comfort by the sparing application of steroid drops once every other day during flare-ups. The specific diagnosis became apparent only after isolation of herpes simplex virus from a conjunctival swab on a routine clinic visit; 1 week later the same eye developed a dendritic ulcer. Curettage of the ulcer was done immediately, and from the epithelial specimen virus was again isolated.

Treatment of complications. The most common complication is permanent stromal scarring with loss of visual acuity. When indicated, penetrating keratoplasty is the only way to restore vision. A severe iritis may lead to acute glaucoma and later to chronic glaucoma secondary to anterior and posterior synechiae. Miotics, as well as carbonic anhydrase inhibitors, usually control the situation. Glaucoma surgery is contraindicated unless there is reasonable hope of restoring vision. Bacterial and fungal infections are treated as outlined in other chapters. Descemetocoele and corneal perforation require emergency keratoplasty or application of tissue adhesives. Uncommon complications include hyphema and occlusion of the nasolacrimal canaliculi.[61]

Recent methods of treatment. Cryotherapy has been greeted with enthusiasm in Europe but is less widely used in the United States. Freezing undoubtedly destroys some virus, but certainly not all, and it is a method used in the laboratory to release virus from infected tissue-culture cells when increased titer of infectious virus is desired. In our hands, cryotherapy has not proved superior to other methods of therapy.

Stimulation of endogenous interferon production by administration of polyinosinic-cytidylic complex (poly IC) has been studied in rabbits and in man, and its use has been suggested as a new therapy.[53] At the present these compounds are not licensed for general human use, and final judgment will have to await laboratory and clinical trials.

VARICELLA-ZOSTER VIRUS INFECTIONS

The varicella-zoster virus (V-Z virus) causes in the nonimmune host a common acute exantheum of childhood, and in the immune host, usually an adult, the herpes zoster syndrome. The close relationship between chickenpox and herpes zoster is shown by epidemiology, by the identity of the two viruses in tissue culture, and by similar immune responses to both infections. V-Z virus can be isolated from skin vesicles in both chickenpox and herpes zoster; and patients with one form of the disease can cause the appearance of the other form to appear in close contacts. For example, a 3-year-old girl with herpes zoster visited a nursery, and 4 other children developed chickenpox.[26] In another report, a nurse with herpes zoster was attended by an intern who developed chickenpox 16 days later. The intern was also taking care of a patient receiving immunosuppressive drugs following kidney transplant. This patient developed herpes zoster.[6]

In children and nonimmune adults the V-Z virus causes chickenpox, a mild but highly contagious disease of childhood characterized by vesicular eruptions in successive crops on the skin and mucous membranes. The peak incidence is in children from 2 to 6 years of age, and transmission of infection is thought to occur by droplet spread followed by infection of the respiratory tract. After an incubation period of 14 to 17 days, malaise, fever, and then the rash make their appearance. The exanthem is diagnosed by (1) rapid evolution of lesions even within a few hours, through states of macular, pustular, and crusting forms; (2) successive crops at 2 to 5 days; and (3) distribution of lesions primarily on the trunk, neck, and face, and proximal but not distal extremities. Although the majority of children recover promptly without sequela, rare but severe complications of chickenpox, such as pneumonia and encephalitis, have been known to occur. Mortality from varicella may be high in neonates.[10]

Corneal and conjunctival manifestations of chickenpox occur in about 4% of the cases.[65] Vesicles may be found on the conjunctiva, particularly on the semilunar fold. Vesicles may occur on the eyelids (Plate 4, *D*) and may lead to eventual scarring of the lid margin and to distortion of the cilia. Limbal phlyctenules and disciform keratitis are occasionally seen on the cornea. Bilateral papilledema has been reported to follow chickenpox.[47] In addition, encephalitis, optic neuritis, oculomotor paralysis, and tonic pupil are occasionally encountered.[28] Although IDU is effective against varicella in vitro, there is little information available that is of benefit in the occasional varicella eye infections. Zoster immune globulin has been recommended to treat severe vaccinia in the newborn or in very ill children.[11]

After primary infection the V-Z virus probably remains in a latent form within the dorsal root ganglions.[14] Reactivation usually occurs without any specific exciting factor, but local pressure on a sensory ganglion from a tumor or a defect in systemic immunity may be responsible for a recurrence. After reactivation the virus spreads peripherally from the dorsal root ganglion or extramedullary cranial nerve ganglion along the sensory nerve; hence, sensory alterations occur before the appearance of vesicles. Occasionally, the virus spreads centrally to cause meningitis, myelitis, and encephalitis, with concomitant paralysis. The skin eruption is limited to the dermatomes corresponding to the involved sensory ganglion and consists of successive crops of maculopapular plaques that eventually crust in 1 to 3 weeks.

Infection of the ophthalmic division of the trigeminal nerve produces the characteristic eruption of skin lesions on the forehead, lids, and nose, as well as damage to the cornea (Plate 4, *E*). The corneal changes range from mild, with punctate staining of the corneal epithelium and no stromal alteration, to severe, with epithelial and stromal ulceration and opacity (Plate 4, *F*). Most of these changes are secondary to the temporary sensory denervation of the cornea, changes also observed when the trigeminal nerve ganglion is sectioned for tic douloureux. In addition, optic neuritis, oculomotor paralysis, levator paralysis, iritis, paralytic mydriasis, and bilateral hemorrhagic retinopathy have been reported.[3,59,62]

Atropine and local steroids are the best treatment for the corneal lesions and iritis. Local treatment with cortisone was shown to be clearly superior in a recent study of 70 patients, one third of whom served as controls.[5] Systemic steroids for a 3-week period during the acute stage of infection were used in one double-blind study; the postherpetic neuralgia was reported to be shortened.[21] In addition, calamine lotion, with 0.25% menthol and 0.25% phenol can be used to dry the skin eruptions. Antibiotics are not usually necessary unless the skin lesions or corneal ulceration becomes infected. The duration of the postherpetic neuralgia may be very long, up to several years, and may require mild analgesics and constant reassurance of the patient.

CYTOMEGALOVIRUS INFECTIONS

Cytomegaloviruses are classified within the herpesvirus group because their morphologic characteristics are identical to those of herpes simplex virus when observed by electron microscopy.[23,30] They also have in common the ability to cause latent or asymptomatic infections; and in both, excretion of infectious virus into urine and saliva may occur for long periods of time in spite of the presence of circulating antibodies. Serologic studies show that 4% of children under age 5, 15% at age 10, and 54% of adults over age 35 have circulating antibodies against the cytomegaloviruses. These data indicate widespread infection of the population, although there is usually no history of a primary illness.[60] However, neonates may develop overt signs of primary infection.

In a prospective study of 185 pregnant women, 6 were found to be excretors of cytomegalovirus.[25] All pregnancies were full term and normal, and only 1 of the 6 neonates yielded virus in urine, throat, and placenta cultures. The only sign of infection was a few petechiae. A study of all babies born during one year in an urban hospital showed that 1.2% were shedding virus.[64] These prospective studies show the relative frequency of mild cytomegalovirus infection at birth without sequelae. However, congenital infection of unborn children by transplacental transfer of cytomegalovirus from their mothers, who may be asymptomatic, can produce a disastrous neonatal illness. The clinical manifestations of cytomegalic inclusion disease are hepatomegaly, splenomegaly, mental retardation, microcephaly, jaundice, petechiae, chorioretinitis, and cerebral calcifications.[23,30,50] The congenital form of infection may also be caused by exchange transfusion immediately after birth when blood carrying cytomegalovirus is inadvertently used. Specific diagnosis requires virologic and serologic data in addition to clinical findings. The presence of infection can be established by (1) isolation of cytomegalovirus, (2) demonstration of specific intranuclear inclusions within markedly enlarged cells, (3) a rising anticytomegalovirus antibody titer, and (4) detection of cytomegalovirus macroglobulin. Diagnosis based on clinical manifestations alone is subject to error because similar illnesses can be produced by congenital toxoplasmosis and congenital rubella; these can be excluded by the toxoplasmosis dye test and the rubella hemagglutination inhibition test. When present, periventricular calcification is strongly suggestive of cytomegalic inclusion disease; however, it is present only in the minority of cases. Treatment is unsatisfactory, although IDU has been used in a few cases. In one 14-week-old girl there was a clinical improvement and marked drop in virus excretion following systemic administration of IDU.[18]

Within the retina of eyes obtained at autopsy of infants who have died of cytomegalic inclusion disease, typical large mononuclear cells with both intranuclear and cytoplasmic inclusions are seen; on electron microscopy, viruses within these inclusions have morphologic characteristics identical to those of herpes simplex virus.[63,71]

Infection acquired after infancy is usually asymptomatic, although a transient hepatitis can often be detected by liver function tests in subclinical cases. Children may remain virus excretors up to 4 years of age. Infection of the adult is rarely diagnosed but may present a clinical picture similar to that of infectious mononucleosis, with predominance of fever and liver disease, and relatively less pharyngitis, lymph node enlargement, and hematologic changes than are usually found in classical infectious mononucleosis.[44] In addition, the heterophil agglutination test is negative for cytomegalic virus–related infectious mononucleosis but positive in most patients with classical infectious mononucleosis. Adults may acquire infection through blood transfusions, particularly after the multiple transfusions required for open heart surgery.[23] The eye is not affected in adult forms of the disease.

INFECTIOUS MONONUCLEOSIS

Infectious mononucleosis is characterized by protracted fever (2 to 3 weeks), enlargement of the lymph glands and spleen, and increased numbers of monocytes and large lymphocytes displaying morphologic abnormalities in the circulating blood.[13,31,58] In addition, 50% to 80% of patients with infectious mononucleosis develop heterophil antibodies. The ocular signs of the disease include periorbital edema, particularly of the upper lid; ocular muscle pain; photophobia; and occasionally a mild conjunctivitis. The relative frequency of the various signs and symptoms are:[13]

	Percent
Adenopathy	100
Malaise and fatigue	90 - 100
Fever	80 - 95
Sweating	80 - 95
Sore throat	80 - 85
Splenomegaly	50 - 60
Periorbital edema	25 - 40
Ocular muscle pain	10 - 20
Photophobia	5 - 10
Conjunctivitis	less than 5

Infectious mononucleosis is included in this chapter because there is considerable evidence that it is caused by the EB virus, a virus indistinguishable under the electron microscope from other human herpesviruses.[13] Antibodies to EB virus are found in populations in many parts of the world and appear early in life. Although the majority of EB virus infections are clinically inapparent, during infectious mononucleosis antibodies to EB virus rise; they also rise in patients with Burkitt's lymphoma. However, the role of EB virus in infectious mononucleosis and Burkitt's lymphoma is still unsettled because of failure to transmit the disease to laboratory animals or human volunteers.

REFERENCES

1. Anderson, S. G., and Hamilton, J.: The epidemiology of primary herpes simplex infection, Med. J. Aust. **1**:308, 1949.
2. Aronson, S. B., and Moore, T. E., Jr.. Corticosteroid therapy in central stromal keratitis, Amer. J. Ophthal. **67**:873, 1969.
3. Bartlett, R. E., Mumma, C. S., and Irvine, A. R.: Herpes zoster ophthalmicus with bilateral hemorrhagic retinopathy, Amer. J. Ophthal. **34**:45, 1951.
4. Bergaust, B., and Westby, R. K.: Zoster ophthalmicus: local treatment with cortisone, Acta Ophthal. **45**:787, 1967.
5. Berkovich, S., and Ressel, M.: Neonatal herpes keratitis, J. Pediat. **69**:652, 1966.
6. Berlin, B. S., and Campbell, T.: Hospital-acquired herpes zoster following exposure to chicken pox, J.A.M.A. **211**:1831, 1970.
7. Bobo, C. B., Antine, B., and Manos, J. P.: Neonatal herpes simplex infection limited to the cornea, Arch. Ophthal. **84**:697, 1970.
8. Brown, D. C., and Kaufman, H. E.: Chronic herpes simplex infection of the ocular adnexa, Arch. Ophthal. **81**:837, 1969.
9. Brown, D. C., Nesburn, A. B., Nauheim, J. S., Pavan-Langston, D., and Kaufman, H. E.: Recurrent herpes simplex conjunctivitis, Arch. Ophthal. **79**:733, 1968.
10. Brunell, P. A.: Varicella-zoster infections in pregnancy, J.A.M.A. **199**:315, 1967.
11. Brunell, P. A., Ross, A., Miller, L. H., and Kuo, B.: Prevention of varicella by zoster immune globulin, New Eng. J. Med. **280**:1191, 1969.
12. Burns, R. P.: A double-blind study of IDU in human herpes simplex keratitis, Arch. Ophthal. **70**:381, 1963.
13. Carter, R. L., and Penman, H. G.: Infectious mononucleosis, Oxford, 1969, Blackwell Scientific Publications.
14. Chang, T.: Recurrent viral infection (reinfection), New Eng. J. Med. **284**:765, 1971.
15. Cibis, A., and Burde, R. M.: Herpes simplex virus-induced congenital cataracts, Arch. Ophthal. **85**:220, 1961.
16. Cogan, D. G., Kuwabara, T., Young, G. F., and Kuck, D. L.: Herpes simplex retinopathy in an infant, Arch. Ophthal. **72**:641, 1964.
17. Coleman, V. R., Thygeson, P., Dawson, C. R., and Jawetz, E.: Isolation of virus from herpetic keratitis, Arch. Ophthal. **81**:22, 1969.
18. Conchie, A. F., Barton, B. W., and Tobin, J. O'H.: Congenital cytomegalovirus infection treated with idoxuridine, Brit. Med. J. **4**:162, 1968.

18a. Darrell, R. W.: Keratitis following penetrating grafts of herpes-convalescent cornea in the rabbit, Arch. Ophthal. In press.

18b. Darrell, R. W., and Vrabec, F.: The corneal stroma in experimental herpetic keratitis in rabbits, Docum. Ophthal. **29**:243, 1971.

19. Dawson, C., Togni, B., and Moore, T. E., Jr.: Structural changes in chronic herpetic keratitis, Arch. Ophthal. **79**:740, 1968.
20. Douglas, R. G., Jr., and Couch, R. B.: A prospective study of chronic herpes simplex infection and recurrent herpes labialis in humans, J. Immun. **104**:289, 1970.
21. Eaglstein, W. H., Katz, R., and Brown, J. A.: The effects of early corticosteroid therapy on the skin eruption and pain of herpes zoster, J.A.M.A. **211**:1681, 1970.
22. Edelhauser, H. F., Schultz, R. O., and Van Horn, D. L.: Experimental herpes simplex keratitis, Amer. J. Ophthal. **68**:458, 1969.
23. Editorial: Diseases caused by cytomegaloviruses, Brit. Med. J. **1**;72, 1968.
24. Ellison, S. A., Carton, C. A., and Rose, H. M.: Studies of recurrent herpes simplex infections following section of the trigeminal nerve, J. Infect. Dis. **105**:161, 1959.
25. Feldman, R. A.: Cytomegalovirus infection during pregnancy, Amer. J. Dis. Child. **117**:517, 1969.
26. Garrett, F. E.:- Herpes zoster ophthalmicus, Amer. J. Ophthal. **46**:741, 1958.

27. Goldman, J. N., Dohlman, C. H., and Kravitt, B. A.: The basement membrane of the human cornea in recurrent epithelial erosion syndrome, Trans. Amer. Acad. Ophthal. Otolaryng. **73**:471, 1969.
28. Goldsmith, M. O.: Tonic pupil following varicella, Amer. J. Ophthal. **66**:551, 1968.
29. Hagler, W. S., Walters, P. V., and Nahmias, A. J.: Ocular involvement in neonatal herpes simplex virus infection, Arch. Ophthal. **82**: 169, 1969.
30. Hanshaw, J. B.: Cytomegaloviruses. In Virology monographs No. 3, New York, 1968, Springer-Verlag New York, Inc., pp. 1-23.
31. Hoagland, R. J.: Infectious mononucleosis, New York, 1967, Grune and Stratton.
32. Hogan, M. J., Kimura, S. J., and Thygeson, P.: Pathology of herpes simplex kerato-iritis, Amer. J. Ophthal. **57**:551, 1964.
33. Irvine, A. R., and Kimura, S. J.: Experimental stromal herpes simplex keratitis in rabbits, Arch. Ophthal. **78**:654, 1967.
34. Jepson, C. N.: Treatment of herpes simplex of the cornea with IDU: a double blind study, Amer. J. Ophthal. **57**:213, 1964.
35. Jones, B.: The management of ocular herpes, Trans. Ophthal. Soc. U. K. **79**:425, 1959.
36. Kaplan, A. S.: Herpes simplex and pseudorabies viruses. In Virology monographs No. 5, New York, 1969, Springer-Verlag New York, Inc.
37. Kaufman, H. E.: Clinical cure of herpes simplex keratitis by 5-iodo-2′-deoxyuridine, Proc. Soc. Exp. Biol. Med. **109**:250, 1962.
38. Kaufman, H. E., Brown, D. C., and Ellison, E. D.: Herpesvirus in the lacrimal gland, conjunctiva and cornea of man—a chronic infection, Amer. J. Ophthal. **65**:32, 1968.
39. Kaufman, H. E., Brown, D. C., and Ellison, E. M.: Recurrent herpes in rabbit and man, Science **156**:1628, 1967.
40. Kaufman, H. E., and Maloney, E. D.: Experimental herpes simplex keratitis, Arch. Ophthal. **66**:99, 1961.
41. Kaufman, H. E., and Maloney, E. D.: IDU and hydrocortisone in experimental herpes simplex keratitis, Arch. Ophthal. **68**:396, 1962.
42. Kaufman, H. E., Martola, E., and Dohlman, C. H.: Herpes simplex treatment with IDU and corticosteroids, Trans. Amer. Acad. Ophthal. Otolaryng. **67**:695, 1963.
43. Kimura, S. J., Diaz-Bonnet, V., Okumoto, M., and Hogan, M. J.: The effect of corticosteroid hormones on experimental herpes simplex keratitis, Amer. J. Ophthal. **75**:945, 1961.
44. Klemola, E., Kaariainen, L., von Essen, R., Haltia, K., Koivuniemi, A., and von Bonsdorff, C. H.: Further studies on cytomegalovirus mononucleosis in previously healthy individuals, Acta Med. Scand. **182**:311, 1967.
44a. Laibson, P. R., and Kibrick, S.: Reactivation of herpetic keratitis in the rabbit, Arch. Ophthal. **77**:244, 1967.
45. Laibson, P. R., and Kibrick, S.: Recurrence of herpes simplex virus in rabbit eyes: results of a three-year study, Invest. Ophthal. **8**:346, 1969.
46. Laibson, P. R., and Leopold, I. H.: An evaluation of double-blind IDU therapy in 100 cases of herpetic keratitis, Trans. Amer. Acad. Ophthal. Otolaryng. **68**:22, 1964.
47. Liioi, J. A., and Aiello, M. V.: Bilateral papilledema following chicken pox, J. Pediat. Ophthal. **7**:155, 1970.
48. Lindgren, K. M., Douglas, R. G., Jr., and Couch, R. B.: Significance of herpesvirus hominis in respiratory secretions of man, New Eng. J. Med. **278**:517, 1968.
49. Luntz, M. H., and MacCallum, F. O.: Treatment of herpes simplex keratitis with 5-iodo-2′-deoxyuridine, Brit. J. Ophthal. **47**:449, 1963.
50. McCracken, G. H., Schinefield, H. R., Cobb, K., Rausen, A. R., Dische, M. R., and Eichenwald, H. F.: Congenital cytomegalic inclusion disease, Amer. J. Dis. Child. **117**:522, 1969.
51. Miller, D. R., Hanshaw, J. B., O'Leary, D. S., and Hnilicka, J. V.: Fatal disseminated herpes simplex virus infection and hemorrhage in the neonate, J. Pediat. **76**:409, 1970.
52. Nesburn, A. B., Elliott, J. H., and Leibowitz, H. M.: Spontaneous reactivation of experimental herpes simplex keratitis in rabbits, Arch. Ophthal. **78**:523, 1967.
53. Park, J. H., Galin, M., Billau, A., and Baron, S.: Prophylaxis of herpetic keratoconjunctivitis with interferon inducers, Arch. Ophthal. **81**:840, 1969.
54. Patterson, A., Fox, A. D., and Davies, G., and others: Controlled studies of IDU in the treatment of herpetic keratitis, Trans. Ophthal. Soc. U. K. **83**:583, 1963.
55. Patterson, A., and Jones, B. R.: The management of ocular herpes, Trans. Ophthal. Soc. U. K. **87**:59, 1967.
56. Pavan-Langston, D., and Brockhurst, R. J.: Herpes simplex panuveitis, Arch. Ophthal. **81**: 783, 1969.
57. Pavan-Langston, D., and Nesburn, A. B.: The chronology of primary herpes simplex infection of the eye and adnexal glands, Arch. Ophthal. **80**:258, 1968.
58. Pejme, J.: Infectious mononucleosis, Acta Med. Scand. Suppl. **413**:1, 1964.
59. Ramsell, T. G.: Complications of herpes zoster ophthalmicus, Amer. J. Ophthal. **63**: 1796, 1967.
60. Rifkind, D.: Cytomegalovirus mononucleosis, Ann. Inst. Med. **69**:842, 1968.

61. Sandford-Smith, J. H.: Herpes simplex canalicular obstruction, Brit. J. Ophthal. **54:** 456, 1970.
62. Singha, S. S.: and Nirankari, M. S.: Herpes zoster ophthalmicus, Orient. Arch. Ophthal. **8**:21, 1970.
63. Smith, M. E., Zimmerman, L. E., and Harley, R. D.: Ocular involvement in congenital cytomegalic inclusion disease, Arch. Ophthal. **76**:696, 1966.
64. Starr, J. G., Bart, R. D., and Gold, E.: Inapparent congenital cytomegalovirus infection, New Eng. J. Med. **282**:1075, 1970.
64a. Stevens, J. G., and Cook, M. L.: Latent herpes simplex virus in spinal ganglia of mice, Science **173**:843, 1971.
64b. Stevens, J. G., Nesburn, A. B., and Cook, M. L.: Recovery of latent Herpes simplex virus from trigeminal ganglia of rabbits with recurrent eye infection, Nature. In press.
65. Stucchi, C. A., and Bianchi, G.: Complications oculaires graves post-varicelleuses chez l'adulte, Ophthalmologica **161**:108, 1970.
66. Tanaka, N., and Kimura, S. J.: Localization of herpes simplex antigen and virus, Arch. Ophthal. **78**:68, 1962.
67. Tanaka, N., and Togni, B.: Further investigations by electron microscopy of herpes simplex virus in the corneal stroma of rabbits with experimental keratitis, Exp. Eye Res. **7**:142, 1968.
68. Thygeson, P.: Chronic herpetic keratouveitis, Trans. Amer. Ophthal. Soc. **65**:211, 1967.
69. Thygeson, P., Hogan, M. J., and Kimura, S. J.: The unfavorable effect of topical steroid therapy on herpetic keratitis, Trans. Amer. Ophthal. Soc. **58**:245, 1960.
69a. Tokumaru, T.: Production of epinephrine-induced skin lesions and fever following local and systemic injections of herpes simplex and vesicular stomatitis viruses in the rabbit, Arch. Ges. Virusforsch. **34**:179, 1971.
70. Torphy, D. E., Ray, C. G., McAlister, R., and Du, J. N. H.: Herpes simplex virus infection in infants: a spectrum of disease, J. Pediat. **76**:405, 1970.
71. Tsukahara, I., Veno, I., and Kawanishi, H.: Retinal changes in human cytomegalovirus infection, Amer. J. Ophthal. **62**:1153, 1966.
72. Vrabec, F., and Darrell, R. W.: The corneal epithelium in experimental herpetic keratitis in rabbits, Docum. Ophthal. **29**:212, 1971.
73. Witmer, R., and Iwamoto, T.: Electron microscope observation of herpes-like particles in the iris, Arch. Ophthal. **79**:331, 1968.

19

Ocular infections caused by the poxvirus, togavirus, myxovirus, paramyxovirus, and picornavirus groups

RICHARD W. DARRELL

Viruses can be grouped together on the basis of similar morphologic characteristics as seen on electron microscopic observation and on the basis of antigenic characteristics shared in common. Although two viruses may be in the same group, the clinical illnesses they produce are often very different from each other. This chapter contains a discussion of ocular infections caused by the following virus groups:

1. Poxvirus group
   a. Variola (smallpox)
   b. Vaccinia
   c. Orf (contagious ecthyma)
   d. Molluscum contagiosum
2. Togavirus group
   a. Rubella (German measles)
   b. Arbovirus disease
3. Myxovirus group (influenza)
4. Paramyxovirus group
   a. Measles (rubeola)
   b. Mumps (epidemic parotitis)
   c. Newcastle disease
5. Picornavirus group

POXVIRUS GROUP

When members of the poxvirus group are observed under the electron microscope in a dry condition, they are found to have a brick-shaped structure; but when observed in thin sections of infected cells, they have an elliptical shape. They all contain DNA and measure 200 to 300 nm. They are dermotropes and develop within the cytoplasm of the infected cell.

Variola (smallpox)

Classical smallpox, or variola major, is characterized by an incubation period of 12 days before the onset of fever and malaise, which last for 1 to 5 days and are followed by the appearance of an exanthem.[14,81] The skin lesions appear all in one crop and are distributed primarily on the face, chest, distal extremities, and palms and soles, all in contrast to the eruption associated with varicella virus infection (chickenpox). The lesions go through papular, vesicular, pustular, and crusting stages before healing, often with residual scarring. There are several types of infection, depending on the virulence of the virus and degree of resistance or immunity of the host. Most severe is hemorrhagic smallpox, in which bleeding appears 2 to 3 days after onset, and death may precede the exanthem. Subconjunctival hemorrhages and bleeding from the mouth and gums are seen. In malignant smallpox at about the tenth day the entire cornea may lose its luster, appear necrotic, and slough, releasing the intraocular contents; death usually follows.[14]

The pocks of classical smallpox may occur on the palpebral or ocular conjunctiva, but they do not develop on the cornea unless the cornea is vascularized. In countries where smallpox is endemic, trachoma is often a common problem and accounts for many vascularized corneal leukomas that subsequently develop pocks during smallpox infection. In nonvascularized corneas, about 2 weeks after onset of smallpox infection a marginal corneal ulcer may develop and proceed to spread across the cornea to the opposite limbus. If the process is slow enough, healing takes place with vascularization following the advancing border of the ulcer; otherwise, perforation of the cornea occurs.[14]

Conjunctivitis may appear 5 days after the skin lesions. In a study of 84 smallpox patients who concurrently developed conjunctivitis, variola virus was isolated from conjunctival swabs in three fourths of the patients.[40] However, if the conjunctivitis persisted longer than 2 weeks, variola virus was not recovered—a finding that suggests that this persistent conjunctivitis was caused by a different infectious agent.

When the virulence of the virus is low or resistance of the patient is high, a mild form of smallpox occurs, with only a limited skin eruption and often without eruption of any kind. A mild conjunctivitis may be the only sign. A study was made of conjunctivitis occurring in relatives or friends of smallpox patients, who brought the patient to the hospital and stayed there during the illness.[40] Of 55 of these family contacts, 21 developed conjunctivitis but no other illness; from over half of these cases of conjunctivitis, variola virus was isolated. These family contacts were presumably protected from severe illness because of previous smallpox infection or vaccination.

Vaccinia

Vaccinia virus is a laboratory virus used for vaccination against smallpox and was originally derived from cowpox or smallpox virus strains. The overwhelming majority of persons vaccinated with vaccinia virus develop no complications. However, since viremia does develop after vaccination, the open skin lesions of children with eczema can become infected and cause severe generalized vaccinia. Postvaccinial encephalitis carries a mortality of up to 40% but occurs rarely—in about 1.9 per million vaccinations.[57] Vaccinia necrosum, or progressive vaccinia, is seen in children undergoing immunosuppressive therapy or otherwise weakened by a chronic illness; this occurs in 1.1 per million vaccinations and is usually fatal.[57] Vaccinia immune globulin is protective when administered promptly.[39] In 1963 there were 7 deaths out of 6 million persons receiving primary vaccinations and 7 million receiving revaccinations in the United States.[57]

Ocular infection occurs when infectious virus is inadvertently transferred from the inoculation site to the eye (autoinoculation), from the vaccination site of a parent or sibling to another person's eye, or rarely, by transfer by unusual means, such as a swimming pool.[20] In 1919 Bedell[5] collected the reports of 91 cases of ocular vaccinia and found one third to have corneal complications; 20 years later Atkinson[2] brought the collection of case reports up to date. Since then several case reports have appeared describing the most common ocular complication, vaccinia of the eyelid (Plate 4, *G*).[9,20,27,55]

Usually the vaccinia vesicle appears on the lid margin, and the conjunctiva becomes markedly swollen; yet there is little pain.[27] Vaccinia of both the eyelids and the vulva occurred in a 3-year-old girl who inoculated herself from her sister's vaccination site.[62] Conjunctivitis alone without lid lesions has also been reported; diagnosis in this case was made by virus isolation.[12] Stenosis of the lacrimal sac can follow ocular vaccinia.[6] Corneal vaccinia takes the form of superficial punctate keratitis, epithelial ulcers, and disciform keratitis. These epithelial ulcers may develop a dumbbell shape superficially resembling herpetic keratitis.[13]

Diagnosis of ocular vaccinia is made by a history of recent vaccination, by isolation of vaccinia virus, and by cytology of infected epithelial cells. In 1892 Guarnieri[28] first described the cytoplasmic inclusions within epithelial cells; these inclusions are still known as Guarnieri bodies. They can be easily seen in cultures of corneal epithelial cells infected with vaccinia virus.[7]

Ocular vaccinia has been treated by idoxuridine,[21,34,37] vaccinia hyperimmune globuline (VIG),[21,23,39] cytosine arabinoside,[26] and monkey interferon.[35] One report suggested that VIG treatment of corneal vaccinia in rabbits caused a larger scar than did treatment with IDU.[24] However, at the present time the accepted treatment is systemic administration of VIG[69] as well as local application of IDU.

Through the assistance of the Red Cross, which provides VIG upon request, Ruben and Lane[69] conducted a retrospective study of ocular vaccinia treated by VIG. Of the 348 cases, only 6% had acute corneal complications, and only 1.2% had permanent corneal scarring. Most of the patients had lid and conjunctival vaccinia; only 2% of them were left with loss of lashes or scarring of the lid margin. Three fourths of the 348 patients were children under 4 years of age who developed ocular vaccinia 7 to 10 days after receiving a primary vaccination.

Orf (contagious ecthyma)

Orf, a viral disease of sheep, is caused by a member of the poxvirus group. Young lambs are most susceptible and develop lesions around their lips, nostrils, and eyes. The infection is occasionally transmitted to persons in contact with infected animals, such as shepherds, veterinarians, butchers, and hunters of wild goats.[10,43,45,60]

In man, the infectious agent probably enters through scratches in the skin. After an incubation period of a few days up to a week, macular lesions appear, the most likely sites being the hands, fingers, wrists, face, and legs. The macular lesions progress through a target stage, an acute vesicular stage, and a regenerative stage, and then regress during a period of 35 to 40 days before healing without scars. Infection of the eyelids is uncommon; the forehead and temple are more usual sites.

Diagnosis is made by history of contact with sheep, by biopsy of a skin lesion, by finding typical intracytoplasmic inclusions on histologic sections, and by noting the 5-week course of the disease.

Molluscum contagiosum

Typical skin lesions are small, waxy, pink tumors with an umbilicated center full of a cheesy material composed of epithelial cell husks. On histologic examination of infected basal epithelial cells, cytoplasmic inclusion bodies are seen, which on electron microscopy can be identified as masses of oval or brick-shaped virus particles typical of the poxvirus group. The virus is spread from person to person by close physical contact; for example, from a baby's face to mother's breast, from sibling to sibling, surgeon to patients, husband to wife, masseuse to clients, prostitutes to soldiers, or in the setting of a swimming pool or Turkish bath.[17] In one family group of 46 people, ranging in age from 10 months to 13 years of age, 25% became infected with molluscum contagiosum; and the tumors lasted from 2 weeks to 1½ years.[59] Transmission of molluscum contagiosum virus by sexual intercourse can be followed by outbreaks of tumors on the skin of the genitalia. This is particularly common in certain military groups.[49] Although the virus has never been cultivated in vitro, transmission is possible by direct skin inoculation of volunteers, with lesions appearing after an incubation period of 16 to 50 days; antibody against molluscum contagiosum virus also appears.[17]

Ocular disease is caused primarily by

the toxic effect of the cheesy material in the center of the molluscum. If a tumor is located on the upper eyelid, this cheesy material may easily fall into the conjunctival fornix and cause a severe follicular conjunctivitis (Plate 4, *H*). If the cause of the conjunctivitis is not recognized, the follicular conjunctivitis can progress to total corneal vascularization.[3,50,78] Treatment by electrocautery, chemical cautery, or excision of the tumor all yield equally good results.

TOGAVIRUS GROUP

Members of this group include rubella virus and many arboviruses. The enveloped virion containing RNA is 50 to 60 nm in diameter, enclosed by a lipid envelope.

Rubella (German measles)

Rubella is a common disease of childhood characterized by low-grade fever, malaise, and morbilliform rash on the face, trunk, and extremities; it is of short duration (3 to 4 days). There are no significant ocular signs.

However, rubella infection during pregnancy can cause persistent virus infection of the fetus and placenta, with devastating effects on the fetus if infection occurs early enough in gestation. During the 1964 to 1965 rubella epidemic, the rate of fetal abnormalities was 50% if infection occurred in the first month of pregnancy, 22% if in the second, and 6% if in the third.[71] Abnormalities include ocular malformation, heart defects, deafness, microcephaly, mental retardation, and chronic infection with virus excretion. Among children who reached their tenth birthday in spite of the fact that their mothers had had rubella during the first 4 months of pregnancy, the frequency of malformation was lower: 15% of these children had permanent abnormalities of the eye, ear, and heart; and 16% were left with minor abnormalities of these organs.[72]

The triad of microphthalmos, iris hypoplasia, and cataract is characteristic of ocular rubella;[68] whereas retinopathy, glaucoma, and strabismus are less common. Rubella retinopathy is not progressive and can help to label other congenital malformations, such as heart disease or cataract, as being of rubella origin.[74] Rubella virus is excreted for as long as 2 years following birth and on many occasions has been isolated from cataractous lenses at surgery; it has also been isolated as long as 3 years after the birth of the child.[52,56,65,70]

Rubella vaccine became possible following the first isolation of rubella virus in tissue culture.[79] In years past, young girls were often exposed to others with German measles in the hope that they might contract the disease and thereafter be protected by complete immunity. Now that rubella vaccine is available, large-scale immunization may prevent rubella in the future. However, rubella will probably not be eradicated, because not everyone will be vaccinated. The question remains whether immunity provided by vaccination is as adequate as natural infection and whether women vaccinated 20 years before will continue to be immune to rubella during pregnancy. Vaccination of women of childbearing age can be hazardous; one mother vaccinated inadvertently at 3 weeks' gestation was later aborted for therapeutic reasons, and rubella virus was recovered from the distorted conceptus.[61] However, given a successful program of vaccination throughout the population, congenital rubella infections should be much decreased.

Arbovirus disease

Over 241 types of viruses have been included in the arbovirus group, so named because arthropods are the principal vectors of infection, and hence the viruses are arthropod borne.[11] In the northeastern United States several varieties of arbovirus encephalitis are recognized: eastern equine, western equine, St. Louis, and Californian encephalitides.[16] Diagnosis is usually made in the context of an epidemic situation, which helps to differentiate the syndrome from aseptic meningitis following mumps, measles, vaccinia, or more rarely, herpes simplex infection. A rash on the eyelids and conjunctivitis occasionally occur. Ocular symptoms are more prominent in dengue and yellow fever, both more prevalent in tropical areas. In particular, dengue fever is characterized by severe deep pain behind the eyes and an erythematous rash affecting the skin of the eyelids as well as other parts of the body.[4,25,66] The illness starts with an acute fever of sudden onset and severe pain in the limbs and trunk, lasting 6 days. The erythema has been compared with that of measles.[66]

Although arbovirus infection during pregnancy has never been associated with congenital malformations, cataracts can be produced in rats by intracerebral inoculation of St. Louis encephalitis virus.[30]

MYXOVIRUS GROUP (INFLUENZA)

The influenza viruses, which comprise the myxovirus group, contain RNA in helical form, enclosed by an ether-sensitive envelope. They vary in shape from 80 to 250 nm in diameter and are found both in spherical and filamentous forms. The presence of 3 distinct antigens serves to classify the viruses into types A, B, and C.

Influenza infection is characterized by a 1- to 4-day incubation period, sudden onset of headache, lassitude, sweating, muscular pain, coryza, cough, congestion of the conjunctiva, and recovery usually within 1 week.[1,32,75] The infection occurs in epidemics, as in 1889, 1918, 1957, and 1968. Ocular symptoms were not significant in the 1918 epidemic, which was noted, however, for causing the deaths of millions of people, including many previously healthy young men. In contrast, during the Asian flu epidemic of 1957, mortality was lower, but ocular symptoms were the rule. In both England and the United States during the 1957 epidemic, conjunctivitis was a frequent sign: 48% of the Royal Air Force personnel contracting influenza during 1957 developed conjunctivitis, as did 60% of the patients studied in Cleveland.[31,36]

Corneal pathology is not usually associated with influenza infection, but there has been one report from the Soviet Union of 87 patients who suffered from a variety of corneal lesions during the Asian flu epidemic; the lesions included superficial punctate keratitis, deep interstitial keratitis, and dendritic keratitis associated with iridocyclitis.[41] Dendritic keratitis may be secondary to the high fever of influenza, a factor known to provoke recurrent herpes simplex virus infection. In Iran during the Asian flu epidemic, follicular conjunctivitis associated with painful preauricular lymphadenopathy was common. Dendritic keratitis, neuroretinitis, vitreous hemorrhage, and ocular muscle paralysis were also reported.[82] Superficial punctate keratitis was seen in 3 cases of influenza in France in 1932.[19]

PARAMYXOVIRUS GROUP

Within this group, viruses causing ocular disease are measles, mumps, and Newcastle disease virus; infections without ocular signs are caused by the parainfluenza and respiratory syncytial viruses. These viruses have an inner helix of RNA 18 nm in diameter and an ether-sensitive envelope 100 to 300 nm in diameter.

Measles (rubeola)

Measles is an acute infectious disease of childhood characterized by a maculopapular, blotchy rash. After an incubation period of about 10 days, fever develops, with the rash appearing 4 days later. During the prodrome, Koplik's spots can be found on the buccal mucosa; and fever, coryza, cough, and red eyes are present.

Photophobia is a characteristic symptom of measles, and children prefer to be in a darkened room. An ophthalmologic examination is rarely done; but when it is, a mild conjunctivitis and epithelial keratitis are nearly always found. Koplik's spots, tiny bluish white spots on a bright red base, may be found on the semilunar fold. Measles virus can be identified within these Koplik's spots as viral microtubular aggregates within nuclei and cytoplasm.[76] The conjunctivitis and keratitis almost always resolve without complication. But in parts of the world where malnutrition is a problem, measles conjunctivitis and keratitis can lead to secondary bacterial infection, perforation of the globe, and blindness. In the Philippines a history of measles preceding or accompanying the corneal lesion has been found in one fifth of the patients with corneal blindness at a general hospital and in one third of the students at a school for the blind. However, none of the patients treated for active cases of measles at the hospital had any ocular complication.[58] The role of malnutrition and poor resistance is pointed out by a report from Zambia, in which measles (50%), chickenpox (25%), or smallpox (25%) shared responsibility for corneal blindness; and three fourths of 686 totally blind persons were associated with these 3 infectious diseases.[51] The epidemic of measles in Haiti during 1966 to 1967 caused severe ocular complications. In 25 patients with corneal ulceration, over half the globes perforated.[21] Reports from different areas in Africa confirm this association between measles and corneal blindness, usually in the context of malnutrition.[42,64]

Even in normally nourished children rare complications of measles can occur. In one case unilateral optic neuritis was the presenting symptom before the rash appeared.[73] Measles virus can pass the placental barrier early in gestation, and the resulting infection may terminate in spontaneous abortion, or the child may be born with congenital measles. Anomalies associated with congenital measles are cataract, dacryostenosis, pigmentary retinopathy, and cardiopathy. Pigmentary retinopathy rarely follows adult measles but is common in congenital measles and must be differentiated from a similar retinopathy caused by chickenpox and influenza viruses.[53] Encephalitis is a very rare complication of measles infection in childhood.

Following administration of measles vaccine, a live attenuated virus strain, clinical measles may develop in about 6 days. Cough, conjunctivitis, rhinorrhea, fever, pneumonia, and thrombocytopenic purpura were noted in one such case.[80] Many people hoped large-scale measles vaccination of the population would eradicate the disease. However, not everyone could be vaccinated; and in 1971 a full-scale measles epidemic was again in progress in the United States.

Mumps (epidemic parotitis)

Mumps is an acute contagious disease characterized by enlargement of one or both parotid and other salivary glands, which become painful. The testicles and ovaries may be affected in adolescents and adults. The major complications of mumps affect the central nervous system and include encephalitis, aseptic meningitis, hemiplegia, quadriplegia, blindness, cranial nerve palsies, deafness, and seizures.[47] Estimates of the frequency of central nervous system complications vary from less than 1% to 30%.[47] Other rare complications of mumps are polyarthritis, pancreatitis, nephritis, and arthritis.

A dramatic keratitis occasionally develops 5 days after onset of parotitis. It is unilateral, causes abrupt loss of visual acuity, and is associated with tearing and photophobia but with little pain; on slit-lamp examination, the keratitis is found to be deep. The entire cornea becomes hazy and gray, with folds in Descemet's membrane. In spite of the dramatic appearance of the keratitis, recovery within 3 weeks is usual.[54,67]

In addition to keratitis, dacryoadenitis occurs in as many as 20% in epidemic situations.[46,47] It is characterized by sudden onset of orbital pain, lid edema, and a mass in the lacrimal fossa. Other rare ocular complications include iritis, conjunctivitis, scleritis, and central retinal occlusion.[67]

Newcastle disease

Newcastle disease, an often fatal pneumoencephalitis of fowl, was first identified at Newcastle-on-Tyne, England.[15] In spite of the neurotropic behavior of the virus in infection of fowls, the virus produces only a self-limited conjunctivitis in man. After the first human case was reported by Burnet[8] in 1943, occasional cases have been reported, usually among poultry workers and laboratory technicians.[23,29,33,38,44,48,63,77] The conjunctivitis is typically unilateral, follicular, and associated with preauricular adenopathy, but without corneal changes (Plate 4, *I*). Recovery is complete in 10 to 14 days.

Diagnosis is made by history of contact with infected birds, isolation of the virus, and by a rise in Newcastle antibodies, which are detected by hemagglutination inhibition, complement-fixation, or neutralization tests.

PICORNAVIRUS GROUP

This group is made up of small ether-resistant RNA viruses. Those of human origin are: (1) enteroviruses (polioviruses, coxsackieviruses, echoviruses, and numbered enteroviruses), and (2) rhinoviruses. Several of these viruses can cause aseptic meningitis and transient or permanent paralysis of the cranial nerves, including the oculomotor nerves. Others are responsible for a variety of upper respiratory infections with predominant involvement of the oropharynx and cervical lymph nodes. Conjunctivitis is not usual, although watery eyes are a frequent occurrence in the common cold. Some of the echoviruses cause aseptic meningitis, rash, and conjunctivitis. However, ocular signs are uncommon in infections caused by the picornavirus group.

Coxsackievirus causes a common infection of cloven-footed animals, the foot-and-mouth disease. Occasionally, infection is transmitted by contact between animal and man, and infection of the human cornea and conjunctiva can occur.

REFERENCES

1. Andrewes, C. H.: Epidemiology of influenza. In Influenza: a review of current research, Geneva, 1954, World Health Organization.
2. Atkinson, W. S., and Scullard, G.: Vaccinia with ocular involvement, Arch. Ophthal. **23**: 584, 1940.
3. Balakrishnan, E.: Molluscum contagiosum conjunctivitis, J. All-India Ophthal. Soc. **12**: 173, 1964.
4. Barkan, H.: The ocular complications of dengue fever, Amer. J. Ophthal. **2**:650, 1919.
5. Bedell, A. J.: Multiple vaccination of the eyelids, Trans. Amer. Ophthal. Soc. **17**:273, 1919.
6. Bill, I.: A case of stenosis in the lacrimal sac caused by vaccinia, Amer. J. Ophthal. **37**:33, 1959.
7. Bland, J. O. W., and Robinow, C. F.: The inclusion bodies of vaccinia and their relationship to the elementary bodies studied in cultures of the rabbit's cornea, J. Path. Bact. **48**:381, 1939.
8. Burnet, F. M.: Human infection with the virus of Newcastle disease of fowls, Med. J. Aust. **2**:313, 1943.
9. Bybee, J. D., Phillips, C. A., Ory, E. M., and Brunschwig, J. P.: Vaccinia of the eyelid, J.A.M.A. **199**:126, 1967.
10. Carr, R. W.: A case of orf (ecthyma contagiosum, contagious pustular dermatitis) contracted by a human from a wild Alaskan goat, Alaska Med. **10**:75, 1968.
11. Catalogue of arthropod-borne viruses of the world, Amer. J. Trop. Med. **19**:1081, 1970.
12. Croffead, G. W., and Harrison, S. W.: Vaccinia conjunctivitis, Amer. J. Ophthal. **53**: 531, 1962.
13. Darrell, R. W., and Vrabec, F.: Vaccinia virus infection of the rabbit cornea, Arch. Ophthal. **86**:568, 1971.
14. Dixon, C. W.: Smallpox, London, 1962, J. & A. Churchill, pp. 94-96.
15. Doyle, T. M.: A hitherto unrecorded disease of fowls due to a filter-passing virus, J. Comp. Path. **40**:144, 1927.
16. Editorial: Arboviruses in the northeastern United States, New Eng. J. Med. **279**:380, 1968.
17. Editorial: Molluscum contagiosum, Brit. Med. J. **1**:459, 1968.
18. Editorial: Prophylaxis against rubella and mumps, Brit. Med. J. **2**:282, 1970.
19. Fradkine, J.: Trois cas de keratite ponctuee superficielle, Soc. Franc. Ophtal. **45**:135, 1932.
20. Frampton, G., and Smith, C.: Primary vaccinia of the eyelid, Brit. J. Ophthal. **36**:214, 1952.
21. Francois, J., De Molder, E., and Gildemyn, H.: Ocular vaccinia, Acta Ophthal. **45**:25, 1967.
22. Frederique, G., Howard, R. O., and Boniuk, V.: Corneal ulcers in rubeola, Amer. J. Ophthal. **68**:996, 1969.
23. Freymann, M. W., and Bang, F. B.: Human

conjunctivitis due to Newcastle virus in the U. S. A., Bull. Johns Hopkins Hosp. **84:** 409, 1949.

24. Fulginiti, V. A., Winograd, L. A., Jackson, M., and Ellis, P.: Therapy of experimental vaccinial keratitis, Arch. Ophthal. **74:**539, 1965.
25. Gill, W. D.: Ocular symptomatology in dengue, Arch. Ophthal. **57:**628, 1928.
26. Gordon, D. M., and Advocate, S.: Vaccinial blepharokeratitis, Amer. J. Ophthal. **59:**480, 1965.
27. Gould, E. L., Havener, W. H., and Andrew, J. M.: Vaccinia lid infection, Amer. J. Ophthal. **56:**830, 1963.
28. Guarnieri, G.: Ricerche sulla patogenesi ed etiologia dell'infezione vaccinica e vaiolosa, Arch. Sci. Med. (Torino) **16:**403, 1892.
29. Gustafson, D. P., and Moses, H. E.: Isolation of Newcastle disease virus from the eye of a human being, J. Amer. Vet. Med. Ass. **118:** 1, 1951.
30. Hanna, C., Jarman, R. V., Keatts, J. G., and Duffy, C. E.: Virus-induced cataracts, Arch. Ophthal. **79:**59, 1968.
31. Holland, W. W.: A clinical study of influenza in the Royal Air Force, Lancet **2:**840, 1957.
32. Hoyle, L.: The influenza viruses. In Virology monographs no. 4, New York, 1968, Springer-Verlag New York, Inc.
33. Ingalls, W. L., and Mahoney, A.: Isolation of virus of Newcastle disease from human beings, Amer. J. Public Health **39:**737, 1949.
34. Jack, M. K., and Sorenson, R. W.: Vaccinial keratitis treated with IDU, Arch. Ophthal. **69:**730, 1963.
35. Jones, B. R., Galbraith, J. E. K., and Al-Hussaini, M. K.: Vaccinial keratitis treated with interferon, Lancet **1:**875, 1962.
36. Jordan, W. S., Jr., Denny, F. W., Jr., Badger, G. F., Curtiss, C., Dingle, J. H., Oseasohn, R., and Stevens, D. A.: A study of illness in a group of Cleveland families, Amer. J. Hyg. **68:**190, 1958.
37. Kaufman, H. E., Nesburn, A. B., and Maloney, E. D.: Cure of vaccinia infection by 5-iodo-2′-deoxyuridine, Virology **18:**567, 1962.
38. Keeney, A. H., and Hunter, M. L.: Human infection with the Newcastle virus of fowls, Arch. Ophthal. **44:**573, 1950.
39. Kempe, C. H., Berge, T. O., and England, B.: Hyperimmune vaccinal gamma globulin, Pediatrics **18:**177, 1956.
40. Kempe, C. H., Dekking, F., St. Vincent, L., Rao, A. R., and Downie, A. W.: Conjunctivitis and subclinical infection in smallpox, J. Hyg. (Camb.) **67:**631, 1969.
41. Kulikova, L. A.: Lesions of the cornea during influenza epidemics, Vestn. Oftal. **79:**72, 1966.
42. Lagraulet, J., and Bard, J.: Lesions oculaires de la rougeole dans les milieux ruraux en Afrique noire, Bull. Soc. Path. Exot. **60:** 203, 1967.
43. Lambie, J. A., and Gustafson, A. A.: Contagious ecthyma in man, J. Lancet **87:**400, 1967.
44. Lamer, L.: Sur un cas conjunctivite de la maladie de Newcastle, Canad. J. Ophthal. **4:**390, 1969.
45. Leavell, V. W., McNamara, M. J., Muelling, R., Talbert, W. M., Rucker, R. C., and Dalton, A. J.: Orf: report of 19 human cases with clinical and pathological observations, J.A.M.A. **204:**657, 1968.
46. Lemke, L., Jütte, A., Oehring, H., and Stelzner, I.: Mumpsinfektion als Ursache der Konjunktivitis Parinaud, Med. Klin. **61:**1107, 1966.
47. Levitt, L. P., Rich, T. A., Kinde, S. W., Lewis, A. L., Gates, E. H., and Bond, J. O.: Central nervous system mumps—a review of 64 cases, Neurology **20:**829, 1970.
48. Lippmann, O.: Human conjunctivitis due to the Newcastle-disease virus of fowls, Amer. J. Ophthal. **35:**1021, 1952.
49. Lynch, P. J., and Minkin, W.: Molluscum contagiosum of the adult: probable venereal transmission, Arch. Derm. (Chicago) **98:**141, 1968.
50. Mathur, S. P.: Ocular complications in molluscum contagiosum, Brit. J. Ophthal. **44:** 572, 1960.
51. McGlashan, W. D.: Measles malnutrition and blindness in Luapula Province, Zambia, Trop. Geogr. Med. **21:**157, 1969.
52. Menser, M. A., Harley, J. D., Hertzberg, R., Dorman, D. C., and Murphy, A. M.: Persistence of virus in lens for three years after prenatal rubella, Lancet **2:**387, 1967.
53. Metz, H. S., and Harkey, M. E.: Pigmentary retinopathy following maternal measles (morbilli) infection, Amer. J. Ophthal. **66:**1107, 1968.
54. Mickatavage, R., and Amdur, J.: A case report of mumps keratitis, Arch. Ophthal. **69:** 758, 1963.
55. Moses, L.: Vaccinia palpebrorum, Amer. J. Ophthal. **60:**331, 1965.
56. Murphy, A. M., Reid, R. R., Pollard, I., Gillespie, A. M., Dorman, D. C., Menser, M. A., Harley, J. D., and Hertzberg, R.: Rubella cataracts, Amer. J. Ophthal. **64:**1109, 1967.
57. Neff, J. M., Levine, R. H., Lane, J. M., and others: Complications of smallpox vaccination in the United States, 1963, Pediatrics **39:** 916, 1967.
58. Ocompo, G., and Olivar, E.: Corneal blind-

ness associated with measles, Philippine J. Ophthal. **1**:5, 1969.
59. Overfield, T. M., and Brody, J. A.: An epidemiologic study of molluscum contagiosum in Anchorage, Alaska, J. Pediat. **69**:640, 1966.
60. Parnell, A. G.: Ecthyma contagiosum (orf), Brit. J. Oral Surg. **3**:128, 1965.
61. Phillips, C. A., Maeck, J. V. S., Rogers, R. A., and Savel, H.: Intrauterine rubella infection following immunization with rubella vaccine, J.A.M.A. **213**:624, 1970.
62. Piazza, M., Piccinino, F., Picciotto, L., and Visconti, M.: Infezione da virus vaccinico a localizzazione palpebrale e vulvare insorta in sequito a contatto indiretto con un soggetto vaccinato di recente, Riv. Ist. Sieroter. Ital. **44**:59, 1969.
63. Pilsworth, R., and Wall, B. J.: The isolation of Newcastle disease virus from human infections, Great Britain Ministry of Health—Monthly Bulletin **23**:122, 1964.
64. Quere, M. A.: Les complications oculaires de la rougeole, cause majeure de cecite chez l'enfant en pays tropical, Ophthalmologica **148**:107, 1964.
65. Rawls, W. E., Phillips, C. A., Melnick, J. L., and Desmond, M. M.: Persistent virus infection in congenital rubella, Arch. Ophthal. **77**:430, 1967.
66. Riad, M.: Some eye complications of dengue fever, Bull. Ophthal. Soc. Egypt **22**:60, 1929.
67. Riffenburgh, R. S.: Ocular manifestations of mumps, Arch. Ophthal. **66**:739, 1961.
68. Roy, F. H., Hiatt, R. L., Korones, S. B., and Roane, J.: Ocular manifestations of congenital rubella syndrome, Arch. Ophthal. **75**: 601, 1966.
69. Ruben, F. L., and Lane, J. M.: Ocular vaccinia: an epidemiologic analysis of 348 cases, Arch. Ophthal. **84**:45, 1970.
70. Scheie, H. G., Schaffer, D. B., Plotkin, S. A., and Kertesz, E. D.: Congenital rubella cataract, Arch. Ophthal. **77**:440, 1967.
71. Sever, J. L.: The epidemiology of rubella, Arch. Ophthal. **77**:427, 1967.
72. Sheridan, M. D.: Final report of a prospective study of children whose mothers had rubella in early pregnancy, Brit. Med. J. **2**:536, 1964.
73. Srivastave, S. P., and Nema, H. V.: Optic neuritis in measles, Brit. J. Ophthal. **47**:180, 1963.
74. Stark, G.: Rubella retinopathy, Arch. Dis. Child. **41**:420, 1966.
75. Stuart-Harris, C. H., and Andrewes, C.: Influenza, London, 1965, Edward Arnold (Publishers), Ltd.
76. Suringa, D. W. R., Bank, L., and Ackerman, A. B.: Role of measles virus in skin lesions and Koplik's spots, New Eng. J. Med. **283**: 1139, 1971.
77. Trott, D. G.: Outbreak of conjunctivitis due to Newcastle disease virus among workers of chicken broiler factory, Brit. Med. J. **5477**: 1514, 1965.
78. Vannas, S., and Lapinleima, K.: Molluscum contagiosum in the skin, caruncle and conjunctiva, Acta Ophthal. **45**:314, 1967.
79. Weller, T. H., and Neva, F. A.: Propagation in tissue culture of cytopathogenic agents from patients with rubella-like illness, Proc. Soc. Exp. Biol. Med. **111**:215, 1962.
80. Wilhelm, D. J., and Peagle, R. D.: Thrombocytopenic purpura and pneumonia following measles vaccination, Amer. J. Dis. Child. **113**:534, 1967.
81. World Health Organization Scientific Group: Smallpox eradication, W. H. O. Techn. Rep. Ser. **393**:1, 1968.
82. Zarrabi: Quelques complications oculaires en Iran pendant la grippe asiatique, Arch. Ophthal. **18**:59, 1958.

20

Ocular syphilis

RANDOLPH WHITFIELD, Jr. AND EMIL WIROSTKO

Following Mahoney's[34] 1943 report on penicillin's great effectiveness for treating syphilis, members of the medical community generally felt that another great affliction of man had finally been conquered by modern medical science. This attitude was strongly reinforced by the dramatic decrease of infectious syphilis following the increase in availability and use of penicillin in the late 1940's. From a high of 106,000 cases of primary and secondary syphilis reported in 1947, the incidence fell to only 6,251 cases by 1957.[57] The results of this apparent success were readily seen in the hospitals and medical schools across the country. The insistence on routine serologic evaluations on all inpatients became so relaxed that these tests often became the exception rather than the rule. In the medical schools the study of syphilis developed such a low priority that the students soon received merely a few hours of instruction in the diagnosis and management of the disease. At present there is a whole generation of medical school graduates who are but vaguely aware of the clinical manifestations and natural course of syphilis. The decrease in routine serologic testing and in physicians' interest in and knowledge of the disease must have had profound, if unmeasurable, effects on the reported incidence of the disease and must have significantly contributed to the sharp decrease in reported cases. In addition, the early indiscriminate use of penicillin for treating many infectious disorders contributed to the apparent decrease in the incidence of clinically recognizable early syphilis. It is a well-known fact that minute amounts of penicillin can alter the natural course of the disease by causing it to evolve directly into the latent stage, aborting the clinically evident early manifestations, with the appearance later of symptomatic late gummatous, cardiovascular, or central nervous system syphilis.

Despite these many factors operating to decrease the reported incidence, the downward trend has reversed itself; and in recent years there has been a marked increase in the number of reported cases of infectious syphilis. In 1970 the figure was 20,186, an increase of 320% over the 1957 level.[57] The significance of the present problem is pointed out by the results of a 1968 report sponsored by the American Public Health Association. This study revealed that private physicians, treating more than 75% of all cases of infectious syphilis in this country, reported only one eighth of the cases to public health authorities.[14] The study concludes that the true incidence of infectious syphilis is actually at least four times the reported incidence, totaling over 80,000 cases in 1970. Syphilis is now far from being under control in this country, and a greater awareness of the problem, especially on the part of physicians, is urgently needed.

Ophthalmologists find themselves in a

unique position concerning the diagnosis and treatment of syphilis. Not only are ocular complaints often the reason for an undiagnosed syphilitic patient to seek medical attention,[62] but in some forms of the disease, such as neurorecurrence and tardive heredosyphilis, ocular lesions are the most common and often the most serious clinical manifestations. In addition, the recent controversial reports of intraocular treponemes in seronegative patients, with the persistence of intraocular treponemes following supposedly adequate therapy, have stimulated a resurgence of basic and clinical research into the nature of the disease, much of which is being conducted by ophthalmologists.

This chapter includes, first, a brief review of the various tests available for the diagnosis of syphilis; second, a presentation of the natural course of the disease and the different ways syphilis may be clinically manifest in the eye; and third, a discussion of some of the more recent research in ocular syphilis and the implications of this research for the clinician as regards diagnosis and treatment of ocular syphilis.

DIAGNOSTIC PROCEDURES

More than 200 different types of serologic tests for syphilis have been developed since August von Wasserman in 1905 described his classical complement-fixing reaction using a syphilitic patient's serum and liver extract from a stillborn syphilitic fetus. All the tests have in common the ability to demonstrate the presence of one or more of the antibodies elicited in the immunologic response of an individual to infection with *Treponema pallidum*. Today there are 2 general types of serologic tests for syphilis: nonspecific reagin tests and specific treponemal tests.

Reagin tests

The Wasserman test and its progeny all detect the presence of the same reactive substance (reagin) found in syphilitic serum. Although reagin antibodies are undetectable in the serum of uninfected individuals, they may occur transiently in acute infections and following inoculations; and, less commonly, they may be found chronically in the serum of some patients suffering with diseases such as systemic lupus erythematosus, lepromatous leprosy, malaria, and other conditions characterized by serum immunoglobulin elevations. The level of reagin in the serum of an infected person varies in a predictable way, corresponding to the clinical stage of the disease. It also falls in a typical manner following adequate therapy, especially in the early stages of the disease (Fig. 20-1). These quantifiable tests, when performed serially, are indispensable in determining the stage of the disease, in detecting reinfection in a patient having had previously adequate therapy, and also in ascertaining the effectiveness of treatment. Because they are inexpensive and simple to perform, they are well suited for routine testing and mass screening of sera. A final use of the reagin test is to examine the cerebrospinal fluid for possible neurologic involvement of the disease. False-positive reactions in the cerebrospinal fluid are quite rare, although false-negative reactions may occur. Thus reagin tests, though not specific for infection with *T. pallidum*, have great value in the diagnosis and management of syphilis. The quantitative reagin tests in common use today are the Venereal Disease Research Laboratory (VDRL) test, the Kahn, Kline, and Mazzini tests, all of which are flocculation tests, and the Kolmer, a complement-fixation test. Of these, the VDRL is the test of choice in the United States because of its reliability, simplicity, and widespread availability.

Treponemal tests

The first serologic test to measure specific antitreponemal antibodies was the *Treponema pallidum* immobilization test (TPI) developed by Nelson[42] in 1949. Although expensive, technically difficult to perform, and lacking sensitivity in early acquired syphilis, it soon became the serologic test against which all others were

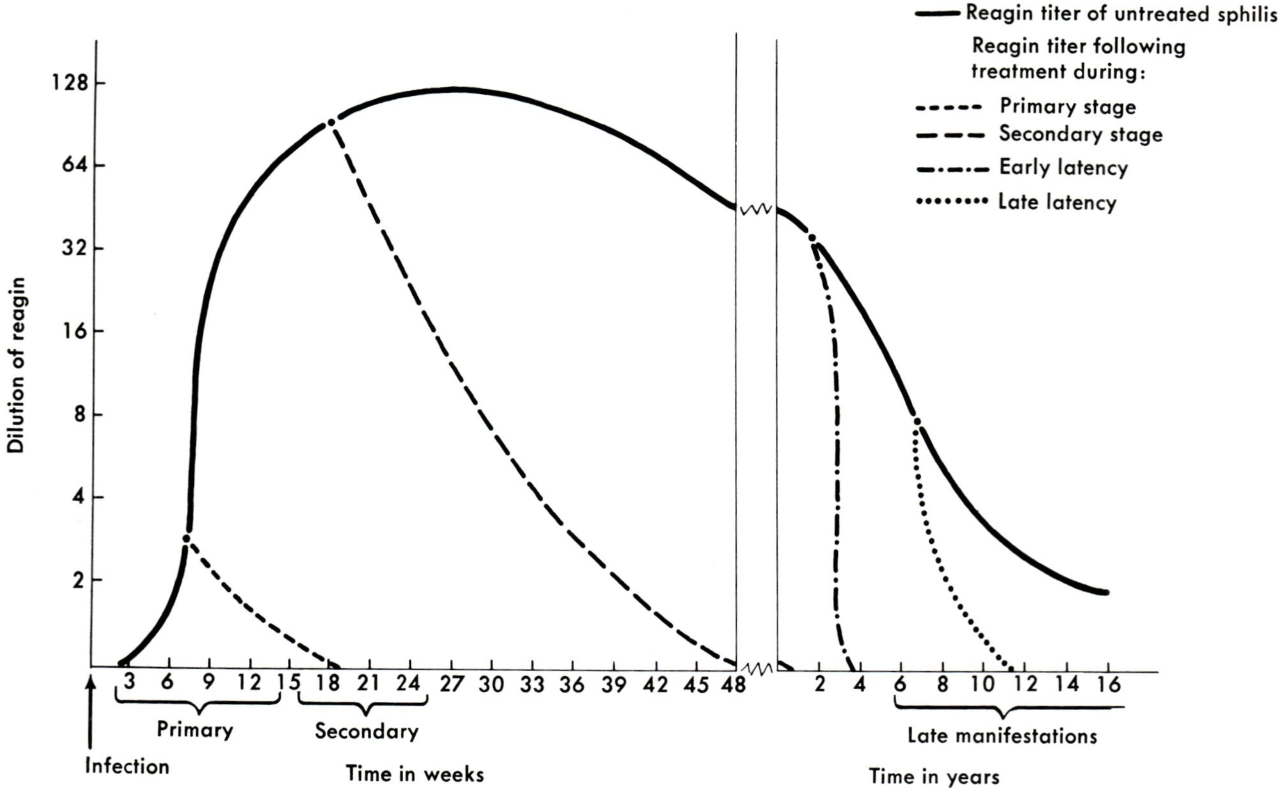

Fig. 20-1. Typical serum reagin titer changes during the course of untreated syphilis and following treatment during the primary, secondary, early latent, and late latent stages. (Adapted from Syphilis—modern diagnosis and management, U. S. Public Health Service Publication No. 743, Washington, D. C., 1961, pp. 17-21.)

measured because of its great specificity and excellent sensitivity in late acquired syphilis. Many treponemal tests quickly followed the TPI, but none of them were able to replace it. However, in 1957 Deacon and his associates[9] at the Venereal Disease Research Laboratories developed an immunofluorescent technique for identifying antitreponemal antibodies. It held great promise as an inexpensive test possessing the specificity and sensitivity of the TPI. It was evaluated and improved over the next several years, and in 1964 the fluorescent treponemal antibody absorption test (FTA-ABS) was presented as a modification of the original FTA test.[21] In its present form the FTA-ABS test is widely available and with its increased sensitivity and specificity is the confirmatory test of choice.[55]

The limitations of the treponemal tests, such as the TPI and the FTA-ABS, should be recognized, however. They are qualitative not quantitative tests, and they do not usually revert to negative following adequate therapy. They have no value in serial use to determine either the stage of disease or the adequacy of treatment. Also, the treponemal tests on the cerebrospinal fluid (CSF) have not been proved reliable.[49]

Table 20-1 is a comparison of the relative sensitivities of the VDRL, the TPI, and the FTA-ABS tests in various stages of syphilis.[33] Because of the greater sensitivity of the FTA-ABS test, it is the test of choice for the ophthalmologist in determining whether syphilis is a possible cause of ocular disease.

CSF examination

The parameters measured in a CSF examination for evidence of neurosyphilitic activity must include cell count, total protein level, and a titered VDRL test. Any cell count above 4 round cells, total protein level above approximately 40 mg/100 ml (depending upon the laboratory), and any reactivity of the VDRL test is considered abnormal. As increased cells and protein in the CSF are nonspecific indications of meningeal inflammation, a reactive VDRL test is the only certain indicator of past or present luetic involvement of the central nervous system (CNS). Soon after infection there is CNS invasion with treponemes in virtually all untreated cases of syphilis. Although the associated involvement of the meninges, vessels, or parenchyma of the CNS may be so slight as to cause no clinical or spinal fluid manifestations, it is known that those who do develop even transient spinal fluid abnormalities at this time have an increased tendency to develop one of the clinical forms of neurosyphilis months or years later. Spinal fluid examination is an essential step in the diagnosis and management of every case of syphilis.

The indications for performing a CSF examination are:

1. Before discharge, following adequate treatment of early acquired or congenital syphilis
2. Before initiating treatment in any patient with late latent, late acquired, or late congenital syphilis
3. Whenever there is clinical or sero-

Table 20-1. Sensitivities of three tests in the various stages of syphilis

Test	Percent reactivity			
	Primary syphilis	Secondary syphilis	Latent syphilis	Late congenital and symptomatic syphilis
VDRL	77	97	75	75
FTA-ABS	85	99	95	96
TPI	56	94	82	93

Adapted from Lucas, J. B.: New developments in venereal disease research, Med. Ann. D. C. **35**:375, 1966.

logic evidence of syphilitic activity or reinfection in a patient having had previous adequate therapy for syphilis

4. In any patient suspected of being a chronic biologic false-positive reactor
5. In any patient being treated for neurosyphilis (Repeated CSF examinations must be performed.)

ACQUIRED OCULAR SYPHILIS

Primary lesions of the eye

Primary syphilis is contracted following prolonged, moist, warm intimate contact with an infectious lesion or with material containing motile treponemes. Following successful inoculation, a generalized spirochetemia ensues within 24 hours. The incubation period preceding the appearance of the chancre is usually 2 to 3 weeks but ranges from 10 to 90 days. The chancre, which is evident in approximately two thirds of all cases, is the first clinical sign of syphilis and appears at the site of original inoculation. It is typically an elevated, eroded, painless papule, associated with rubbery, nontender enlargement of the lymph nodes draining the area of the chancre. Extragenital chancres are not uncommon. The lesion lasts 1 to 5 weeks and then disappears spontaneously. It is infectious, and a properly performed darkfield examination usually reveals a large number of motile treponemes. At the first appearance of the chancre the serologic tests may or may not be reactive, though they rapidly become so during the following month.

Although the primary chancre is usually genital, it may occur almost anywhere on the body; and conjunctival primary lesions have been reported repeatedly since the first written description by Desmarres in 1854.[11] The conjunctival chancre, typically presenting as a nontender, firm, eroded papule, associated with enlarged, painless, preauricular and submandibular lymph nodes, is not different from one in any other location. It may arise from the bulbar or palpebral conjunctiva, with a predilection for the lower fornix. Stokes makes special mention of the conjunctiva as a common site for nonvenereally acquired chancres in physicians: "Two of four such lesions . . . were in physicians, and in none did the ophthalmologist consulted make or even suggest the diagnosis."[54] History and darkfield and serologic examination, combined with physical findings, usually make the diagnosis a simple one. The problem of diagnosis is that one must be aware of the possibility of syphilis in the first place.

Secondary lesions of the eye

The secondary, or mucocutaneous, stage of the disease has its onset within 6 months of the inoculation, occurring usually within a few weeks of and occasionally concomitant with the regression of the chancre. The signs and symptoms of the secondary disease may be pronounced or may be so slight as to pass unnoticed by the patient. Fever, headache, alopecia, iritis, and malaise may be prominent heralding symptoms; but the hallmarks of secondary syphilis are generalized lymphadenopathy and papulosquamous lesions of the skin and mucous membranes. These lesions are infectious, darkfield positive for treponemes, and in early secondary syphilis are usually discrete, generalized, and bilaterally symmetrical. Antibody production is at its height, and the serologic tests are all strongly reactive. The signs and symptoms of this stage regress slowly over a period of several weeks, and the patient thereafter becomes completely asymptomatic.

Ocular complications occur in 4.5% of all patients with secondary syphilis and in 9.3% of those with relapsing secondary syphilis.[61]

LIDS AND CONJUNCTIVA. The skin of the lids is often involved in the generalized mucocutaneous eruption, which is so typical of secondary syphilis with macular, papular, squamous, and pustular eruptions, or any combination of these. The lesions are usually dry, nonpruritic, and bilaterally symmetrical. They are darkfield positive and infectious. The alopecia of secondary syphilis may be manifest by the temporary loss of the eyebrows, especially a bilaterally symmetrical loss of the outer portions.

A transient nonspecific conjunctivitis often appears concomitantly with the development of systemic symptoms and skin rash. It may vary from mild to severe and usually lasts only a few days.

Specific luetic conjunctivitis is much less common, occurs later in the secondary stage, and has three forms. The most common form is that of diffuse papillary conjunctivitis, with the palpebral conjunctiva involved in a hypertrophic papillary inflammatory process. Its frequent association with a pannus and its granular configuration bring trachoma into the differential diagnosis. However, scrapings reveal motile treponemes on darkfield examination; results of serologic tests are strongly positive; and no follicles are present on examination of the conjunctiva.

Syphilitic mucous patches, commonly found on other mucous membranes in this stage of the disease, form the second, much less common, form of specific syphilitic involvement of the conjunctiva. The patches vary from 2 to 10 mm in diameter, are slightly elevated with an erythematous base, and have an overlying pearly gray membrane. These may occasionally develop into papules or, rarely, into frankly flowering condyloma lata. The third form of specific luetic conjunctivitis, called syphilitic scleroconjunctivitis, is extremely rare.[11] It is a perilimbal inflammation, with edema, injection, and elevation of the perilimbal conjunctiva, and with involvement of the episclera as well. It may be associated with a mild iritis or iridocyclitis.

A final form of mucous membrane inflammation that may affect the ocular adnexa is the rare extension of secondary rhinitis to involve the tear sac, causing an acute obstructive dacryocystitis. All these forms of early inflammation respond dramatically to specific antisyphilitic therapy.

CORNEA AND SCLERA. Simple scleritis occurs rarely, and episcleritis occurs only slightly less rarely in secondary syphilis. Interstitial keratitis is a rare complication of acquired early syphilis, accounting for less than 3% of all cases of the disorder. It is often associated with anterior uveitis, and but for its tendency to be unilateral, its rapid evolution, and relatively benign course, is quite similar to the interstitial keratitis of congenital syphilis.

IRIS AND CILIARY BODY. According to Hogan and Zimmerman,[20] the most common syphilitic eye lesion is the iritis of secondary syphilis, and it comprises about 75% of all the eye lesions of the early acquired disease. Approximately 4% of those in the secondary stage develop iritis. It is slightly more common in males than in females and occurs twice as frequently in Negroes as in Caucasians.[40] In 1943 Woods[61] reported that between 30% and 40% of all cases of iritis were syphilitic in origin, but with the decrease in the incidence of syphilis its importance as a cause of iritis also diminished. However, serologic determinations are certainly indicated in any case of iritis of unknown or doubtful cause. Usually the diagnosis is not difficult, as the iritis is associated with florid mucocutaneous lesions in 75% of the cases, and in every case there usually is other evidence of early syphilis.[40]

There are two special types of iritis that deserve mention. The first is recurrent iridocyclitis, called iridorelapse, which follows inadequate therapy for early syphilis. Although morphologically nonspecific and usually quite responsive to specific antiluetic therapy, iridorelapse is important because it is associated with concomitant neurorecurrence in about 25% of the cases and is thought to indicate a predisposition to the development of symptomatic late neurosyphilis.[39] It is usually unilateral and occurs within 4 months of antiluetic therapy.

Iritis may also develop as a complication following antisyphilitic therapy in the unusual systemic reaction called the Jarisch-Herxheimer reaction. This generalized reaction occurs within 24 hours after treatment of a syphilitic patient with even small amounts of penicillin and is thought to be a reaction to the systemic release of toxins following the rapid destruction of large numbers of treponemes throughout the body. It is characterized by low fever, chills, and generalized malaise lasting 24 to 36 hours, and occasionally by sudden inflammatory activation of previously quiescent syphilitic lesions. Sudden loss of vision following initial treatment of syphilitic optic neuritis has been reported, and even more calamitous reactions following initial treatment of cardiovascular or central nervous system syphilis are on record. However, the iritis of the Jarisch-Herxheimer reaction, though occasionally intense, is typically self-limited, responds well to the usual therapeutic measures, and rarely results in permanent ocular damage.

In addition to iridorelapse and the iritis of the Jarish-Herxheimer reaction, there are two general types of iritis in early acquired syphilis. The first is roseola of the iris, often a symptom heralding secondary syphilis and occurring within the first few months after infection. It is acute in onset, bilateral in about one half of the cases, is manifested by engorgement of the superficial iris vessels, and is accompanied by photophobia and circumcorneal injection. It is usually mild, responds well to specific antiluetic therapy and does not recur.

The second type is the plastic iritis of secondary syphilis. It is often bilateral, but in contrast to roseola occurs later in the secondary stage, and is often quite severe, producing marked decrease in visual acuity, intense pain, and photophobia. Slit-lamp examination reveals a violent anterior chamber reaction with a copious cellular, fibrinous, and occasionally hemorrhagic exudate. Ocular hypotony with inflammation in the anterior vitreous is commonly associated with severe iritis, indicating a significant cyclitis. The process may remain simple and plastic, or may, in a more typically syphilitic reaction, include the development of nodules on the surface of the iris. The iris lesions in this papular iritis vary in size from 0.5 to 3 or 4 mm and range in appearance from multiple, slightly elevated, pink nests of newly formed capillaries to isolated, large, fleshy, elevated yellowish papules. If untreated, the eye may develop extensive posterior synechiae with iris bombé and secondary glaucoma as frequent complications. If the patient receives prompt specific antiluetic therapy, along with topical mydriatics and steroids, the prognosis is usually good, with permanent severe sequelae uncommon. Asymptomatic isolated grayish patches of atrophic iris at the site of previous iris nodules are occasionally found as the sole sign of previous papular iritis.

Other than the extremely rare occurrence of a ciliary syphiloma in late secondary syphilis, the ciliary body is rarely involved alone but is frequently associated with any intense and extensive iritis described above.

CHOROID AND RETINA. Although the choroid or retina may occasionally be independently affected as a complication of secondary syphilis, they are typically involved together in various forms of chorioretinitis, which depending upon the investigator, are reported to account for 8% to 16% of all cases of chorioretinitis arising in adults.[3] There are no typical morphologic characteristics of syphilitic chorioretinitis, but when it occurs as a complication of acquired syphilis it is usually restricted to the posterior pole and the midperiphery, whereas the more frequent chorioretinitis of congenital syphilis involves the midperiphery and far periphery. It characteristically has its onset in the late secondary stage, though it may appear as late as 10 years after the initial infection.

The diffuse chorioretinitis of Förster is by far the most common form of acquired syphilitic chorioretinitis. Bilateral in about 50% of the cases, this diffuse syphilitic chorioretinitis is usually restricted to the posterior segment, involving the macula and peripapillary areas most frequently and the far periphery only rarely. The initial symptoms include diminished visual acuity, flashes of light, and metamorphopsia. There is often an associated ring scotoma, which is so typical of acute syphilitic chorioretinitis that, when present, it should suggest a syphilitic cause of the disorder.[12] Although there is no diagnostic ophthalmoscopic appearance, there is typically a dense vitreous haze through which slight blurring of the disc margins may be seen. In the posterior pole a grayish edematous retina overlies multiple areas of yellowish, deep inflammatory infiltrates of varying sizes. Abundant superficial perivascular exudates and scattered flame-shaped hemorrhages in the posterior pole are also common findings. The course of the untreated disease is prolonged, remittent, unpredictable, and is characterized by progression, with enlargement and coalescence of the inflammatory patches and the almost invariable exuberant reaction of the retinal pigment epithelium with peripheral pigment aggregates. Occasionally, a secondary anterior uveitis may complicate the picture, resulting in a chronic degenerative panuveitis that is refractory to all therapy. One may see perivascular and midzone diffuse pigmentary deposits, patchy areas of chorioretinal atrophy, with variable subretinal gliosis and occasionally varying degrees of optic atrophy in the end stage of the disease. The ring scotoma is rarely present in the late stages, having either progressed to marked field contracture by breaking through to the periphery if the disease was severe and generalized or regressed to irregular scotomas corresponding to the areas of scarring and atrophy. The severe atrophic form with marked field contracture is easily confused with primary retinal pigmentary degeneration, although the optic atrophy and vascular atresia in the syphilitic disease is not as pronounced as in the hereditary disorder. The history of a chancre and a highly reactive serologic test, with the presence of other signs and symptoms of secondary syphilis, make the diagnosis relatively straightforward. Visual loss is highly variable, rarely complete, and often significant.

Several other forms of chorioretinitis have been described as occurring within 2 years of infection with the spirochete. All of these forms probably represent clinical variations of Förster's chorioretinitis and are not important as distinct clinical entities. However, they do have value in indicating the range of host response to infection by *T. pallidum*. Many of these various types of chorioretinitis may be grouped together conveniently under the term focal disseminated chorioretinitis. They differ from Förster's chorioretinitis in that only a few circumscribed areas become inflamed in these forms. All of these forms are rare. Included in this category are chorioretinitis juxtapapillaris, central chorioretinitis, and anterior chorioretinitis; the names indicate the location of the majority of the lesions. Anterior chorioretinitis, certainly atypical in acquired syphilis, is interesting in that it is occasionally associated with iridocyclitis and interstitial keratitis.

A rare but distinct syphilitic entity is the neuritis papulosa of Fuchs. It occurs within 2 years of infection and is unilateral. It is an intense exudative papillitis, with peripapillary chorioretinitis occurring with a marked vasculitis and dense vitreous reaction. The exudate arises from the disc and blooms up into the vitreous, obscuring the disc in the acute phase. Early visual loss is the rule; but if the patient receives prompt penicillin therapy, the inflammation recedes, with fair return of vision, leaving an atrophic band of scar tissue extending from the disc to the area where chorioretinitis had occurred.

The retina is occasionally involved in a discrete inflammatory process in which the choroid remains essentially free of disease. The inflammation begins as a retinal vasculitis at the posterior pole, with associated papillitis and retinitis. It may remain confined to the area around the disc (retinitis circumpapillaris),[26] or the retinitis may extend diffusely to the equator and beyond. Marked retinal edema, macular star formation, perivascular exudates with sheathing, and superficial, intraretinal, and vitreous hemorrhages are prominent features. A secondary iridocyclitis may complicate the process. Visual loss is quite variable. If the patient receives adequate specific antisyphilitic therapy, recurrences are rare. The response of the retinal pigment epithelium varies from the formation of occasional spicule-shaped pigment clumps following the milder forms of inflammation associated with little retinal or optic atrophy to widespread disorganization of the pigment epithelium, with extensive diffuse pigment mobilization and clumping found with significant retinal and optic atrophy in the severe inflammations.

Several other forms of syphilitic retinal involvement have been described. Syphilitic retinal perivasculitis is simply a mild form of inflammation in which the process does not spread from the vessels to cause a significant retinitis or retinochoroiditis. The arteries are more often involved than the veins, and the process includes vascular sheathing, perivascular exudates, occasionally intraretinal hemorrhages, and rarely vitreal hemorrhage with the development of retinitis proliferans. A rare complication of syphilitic retinal vascular inflammation is thrombosis of the central retinal artery or vein, though branch occlusions of either the artery or vein are not rare.

A final form is recurrent central syphilitic retinitis, also called toxic exudative syphilitic retinitis. It is characterized by recurrent, often bilateral, macular edema, indistinguishable clinically from central serous retinopathy. Indeed, Woods[61] doubts that the cases reported in the literature are syphilitic in origin at all and believes that they represent idiopathic central serous retinopathy. Specific antiluetic therapy, always indicated to prevent later syphilitic systemic complications, may be curative in the above forms of chorioretinal complications, although these complications may be refractory to even the most intensive specific and nonspecific measures. Förster's chorioretinitis and simple retinitis usually respond in the most satisfactory manner.

OPTIC NERVE. Mention should be made here of neurorecurrence and early neurosyphilis, as they occur within the first 2 years after infection. As a result of the generalized spirochetemia following infection, treponemes are distributed widely throughout the body; and the central nervous system is no exception. Stokes[54] states that involvement of the CNS occurs in an "overwhelming proportion of early cases of syphilis." The involvement is usually transitory and asymptomatic and is associated with similarly transient abnormalities in the CSF. Woods indicates that abnormal results of spinal fluid examinations occur in 28% to 56% of all cases of early syphilis.[59] Indeed, treponemes may be found in the spinal fluid sometime during the course of early syphilis in over 40% of all cases.[54] In about 25% of all cases of early syphilis (meaning primary, secondary, and early latent stages), the involvement of the CNS is sufficient to cause some clinical signs and symptoms, usually those of transient mild meningeal irritation. In a much smaller percentage gross signs of CNS disease develop and almost invariably indicate "serious damage, not infrequently irreparable."[54]

The only other form of early neurosyphilis is called neurorecurrence. Although uncommon, it is important because it occurs following inadequate therapy for primary or secondary syphilis. In fact, those receiving inadequate therapy for early syphilis have a much greater chance of developing neurosyphilis than those not treated at all.[39] Neurorecurrence is typically meningovascular in type, often presenting as a sudden cranial nerve palsy or hemiplegia within the first 2 years of the disease. The prognosis is usually good with prompt therapy because the signs and symptoms are caused by acute, potentially reversible, lesions rather than by old scarred changes of late neurosyphilis. Neurorecurrence definitely predisposes the patient to the later development of symptomatic late neurosyphilis. Thus, it is imperative that a normal result of a CSF examination be obtained before a patient is discharged as having been adequately treated for early syphilis.

Changes occurring in the optic nerve in early acquired syphilis include papilledema, optic neuritis (called neuroretinitis when the retina is extensively involved, as described above), and retrobulbar neuritis.

Papilledema is only occasionally seen in early acquired syphilis and is usually a complication of acute extensive syphilitic meningitis. Occurring as a result of increased intracranial pressure, it is typically associated with other obvious signs of acute meningitis, such as severe frontal headache, meningismus, and sudden cranial nerve palsies, which are often manifest as acute diplopia, ptosis, or unilateral central deafness. Choked discs are usually bilateral and often cause little loss of vision unless present for a long time. The prognosis for vision is excellent, if therapy is promptly instituted.

Inflammation of the optic nerve, occurring anywhere from the optic disc to the chiasm, is common in late secondary syphilis and is one of the most frequent manifestations of early neurosyphilis and of neurorecurrence. Minimal degrees of optic neuritis may be the only manifestation of early involvement of the central nervous system by the treponeme. Stokes[54] states that 13% of all those with secondary syphilis develop some degree of optic neuritis, though it may be transient and slight, and he also reports that involvement of the optic nerve in early syphilis accounts for 11.1% of all syphilitic eye complications. Moore emphasizes the importance of ruling out optic neuritis in early syphilis because of its prognostic significance. When present, optic neuritis indicates greatly increased chances of developing late symptomatic neurosyphilis.[39] It is interesting that minimal changes in the optic nerve are the most common signs of CNS involvement in early syphilis. Therefore, careful ophthalmologic examination is mandatory in every case.

Optic neuritis, or inflammation of the intraocular portion of the optic nerve, may range in severity from a common evanescent hyperemia of the disc to a rare severe neuroretinitis. It usually occurs in the late secondary stage, often is bilateral, and may occur as an isolated ocular lesion in conjunction with syphilitic meningitis or as a manifestation—occasionally the sole manifestation—of neurorecurrence. Clinical symptoms may be minimal, but diminished visual acuity of varying degree is commonly reported. The ophthalmoscopic appearance is typical for optic neuritis with blurred disc margins, hyperemia, and edematous elevation of the disc, which is occasionally obscured by an overlying vitreous reaction. In the severe cases there is edema of the surrounding retina, perivascular sheathing at the nerve head, and superficial hemorrhages in the retina and disc. The mild forms display no visual field changes. In moderately severe cases there is usually enlargement of the blind spot, and with severe inflammation there is often a dense central or paracentral scotoma with peripheral contraction of the fields.

Syphilis causes 4% to 7% of all cases of retrobulbar neuritis.[6,58] Retrobulbar neuritis is rare in congenital syphilis and only slightly more common in late acquired neurosyphilis, occurring usually in the secondary stage of the disease. Symptoms include pain on movement of the eye and visual loss proportional to the severity of the disease. There are usually no ophthalmoscopic signs of the neuritis, though other syphilitic ocular lesions may be found. Central, paracentral, and sector scotomas, with peripheral loss of vision, also may occur. All forms of optic nerve inflammation in early acquired syphilis respond rapidly to early antiluetic therapy.

LATENT SYPHILIS

The period from the disappearance of the secondary signs and symptoms to 4 years after original infection is arbitrarily called early latent syphilis. During this time the patient remains potentially infectious. This stage is characterized by the recurrence of secondary lesions in approximately 25% of the cases. As time passes, recurrences become less symmetrical, more sporadic and isolated, and begin to assume the arciform configuration typical of the skin lesions of late gummatous syphilis, though they usually remain darkfield positive. Between secondary relapses, which become uncommon after the first year, the patient is completely asymptomatic. The only indication that he is infected with *T. pallidum* is a reactive serologic test, with both reagin and treponemal tests being uniformly strongly reactive.

Four years after infection the patient is said to enter the late latent stage, having a reactive serologic test as the only evidence of infection. The period of late latency may last a lifetime or be followed 1 to 20 years later by the appearance of late symptomatic syphilis. Of those persons remaining untreated, approximately one third will slowly revert to a negative serologic reaction over the years, with no other signs or symptoms of syphilis. One third will retain a positive serologic reaction but remain asymptomatic. The final third will go on to develop one or a combination of the forms of late symptomatic syphilis, including gummatous (15%), cardiovascular (10%), and symptomatic central nervous system syphilis (8%).

ACQUIRED LATE SYMPTOMATIC SYPHILIS

Gummatous syphilis is also known as late benign cutaneous syphilis because one who develops late lesions in the skin often does not develop the other two potentially more serious forms of late syphilis. The gumma may involve practically any tissue in the body. Skin, bone, and the liver are affected most frequently. Gummas of the central nervous system, heart, and lungs occur uncommonly but are potentially more dangerous. The gumma, thought to be a manifestation of hypersensitivity to the spirochete, is essentially a granuloma composed of round cells and giant cells with central necrosis. It may occur as a caseating tumor or as a destructive infiltrative lesion. Treponemes are present, though scarce, and the serologic tests are strongly reactive.

Gummatous lesions of the eye

ORBIT. Gummatous disease of the orbit is rare, accounting for less than 1% of all ocular syphilis.[58] It may occur as early as the late secondary stage but usually has its onset several years following infection. Gummatous periostitis or osteitis in the bones of the orbit is the most frequent form, producing local pain, especially at night, and tenderness of the orbital rim to palpation. Exophthalmos with diffuse gummatous infiltration of the retrobulbar tissues and extraocular muscle palsies is not uncommon. If the infiltrative process is pronounced, any of the intraorbital structure may be invaded, including the muscles, nerves, and the globe itself. When the process is located in the apex of the orbit, painful ophthalmoplegia, ptosis, and paresis of the trochlear and abducens nerves along with corneal hypesthesia may occur, forming the clinical entity known as the superior orbital fissure, or Tolosa-Hunt syndrome.[28]

Other causes of this syndrome include other inflammatory disease processes, tumor, hemorrhage, and fracture. The diagnosis of syphilis in any form of orbital gumma is made by the presence of a reactive serologic test and prompt regression of signs and symptoms with luetic therapy. Conjunctival gummas are also rare, occurring predominantly on the perilimbal bulbar conjunctiva. The initial lesion is a small, nontender, pink limbal nodule associated with painless preauricular and submandibular lymphadenopathy. It responds well to penicillin; untreated it may continue to enlarge, breaking down to form a chronic, painless ulcer penetrating the globe. Gummas of the lids have been reported and may involve the skin alone or begin as an infiltrative tarsitis. The skin lesions are typical of skin gummas elsewhere, being asymmetrical, arciform, destructive lesions, which spread peripherally, leaving either indolent painless ulcers or atrophic "cigarette paper" scarring. Gummatous tarsitis is quite rare, presenting initially as a painless thickening of the lid, and without treatment it progresses to ulceration and extensive destruction of the lid structures.

CORNEA AND SCLERA. The scleritis of late

acquired syphilis may take many forms, all of which are felt to be essentially gummatous in nature. Isolated gummas of the sclera do occur, though they are usually extensions through the sclera of a ciliary gumma.[11] Also, diffuse or localized scleritis or episcleritis may occur on the basis of gummatous infiltration. The response to penicillin is rapid.

The several corneal complications of late acquired syphilis may all be described as gummatous lesions, though the pathogenesis is obscure in some complications. All have in common a frequent association with anterior uveitis, and all are felt to be late allergic reactions to the treponeme. The first is the isolated corneal gumma, which is quite rare and is similar to isolated gummas of the conjunctiva and sclera, described above, appearing as a slowly enlarging nodular opacity anywhere on the cornea. Prompt diagnosis and antibiotic therapy are needed because of the tendency of the gumma to perforate the cornea.

Interstitial keratitis of late acquired syphilis is similar to the rare interstitial inflammation occurring in secondary infection mentioned above, although it is somewhat more frequent. The time from infection to onset is usually 8 years or longer. Unilateral and segmental involvement limited to the periphery is the rule, though occasionally, when associated with an intense iritis, the lesion may be fulminant, with severe residual scarring. An unusual complication of this latter form is the development of a posterior corneal abscess, which ruptures through Descemet's membrane into the anterior chamber. This is keratitis pustuliformis profunda, which is associated with a severe gummatous iridocyclitis, and has single or multiple peripheral infiltrates in the posterior layers of the stroma.[56] The uveitis is severe and is accompanied by marked pain, photophobia, and diminution of vision. The response to antisyphilitic therapy is prompt, the amount of disability depending on how long the process was allowed to continue before treatment.

A final form of syphilitic keratitis is the keratitis punctata profunda of Mauthner. Occurring in association with syphilitic iritis, it is characterized by multiple small, round, deep stromal opacities. There is little associated corneal inflammatory reaction, and with control of the iritis the opacities usually regress rapidly, leaving little or no scarring.[56]

IRIS AND CILIARY BODY. Gummas of the ciliary body, though uncommon, have been reported in the literature regularly since the first description by von Arlt in 1853.[12] They may occur as an isolated phenomenon or, as in the usual case, in association with a severe iridocyclitis or anterior uveitis. They are usually first seen as they protrude into the anterior chamber at the angle, appearing as a pale gray or pinkish globular tumor. Untreated they go on to necrosis, greatly exacerbating the uveitis, with penetration of the globe and endophthalmitis as late sequelae. Primary iris gummas are a great rarity. The clinical appearance and course is similar to those of ciliary gummas.

The most common ocular inflammatory lesion of late acquired syphilis is chronic gummatous iritis, or more properly, uveitis, with an incidence of 3.1%.[40] It occurs as an isolated lesion only 25% of the time, complicated most often by an accompanying keratitis as mentioned above and slightly less frequently with an extensive posterior uveitis or chorioretinitis. The average time between infection and onset is 9 years. As in early luetic iritis, uveitis is more common in males than in females and is twice as prevalent among Negroes as it is among Caucasians. It is associated with extraocular manifestations of late syphilis in about one half the cases. Its onset is typically abrupt, with pain and redness of the eye and sudden decrease in vision. The slit lamp reveals a violent anterior chamber reaction, a copious fibrinous exudate, extensive mutton-fat precipitates on the corneal endothelium and anterior lens capsule, and occasionally hypopyon or hyphema. There is an early tendency to extensive posterior synechiae formation, though the cyclitis is often so severe as to cause a prolonged secondary ocular hypotension. Unlike the iritis of early syphilis, the tendency in late syphilis is for remission and relapse with progressive damage to the eye. Cataract, secondary glucoma, retinal detachment, and occasionally phthisis bulbi are the serious sequelae that occur in approximately 25% of all cases. Significant permanent visual loss occurs in over 50% of the patients.[40] The diagnosis may be difficult because of the nonspecific nature of the inflammation. The VDRL test is reactive in approximately 40% to 50% of the cases, though the FTA-ABS test should be positive in over 90%. The therapeutic response to antibiotic treatment is variable as in many other forms of ocular syphilis. Therapy may hasten the resolution of an acute episode and decrease the chances for recurrence, but late luetic uveitis is often refractory to penicillin and all other therapy, including atropine and steroids. Primary isolated gummas of the retina, choroid, and optic nerve have been reported but are so rare as to warrant only passing mention.

LENS. Although primary involvement of the lens in a luetic process is not known, secondary cataracts are common. In addition, lenticular dislocation, whether or not associated with trauma, is associated with a reactive FTA-ABS test in over 50% of the cases.[49] The pathologic mechanism is not known.[23]

Neurosyphilitic lesions of the eye

In all forms of neurosyphilis, ocular examination is a most valuable clinical tool for evaluating neurologic involvement. The following list* indicates the great frequency of eye signs in neurosyphilis.

Some syphilitic ocular complications	63%
Argyll Robertson pupils	35%
Irregular pupils	21%
Anisocoria	19%
Fundus changes	15%
Muscular paralysis	12%

*Modified from Stokes, J. H., Beerman, H., and Ingraham, N. R.: Modern clinical syphilology, Philadelphia, 1945, W. B. Saunders Co., p. 980.

The ocular lesions of neurosyphilis are usually limited to pupillary changes, extraocular muscle palsies, and retinal, optic nerve, and optic radiation involvement. Other ocular structures may be involved concomitantly in distinct luetic processes unrelated to the neurosyphilitic disease.

The pathologic process common to all types of neurosyphilis and indeed basic to the production of almost all syphilitic lesions is perivascular inflammation, with round cell cuffing of small vessels and a concomitant obliterative endarteritis. If this process is so slight as to cause changes in the CSF only, with no clinical manifestations of the disease, asymptomatic neurosyphilis is said to be present. If the involvement is chiefly limited to the meninges and the vessels of the central nervous system, the disease is called meningovascular syphilis; and if the pathologic changes involve primary destruction of the neural tissue of the brain or spinal cord, the process is labelled parenchymatous neurosyphilis. Often the types are not easy to distinguish, but as a general classification they have both clinical and pathologic validity.

Asymptomatic neurosyphilis, comprising about one third of all cases of neurosyphilis, differs from latent syphilis only in that the CSF is abnormal. There are no signs or symptoms by definition. The disease is important because it predisposes the patient to later serious CNS involvement. When the CSF is abnormal, it should be repeatedly studied after adequate therapy until it reverts to normal.

MENINGOVASCULAR NEUROSYPHILIS. The signs and symptoms of meningovascular neurosyphilis are referable to meningeal inflammation and vascular occlusion. As indicated above, they may have their onset as early as the late primary stage but usually occur several years after infection. Three major types recognized are cerebral meningeal, cerebral vascular, and meningovascular syphilis of the spinal cord.

Cerebral meningeal neurosyphilis, which may appear within the first 2 years of infection, is not common. The meningeal involvement may be diffuse or restricted to the convexity or basilar areas of the brain. The signs and symptoms relate to meningeal inflammation above the foramen magnum, secondary hydrocephalus, cranial nerve damage, and focal cortical injury. They include stiff neck, papilledema, diplopia, facial palsy, confusion, delirium, and seizures.

Cerebral vascular neurosyphilis comprises about 10% of all cases of neurosyphilis and appears, on the average, 7 years after infection. The common pathologic process is syphilitic arteritis. The signs and symptoms depend upon the particular vessel or vessels involved and are indistinguishable from cerebral thrombosis from other causes.

Spinal meningovascular syphilis is simply a grouping of those patients having signs and symptoms referable to vascular occlusion and meningeal involvement of the cord. Symptoms include peripheral motor weakness and sensory loss. In all forms of meningovascular syphilis, CSF changes and reactive serologic tests are the rule.

Cranial nerve palsies are so frequent in meningovascular syphilis as to be its most characteristic feature. Table 20-2 shows the relative frequency of individual cranial nerve involvement in the meningeal form of the disease.

Table 20-2. Cranial nerve involvement in meningeal neurosyphilis

Cranial nerve	Percent involvement
I	1.5
II	26
III	23
IV	2.5
V	11
VI	21
VII	40
VIII	41
IX and X	6
XI	0.5
XII	3.5

Adapted from Stokes, J. H., Beerman, H., and Ingraham, N. R.: Modern clinical syphilology, Philadelphia, 1945, W. B. Saunders Co., p. 998.

Of the nerves serving the extraocular muscles, the third nerve is most frequently involved, followed closely by the sixth, with the trochlear nerve being much less commonly affected. Acute ptosis is said to be the most frequent symptom.[58] The more important associated symptoms include severe headache, diplopia, and often sudden unilateral or bilateral deafness. Cranial nerve palsies may be isolated or multiple, depending on the location and extent of involvement. An interesting collection of signs and symptoms called Roger's syndrome is occasionally seen in which there is pain and hypesthesia over the distribution of the first two divisions of the fifth cranial nerve, associated with homolateral abducens paresis and Horner's syndrome. The causative lesion is an area of syphilitic meningeal inflammation localized to the tip of the petrous bone.[58]

Pupillary changes are common in meningovascular syphilis, with an incidence of approximately 30%. Argyll Robertson pupils are a rarity in the meningeal form and are only slightly more common in the vascular form. The typical pupillary changes are anisocoria and occasionally bilaterally dilated unresponsive pupils. This is easily understandable in view of the high frequency of third nerve involvement and the fact that the pupillomotor fibers run peripherally in the nerve and are thus subject to early involvement in meningeal disease.

As is seen in Table 20-2, the optic nerve is the most frequently involved cranial nerve, except for the facial and acoustic nerves. Primary optic neuritis probably does not occur in neurovascular syphilis. The changes in the optic nerve, chiasm, optic tract, and optic radiation are secondary to local inflammatory or infiltrative meningeal disease and vascular occlusion of small or large vessels and occur less commonly from increased intracranial pressure. In the rare acute meningeal form of this disease papilledema is quite common. Visual field changes occur frequently in both the meningeal and vascular forms. When the meningeal involvement is predominantly basilar, chiasmal and optic tract damage occurs, frequently leading to variable central scotomas and peripheral field changes and occasionally to loss of vision in one eye and peripheral field defects in the other. Hemianopsia occurs much less frequently and is usually homonymous, with bitemporal defects occurring in less than 20% of the cases.[58] In the vascular form field defects are common and are enormously variable. Merritt[35] reports that the middle cerebral artery or one of its branches is occluded in the great majority of cases. Thus, total homonymous hemianopsia is the predominant defect, although partial or quadrantic defects frequently occur, their congruity increasing with the proximity of the involved area to the occipital pole. Optic atrophy is unusual in meningovascular syphilis but occurs occasionally secondary to prolonged papilledema or to involvement of the intracranial portion of the optic nerve or chiasm, with scarring from extensive meningeal inflammation. The typical appearance of secondary optic atrophy includes blurring of disc margins and obliteration of the normal optic cup with proliferation of gray glial tissue. The response of the meningeal form to penicillin is usually rapid, with prompt remission of symptoms. The progress of the vascular form will be arrested with treatment, though the neurologic deficit produced by the occlusive disease is often permanent.

PARENCHYMATOUS NEUROSYPHILIS. In parenchymatous neurosyphilis the major changes are within the neural substance of the brain and spinal cord. The two major types are tabes dorsalis and general paresis.

Tabes dorsalis. Tabes dorsalis accounts for about one third of all cases of neurosyphilis. The major pathologic changes in tabes consist of degeneration in the optic nerves, posterior columns, and dorsal roots of the spinal cord, with signs and symptoms of optic atrophy, ataxia, lancinating pains, areflexia, bladder dysfunction, and Argyll Robertson pupils. The pathogenesis of tabes remains obscure. The period between infection and onset is much greater than for any other form of late syphilis, with an average of 15 years and a range of 5 to 50 years. Unlike paresis, in which many treponemes are found in the brain substance surrounded by profuse inflammation, in tabes treponemes are not present in the involved nerves and tracts, and extensive degeneration often occurs in the absence of any signs of inflammation. In addition, serum and CSF reagin titers are typically low. The CSF shows some abnormalities in 90% of the cases, with the VDRL test reactive in 75%. The progress of the disorder can usually be halted with the use of large amounts of penicillin.

Ocular complications of tabes are frequent and often severe. Extraocular muscle paresis occurs in 12% to 25% of the cases,[35,54] with the third nerve most often involved and less commonly the sixth and the fourth. Bilateral permanent ptosis is a frequent presenting sign, and when associated with pupillary signs, syphilis is the most probable diagnosis. Transient diplopia may be an early symptom and precedes the development of frank tabes by many years. Whether cranial nerve involvement in tabes is secondary to nuclear damage or to basilar meningitis is not known.

Pupillary abnormalities occur in over 90% of tabetic patients, with the incidence of Argyll Robertson pupils reported to be 48% to 80%.[35,54] Pupillary changes other than light-near dissociation include atrophy, fixed miotic pupils, anisocoria, irregular pupils, and dilated pupils unresponsive to light or accommodation. Pupillary atrophy in tabes may be secondary to previous luetic uveitis or may be neurogenic in origin. Neurogenic tabetic pupillary atrophy may occur concomitantly with pupillomotor paresis or light-near dissociation or may occur as an independent phenomenon. The iris atrophy may be generalized or segmental. There is usually depigmentation and stromal atrophy with marked thinning and loss of normal surface details, all resulting in a grayish, smooth iris often with a small irregular pupil.

The Argyll Robertson pupil has long been regarded as a pathognomonic sign of late CNS syphilis, and indeed in over 90% syphilis is the cause of this abnormality.

Four criteria must be found for the complete Argyll Robertson pupil syndrome to be present.

1. No reaction to light, either by direct or consensual stimulation
2. Intact near synkinesis
3. Miosis
4. Enough light perception to assure that loss of the light reflex is not on the basis of amaurosis

Poor response to mydriatics has often been added as a fifth criterion because Argyll Robertson[45] in his original description of four patients noted that there was poor dilatation from atropine in all cases. Loewenfeld in her recent elegant and extensive review of the subject has shown that poor response to mydriatics is a feature that, though often present, is not related to the neurologic defect but is secondary to the frequently associated iris atrophy.[32] Several other observations that have importance in the Argyll Robertson syndrome as a diagnostic sign of neurosyphilis were made by Loewenfeld. Perhaps the most important suggestion, supported by other authors,[49] is that if the criterion of absolutely no response to light is strictly adhered to, many cases of neurosyphilis will be missed. The major feature of the phenomenon is light-near dissociation, and even in the presence of a "fairly ample" response to light a partial Argyll-Robertson syndrome exists if a "clear-cut dissociation" can be demonstrated.[32] The partial syndrome is just as important a sign of neurosyphilis as is the fully developed form in which there is absolutely no movement of the pupil to light. It must be kept in mind, however, that an intense light source must be used before light-near dissociation can be said to exist. The phenomenon is bilateral in the majority of cases but may exist as a strictly unilateral phenomenon. Loewenfeld also mentions the fact that though small pupils are the rule, the intense meiosis is not a strict criterion. In bright light the Argyll Robertson pupil may actually be larger than a normal one; however, in dim illumination the normal pupil promptly dilates, while the Argyll Robertson pupil remains stationary.[32]

Loewenfeld suggests that the site of the lesion responsible for the Argyll Robertson syndrome is a small area immediately rostral to the Edinger-Westphal nucleus where the intercalated light reflex fibers from the pretectum and supranuclear inhibitory pathways from the cortex are in close proximity.[32] Interruption of the intercalated light reflex fibers would abolish the homolateral light reflex, and interruption of the inhibitory pathways from above would account for the meiosis. A lesion confined to this site would spare the near reflex fibers and the oculomotor outflow, which are situated ventrally.

Several other conditions have been reported to cause the Argyll Robertson syndrome; these include diabetes, multiple sclerosis, chronic alcoholism, encephalitis, mesencephalic tumor, and trauma. However, as neurosyphilis causes over 90% of the cases, great effort must be made to exclude that diagnosis before another process is accepted as the cause. An entity that may easily be confused with the Argyll Robertson syndrome is the tonic pupil of Adie. It reacts so slowly to light that a mistaken diagnosis of Argyll Robertson syndrome may be made on brief examination. Adie's pupil is unilateral in 80% of the cases, is usually dilated rather than meiotic, contracts slowly to light, and constricts promptly with a dilute (2.5%) solution of methacholine (Mecholyl).[46]

Optic atrophy may be the only manifestation of CNS syphilis; it is the most common ocular sign of tabes after pupillary changes. It occurs in 15% to 20% of all tabetic patients[22] and is the most serious ocular complication of neurosyphilis, resulting in total blindness in the great majority of untreated cases.[58] It is more common in men than in women and in Caucasians than in Negroes. Woods[61] proposed a luetic cause in 23.3% of all optic neuropathies and in 51% of all cases of primary optic atrophy. Although this may be a bit higher than is acceptable today, syphilis remains the most common cause of optic atrophy, and serologic studies are indicated in every case.[5] Tabetic optic atrophy is primary in type and is called "interstitial neuritis" by Merritt.[35] The time from primary infection to development of optic atrophy is quite long, averaging 24 years.[41] It does not result from syphilitic arachnoiditis or basilar meningeal inflammation but is a primary process occurring in the intracranial portion of the nerve anterior to the chiasm. Loss of myelin sheaths occurs early, followed by degeneration of nerve fibers. Glial scarring occurs late in the disease.

There are three general patterns of degeneration of the optic nerves resulting in distinctive visual field changes. The first is progressive concentric atrophy, which arising at the periphery of the nerve results in slow, progressive contraction of peripheral fields and terminates in extremely small central fields often with surprisingly good acuity. The second form is degeneration of wedge-shaped sectors of the nerve, giving rise to localized peripheral scotomas, often with normal central vision unless the papillomacular bundle is involved. The third form is diffuse degeneration of the entire thickness of the nerve, causing central, paracentral, and centrocentral scotomas, associated with peripheral contracture. Altitudinal, binasal, bitemporal and homonymous defects may rarely be produced. The clinical appearance includes a slowly developing bluish pallor of the discs, with no associated fundus lesions or other evidence of inflammatory disease. The margins are quite sharp, and the cup may have a slight atrophic accentuation. Attenuation of the vessels occurs in the late stages, perhaps from glial proliferation and constriction of the vessels centrally. Prognosis must be guarded in every case, for despite antisyphilitic therapy, significant visual loss is common. Treatment must be prompt and vigorous. In a series of 249 untreated cases reported by Moore and Woods[41] all patients lost their vision within 9 years after onset of symptoms.

Paresis. General paralysis of the insane, or paresis, is chronic syphilitic meningoencephalitis, resulting in diffuse extensive parenchymal damage to the brain. The clinical manifestations are enormously variable. Common signs include facial and tongue tremors, dysarthria, hyperactive deep tendon reflexes, and pupillary changes. Early symptoms are usually quite nonspecific, often including minor personality changes with progress within months to psychosis and dementia. It is a fatal disease if untreated, the late stages made manifest by dementia and paralysis. The spinal fluid is almost invariably indicative of infection, and the VDRL test is reactive in the blood and spinal fluid in approximately 90% of all cases.

Extraocular muscle palsies and optic atrophy are rare in the pure form of paresis, though in the mixed disorder, known as taboparesis, both occur not infrequently. Pupillary changes are the most common ocular manifestation of paresis. The list below indicates the frequency of various pupillary changes.*

Altered light reflex	78%
Anisocoria	68%
Lost light reflex	52%
Irregular pupils	39%
Diminished accommodation reflex	17%
Mydriasis	13%

As can be seen in the list, complete loss of light reflexes is present in 52%, but some diminution of light reflex can be detected in 78%, thus emphasizing the importance of the partial Argyll Robertson syndrome, or light-near dissociation, in making the diagnosis of CNS syphilis.

CONGENITAL SYPHILIS

Heredosyphilis is in the main quite similar to acquired syphilis, although there are

*Adapted from Stokes, J. H., Beerman, H., and Ingraham, N. R.: Modern clinical syphilology, Philadelphia, 1945, W. B. Saunders Co., p. 1002.

enough differences to warrant a separate description. The fetus is infected transplacentally, and as in early acquired syphilis a generalized spirochetemia rapidly ensues, with all tissues of the body invaded by treponemes. Symptoms may be present at birth, or it may be several years before the infection becomes manifest.

There are two clinical forms of congenital syphilis: infantile and tardive.

Early congenital syphilis

Infantile, or early congenital, syphilis makes its appearance within the first 2 years of life. The skin lesions are usually infectious and correspond to secondary lesions in the acquired form. The signs and symptoms of early congenital syphilis include skin and mucous membrane lesions, widespread osteoperiostitis, anemia, and hepatosplenomegaly. The earlier the infantile disease becomes manifest, the poorer are the infant's chances for survival. If symptomatic at birth, the infant is usually desperately ill and often does not survive despite intensive therapy. As both reagin and treponemal antibodies cross the placenta, the newborn will have a reactive serologic test if the mother does. A diphasic VDRL titer over the first 3 months of life is diagnostic of infection in the newborn as the infant clears the passively acquired maternal antibodies and begins to produce his own. After the first few months of life the serologic tests are typically strongly reactive in early congenital syphilis. As in early acquired syphilis the CSF must be evaluated, for a significant percentage will develop asymptomatic neurosyphilis.

Ocular lesions of early congenital syphilis are uncommon and are even less commonly observed or reported because those that do occur are predominantly intraocular and therefore rarely visualized and recognized in the infant. The lids and conjunctiva may occasionally be involved in the generalized cutaneous eruptions. These lesions are infectious and are similar to the well-known rash of secondary syphilis, except for the occurrence of bullae, which are peculiar to congenital syphilis and are not seen in the acquired disease.

The most common cause of acute iritis in infancy is reported to be early congenital syphilis.[12] Reliable estimates of its incidence are not available, and it is probable that the majority of cases escape diagnosis unless the iritis is quite severe. Typically, the iritis begins late in the first year of life, with a variable outcome; it responds well to antisyphilitic therapy.

Interstitial keratitis and anterior uveitis may also occur within the first 2 years of life and have even been reported to be present at birth,[11] but these are distinct rarities. Extraocular muscle palsies and secondary optic atrophy are each thought to occur in approximately 1% of the cases.[54] The two important ocular lesions of infantile heredosyphilis are optic neuritis and chorioretinitis.

Carroll reported that in a series of 41 cases of optic neuritis in children 2 were caused by congenital syphilis; the incidence of optic neuritis among congenial syphilitic patients has been reported to be approximately 5%.[29] The clinical appearance is in no way different from the optic neuritis of the acquired disease and if untreated may progress to secondary optic atrophy in a small percentage of cases.

Although the chorioretinitis of congenital syphilis is usually not discovered until after the first several years of life, it is thought to begin during infancy.[25] Its incidence among congenital syphilitic patients is approximately 14%, and it accounts for over 80% of all cases of chorioretinitis in children.[58] There is a much higher incidence of chorioretinitis, especially the peripheral form, in congenital syphilitic patients with interstitial keratitis. The course of the acute disease is probably similar to that of the chorioretinitis of acquired syphilis; but since chorioretinitis is only rarely observed in its active stages, this hypothesis is speculative. When discovered, the chorioretinitis is usually old and inactive; and though it may take many different forms, there are some morphologic characteristics that are helpful in establishing the cause. The typical form of heredosyphilitic chorioretinitis is the salt-and-pepper fundus in which the changes are predominantly confined to the peripheral retina. Examination of the fundus reveals granular areas of diffusely distributed fine dots of pigment interspersed among similarly sized pale yellow lesions on a reddish yellow background. The process, which is invariably bilateral, may be segmental or may involve the full circumference of the periphery and is associated with perivascular sheathing and narrowing of both arteries and veins over and around the disc in a high percentage of cases.[25] There may occasionally be an accompanying pallor or frank atrophy of the disc. An important associated finding is the frequently occurring fine punctate haze in the anterior vitreous. Variations on the typical configuration occur frequently. Isolated, sparse pigment clumps of varying size scattered from the midzone to the periphery may be the only manifestation of a previous chorioretinitis. Scattered peripheral yellowish red areas of chorioretinal atrophy with sparse central or peripheral pigment depositions are seen less frequently; and the typical retinitis pigmentosalike fundus with midzone pigmentary degeneration, prominent bone spicule pigment forms, vascular atresia, and beeswax pallor of the disc is now felt to be a rare manifestation.[25] A mixture of the various forms is seen in the majority of cases. The diagnosis of syphilis is suggested by the predominantly peripheral location of the involvement, the occurrence of pepper-and-salt changes alone or in association with other types of lesions, and finally by the presence of perivascular sheathing, especially at the posterior pole.[25] The syphilitic cause is best determined by a history of syphilis in the parents, corneal changes of interstitial keratitis, or other stigmata of heredosyphilis rather than by any specific fundus abnormality. The VDRL test may be nonreactive in 25%, though the FTA-ABS test will be positive over 90% of the time. Vision is often unimpaired, but optic atrophy or macular involvement may cause severe visual loss in a small percentage of cases.

Tardive heredosyphilis

Late, or tardive, congenital syphilis is that which has persisted past the first 2 years of life. In over half the cases it is asymptomatic, detectable only serologically. It roughly corresponds to the late forms of acquired syphilis and is noninfectious. A large percentage of late congenital syphilitic patients have one or more stigmata of the disease without ever developing active late destructive lesions. Typical stigmata are caused by osteoperiostitis, the hallmark of congenital syphilis. These lesions may be hypertrophic and sclerotic with frontal bossing, saber shins, and clavicular swellings, or destructive, as in the saddle nose deformity and palate perforations. Various ectodermal defects are common, including dental dystrophies, hypertrichosis, and perioral scarring. Approximately 26% of untreated late congenital syphilitic patients will develop neurosyphilis,[54] usually paretic in type. In addition, isolated neural deafness is seen in 10%, and interstitial keratitis is seen in 52%.[54] Gummas, especially of bone and nasopharynx, are common serious late sequelae. Late congenital cardiovascular syphilis is a great rarity. Serologic tests in untreated late congenital syphilis are unusual, with great fluctuations in reagin titer when the VDRL test is reactive. In 25% of the cases the VDRL test is nonreactive. The FTA-ABS test is reactive 96% of the time in late congenital syphilis. Again, a CSF evaluation is imperative.

Ocular complications occur in over 75% of patients with late congenital syphilis.[54] Gummatous involvement of the lids, conjunctiva, and orbit occurs in a small percentage of patients with late heredosyphilis and is similar to the acquired disease in all respects, except that obstructive gummatous dacryocystitis is much more common in congenital syphilis, with an incidence of 2%.[54] Chronic late uveitis occurs in 7% to 10% of the cases and corresponds to late acquired luetic uveitis. The ocular signs and complications of the various forms of congenital neurosyphilis are no different from those occurring in the corresponding acquired forms. Paresis accounts for one fifth of all cases of congenital neurosyphilis. Almost all congenital paretic patients have abnormal pupils, and light-near dissociation is frequent. Optic atrophy, the most serious ocular complication of syphilis, occurs in 6% of all cases of congenital syphilis.[29] Pure tabes dorsalis is an uncommon complication of heredosyphilis, accounting for about 10% of all cases of hereditary neurosyphilis. It is typically mild in its manifestations, except for its ocular complications. Essentially all have abnormal pupils; extraocular muscle palsies and progressive primary optic atrophy each occur in 50% of the cases.[35] Treatment of congenital neurosyphilis is the same as for the acquired disease, though the results are often less satisfactory, especially in juvenile tabes.

Interstitial keratitis is the most common lesion of late congenital syphilis, occurring in approximately one half of all untreated patients. Although it may not appear until the patient is 30 years old, and although it has also been reported to be present at birth, interstitial keratitis typically occurs in the early teens, with the vast majority of cases occurring in patients between the ages of 5 and 20. It is more common in females than in males, with a ratio of 3:2. Approximately 95% of all cases of interstitial keratitis is caused by syphilis, the congenital form accounting for over 90%, whereas only 3% is seen in the acquired disease. Mycobacteria and other bacteria rarely cause a similar keratitis. Syphilis is the cause of such an overwhelming majority of cases that it must be carefully excluded before another cause can be considered. The pathogenesis of the disease is not understood, but it is felt to be a manifestation of allergy to the treponeme. Supporting the theory of allergic reaction are the facts that it is quite rare in the early stages of both congenital and acquired syphilis where there are great numbers of treponemes throughout the tissues and in the general circulation, that it occurs approximately 10 years after infection in both the congenital and acquired disease at a time when treponemes are rarely found in the blood or tissues, and that it is refractory to any antiluetic treatment. However, it responds well to the corticosteroids. It is felt that the cornea is sensitized to treponemes during the initial spirochetemia following infection and becomes the site of an acute anamnestic allergic response years later with the release of treponemes into the general circulation. Why there should be a release of treponemes years later has never been adequately explained. It is a bilateral disease in most untreated cases; initially one eye may be involved with an interval of weeks to months before the second eye becomes affected.

The disease begins typically with an initial infiltrative stage, characterized by decreased acuity, redness, pain, lacrimation, photophobia, and blepharospasm. Slit-lamp examination reveals a rapidly progressing stromal haze, which may begin peripherally, centrally, or in scattered patchy areas. Within a few days the stroma is involved in all of its layers, with a diffuse infiltrate resulting in a generalized ground-glass haze and visual acuity often reduced to hand movements or light perception. In practically every case a severe iritis or anterior chorioretinitis develops concomitantly with the initial stages. It is severe, with turbid aqueous, extensive plastic keratic precipitates on the endothelium, and often with ocular hypotony indicative of ciliary body involvement. Widespread necrosis of the corneal lamellae may occur, with stromal edema and folds in Descemet's membrane occurring as prominent secondary changes. New blood vessels make their appearance in all levels of the stroma at the periphery, heralding the stage of vascularization. The new vessels grow slowly inward from the periphery over a period of months; during this time the eye remains acutely inflamed, red, painful, and functionally blind. This invasion of the cornea, with inward progression of straight, radially oriented vessels at all stromal levels, forming rich anastomoses in the areas of denser stromal haze and necrosis, is characteristic of the disease. The central ends of the vessels branch out to form fine brushlike vascular structures. When the vessels finally meet axially, there is a dramatic regression of the disease; and the patient enters the final stage of the process, in which the corneal infiltrates are resorbed and the vessels are obliterated. This final process may take many months, the entire course lasting 1½ to 2 years. There is often a remarkable repair and clearing of the cornea. The vessels never disappear completely but become atretic and persist as fine lines or ghost vessels. Patches of deep stromal opacities may remain and if central can significantly reduce vision. The folds in Descemet's membrane may persist to form typical hyaline ridges, which are most often vertical or radial in orientation. Permanent linear or concentric splits in the membrane occur, as do localized areas of thickening where extensive keratic precipitates have become organized into plaques, often with small flecks of inspissated pigment. Rarely are the changes so severe as to lead to eventual degeneration of the cornea, with loss of substance, band keratopathy, persistent discomfort, and eventual perforation as the final outcome. Intractable glaucoma occasionally may also occur, secondary to severe iritis.[31] In general, however, the outlook is surprisingly good for vision, with 70% of these patients having 20/20 to 20/100 acuity and only 10% having poorer than 20/200 acuity.[11]

Without treatment the disease recurs in 27% of such cases, and eventual bilateral involvement is the rule.[54] Although specific antisyphilitic therapy does not greatly affect the course of the acute inflammation, it does reduce the chances for recurrence in the same eye to 3.6%; and when instituted during the involvement of the first eye, therapy significantly decreases the occurrence of bilateral disease.[54] Topical steroids have a definite place in the management of the acute process. They only suppress the inflammatory response, which will reappear upon cessation of therapy. If steroids are used continuously for 1½ to 2 years, the disease may run its course suppressed; and the severe sequelae will be avoided.[11] The most effective treatment, of course, is prevention by treating the infected mother during her pregnancy. If this is accomplished, the later development of active interstitial keratitis in the child is a rare phenomenon.

• • •

Before some of the recent research in ocular syphilis is discussed, a summary of the more important ocular lesions of syphilis and an outline of antibiotic therapy is presented.

The following list indicates the reactivity of the FTA-ABS test in patients with various types of ocular disease seen in a large municiple eye clinic.[47]

Any pupillary abnormality	46%
Pupillary light-near dissociation	67%
Interstitial keratitis	100%
Chronic uveitis	30%
Primary optic atrophy	67%
Dislocated lens	53%

The importance of any reactivity of the FTA-ABS test, including a borderline positive reaction, has recently been emphasized by Seeley and his associates[46a] as a significant indicator of luetic involvement. Although the FTA-ABS test is the most sensitive and specific serologic test that is available for syphilis, great efforts should be made to rule out syphilis in a patient having any one of the above findings, even in the face of a negative FTA-ABS test. Despite reports to the contrary, Smith[49] estimates that the FTA-ABS test is nonreactive in 40% to 50% of all cases of tardive heredosyphilis. In addition, the possibility of syphilis should be carefully evaluated in a patient with any of the following ocular findings that are not obviously caused by another process.

1. Pigmentary chorioretinal changes, especially of the salt-and-pepper type or if predominantly anterior in location
2. Acute iritis
3. Marked visual field changes, particularly extensive contracture of field
4. Ptosis or other extraocular muscle palsy
5. Significant active perivasculitis or old perivascular sheathing

Penicillin is the drug of choice in the treatment of all stages of syphilis. Tetracycline and erythromycin have also been extensively evaluated in early syphilis and have been found to be effective substitutes when penicillin cannot be used. The following dosage schedules are recommended by the Venereal Disease Program of the National Center for Disease Control.[55]

Primary, secondary, and latent syphilis

Benzathine penicillin G—2.4 million units IM at one session

Procaine penicillin G with 2% Aluminum Monostereate in Oil (PAM)—4.8 million units IM total dose; give 2.4 million units initially, followed by 1.2 mμ given twice at 3-day intervals

Aqueous procaine penicillin G (APPG)—4.8 million units IM total dose, given in eight 600,000 unit daily injections

Tetracycline HCl—total oral dose of 30 to 40 gm, given in 4 equally divided doses daily over a period of 10 to 15 days

Erythromycin—same as for tetracycline

Congenital syphilis

If patient is an adult, then treatment is the same as for late syphilis. If patient is a child, then use:

Benzathine penicillin G—50,000 μ per kg of body weight in single treatment

APPG—100,000 μ per kg of body weight, given in 10 equally divided daily doses

Late syphilis (includes asymptomatic and symptomatic neurosyphilis and cardiovascular and gummatous syphilis)

Benzathine penicillin G—6 to 9 million units IM total dose, given as 2 or 3 injections of 3.0 million units each given 7 days apart

PAM—6 to 9 million units IM total dose, given as repeated injections of 1.2 million units at 3-day intervals

APPG—6.0 to 9.0 million units total IM dose, given in daily injections of 600,000 units

Tetracycline and erythromycin—total oral dose of 60 to 80 gm, given in equally divided 4 doses daily over a period of 20 to 30 days

If the above treatment schedules are adhered to, success in treating syphilis in the infectious stages is reported to be effective in over 95% of the cases,[48] with rapid disappearance of signs and symptoms and a return of the serum to a nonreactive state when tested by reagin and treponemal tests. Treatment of late symptomatic syphilis has proved to be somewhat less effective. Adequate treatment does eradicate all signs of active clinical infection and arrests the progress of the disease in the great majority of cases. However, it has long been recognized that clinical progression of ocular and central nervous system syphilis occasionally occurs despite intensive antibiotic therapy. In addition, permanent sequelae of late symptomatic syphilis secondary to the irreversible damage of tissues before treatment are not ususual. Finally, measurable levels of specific antitreponemal antibodies typically persist indefinitely, and detectable levels of reagin may sometimes remain.

Despite the occasional exceptions, penicillin has over the years continued to have undiminished treponemicidal effects; no strain of *T. pallidum* has yet been reported to be resistant to penicillin, and its clinical efficacy in early syphilis has remained unchallenged. What, then, is the significance of the recent work indicating persistence of treponemes in human beings and in laboratory animals that have received supposedly adequate penicillin therapy?

It should first be emphasized that this is not a new finding. In 1945 Levaditi and Vaisman[30] reported the persistence of treponemes in rabbits, following both penicillin and heavy metal therapy. This work did not stimulate much interest, because effective therapy was determined in the main on clinical grounds alone and because sensitive techniques for detecting the presence of low concentrations of treponemes in tissues were lacking. The decreased effectiveness of penicillin in curing previously untreated cases of long-standing syphilis and the persistence of reactive specific treponemal tests in these patients following supposedly adequate penicillin therapy prompted a French worker, Pierre Collart, to search for treponemes in syphilitic patients and in rabbits treated with penicillin. In 1962 he reported finding viable treponemes in rabbits and human beings treated with massive doses of penicillin (one rabbit had received 9 million units of penicillin per kg of body weight, and a syphilitic patient had been treated with 151,000,000 units of the drug).[8] He was also able to demonstrate the infectivity of these persistent organisms by passive transfer to rabbits. He concluded that:

> 1. Therapy administered long after contraction of syphilis cannot destroy the Treponema that have been longtime residents in the host body.
> 2. The presence of spirochetes is the determining factor in the persistence of antibodies in the blood serum.
> 3. The Treponema discovered were still viable, but had lost all or part of their virulence in the tissues in the state of commensal organisms.
> 4. Under biological conditions still not ascertained, these organisms can revert and become pathogenic, at least to the host that shelters them.
>
> Hence the behavior of syphilis can be likened to that of other long term infectious diseases.[8]

Because of penicillin's great clinical value and of the fact that Collart's technique for locating the sparse organisms entailed significant technical difficulty in recognizing persisting organisms with altered morphologic characteristics, his work was doubted by other workers in the field, especially in this country where penicillin's effectiveness had been discovered. His results were confirmed by the work of Del Carpio[10] in 1963 and Boncinelli[4] in 1966, both in Italy. At the Venereal Disease Research Laboratories Yobs and her associates[63] in 1968 reported finding treponemes in lymph nodes from 11 of 45 TPI-reactive male volunteers who had been treated for syphilis in the past. By passage to animals these organisms proved to be infectious treponemes. After retreatment 3 out of 5 patients continued to harbor treponemes.

In 1967 Smith and Israel[51] reported finding motile treponemes in aqueous humor, spinal fluid, and liver biopsy specimens from 4 patients with signs and symptoms of late syphilis and negative reagin serologic tests. Three of the four patients had reactive or weakly reactive FTA-ABS tests but completely normal spinal fluids. The fourth patient's serum and spinal fluid remained nonreactive to VDRL, TPI, and FTA-ABS tests on repeated occasions, though his spinal fluid did exhibit an elevated protein level. The organisms from all of the patients took up the specific antitreponemal fluorescent antibody stain and fluoresced on ultraviolet darkfield microscopy (FADF). In another paper published a month later Smith and Israel[51] further described the findings in one of the four original patients. The patient had bilateral anterior uveitis and neuroretinitis. She gave no history of syphilis and had repeatedly negative TPI tests but had weakly reactive VDRL and FTA-ABS tests on several occasions. The organisms were motile, morphologically identical to *T. pallidum*, took up the specific fluorescent antibody stain, and were found in the aqueous both before and after treatment with 9,200,000 units of benzathine penicillin G. The two reports not only confirmed the earlier work of Collart but reaffirmed the position of many of the earlier syphilologists that active and progressive late syphilis, especially ocular syphilis and neurosyphilis, could exist in the presence of negative reagin tests and normal spinal fluid examinations.

The presence of intraocular treponemes was not a new finding,[1,2] but the use of the highly specific FADF technique for aqueous examination and the intraocular presence of treponemes after therapy had not been reported previously. Confirmatory reports soon appeared. Goldman and

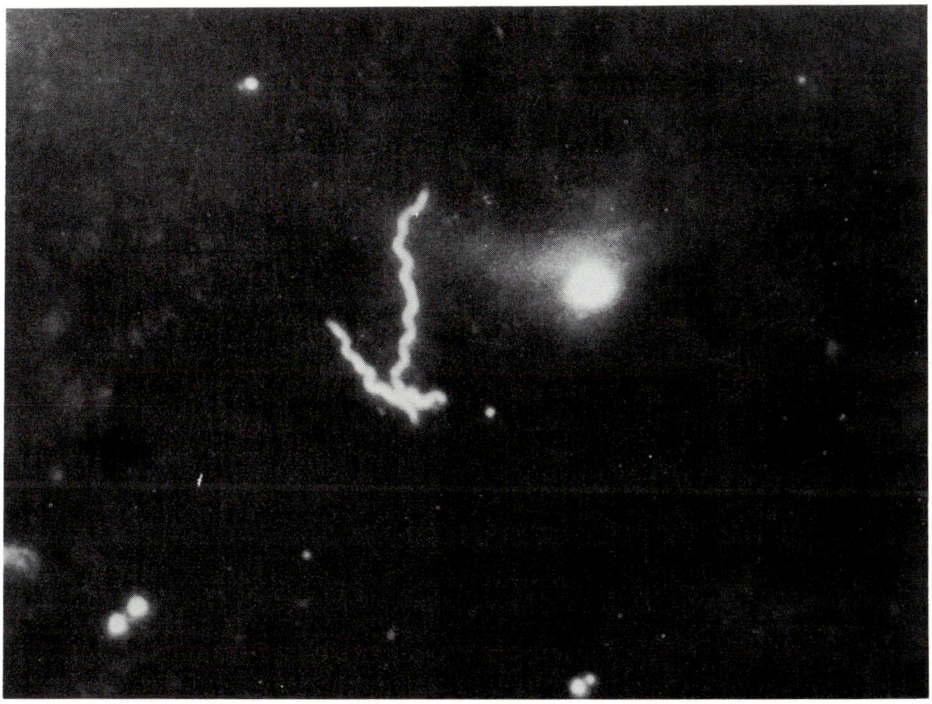

Fig. 20-2. Darkfield preparation of aqueous fluid from patient with uveitis. These spirochetes reacted specifically with fluorescein-labeled rabbit antibody to *T. pallidum.*

Girard[17] reported finding motile, FADF-positive treponemes in the aqueous of 2 congenital syphilitic patients who had been repeatedly treated with penicillin. Christman and his co-workers[7] found similar organisms in 12 of 36 patients thought to have ocular syphilis. Six of the 12 had uveitis. Intensive therapy of these 6 patients, using ampicillin and probenecid, a regime reported to produce significantly elevated intraocular levels of the treponemicidal antibiotic,[16] resulted in the temporary resolution of the uveitis, with concomitant disappearance of the intraocular treponemes in 5 of the patients; 2 of the 5 patients had subsequent recurrence of uveitis and treponemes. Dunlop and his associates[13] and Rice and his associates[44] found treponemes in the aqueous humor of 5 of 9 patients having late syphilis and ocular inflammatory disease. More recently, Whitfield and Wirostko,[59] in a controlled study of 50 patients with uveitis of unknown cause, found 6 to be harboring organisms morphologically indistinguishable from *T. pallidum.* Fig. 20-2 is a microphotograph of organisms found in the aqueous of one of these patients. The organisms from 5 of the 6 reacted specifically with fluorescein-labeled anti–*T. pallidum* rabbit globulin. No organisms resembling *T. pallidum* were found in aqueous specimens obtained at cataract surgery from a control group of 50 patients having senile cataracts, negative serologic tests, and no other clinically evident ocular disorder. Three of the 6 patients harboring treponemes had weakly reactive VDRL or FTA-ABS tests. Serologic tests on the remaining 3 were repeatedly nonreactive. Subsequent treatment of 3 of the 6 patients with a full course of ampicillin and probenecid had no clinically evident effect on the course of their disease.[60] Rice and his co-workers[43] found treponemelike forms in the aqueous or spinal fluid in 33 of 75 patients. Eight of the 33 had previously been treated for syphilis.

The above reports have not been accepted without controversy. In 1969 Montenegro and his associates[38] presented an interesting report of the various artefacts that may closely mimic treponemes on darkfield examination. Problems with artefacts on darkfield examination are certainly not new, Stokes wrote in 1944: "Certain artefacts in the darkfield have caused inexperienced observers a good deal of difficulty at times."[54] For an experienced darkfield microscopist artefacts are a nuisance but present no major problem. In the FADF test, use of identically processed known *T. pallidum* controls for comparison, scrupluously cleaned slides, and frequent alternation of white light with an ultraviolet source ensure that the microscopist will have no difficulty distinguishing organisms from artefacts.

It has also been suggested that the treponemelike forms are not *T. pallidum* but are saprophytic organisms, perhaps from the mouth.[15] There are some data to support the contention that in a small percentage of cases some gingival treponemes may fluoresce on FADF testing.[18] However, the specificity of the fluorescent antibody staining technique has been extensively investigated, and it has been confirmed that when properly used, the FADF test has a very high degree of specificity.[37] It is entirely possible that organisms that have been indistinguishable morphologically from *T. pallidum* and that take up the specific anti–*T. pallidum* fluorescent stain but that are other than *T. pallidum* have on occasion been found in the eye and elsewhere, but it is highly unlikely that this has occurred in more than a small percentage of cases. Typical morphologic characteristics, specific antibody staining, and on occasion typical motility on wet darkfield examination have been repeatedly found; and all support the thesis that *T. pallidum* does persist in the aqueous humor, spinal fluid, and other tissues after treatment.

Perhaps the strongest evidence that these organisms are *T. pallidum* has come from successful passive transfer to laboratory animals. Collart, Boncinelli and his associates, and Yobs and her associates all successfully infected rabbits, using the persisting treponemes they found in the lymph nodes of previously treated rabbits and human beings. Hardy and his co-workers[19] found pathogenic *T. pallidum* in the ocular tissues of a newborn who had been unsuccessfully treated for congenital syphilis with huge doses of penicillin, and they were able to infect a rabbit with the material. In his extensive monograph on the subject of seronegative late syphilis and in other publications Smith has reported successfully infecting rabbits and primates with syphilis on multiple occasions, using specimens of aqueous humor and spinal fluid from patients with treated syphilis.[49,52,53]

There appears to be substantial evidence that *T. pallidum* may persist in the eye and other tissues following even massive antibiotic therapy, especially in late ocular and central nervous system syphilis. This probably has not occurred as the result of the development of penicillin-resistant strains, but rather by using new and more sensitive techniques we have become aware of a process that is integral to the disease. It is likely, as Collart suggests, that a persistent reactive serologic test following treatment indicates the continued presence of treponemes stimulating antibody production. There is no reason to think that syphilis is uniquely different from other infectious diseases nor that treatment with penicillin can completely eradicate all treponemes. All that is needed is antibiotic assistance to eradicate enough organisms to allow the host's protective apparatus to take over. The relative isolation of the eye and central nervous system from the general circulation is likely quite important in the occasional persistence of treponemes in the aqueous humor and spinal fluid following treatment.

We also have good evidence that treponemes may persist and that active ocular syphilis or neurosyphilis may be present despite negative reagin and treponemal tests of the blood and spinal fluid.[52]

Yobs and her associates[63] and Collart[8] point out that the persisting organisms often have lowered virulence and modified antigenic structure as a result of their long and intimate association with the host tissues, perhaps as a direct effect of the host's antibodies developed during that association. It is certainly a possibility that the antigenic structure of the treponemes might become so altered that it no longer stimulates measurable treponemal or reagin antibody production in the host nor strongly takes up specific antibody stains itself. This is a possible explanation for both the phenomenon of late seronegative syphilis and for the presence of variably staining organisms occasionally found in late ocular syphilis, especially in late congenital syphilis.[18]

The major import of this recent finding is to underscore strongly the old dictum that the diagnosis of syphilis is a clinical one. Although the myriad new and complex laboratory tests are often of great assistance and their intelligent use is important, the disease must first be considered in the differential diagnosis, and the appropriate tests must be decided upon. There is no substitute for careful history and physical examination. The FTA-ABS test is the most sensitive and specific serologic procedure available for the diagnosis of syphilis and should be used whenever the diagnosis is considered; yet it has its occasional false-negative results, and false-positive results may also, although rarely, occur. Fresh darkfield and FADF studies of the aqueous can be quite helpful in difficult cases, though the procedures are technically demanding.

The treatment of early syphilis, using the currently accepted modes of therapy, achieves excellent clinical results; and there are no indications to modify it. The treatment of late syphilis continues to be unsatisfactory, though the above guidelines have proved to be effective in the great majority of cases. There appears to be good evidence for the persistence of pathogenic *T. pallidum* in a small percentage of patients thought to have received adequate treatment. Efforts to determine the effects of the persistent organism on the eye and other tissues and to develop appropriate effective therapy must continue. In such cases a trial of intensive retreatment is certainly indicated. Meyer, Boudin, and Collart[36] recently suggested using 1,000,000 units of aqueous penicillin G daily for 30 days. Other regimens, including those utilizing antibiotics alternated with intensive steroid therapy, are being tried; but these remain in the experimental stage. The best treatment of the complications of late syphilis continues to be prevention, in the form of epidemiologic tracing of contacts of infectious individuals, early diagnosis, and adequate therapy of the disease in its early stages.

REFERENCES

1. Agarwal, L. P.: Aqueous humor examination in granulomatous iridocyclitis, Docum. Ophthal. **14**:97, 1960.
2. Amsler, M., and others: L'Humeur aqueuse et ses fonctions, Paris, 1955, Masson et Cie.
3. Balentyne, H. J., and Michaelson, I. C.: The fundus of the eye, Baltimore, 1963, The Williams and Wilkins Co., p. 564.
4. Boncinelli, U., and others: Richerche sulla persistenza del Treponema pallidum, nelle linfoghiandole di luetici trattati, G. Ital. Derm. **107**:1, 1966.
5. Carrol, F. D.: Optic atrophy, Trans. Pacif. Coast Otoophthal. Soc. **31**:36, 1950.
6. Carrol, F. D.: Retrobulbar neuritis, Arch. Ophthal. **24**:44, 1970.
7. Christman, E. H., Hamilton, R. W., Heaton, C. L., and Hoffmeyer, I. M.: Intraocular treponemes, Arch. Ophthal. **80**:303, 1968.
8. Collart, P.: Persistence of T. pallidum in late syphilis in rabbits and humans, notwithstanding treatment: 1962 proceedings of the World Forum on Syphilis and Other Treponematoses, U. S. Public Health Service Publication No. 997, Washington, D. C., 1964, U. S. Government Printing Office, pp. 289, 291.
9. Deacon, W. E., Falcone, V. H., and Harris, A.: A fluorescent test for treponemal antibodies, Proc. Soc. Exp. Biol. Med. **96**:477, 1957.
10. Del Carpio, C.: Effetti di un trattamento massiccio con penicillina nella sifilide sperimentale de coniglio a diversa distanza dall'

infezione, Riv. Ist. Sieroter. Ital. **38**:166, 1963.

11. Duke-Elder, S.: System of ophthalmology. Diseases of the outer eye, vol. 8, St. Louis, 1965, The C. V. Mosby Co., pp. 237, 239, 539, 828, 829, 1032.
12. Duke-Elder, S.: System of ophthalmology. Diseases of the uveal tract, vol. 9, St. Louis, 1966, The C. V. Mosby Co., pp. 300, 306, 307.
13. Dunlop, E. M. C., King, A. J., and Wilkinson, R. E.: Study of late ocular syphilis: demonstrations of treponemes in aqueous humor and cerebrospinal fluid. III. General and serological findings, Trans. Ophthal. Soc. U. K. **88**:275, 1968.
14. Fleming, W. L., Brown, W. J., Donohue, F., and others: National survey of venereal disease treated by physicians in 1968, J.A.M.A. **211**:1827, 1970.
15. Golden, B., and Thompson, H. S.: Implications of spiral forms in the eye, Survey Ophthal. **14**:179, 1968.
16. Goldman, E. E., McClean, J. H., and Smith, J. L.: Penicillins and aqueous humor, Amer. J. Ophthal. **65**:717, 1968.
17. Goldman, J. N., and Girard, K. F.: Intraocular treponemes in treated congenital syphilis, Arch. Ophthal. **78**:47, 1967.
18. Goldman, J. N., and Girard, K. F.: Fluorescent staining of treponemes in uveitis, Arch. Ophthal. **79**:716, 1968.
19. Hardy, J. B., Hardy, P. H., Oppenheimer, E. H., Ryan, S. J., and Sheff, R. N.: Failure of penicillin in a newborn with congenital syphilis, J.A.M.A. **212**:1345, 1970.
20. Hogan, M. J., and Zimmerman, L. E.: Ophthalmic pathology, Philadelphia, 1968, W. B. Saunders Co., p. 397.
21. Hunter, E. F., Deacon, W. E., and Meyer, P. E.: An improved FTA test for syphilis, the absorption procedure (FTA-ABS), Public Health Rep. **79**:410, 1964.
22. Igersheimer, J.: Optic atrophy in tabes, Arch. Ophthal. **42**:170, 1949.
23. Jarrett, W. H.: Dislocation of the lens, Arch. Ophthal. **78**:290, 1967.
24. Kennedy, C., and Carrol, F. D.: Optic neuritis in children, Arch. Ophthal. **63**:748, 1960.
25. Klauder, J. V., and Meyer, G. P.: Chorioretinitis of congenital syphilis, Arch. Ophthal. **48**:147, 1953.
26. Knapp, A.: Bilateral circumpapillary chorioretinitis with detachment of the retina in syphilis, Trans. Amer. Acad. Ophthal. Otolaryng. **25**:132, 1920.
27. Knox, J. M., and Glicksman, J. M.: The FTA-ABS test for syphilis: performance in 1033 patients, Brit. J. Vener. Dis. **42**:18, 1966.
28. Lakke, J. P. W. F.: Orbital fissure syndrome, Arch. Neurol. (Chicago) **7**:289, 1962.
29. Lennarson, V. E., and Jeans, P. C.: Congenital syphilis of the eye, Amer. J. Syph. Gon. Vener. Dis. **21**:90, 1937.
30. Levaditi, C., and Vaisman, A.: Sort des treponemes syphilomateux chez les lapins traites par la penicilline, Bull. Acad. Nat. Med. (Paris) **129**:394, 1945.
31. Licher, P. R., and Shaffer, R. N.: Interstitial keratitis and glaucoma, Amer. J. Ophthal. **68**:241, 1969.
32. Loewenfeld, I. E.: The Argyll Robertson pupil 1869-1969: a critical survey of the literature, Survey Ophthal. **14**:199, 1969.
33. Lucas, J. B.: New developments in venereal disease research, Med. Ann. D. C. **35**:375, 1966.
34. Mahoney, J. F., and others: Penicillin treatment of early syphilis: a preliminary report, Amer. J. Public Health **33**:1387, 1943.
35. Merritt, H. H.: Textbook of neurology, ed. 3, Philadelphia, 1963, Lea and Febiger, pp. 128, 134, 137, 153.
36. Meyer, J., Boudin, G., Collart, P., and others: Latent syphilis, Concours. Med. **91**:4651, 1969.
37. Meyer, P. E., and Hunter, E. F.: Antigenic relationships of 14 treponemes by immunofluorescence, J. Bact. **93**:784, 1967.
38. Montenegro, E. N. R., Nicol, W. G., and Smith, J. L.: Treponemalike forms and artifacts, Amer. J. Ophthal. **68**:197, 1969.
39. Moore, J. E.: The relation of neurorecurrences to late syphilis, Arch. Neurol. Psych. **21**:117, 1929.
40. Moore, J. E.: Syphilitic iritis, Amer. J. Ophthal. **14**:121, 1931.
41. Moore, J. E., and Woods, A. C.: The pathology and pathogenesis of syphilitic primary optic atrophy, Amer. J. Ophthal. **23**:4, 1940.
42. Nelson, R. A., and Mayer, M. M.: Immobilization of T. pallidum in vitro by antibody produced in syphilitic infection, J. Exp. Med. **89**:369, 1949.
43. Rice, N. S. C., Dunlop, E. M. C., Jones, B., Hare, M. J., and others: Demonstration of treponema-like forms in cases of treated and untreated late syphilis, and of treated early syphilis, Brit. J. Vener. Dis. **46**:1, 1970.
44. Rice, N. S. C., Jones, B., and Wilkinson, A. E.: Study of late ocular syphilis, Trans. Ophthal. Soc. U. K. **88**:259, 1968.
45. Robertson, D. A.: Four cases of spinal myosis: with remarks on the action of light on the pupil, Edin. Med. J. **15**:487, 1869.
46. Scheie, H. G.: Site of disturbance of Adie's syndrome, Arch. Ophthal. **24**:225, 1940.

46a. Seeley, R. L., Sarker, M., and Smith, J. L.: The borderline fluorescent treponemal anti-

body absorption test reactor, Arch. Ophthal. **87**:16, 1972.
47. Slight, J. R.: Personal communication, 1967.
48. Smith, C. A., and others: Benzathine penicillin G in the treatment of syphilis, Bull. W.H.O. **15**:1087, 1956.
49. Smith, J. L.: Spirochetes in late seronegative syphilis, penicillin notwithstanding, Springfield, Ill., 1969, Charles C Thomas, Publisher, pp. 30, 90, 124, 255, 261, 305.
50. Smith, J. L., and Israel, C. W.: Spirochetes in the aqueous humor in seronegative ocular syphilis: persistence after penicillin therapy, Arch. Ophthal. **77**:474, 1967.
51. Smith, J. L., and Israel, C. W.: The presence of spirochetes in late seronegative syphilis, J.A.M.A. **199**:980, 1967.
52. Smith, J. L., and Israel, C. W.: Recovery of spirochetes in the monkey by passive transfer from human late seronegative syphilis, Brit. J. Vener. Dis. **44**:109, 1968.
53. Smith, J. L., Israel, C. W., and McCrary, J. A.: Recovery of T. pallidum from aqueous humor removed at cataract surgery in man by passive transfer to rabbit testes, Amer. J. Ophthal. **65**:242, 1968.
54. Stokes, J. H., Beerman, H., and Ingraham, N. R.: Modern clinical syphilology, Philadelphia, 1945, W. B. Saunders Co., pp. 59, 504, 604, 607, 609, 1010, 1011, 1113, 1114, 1115, 1117.
55. Syphilis—a synopsis, U. S. Public Health Service Publication No. 1660, Washington, D. C., 1967, U. S. Government Printing Office.
56. Thomas, C. I.: The cornea, Springfield, Ill., 1955, Charles C Thomas, Publisher, p. 581.
57. Venereal disease fact sheet, U. S. Public Health Service Publication, Washington, D. C., 1970, U. S. Government Printing Office.
58. Walsh, F. W., and Hoyt, W. F.: Clinical neuro-ophthalmology, vol. 2, ed. 3, Baltimore, 1969, The Williams and Wilkins Co., pp. 1578, 1583, 1592, 1593, 1605, 1959.
59. Whitfield, R., and Wirostko, E.: Uveitis and intraocular treponemes, Arch. Ophthal. **84**:12, 1970.
60. Whitfield, R., and Wirostko, E.: Unpublished data.
61. Woods, A. C.: Syphilis of the eye, Amer. J. Syph. Gon. Vener. Dis. **27**:133, 1943.
62. Wuepper, K. D.: Red eye as the presenting sign of syphilis d'emblee, Calif. Med. **107**:518, 1967.
63. Yobs, A. R., Clark, J. W., Jr., Mothershed, S. E., and others: Further observations on the persistence of T. pallidum after treatment in rabbits and humans, Brit. J. Vener. Dis. **44**:116, 1968.

Index

A

Abscess
  in dacryocystitis, staphylococcal, 73
  lid, 71
Acid-fast bacilli in tuberculosis, 53
Acremonium, 221
Actinomyces israelii, 227
Adenovirus, 278-296
  discovery of, 278-280
  epidemiology of infections due to, 285-286
  groups, characterization of, 283-285
  infection, HeLa cells after, 295
  keratitis, 176-177
  laboratory identification, 294-296
    fluorescein-labeled antibody for, 295-296
    isolation of virus, 294
    tests of rising antibody titer in serum from convalescent patients, 295
  ocular diseases associated with, 280
  ocular infections induced by, 280-283
    production in human volunteers, 281
Air
  cleaning, 110-111
  conditioning, and asepsis, 109
  current tracing, and asepsis, 108-109
  filters, efficiency ratings of, 110-111
  hygiene for hospitals, 106-112
Airborne contaminants
  counts of, 109
  origin, nature, and fate of, 107-108
Airborne organisms, collection of, 109
Alkaloids, allergenic, 163-164
Allergen(s), 156-157
Allergenic drugs, 162-164
Allergy, 156-184
  autogenous, 158
  of conjunctiva, 158-167
  of cornea; *see* Cornea, allergy of

Allergy—cont'd
  in dermatoconjunctivitis; *see* Dermatoconjunctivitis, allergic
  general concepts, 156-158
  of lid; *see* Lid, allergy of
  microbiallergic reactions, 157
  of optic nerve; *see* Nerve, optic, allergy of
  response, immediate, 157
  of retina; *see* Retina, allergy of
  of sclera; *see* Sclera, allergy of
  syndrome of drug irritation, 164-165
  of uvea; *see* Uvea, allergy of
Alternaria
  in corneal ulcer, 237
  keratitis due to, 229
Ammonium compounds, quaternary, 97
Anesthetics, local, allergenic, 162-163
Antibacterial spectra of inhibitory flora, 30-32
Antibiotic(s)
  activities of organisms, 32
  allergenic, 163
  before cataract surgery, infection after, 78
  mycotic flora and, 215
  partially purified, of *Staphylococcus*, 38
  produced by inhibitory flora, 26-30
  -producing micrococci, bacterial susceptibility to, 31
  -producing organisms in conjunctivitis, 33
  production in staphylococcal cultures, 28
  prophylactic, 87
Antibody(ies)
  fluorescein-labeled, to identify adenovirus, 295-296
  titer, in adenovirus infection, 295
  viral, 270-272
Antigens, viral, 270-272
Antiseptic(s)
  definition, 91-92

Antiseptic(s)—cont'd
  skin, 102
  technique, development of, 88-89
Arbovirus disease, 316-317
Asepsis, 86-118
  air hygiene for hospitals, 106-112
  antibiotics and, prophylactic, 87
  antiseptic era, 88-89
  beginnings of, 89
  contaminants, 103-104
  disinfectants, 97-98
  foundations of, 86
  infection, concepts concerning, before 1850, 88
  medications, 98-103
  misconceptions concerning, 87
  pitfalls related to, 87
  preantiseptic era, surgery in, 88
  responsibility for, 87-88
  solutions, 98-103
  surgical scrub routine, 104-106
  susceptibility of ocular tissues, 86-87
  technique, development of, 88-89
  terms used in, definition, 91-92
Aspergillus, 216, 221, 226, 227
  keratitis due to, 222
    mycotic, 232-235
  niger, involving punctum, canaliculus, and conjunctiva, 219
Axenfeld, Theodor, 8-9

B

Bacillus(i)
  acid-fast, in tuberculosis, 53
  in conjunctivitis
    epidemic, 6
    follicular, fusospirochetal and fusiform, 68
  Koch-Weeks, causing conjunctivitis, smear from, 42
  Morax-Axenfeld, causing conjunctivitis, 53
Bacteria
  acid-fast, atypical, role in ocular disease, 127-129
  in conjunctivitis, microbiallergic, 160-162
  in eye of newborn, 13
  flora; *see* Flora, bacterial
  infections due to; *see* Infections, bacterial
  in normal eye at various ages, 14
  spore-forming, 92-93
  susceptibility to antibiotic-producing micrococci, 31
  vegetative, 93
Basophils, 48
Beauveria brumptii, 221
Bedding
  in operating room, and asepsis, 111-112
  precautions in hospital hygiene, 116
Benzalkonium chloride, allergenic, 164
Bitot spots, 57
Blankets in operating room, and asepsis, 111-112
Blastomyces, 223, 227
Blepharitis, seborrheic, 224
Blepharochalasis in leprosy, 142
Blood agar plate, inoculation of, 20
Boutonneuse fever, 261-262
Brow in leprosy, 141

C

Canaliculus
  in conjunctivitis, palpebrae, due to Vincent's infection, 55
  infections, 72-73
  inferior, and *Aspergillus niger,* 219
Candida, 216, 226, 227
  albicans, 228
    hypopyon ulcer due to, 219
  in mycotic keratitis, 234, 235
  parapsilosis, causing conjunctivitis and meibomitis, 54
  tropicalis, causing keratitis, 229
Cataract extraction
  antibiotics before, infection after, 78
  endophthalmitis after, 78, 90
    Neurospora sitophila causing, 226
    Staphylococcus study before and after surgery, 81
Catarrh, vernal, and keratitis, 177
Cells
  epithelial
    granules seen in scrapings, 47
    multinucleated, 50-51
    normal, 46
    vacuolated, in keratoconjunctivitis sicca, 50
  HeLa; *see* HeLa cells
  in inflammation of conjunctiva and cornea, 47-51
  plasma, 49-50
Cellulitis of orbit, 73
  bacterial agents in, 74
Cephalosporium, 219, 223, 226, 228
  in mycotic keratitis, 236, 238
Cerebrospinal fluid exam in syphilis, 325-326
Chancre of lid, scraping in, 43
Chlamydia, 56, 241-252
Choroid in syphilis, 328-330
Ciliary body in syphilis, 327-328, 333-334
Cladosporium, 226
Clostridium septicum, in mice, 35-37, 38
Coccidioides immitis, 227
Colitis, ulcerative, complicated by keratoconjunctivitis, 175
Collagen diseases, scleritis in, 179
Collyria, 100-101
  handling of, 101
  preservation of, 100-101
  sterile, preparation of, 100
  sterility testing of, 101
  sterilization in final container, 100
Complement-fixation test in toxoplasmosis, 191
Conjunctiva
  allergy of, 158-167

Conjunctiva—cont'd
Aspergillus niger and, 219
cultures
comparison of dry and wet swabs, 21
technique, 19-22
flora
effect of surgical dressing on, 83
worldwide study of, 16
fungi in, incidence, 214
infections
bacterial, 51-56
mumps virus causing, 271
viral, lymphocytes in scrapings, 49
inflammation, smears and scrapings in, 47-51
microorganisms in, 14
pharyngoconjunctival fever; *see* Pharyngoconjunctival fever
sac, and asepsis, 106
scrapings, 60
in conjunctivitis due to *Candida parapsilosis,* 54
in conjunctivitis due to Morax-Axenfeld bacillus, 53
in conjunctivitis due to *Staphylococcus aureus,* 51
in keratoconjunctivitis sicca, 50
in trachoma, 247
Staphylococcus aureus culture from, 171
subconjunctival hemorrhages in scrub typhus, 264
in syphilis, 326-327
in trachoma, 50
tubercles in, 123
tuberculosis
incidence, 120
in vitamin A deficiency, 57
Conjunctivitis
allergic, differentiation of chronic types, 160
antibiotic-producing organisms in, 33
atopic, 158-160
bacterial
acute, 63-65
acute, etiologic agents in, 64
chronic, 65-69
chronic, etiologic agents in, 67
bacterial flora in, 33
Candida parapsilosis causing, scraping in, 54
dermatoconjunctivitis; *see* Dermatoconjunctivitis
epidemic, bacillus in, 6
etiologic agents in, 66
experimentally induced in hay fever patient, 159
exudate in, nature of, 66
follicular, 294
bacillus, fusospirochetal and fusiform, 68
in pharyngoconjunctival fever, 292
fusospirochetal infection causing, 68
gonococcal, 48
in newborn, 45
inclusion, 241-252
diagnosis, clinical, 247-248

Conjunctivitis—cont'd
inclusion—cont'd
diagnosis, differential, 249
diagnosis, laboratory, 250
epidemiology, 243-244
etiology, 244-245
incidence, 249
prophylaxis, 250-251
therapy, 250-251
keratoconjunctivitis; *see* Keratoconjunctivitis
Koch-Weeks bacillus causing, smear in, 42
membranous
etiologic agents in, 65
Streptococcus hemolyticus causing, scraping in, 52
microbiallergic, 160-162
bacteria in, 160-162
Staphylococcus causing, 161
Morax-Axenfeld bacillus causing, scraping in, 53
palpebral, Vincent's infection causing, 55
pneumococcal, scraping in, 44
pseudomembranous, etiologic agents in, 65
sites of lesions, 66
Staphylococcus aureus causing, scrapings in, 51
subacute, diplobacilli in, 8
vernal, 49, 165-167
clinical aspects, 165-166
corneal lesions in, 167
etiology, 167
mixed type, 166
objective findings in, 166-167
symptoms, 166
Contact lenses
saline for, 100
solutions for, 103
Contaminants, 103-104
airborne
counts of, 109
origin, nature, and fate of, 107-108
respiratory, in operating room, 111
Contamination, sources of, in operating room, 111
Cornea
allergy of, 172-178
atopic, 173-174
classification, 173
contact, 174
to dusts, 173-174
to ingestants, 174
to pollen, 173-174
in transplant, 177-178
ulcer and, marginal, 175-176
ulcer and, ring, 176
in conjunctivitis, vernal, 167
edema, disciform, of stroma, 176
graft, keratitis of, 177
infections, bacterial, 51-56
type of injury causing, 69
inflammation, smears and scrapings in, 47-51
leproma, 148-149
nerves, in leprosy, 144

Cornea—cont'd
scar, in leprosy, 150
scrapings, 60
female sex chromatin mass in, 47
serious injuries, causes of, 211
in syphilis, 327, 332-333
transplants, allergic reactions in, 177-178
ulcer; *see* Ulcer, cornea
Corticosteroids, allergenic, 164
Cortisone causing allergic dermatoconjunctivitis, 169
Cosmetics causing lid allergy, 169-170
Coxiella burnetti, 264
Credé, Karl, 4
Cryotherapy, 307
Cryptococcus, 227
CSF exam in syphilis, 325-326
Cultures
conjunctiva
comparison of dry and wet swabs, 21
technique, 19-22
equipment for, 20
lid, technique, 19-22
staphylococcal, antibiotic production in, 28
Cyst in toxoplasmosis, 189
Cytology, 41-62
history of, 41-44
scrapings, normal, 44-47
Cytomegalovirus infections, 308-309

D

Dacryocystitis, staphylococcal, with abscess, 73
Degerming the skin, 103-104
Dermacentor andersoni, 261
Dermatitis
atopic, and keratitis, 177
lid, infectious eczematoid, 170-171
Dermatoconjunctivitis, allergic, 162-165
cortisone causing, 169
eserine causing, 163
hyoscine causing, 163
Diphtheria
mixed, 40
-*Staphylococcus* infection, in guinea pigs, 39
Diplobacilli in subacute conjunctivitis, 8
Diplococcus pneumoniae and trachoma, 249
Disinfectants, 97-98
instrument, 102-103
Disinfection
comparison with sterilization, 114
definition, 91
Dressings
postoperative, saline for, 100
surgical, effect on flora in conjunctiva, 83
Drug(s), 98-103
allergenic, 162-164
in infections, 98-99
irritation, syndrome of, 164-165
lid allergy due to, 169
Dry heat for sterilization, 95-96
Dust
control, in hospital hygiene, 116
corneal reactions to, 173-174

E

Ear, lepromatous nodules of, 135
Ecthyma, contagious, 315
Eczema of lid
dermatitis and, infectious, 170-171
staphylococcal, 171-172
Edema
cornea, disciform, of stroma, 176
lid, allergic, 167
Endodyogeny in *Toxoplasma,* 187
Endophthalmitis, 73-74
after cataract extraction, 78, 90
Neurospora sitophila causing, 226
causative agents in, 75
after injury, 75
Entropion, lid, in leprosy, 142
Environmental
factors in resistance of organisms, 92
sanitation in hospital hygiene, 116
Eosinophils, 48
Episcleritis in leprosy, 143
Epithelium; *see* Cells, epithelial
Equipment for cultures, 20
Erythromycin in syphilis, 343
Eserine causing allergic dermatoconjunctivitis, 163
Exudates
in conjunctivitis, nature of, 66
cytology, 41-62
smears from, techniques for preparing, 58-61
Eye
flora; *see* Flora
infections; *see* Infections
leprosy; *see* Leprosy
susceptibility of tissues and asepsis, 86-87
tuberculosis; *see* Tuberculosis
Eyebrow in leprosy, 141
Eyelid; *see* Lid

F

Face
in leprosy, 141
tuberculoid, 151
powders and creams causing lid allergy, 170
Fever
boutonneuse, 261-262
pharyngoconjunctival; *see* Pharyngoconjunctival fever
Q, 264-265
rickettsiae of, 254
Rocky Mountain spotted, 260-261
fundus in, 261
South African tick bite, 261-262
trench, 265
typhus, 259-260
Fite-Faraco stain in mycotic keratitis, 232
Flaming for sterilization, 96

Flocculation test in toxoplasmosis, 196
Flora
bacterial
in conjunctivitis, 33
of healthy eye, 13-23
prior to surgery, 15
sources of, 17-18
cadaveric eyes, 18
conjunctiva
effect of surgical dressing on, 83
worldwide study, 16
inhibitory
antibacterial spectra of, 30-32
antibiotics produced by, 26-30
characteristics, 26-30
clinical observations relating to, 32-34
in vivo significance in experimental infections, 34-40
potential protective role of, 24-26
inhibitory properties of, 24-40
normal, 13-17
comparison with postmortem donor eyes, 19
relationship to infections, 18-19
skin, 103
successful cultivation of, 74-75
Fluorescein
-labeled antibody to identfy adenovirus, 295-296
techniques in ocular toxoplasmosis, 196-198
Fuchs, Ernest, 288
Fundus
in Rocky Mountain spotted fever, 261
in toxoplasmosis, 199
Fungi, 93
in conjunctiva, incidence, 214
in healthy man, 211-216
infections, 208-240
in keratomycosis, 209
in normal eyes, 212
incidence, 213
Fusarium, 219
keratitis due to, 229
mycotic, 236

G

Gaseous sterilization, 96
German measles, 316
Glenospora, 223
Gomori silver methenamine stain in mycotic keratitis, 232
Gonioscopy, saline for, 100
Gonococcal conjunctivitis, 48
Gonococci in ophthalmia neonatorum, smear from, 43
Gonorrhea
conjunctivitis due to, in newborn, 45
smears in, 42
Gram stain in mycotic keratitis, 232
Granules in epithelial cells
"green," 46
in scrapings, 47
Gummatous lesions of eye, 332-334

H

Hair preparations causing lid allergy, 170
Halberstaedter, 243
Hay fever and atopic conjunctivitis, 159
Heat, dry, for sterilization, 95-96
HeLa cells
after adenovirus infection, 295
electron micrograph of nucleus, 285
normal, 284
Toxoplasma multiplication in, 188
Hemagglutination test in toxoplasmosis, 192-194
Hemorrhages, subconjunctival, in scrub typhus, 264
Heredosyphilis, tardive, 340-342
Herpes simplex infections, 302-307
primary, 302-303
recurrent, 303-305
treatment, 305-307
Histoplasma, 227
History
of cytology, 41-44
of development of aseptic technique, 88-89
of microbiology of eye, 1-12
Hospital
hygiene, 114-116
air, 106-112
bedding precautions, 116
dust control, 116
environmental sanitation, 116
role of laboratory in, 115
routine controls, 115
staff attitudes toward, 114-115
sterility surveys, 115-116
infections, committee on, 115
Hot air for sterilization, 95-96
Howe, Lucien, 4, 5
Humidity in hospital and asepsis, 108
Hyalopus, 223, 226
Hydrocortisone in colitis and keratoconjunctivitis, 175
Hygiene; *see* Hospital hygiene
Hyoscine causing allergic dermatoconjunctivitis, 163
Hypertrophy in tuberculosis, 122
Hypopyon ulcer due to *Candida,* 219

I

Infections, 89-91
agents responsible for, early observations on, 2-3
bacterial, 63-76
conjunctiva, 51-56
cornea, 51-56
cornea, type of injury causing, 69
lacrimal, 72-73
lacrimal apparatus, etiologic agents in, 72
canaliculi, 72-73

Infections—cont'd
  concepts concerning, before 1850, 88
  conjunctiva; *see* Conjunctiva, infections
  epidemiology, 90
  etiology, 89-90
  experimental, in vivo significance of inhibitory microorganisms in, 34-40
  fungal, 208-240
  hospital, committee on, 115
  lid, 71-72
    bacterial agents in, 71-72
    dermatitis, eczematoid, 170-171
  medications in, 98-99
  mycobacteria causing, atypical pathogenic, 126-127
  postoperative; *see* Postoperative infections
  relationship to normal flora, 18-19
  socket, 73, 74
  sources of, 91
  superficial, factors in resistance to, 24
  Vincent's causing palpebral conjunctivitis, 55
  viral, 56
    lymphocytes in conjunctival scrapings in, 49
Infectious mononucleosis, 309-310
Inflammation
  conjunctiva, smears and scrapings in, 47-51
  cornea, smears and scrapings in, 47-51
  noninfectious, 56-58
Influenza, 317
  virus, 272, 273
Ingestants, corneal reactions to, 174
Injury; *see* Trauma
Inoculation of blood agar plate, 20
Instrument(s)
  cutting-edge, sterilization of, 113
  disinfectants, 102-103
Iris
  pearls in leprosy, 150
  in syphilis, 327-328, 333-334
Iritis
  herpetic
    complications, treatment of, 307
    treatment, 306
  in leprosy, 150

K

Keratinization and Bitot spots, 57
Keratitis
  adenovirus, 176-177
  Aspergillus causing, 222
  catarrh and, vernal, 177
  dendritic
    complications, treatment of, 307
    treatment, 305-306
  dermatitis and, atopic, 177
  fungi causing, 229
  herpes simplex, of graft, 177
  interstitial, 174
Keratitis—cont'd
  in leprosy, 145-146
    exposure keratitis, 152
    pannus after, 147-148
  metaherpetic
    complications, treatment of, 307
    treatment, 306
  microbiallergic, 174-177
  mycotic, laboratory diagnosis, 230-238
    Aspergillus in, 232-235
    Candida in, 234, 235
    Cephalosporium in, 236, 238
    cultural characteristics of fungi in, 232-238
    cultures, identification of, 232
    cultures, primary, 232
    cultures, purification of, 232
    Fusarium in, 236
    microscopic exam, direct, 230-231
    Penicillium in, 238
    specimen collection, 230
    stains, special, 231-232
  mycotic, treatment, 230
  in periarteritis nodosa, 177
  rosacea, 177
  stromal
    complications, treatment of, 307
    treatment, 306-307
Keratoconjunctivitis
  epidemic, 286-291
    contrasted with pharyngoconjunctival fever, 293
    early records in U. S., 289
    early records in various countries, 287
    first pictorial representation of opacities in, 288
    isolation of causative agent in, 291
  phlyctenular, 174-175
  sicca, vacuolated epithelial cells in, 50
Keratomycosis
  fungi in, 209
  by geographic area of world, 220
  incidence, Armed Forces study, 222
Keratoplasty, keratitis after, 177
Klebsiella pneumoniae
  in corneal ulcer, 52
  trachoma and, 249
Koch, Robert, 4-5
Koch-Weeks bacillus, causing conjunctivitis, smear from, 42

L

Laboratory, role in hospital hygiene, 115
Lacrimal
  apparatus, bacterial infections, etiologic agents in, 72-73
  obstruction due to *Nocardia* species, 73
  sac
    asepsis and, 106
    infections, 72-73
Lanolin, allergenic, 164

Leber, Theodor, 210
Lens(es)
  contact; *see* Contact lenses
  in syphilis, 334
Lepra reaction, 139
Lepride, 138
Leproma
  cornea, 148-149
  miliary, 150
Leprosy, 131-155
  acute exacerbations, 138-139
  blepharochalasis in, 142
  brow in, 141
  clinical types, 135-139
  corneal nerves in, 144
  corneal scar in, 150
  dimorphous, 138
  distribution of, 132
  ear in, 135
  episcleritis in, 143
  etiology, 132-135
  face in, 141, 151
  history, 131-132
  indeterminate, 135
  iritis in, 150
  keratitis in, 145-146
    exposure, 152
    pannus after, 147-148
  lepromatous, 135-137
  lid in, 141
    entropion, 142
  ocular manifestations of, 139-153
  phalanges in, 136
  pterygium in, 150
  retina in, 152
  therapy, 153-154
  trichiasis in, 143
  tuberculoid, 137-138
    facies in, 151
Lid
  abscess, 71
  allergy of, 167-172
  allergy of, contact, 167-170
    cosmetics causing, 169-170
    drugs causing, 169
    witch hazel causing, 168
  allergy of, margin affections, 172
  chancre of, scraping in, 43
  cultures, technique, 19-22
  dermatitis, infectious eczematoid, 170-171
  eczema, staphylococcal, 171-172
  edema, allergic, 167
  entropion in leprosy, 142
  infections, 71-72
    bacterial agents in, 71-72
    dermatitis, eczematoid, 170-171
  in leprosy, 141, 142
  margin, 172
    microorganisms in, 14
    scrapings, 60
Lid—cont'd
  pediculosis of, 258
  in scrub typhus, 264
  Staphylococcus aureus culture from, 171
  in syphilis, 326-327
  verrucae of, 297
Lipstick causing lid allergy, 170
Lymphocytes, 48
  in conjunctival scrapings in viral infections, 49

M

Macrophage, 48
Macule, tuberculoid, 137
Masking technique for surgery, 111
Measles, 317-318
  German, 316
Medicaments; *see* Drugs
Medications; *see* Drugs
Meibomitis due to *Candida parapsilosis*, scraping in, 54
Meningovascular neurosyphilis, 334-336
Mercurials, allergenic, 164
Microbiallergic reactions, 157
  conjunctivitis, 160-162
    bacteria in, 160-162
    Staphylococcus causing, 161
  keratitis, 174-177
  optic nerve, 183
  retina, 183
  sclera, 178-179
  uvea, 180
Microorganisms
  in conjunctiva, 14
  in eyelid margins, 14
  inhibitory
    clinical observations related to, 32-34
    in vivo significance in experimental infections, 34-40
Microsporum, 227
Miotic alkaloids, allergenic, 163-164
Molluscum contagiosum, 315-316
Monocyte, 48
Mononucleosis, infectious, 309-310
Monosporium apiospermum
  in corneal ulcer, 237
  keratitis due to, 229
Morax-Axenfeld bacillus causing conjunctivitis, 53
Morax, Victor, 7, 8
Moraxella and trachoma, 249-250
Mucor, 229
Mumps, 318
  virus causing conjunctival infection, 271
Murine typhus, 260
Mycobacteria
  discovery of, 119-120
  pathogenic, atypical, infections due to, 126-127
Mycotic disease
  clinical aspects, 227-230
  factors that may promote, 210

Mycotic disease—cont'd
incidence
external eye, 216-226
internal eye, 226-227
after surgery, 225
Mycotic flora, steroids and antibiotics, 215
Mycotic keratitis; *see* Keratitis, mycotic
Mydriatic alkaloids, allergenic, 163-164
Myxovirus group, 317

N

Nail polish and lacquer causing lid allergy, 169-170
Nerves
corneal, in leprosy, 144
cranial, in meningeal neurosyphilis, 335
optic, allergy of, 182-183
atopic, 182-183
microbiallergic, 183
optic, in syphilis, 330-331
Neurospora, 226
sitophila causing endophthalmitis after cataract extraction, 226
Neurosyphilis
cranial nerve in, 335
lesions of eye, 334-338
meningovascular, 334-336
parenchymatous, 336-338
Neutralization test in toxoplasmosis, 191
Neutrophils, polymorphonuclear, 48
in chancre of lid, 43
Newborn
bacteria in eye of, 13
conjunctivitis, gonorrheal, 45
ophthalmia, gonococci in, smear from, 43
Newcastle disease, 318-319

O

Ocular; *see* Eye
Ointments, 101-102
handling of, 102
preparation, 101-102
selection of vehicle, 102
sterilization, 101-102
Operating room, organisms liberated in, 111-112
Operative field and asepsis, 105-106
Ophthalmia neonatorum, gonococci in, smear from, 43
Optic nerve; *see* Nerves, optic
Orbit
cellulitis, 73
bacterial agents in, 74
in syphilis, 332
Orf, 315

P

Palpebral conjunctivitis, Vincent's infection causing, 55
Pannus
formation, early, 247
after keratitis in leprosy, 147-148
Papovavirus ocular infection, 296-298
Paramyxovirus group, 317-319
Parenchymatous neurosyphilis, 336-338
Paresis, 338
Parotitis, epidemic, 318
virus causing conjunctival infection, 271
Pathogens, in patients awaiting surgery, 79
Pearls in leprosy
iris, 150
retina, 152
Pediculosis of lid, 258
Penicillin in syphilis, 343
Penicillium, 219, 226
in mycotic keratitis, 238
Perfume causing lid allergy, 170
Periarteritis nodosa, 183
keratitis in, 177
Periodic acid, Schiff reagent stain in mycotic keratitis, 232
Petit, Paul J., 9, 10
Petrolatum, allergenic, 164
Phalanges in leprosy, 136
Pharyngoconjunctival fever, 291-294
conjunctivitis in, follicular, 292
contrasted with epidemic keratoconjunctivitis, 293
Phenolic compounds, synthetic, 98
Picornavirus group, 319
Pieringer, Joseph F., 1, 3-4
Pityrosporum orbiculare, 223, 224, 226, 227
Plasma cells, 49-50
Pneumococcal conjunctivitis, scraping in, 44
Pollens, corneal reactions to, 173-174
Postoperative dressings, saline for, 100
Postoperative infections, 77-85
after antibiotics before cataract surgery, 78
endophthalmitis after cataract extraction, 78
incidence, 80, 90
Pott's disease, mummy with, 120
Poxvirus group, 313-316
Precipitin(s)
test in toxoplasmosis, 194-196
testing for, by agar-diffusion technique, 195
Pseudoinclusion bodies, 46
Pterygium in leprosy, 150
Pullularia, 226
Punctum, lower, and *Aspergillus niger,* 219

Q

Q fever, 264-265
rickettsiae of, 254

R

Radiation and sterilization, 96-97
Radioactive methods in toxoplasmosis, 198
Reagin tests in syphilis, 323
Resistance of organisms, 92-93
environmental factors in, 92
natural vs. acquired or induced, 92
Respiratory contaminants in operating room, 111

Retina
allergy of, 182-183
atopic, 182-183
detachment and, 183
microbiallergic, 183
pearls in leprosy, 152
in syphilis, 328-330
Retinopathy, angiospastic, central, 183
Rhinosporidium, 223, 227
Ricketts, Howard Taylor, 254
Rickettsiae, 253-266
discussion of, 253-259
producing ocular disease, 255, 257
of Q fever, 254
typhus, electron micrographs of, 256
Ring ulcer and corneal allergy, 176
Rocky Mountain spotted fever, 260-261
fundus in, 261
Rosacea keratitis, 177
Rubber bulbs and droppers, sterilization of, 113
Rubella, 316
Rubeola, 317-318

S

Saline
for contact lenses, 100
for gonioscopy, 100
for postoperative dressings, 100
solutions, 99-100
for intraocular surgery, 99-100
Sanitization, definition, 92
Sclera
allergy of, 178-180
atopic, 178
microbiallergic, 178-179
in syphilis, 327, 332-333
Scleritis in collagen diseases, 179
Scrapings
conjunctiva, 60
in conjunctivitis due to *Candida parapsilosis,* 54
in conjunctivitis due to Morax-Axenfeld bacillus, 53
in conjunctivitis due to *Staphylococcus aureus,* 51
in inflammation, 47-51
in keratoconjunctivitis sicca, 50
lymphocytes in viral infection, 49
in trachoma, 247
in conjunctivitis
pneumococcal, 44
Streptococcus hemolyticus causing, 52
cornea, 60
female sex chromatin mass in, 47
inflammation, 47-51
ulcer, *Klebsiella pneumoniae* in, 52
cytology, 41-62
normal, 44-47

Scrapings—cont'd
lid
in chancre, 43
margin, 60
pseudoinclusion bodies in, 46
smears from, techniques for preparing, 58-61
Scrub routine, surgical, 104-106
Scrub typhus; *see* Typhus, scrub
Sex chromatin mass, female, in corneal scraping, 47
Skin
antiseptics, 102
degerming of, 103-104
flora, 103
of hands as contaminants, 103-104
Smallpox, 313-314
Smears
conjunctiva, inflammation, 47-51
in conjunctivitis, in Koch-Weeks bacillus, 42
cornea, inflammation, 47-51
in gonorrhea, 42
in ophthalmia neonatorum, gonococci in, 43
pseudoinclusion bodies in, 46
techniques for preparation, 58-61
tray equipped for, 59
Socket infections, 73, 74
Solutions, 98-103
for contact lenses, 103
saline, 99-100
for intraocular surgery, 99-100
South African tick bite fever, 261-262
Spirochetes in chancre of lid, 43
Sporotrichum, 223
Stainless steel, sterilization of, 112
Staphylococcus
albus, 26
antibiotic of, partially purified, 38
aureus
culture from conjunctiva and lids, 171
in noninfected eyes, 18
trachoma and, 249
conjunctivitis due to
microbiallergic, 162
scrapings in, 51
cultures, antibiotic production in, 28
dacryocystitis due to, with abscess, 73
-diphtheria infection, in guinea pigs, 39
identification in relation to inhibitory activites, 28
lid eczema due to, 171-172
study before and after cataract extraction, 81
Steam under pressure for sterilization, 95
Sterility surveys in hospital hygiene, 115-116
Sterilization, 112-114
cleaning in, 94
collyria, 100
comparison with disinfection, 114
cutting-edge instruments, 113
definition, 91
heat-sensitive items, 113

Sterilization—cont'd
  incomplete, 94
  methods, 95-97
    dry heat, 95-96
    flaming, 96
    gaseous, 96
    gaseous, merits of, 114
    ionizing radiations, 96-97
    steam, merits of, 114
    steam under pressure, 95
  ointments, 101-102
  packaging in, 94-95
  principles of, 93-95
  processing in, 94
  rubber, 113
  stainless steel, 112
  time factor in, 94
  tonometers, 114
Steroids and mycotic flora, 215
Streptococcus hemolyticus causing conjunctivitis, scraping in, 52
Stromal keratitis
  complications, treatment of, 307
  treatment, 306-307
Sulfonamides, allergenic, 163
Surgery
  masking technique for, 111
  mycotic disease after, 225
  organisms liberated in operating room, 111-112
  pathogens in patients awaiting, 79
  in preantiseptic era, 88
  saline for, 99-100
  scrub routine for, 104-106
Surgical dressing, effect on flora in conjunctiva, 83
Syphilis, 322-349
  congenital, 338-342
    drug dosage schedule in, 343
    early, 339-340
    tardive heredosyphilis, 340-342
  CSF exam in, 325-326
  diagnostic procedures, 323-326
  erythromycin in, 343
  late, drug dosage schedule in, 343
  latent, 331-332
    drug dosage schedule in, 343
  neurosyphilis; *see* Neurosyphilis
  ocular, 322-349
  ocular, acquired, 326-331
    choroid in, 328-330
    ciliary body in, 327-328
    conjunctiva in, 326-327
    cornea in, 327
    iris in, 327-328
    lid in, 326-327
    optic nerve in, 330-331
    primary lesions, 326
    retina in, 328-330
    sclera in, 327
    secondary lesions, 326-331
  ocular, acquired, late symptomatic, 332-338
    ciliary body in, 333
Syphilis—cont'd
  ocular, acquired, late symptomatic—cont'd
    cornea in, 332-333
    gummatous lesions, 332-334
    iris in, 333-334
    lens in, 334
    neurosyphilitic lesions, 334-338
    orbit in, 332
    sclera in, 332-333
  penicillin in, 343
  primary, drug dosage schedule in, 343
  reagin titer changes, typical serum, during course of, 324
  secondary, drug dosage schedule in, 343
  tests in
    reagin, 323
    sensitivities in various stages of syphilis, 325
    treponemal, 323-325
  tetracycline in, 343

T

Tabes dorsalis, 336-338
Temperature in hospital and asepsis, 108
Tenonitis, 179
Tetracycline in syphilis, 343
Togavirus group, 316-317
Tonometers, sterilization of, 114
Torulopsis, 223
Toxocariasis, ocular, 203-207
  in children, 206
  contrasted with visceral larva migrans, 205
  diagnosis, 205-206
  pathology, 203-205
  prevention, 207
  therapy, 206-207
Toxoplasma
  division by internal budding, endodyogeny, 187
  dye test in toxoplasmosis, 191-192
  multiplication in HeLa cell, 188
  organisms in peritoneal exudate (in mice), 186
  two recently divided organisms, 187
Toxoplasmosis, ocular, 185-202
  cyst, 189
  diagnosis, 191-201
    conclusions concerning, 198-201
  fundus in, 199
  history, 190-191
  tests in
    complement-fixation, 191
    flocculation, 196
    fluorescein techniques, 196-198
    hemagglutination, 192-194
    neutralization, 191
    precipitin, 194-196
    radioactive methods, 198
    toxoplasma dye, 191-192
Trachoma, 241-252
  conjunctiva in, 50
    scrapings, 247
  diagnosis
    clinical, 245-247

Trachoma—cont'd
  diagnosis—cont'd
    differential, 248-249
    laboratory, 250
  epidemiology, 241-243
  etiology, 244-245
  geographic distribution, 242
  incidence, 249
  prophylaxis, 250-251
  stage I, 246
  stage IIa, 246
  stage III, cicatrizing, 248
  therapy, 250-251
  TRIC agents and, 249-250
Transplants, corneal, allergic reactions in, 177-178
Trauma
  cornea, bacterial infection after, 69
  endophthalmitis after, 75
Trench fever, 265
Treponema pallidum, 323, 329, 343-347
  uveitis and, 345
Treponemal tests in syphilis, 323-325
TRIC agents, 249-250
Trichiasis in leprosy, 143
Trichophyton, 223, 227
Tubercles in conjunctiva, 123
Tuberculoid leprosy, 137-138
Tuberculosis, 119-130
  acid-fast bacilli in, 53
  areas of eye involved in, 124
  primary, 120-124
    conjunctiva, incidence, 120
    hypertrophic, 122
    nodular, 121
    polypoid, 122
    ulcerative, 121
  secondary, 124-127
Typhus
  fever, 259-260
  murine, 260
  rickettsiae, electron micrographs of, 256
  scrub, 262-264
    lid in, 264
    subconjunctival hemorrhages in, 264
  South African tick, 262

U

Ulcer
  cornea, 69-71
    Alternaria in, 237
    etiologic agents in, 69
    Klebsiella pneumoniae in, 52
    Monosporium apiospermum in, 237
    tuberculous, 121
    Verticillium causing, 219
    Verticillium in, 237
  hypopyon, due to *Candida,* 219
  marginal, and corneal allergy, 175-176
  ring, and corneal allergy, 176
Ulcerative colitis complicated by keratoconjunctivitis, 175
Uvea, allergy of, 179-182
  atopic, 180
  autogenous, 180-182
  microbiallergic, 180
Uveitis
  phacoanaphylactic, 181
  sympathetic, 181-182
  Treponema pallidum and, 345

V

Vaccinia, 314-315
Varicella
  virus particle, 269
  -zoster virus infections, 307-308
Variola, 313-314
Ventilation and asepsis, 109
Vernal conjunctivitis, 49
Verrucae of lid, 297
Verticillium, 216
  in corneal ulcer, 219, 237
Vincent's infection causing palpebral conjunctivitis, 55
Viral antibodies, 270-272
Viral antigens, 270-272
Virion, 269
Viruses, 93, 267-277
  adenovirus; *see* Adenovirus
  animal, relative sizes of, 270
  arbovirus, 316-317
  classification by chemical and physical properties, 268
  complete virus particle, components of, 269
  cytomegalovirus, 308-309
  discussion of, 267-269
  infections, 56
    lymphocytes in conjunctival scrapings in, 49
    pathogenesis, 272-275
  influenza, 272, 273
  mumps, causing conjunctival infection, 271
  myxovirus group, 317
  ocular infection due to, 274-276
    diagnosis, 275-276
  papovavirus, 296-298
  paramyxovirus group, 317-319
  picornavirus group, 319
  poxvirus group, 313-316
  structure of, 269-270
  togavirus group, 316-317
  varicella virus particle, 269
  wart, 297
Visceral larva migrans contrasted with toxocariasis, 205
Vitamin A deficiency, conjunctiva in, 57
Volutella, 226, 236, 238
von Prowazek, 243
Varicella-zoster (V-Z) virus, 307-308

W

Wart virus, 297
Weeks, John Elmer, 5-6
Witch hazel causing lid allergy, 168